Handbook of Diabetes

Editor: Edwina Orion

AMERICAN
MEDICAL PUBLISHERS
www.americanmedicalpublishers.com

AMERICAN
MEDICAL PUBLISHERS
www.americanmedicalpublishers.com

Cataloging-in-Publication Data

Handbook of diabetes / edited by Edwina Orion.
p. cm.
Includes bibliographical references and index.
ISBN 978-1-63927-118-4
1. Diabetes. 2. Diabetes--Diagnosis. 3. Diabetes--Treatment. 4. Diabetes--Complications. 5. Endocrine glands--Diseases.
6. Carbohydrate intolerance. I. Orion, Edwina.
RC660 .H36 2022
616.462--dc23

American Medical Publishers,
41 Flatbush Avenue,
1st Floor, New York,
NY 11217, USA

ISBN 978-1-63927-118-4 (Hardback)

Contents

Preface

Diabetes, also known as diabetes mellitus, is a set of metabolic disorders which are distinguished by high blood sugar levels for a long period. There are three major types of diabetes, named as type 1, type 2 and gestational diabetes. Type 1 is managed with insulin injections and type 2 is treated with medications with or without insulin. Gestational diabetes is treated through a diabetic diet along with exercise. The symptoms of diabetes include frequent urination, increased hunger and thirst. If the proper treatment is not provided, it can cause various serious complications such as stroke, chronic kidney disease, cardiovascular diseases, damage to the eyes and foot ulcers. The prevention of diabetes include the intake of a healthy diet, regular physical exercise and avoiding the use of tobacco. The topics included in this book on diabetes are of utmost significance and bound to provide incredible insights to readers. It unravels the recent studies in this field. Coherent flow of topics, student-friendly language and extensive use of examples make this book an invaluable source of knowledge.

The information shared in this book is based on empirical researches made by veterans in this field of study. The elaborative information provided in this book will help the readers further their scope of knowledge leading to advancements in this field.

Finally, I would like to thank my fellow researchers who gave constructive feedback and my family members who supported me at every step of my research.

Editor

1

Bidirectional Relationship between Gastric Emptying and Plasma Glucose Control in Normoglycemic Individuals and Diabetic Patients

Bogdan Mircea Mihai,[1] Cătălina Mihai,[2] Cristina Cijevschi-Prelipcean,[2] Elena-Daniela Grigorescu,[1] Mihaela Dranga,[2] Vasile Drug,[2] Ioan Sporea,[3] and Cristina Mihaela Lăcătuşu[1]

[1]*"Grigore T. Popa" University of Medicine and Pharmacy, Clinical Centre of Diabetes, Nutrition and Metabolic Diseases, "Sf. Spiridon" Clinical Hospital, Iaşi, Romania*
[2]*"Grigore T. Popa" University of Medicine and Pharmacy, Institute of Gastroenterology and Hepatology, "Sf. Spiridon" Clinical Hospital, Iaşi, Romania*
[3]*Gastroenterology, "Victor Babes" University of Medicine and Pharmacy Timişoara, Romania*

Correspondence should be addressed to Cătălina Mihai; catalinamihai@yahoo.com

Academic Editor: Patrizio Tatti

Gastric emptying and glycemic control pathways are closely interrelated processes. Gastric chyme is transferred into the duodenum with velocities depending on its solid or liquid state, as well as on its caloric and nutritional composition. Once nutrients enter the intestine, the secretion of incretins (hormonal products of intestinal cells) is stimulated. Among incretins, glucagon-like peptide-1 (GLP-1) has multiple glycemic-regulatory effects that include delayed gastric emptying, thus triggering a feedback loop lowering postprandial serum glucose levels. Glycemic values also influence gastric emptying; hyperglycemia slows it down, and hypoglycemia accelerates it, both limiting glycemic fluctuations. Disordered gastric emptying in diabetes mellitus is understood today as a complex pathophysiological condition, with both irreversible and reversible components and high intra- and interindividual variability of time span and clinical features. While limited delays may be useful for reducing postprandial hyperglycemias, severely hindered gastric emptying may be associated with higher glycemic variability and worsened long-term glycemic control. Therapeutic approaches for both gastric emptying and glycemic control include dietary modifications of meal structure or content and drugs acting as GLP-1 receptor agonists. In the foreseeable future, we will probably witness a wider range of dietary interventions and more incretin-based medications used for restoring both gastric emptying and glycemic levels to nearly physiological levels.

1. Introduction

Gastric emptying and glycemic variations are interdependent processes influenced by the incretin system, the solid or liquid state of ingested nourishment, and the macronutrient composition of food [1–3]. In diabetic patients, gastric emptying may be either accelerated or delayed, with irregular intra- and interindividual fluctuations in the rate and clinical expression [4, 5]. Gastric emptying also interacts with overall and postprandial glycemic control [6, 7]. Therapeutic approaches aiming to correct both gastric emptying and variations of serum glucose levels include diet changes in meal sequence or content and incretin-based medications [8–11].

The relation between the stomach and diabetes mellitus was alleged ever since ancient times. In the first century AD, Aretaeus of Cappadocia, whose reputation is due to his work related to diabetes more than any other physician in antiquity, would say "We must, therefore, strengthen the stomach by all means, which is the fountain of thirst" when speaking of diabetes mellitus treatment [12]. This hypothesis is obviously no longer valid in the 21st century, but the close bond between gastric emptying and glycemic control is recognized today as a reality beyond any doubt. This relationship is bidirectional; on the one hand, gastric emptying is influenced by glycemic control (as hyperglycemic values slow it down and hypoglycemia accelerates it), while on the other hand, gastric emptying may influence glycemic values, particularly postprandial ones [13, 14].

This review focuses on the current knowledge of the influences gastric emptying and glycemic fluctuations exert upon each other. The paper outlines the physiology and assessment of gastric emptying, diabetes-induced disorders of this relationship, but also the influence of nutrients and GLP-1 receptor agonists on gastric emptying and glycemic control.

2. Physiologic Control of Gastric Emptying

When foods enter the stomach, the proximal gastric region initially relaxes in order to "accommodate" the ingested nourishments. They subsequently reach the distal areas of the stomach and, by means of antral contractions, are ground and mixed with the gastric hydrochloric acid secretion. Gastric chyme (Greek: *khymos* = juice), a semifluid mass, is thus formed. When the resulting particles are less than 1–2 mm in diameter, they go through the pylorus into the duodenum. Their transit is backed by antral contractions and relaxation of the pyloric sphincter. In normal conditions, the rate of gastric emptying may vary between 1 to 4 kcal/min [1], depending on the composition of gastric content (solids or liquids) and the macronutrient type [2]. As a result of their high caloric content, lipids are evacuated more slowly from the stomach than carbohydrates or proteins [15]. Digestion of solids begins after feeding with a lag time of 20 to 40 minutes, required for their grounding into 1–2 mm diameter particles, and then, a quasilinear gastric emptying begins. Therefore, their evacuation from the stomach begins approximately 40 minutes after food intake and may last for a few hours. Evacuation of liquids is immediate (without any lag phase) and usually monoexponential. The more nutritionally dense the liquids are, the slower the gastric emptying becomes [3]. In fact, caloric content of foods may exert a greater influence on gastric emptying than previously thought. Some recent results suggest not only liquids of equal energetic densities are evacuated from the stomach with similar speeds, but meals with the same caloric content given with equal amounts of water have nearly identical gastric emptying curves, no matter if their initial form was solid or liquid [16–18].

Nearly thirty years ago, Malbert and Ruckebusch described an intermittent transpyloric flux, with antral contractions and pyloric relaxation turning up at approximately 20-second intervals, while duodenal flux was continuous and uniform [19]. At that moment, the mechanical function of the duodenal bulb was thought to be the only factor to transform this flux from intermittent to continuous. The mechanism is in fact far more complex. When nutrients reach the intestine, they become a signal stimulating the blood release of intestinal hormones known as the incretin system. K cells from the upper intestine (duodenum) secrete *glucose-dependent insulinotropic peptide* (GIP); in the distal segment of the intestine, L cells secrete *glucagon-like peptide-1* (GLP-1). Both GLP-1 and GIP have glucose-dependent insulin secretion effects; GLP-1 inhibits glucagon secretion, and GIP exerts glucagonotropic actions [3, 20–22]. While it was demonstrated that GIP has no effect on gastric emptying, GLP-1 induces an inhibitory feedback effect, delaying gastric emptying [22]. Recent data also suggest a relation between glycemic values and stomach emptying [13, 23]. High velocity gastric emptying allows nutrients to reach the intestine more rapidly, thus increasing postprandial glycemia; on the other hand, hyperglycemia delays stomach emptying, so the nutrients are propelled more slowly for absorption at the intestinal level [14]. Hypoglycemia induces reverse effects, by accelerating gastric emptying and increasing the nutrient absorption speed, thus allowing for a more prompt correction of glycemic levels [1]. The ability to increase gastric emptying was found to persist in healthy individuals even after repeated hypoglycemic episodes [24]. This is in contrast to other hypoglycemia-induced reactions, such as the clinical signs induced by adrenergic response, which are subdued by impaired hormonal counterregulation and tend to fade out during recurrent hypoglycemias.

3. Assessment of Gastric Emptying

The first measurement of gastric emptying dates back to the Middle Ages, when Frederic II Hohenstaufen, the leader of the Holy Roman Empire, ordered two prisoners to be well fed and then sent one of them to hunt and let the other one rest. The two men were then executed, and gastric content was analysed in both cases; the man who went hunting had a full stomach, while the second man's stomach was empty [25]. Activity of the sympathetic nervous system had been predominant in the man who went hunting and had physical exercise, inducing relaxation of gastrointestinal muscularity and sphincter contraction, while the other showed a predominance of the parasympathetic nervous system, with opposite effects.

At present, multiple methods of measuring gastric emptying exist. As a general condition, temporary discontinuation of prokinetics, anticholinergics, opiates, or any other medication exerting an influence on gastric motility is needed whenever possible; in order to avoid the delaying effect of high glycemic values, some investigation protocols require the procedures to be performed at fasting glucose levels below 15.3 mmol/L (275 mg/dL) [26, 27]. Among these methods, the golden standard is scintigraphy performed after labelling solid and/or liquid food with radiotracers (technetium, indium) [28]. However, standardization of the method was only recently accomplished, with current guidelines advising for the administration of a specified low-fat meal (egg white from two large eggs, two slices of bread with jam and water) labelled with ^{99m}technetium sulphur colloid and for the measurement of gastric content after 1, 2, and 4 hours. These technical conditions were fulfilled, and a gastric retention of more than 60% after 2 hours or 10% after 4 hours is considered pathological [29, 30].

Breath tests are methods seemingly as good as scintigraphy [31]. Food is labelled with ^{13}carbon (^{13}C); after food is evacuated from the stomach, ^{13}C enters the intestine, is absorbed into bloodstream, and reaches the liver, being transformed into $^{13}CO_2$. Determination of $^{13}CO_2$ in exhaled air provides indirect data on gastric emptying. This method has the advantage of not involving radiations, thus being allowed in children and pregnant women [31].

2D or 3D ultrasonography is a useful method, but it requires considerable amounts of patience and experience from the examiner [32, 33].

Another modern alternative is the use of a wireless motility capsule, a 26 × 13 mm medical device with pressure, temperature, and pH-measuring sensors, approved in 2006 by the Food and Drug Administration for the study of gastric emptying when gastroparesis is suspected. A sudden increase in pH values marks the moment when the capsule exits the stomach and enters the duodenal region; values greater than 5 hours are considered representative for delayed gastric emptying. The wireless motility capsule may be used in ambulatory settings; it has the advantage of avoiding exposure to radiations, but its use is limited in dysphagia or possible bowel obstruction, due to its size [26]. Comparison between gastric emptying time measured by the wireless motility capsule and the golden standard of scintigraphy yielded good results in healthy individuals and patients with gastroparesis [34].

4. Causes of Gastric Emptying Disorders in Diabetes

Disordered gastric emptying in diabetic patients must be understood in terms of factors controlling gastrointestinal motility. A normal evacuation of the stomach involves coordination between contractile activities of its proximal and distal regions, pylorus, and proximal duodenum. These movements are controlled by the enteric and autonomic nervous systems, as well as by neurohormonal pathways. The enteric nervous system is represented by Cajal interstitial cells, belonging to the Auerbach nerve plexus within the muscle layer of the digestive tube. The enteric nervous system comprises over 10^8 neurons, thus being considered an authentic brain of the digestive tract; Cajal interstitial cells operate as a pacemaker. The motor activity of the digestive tube is modulated by the autonomic (extrinsic) nervous system; the parasympathetic nervous system induces the contraction of intestinal musculature and sphincter relaxation, while the sympathetic nervous system elicits opposite actions. Among neurohormonal pathways, acetylcholine and substance P promote muscular contraction, while nitric oxide, carbon monoxide, and vasoactive intestinal polypeptide exert inhibitory actions [35, 36].

Until a few years ago, the traditional paradigm on delayed gastric emptying in diabetic patients considered it to be induced exclusively by vagal neuropathy and to be irreversible. Recent data suggest a much more complex process, influenced by multiple pathophysiologic mechanisms which are not yet completely understood; some are reversible, and some are not [32, 37]. Loss or dysfunction of Cajal interstitial cells plays a major pathophysiologic part in the induction of abnormal gastric emptying under diabetic conditions. Anomalies of enteric nerves, immune system, or nitric oxide synthase (inducing low nitric oxide levels) and low levels of carbon monoxide-producing heme oxygenase, which protects Cajal interstitial cells from oxidative stress, are also involved [3, 38]. Recent experimental data attribute damage of myenteric cholinergic neurons and interstitial cells of Cajal to impaired signalling through the axes of insulin and insulin-like growth factor-1 receptors [32, 39].

The term *gastroparesis diabeticorum* was coined by Kassander in 1958 [40]. Recent publications shed new light on our knowledge about this complication of diabetes mellitus. Delayed gastric emptying in diabetic patients may often be merely mild or moderate, and some persons may even exhibit accelerated propulsion of the stomach content into the duodenum. Considering this, the term *gastroparesis* should be limited to those severe clinical forms displaying symptoms and an important delay of gastric emptying, where food consumed many hours or days before is found in vomit or in aspiration liquid [38]. The relationship between the speed of gastric emptying and the symptoms is weak, with some patients having severe symptoms but only minor delays in stomach emptying, while others may have a severely delayed gastric emptying and no symptoms at all [41]. Moreover, it is commonly acknowledged today that more severe delays in gastric emptying or aggravations of symptoms may not appear even after many years of evolution [42].

More than 20 years ago, Horowitz et al. described a delayed gastric emptying for solids as well as liquids in patients with diabetic gastroparesis [43]. His team reported an increased prevalence of delayed gastric emptying in individuals with long-term type 1 or type 2 diabetes, despite significant fluctuations in gastric emptying from one individual to another, both in diabetic patients and in nondiabetic control subjects [4].

Recent research brought forth a change in paradigm on delayed gastric emptying. If this delay is limited, its effects may even be beneficial by the protection it offers against glycemic variations. This concept is not entirely new; glucose perfusions were reported to suppress "hunger" contractions ever since 1956 [44]. Results of scintigraphic measurements published during the 90s showed that hyperglycemia delays gastric emptying in patients with type 1 diabetes for both solids and liquids [27]. In diabetic conditions, these variations act as a buffer against serum glucose fluctuations; when glycemic values are elevated, gastric emptying is delayed in order to avoid supplementary amounts of glucose reaching the intestine in a short time, thus increasing glycemia even more. On the contrary, hypoglycemia would need more glucose entering the bloodstream as quickly as possible; therefore, a faster gastric emptying, rapidly sending glucose into the duodenum for absorption, is beneficial for the organism. Scintigraphic measurements also proved the validity of such a mechanism in various clinical settings. Glycemic values of approximately 2.8 mmol/L (50 mg/dL) increase the rate of gastric emptying in patients with type 1 diabetes [5]. Delayed gastric emptying was also described in individuals recently diagnosed with type 2 diabetes and with mean HbA_{1c} values of 10.5%; after 3 months of antihyperglycemic therapy, allowing HbA_{1c} values to be reduced at approximately 5%, a new scintigraphy was performed, showing an increase in gastric emptying nearing the evacuation speed of nondiabetic persons [45].

5. Glycemic Responses Induced by Fluctuations of Gastric Emptying

As mentioned before, gastric emptying establishes a bidirectional relationship with glycemic levels: glycemia influences gastric emptying, while the latter may also influence the value of postprandial glycemia. Postprandial serum levels of glucose are essential in diabetic patients. First, postprandial hyperglycemia is associated with increased oxidative stress and thus directly involved in the pathogenesis of chronic micro- and macrovascular complications of diabetes mellitus [46]. Second, data published by Monnier et al., showing postprandial hyperglycemia to be an important constituent of glycemic control, particularly in patients with only slightly increased HbA_{1c} values, are seen today as undisputed common knowledge [47]. Third, lifestyle in developed industrialized countries involves the ingestion of approximately 2500 kilocalories per day, split in 2 or 3 daily meals. Since the rate of gastric emptying is 1 to 4 kilocalories/minute, it results that modern mankind spends almost all the time in a postprandial or postabsorptive state, with only 3 or 4 hours early in the morning spent in an authentic fasting state [38]. All these considerations highlight the importance of postprandial hyperglycemia.

Several research teams found a direct relationship between the rate of gastric emptying and postprandial serum glucose levels [6, 7, 48, 49]. In patients with type 1 diabetes, altered rates of gastric emptying may impair efforts to adjust doses of prandial insulin according to the amounts of ingested nutrients. The most difficult problem in patients with type 1 diabetes is not the issue of too high or too low speeds of gastric emptying but its unpredictability. Most authors found that gastric emptying is increased even after recurrent episodes of hypoglycemia, not only in healthy individuals [24] but also in diabetic patients [50]. On the contrary, Lysy et al. evaluated gastric emptying in insulin-treated diabetic persons with frequent hypoglycemia and found it to be delayed in most situations [51]; in fact, such individuals exhibit discrepancies between the action of prandial insulin and the rates of gastric emptying [52]. Moreover, Parthasarathy et al. found delayed gastric emptying (even though associated with lesser postprandial hyperglycemia) to paradoxically induce a tendency towards higher glycemic levels throughout the day at continuous glucose monitoring measurements and therefore to favour, in time, a worsened glycemic control [53]. Hereupon, the evaluation of diabetic patients with frequent hypoglycemia should best include the assessment of gastric emptying; the "gastric hypoglycemia" (by delayed gastric emptying) proves to be an important concept in the management of diabetes mellitus [53].

6. Effects of GLP-1 on Gastric Emptying

As seen before, GLP-1 is an incretin hormone secreted by L cells in the distal intestine and having both the roles of increasing insulin secretion (secretagogue) and reducing glucagon secretion, as well as the effect of delaying gastric emptying [54–56]. When gastric emptying is fast, high amounts of GLP-1 are synthesized and bring it back to normal by a mechanism of inhibitory feedback. In the postprandial state, the main effect of GLP-1 is not the stimulation of insulin secretion but lowering of postprandial glycemia by means of delayed gastric emptying [57]. When intravenous erythromycin was used to counteract the delayed gastric emptying induced by a GLP-1 infusion in healthy individuals after a liquid test meal, the insulin secretory response and postprandial glucose concentrations were reversed and brought close to the levels seen during placebo administration, thus proving its main effect on gastric emptying [58].

GLP-1 effect on gastric emptying after a long-term, continuous use was proven recently to fade by a phenomenon of tachyphylaxis. On the contrary, insulinotropic and glucagonostatic actions of GLP-1 are not modified even after a long-term use. The mechanism causing the difference between the evolution of GLP-1 effects over time is not known [59, 60].

7. Influence of Nutrients on Gastric Emptying and Glycemic Levels

Nutritional factors are frequently overlooked, and discussion is often limited to other physiological or pharmacological issues in publications analysing the correlations between gastric emptying and glycemic values. However, effects exerted by the main nutrients or other food components on both these aspects can in fact hardly be separated from other perspectives, given that both gastric emptying and postprandial glycemic values imply the coexistence of meals and therefore nutrients. It is our team's opinion, supported by our double professional expertise in the fields of both clinical nutrition and diabetes care, that a complete description of the multilateral relationship existing between gastric emptying and glycemic levels and regulation should always include referrals to the influence exerted by food principles.

Adding sources rich in proteins to carbohydrate-based meals determines a 20% to 30% reduction in postprandial glucose levels [61]. Besides the stimulation of insulin secretion (driven by direct stimulatory effects, but also indirectly, through an increased incretin response), underlying pathways include delayed gastric emptying under the influence of the same incretin hormones [62]. Whey or soy proteins seem to give the best responses [8, 63], but favourable effects on postprandial glycemic levels were also reported for rice, pea, and oat proteins [64]. Giezenaar et al. found whey protein drinks to slow gastric emptying and alter insulin, glucagon, GLP-1, and GIP secretions in older men and women [65]. The structure of whey and soy proteins is rich in branched-chain amino acids, allowing faster digestion and absorption times, and therefore a quicker insulin release from pancreatic beta cells [66]. Ma et al. administered whey-based drinks to type 2 diabetes patients and proved a reduction of 50% or 40% in postprandial blood glucose areas under the curves if drinks were ingested 30 minutes before meals or when meal began, respectively [67]. Jakubowicz et al. found a 28% reduction in postprandial glycemic levels and increased responses in insulin, C-peptide, GLP-1, and GIP secretions when a whey preload was administered before a high glycemic index breakfast to a group of well-controlled type 2 diabetic patients [68].

In contrast with whole-structure proteins, intragastric administration of isolated amino acids such as lysine, leucine, or isoleucine does not seem to influence gastric emptying, even though it may reduce postprandial glycemic levels, most probably by direct stimulation of insulin secretion [69, 70]. However, paradoxical results are also published, leaving the debate about free amino acid effects on gastric emptying still open [71, 72]. Other three amino acids, histidine, glutamate, and aspartate, were reported to increase both postprandial glycemic levels, velocity of gastric emptying, and GLP-1 serum concentrations [71]. L-Tryptophan isomeric form was found to significantly delay gastric emptying, even though the effect on GLP-1 secretion was minimal [72].

Classical nutrition information considers that meals with high lipid content reduce the velocity of gastric emptying [15]. Recent data seem to confirm this theory by showing, for example, that high-fat meals may worsen symptoms of diabetic gastroparesis when compared to low-fat ones [73]. More than the absolute lipid load, the degree of emulsification and the lipid droplet size seem to influence gastric emptying. Tan et al. showed that fine emulsions of olive oil in water slowed gastric emptying more than a coarse emulsion or a nonemulsified mixture of olive oil and water [9].

Dietary fiber-rich foods are also able to reduce postprandial glycemia, with soluble fiber exerting the most pronounced effect. Most common explanations usually refer to an unmediated ability of soluble fiber to delay glucose absorption [74]. However, Repin et al. recently found that multiple types and doses of soluble fiber are able to induce similar reductions in postprandial glycemia and insulinemia, concluding that a modified meal viscosity and maybe a slower gastric emptying are involved [75]. Steinert et al. reported the use of oat bran mixed in water as a preload before a white bread test meal to efficiently reduce the postprandial glycemic area under curve and speculated it may be correlated to a delayed gastric emptying [76]. The comparison between effects induced by ingestion of proportional amounts of porridge based on either oat flakes or oat flour with the same protein, fat, and carbohydrate content showed lower levels of postprandial glycemia and a slower gastric emptying for oat flake porridge, explained by its conserved fiber structure [77]. However, the exact magnitude and conditionality of the effect fibers may exert on gastric emptying are still debatable. Contrary to previous evidences, a small study found that polydextrose, a low-viscosity soluble fiber, was able to reduce energy intake and postprandial glycemic and insulinemic responses but not to significantly modify gastric emptying [78].

8. Effects of GLP-1 Receptor Agonists on Gastric Emptying and Glycemic Levels

New knowledge on incretin hormones allowed the development of new drug therapies including GLP-1 receptor agonists. This class currently includes multiple representatives, some in clinical use and others in various stages of development [79]. GLP-1 receptor agonists are classified based on their half-life; the short-acting agents are designated as prandial agonists (exenatide BID, lixisenatide), while long-acting agents are considered nonprandial agonists (exenatide QW, liraglutide). Their glycemic effects differ, as prandial agonists mostly influence postprandial glycemia and nonprandial agonists exert a greater effect on fasting glycemia [10, 11, 80]. As nonprandial GLP-1 receptor agonists have longer half-lives and prolonged action, the gastric emptying effect is reduced by tachyphylaxis and their influence on postprandial glycemia is thus diminished by comparison with prandial agonists [81–84]. However, effects of short-acting and long-acting GLP-1 receptor agonists on postprandial glycemia are not always different, since semaglutide, a longer-duration GLP-1 receptor agonist recently approved in the United States by Food and Drug Administration, seems able to lower postprandial glycemia and the velocity of gastric emptying in obese subjects [85].

Novel therapeutic guidelines for type 2 diabetes recommend the association of prandial GLP-1 receptor agonists to basal insulin; benefits of such pharmacologic combinations bring together the predominant effect of basal insulin on fasting glycemia and the effect of prandial GLP-1 receptor agonists on postprandial glycemia, based on their ability to inhibit gastric emptying [86, 87]. This association between basal insulin and prandial GLP-1 receptor agonists is preferred today to the classical intensification of basal insulin therapy by adding prandial insulins, as it offers advantages of both a lower risk for hypoglycemia and a reduced weight gain [88, 89].

The effect of GLP-1 receptor agonists in diabetic patients with autonomic neuropathy and delayed gastric emptying, even though less studied, is usually feared to be deleterious in clinical practice by inducing or aggravating digestive intolerance, and therefore, their administration is intuitively avoided by most physicians in the case of patients with diabetic gastroparesis. However, treatment with long-acting GLP-1 receptor agonist liraglutide was found to have minor or no effects on gastric motility in the recent study on subjects with diabetic neuropathy [84]. Beyond its usual indications in type 2 diabetes therapy, a trial also using liraglutide, this time in type 1 diabetic patients submitted to a hypoglycemic clamp, found no effect of this GLP-1 receptor agonist on gastric emptying or on recovery from hypoglycemia. However, gastric emptying was measured in this study by the less-used method of an absorption test of paracetamol given within a liquid meal [90]. Nevertheless, even if no detrimental effects would occur, choosing short-acting GLP-1 receptor agonist therapies in patients with diabetic gastroparesis seems an illogical and useless option, since their benefits are based on delay of gastric emptying. Patients with type 2 diabetes and slow gastric emptying at baseline may benefit more from treatment with long-acting GLP-1 receptor agonists, while in those with preserved gastric emptying, short-acting GLP-1 receptor agonists may be preferable. Although not yet tested, this hypothesis warrants further investigation.

9. Conclusion

Gastric emptying and glycemic control exert an ongoing influence upon each other. Normal rates of gastric emptying, of 1 to 4 kcal/min, correspond to the best balance between intestinal propulsion and absorption of macronutrients (especially carbohydrates), incretin hormone secretion, and postprandial glycemic levels. Contrary to this equilibrium state, higher rates of gastric emptying may induce postprandial hyperglycemia but also represent a compensatory mechanism intervening when hypoglycemia occurs, while slower gastric emptying limits postprandial glycemic excursions or even acts as compensator under hyperglycemic conditions. In diabetic patients, fluctuations in gastric emptying are induced by complex pathophysiological pathways; these fluctuations may have a highly variable, unpredictable time pattern and limited correlations with the severity of clinical manifestations but strongly associate with variations in postprandial glycemic levels. Increased knowledge of this relation between gastric emptying and postprandial glycemic values allowed therapies targeting both factors to be updated, including diets with modified content or incretin-based medications. Future research and development will probably expand the range of both types of interventions, with diets based on reconsidered meal content or sequence and more GLP-1 receptor agonists approved for clinical use.

Conflicts of Interest

The authors declare that there is no conflict of interest.

References

[1] C. S. Marathe, C. K. Rayner, K. L. Jones, and M. Horowitz, "Relationships between gastric emptying, postprandial glycemia, and incretin hormones," *Diabetes Care*, vol. 36, no. 5, pp. 1396–1405, 2013.

[2] J. E. Stevens, K. L. Jones, C. K. Rayner, and M. Horowitz, "Pathophysiology and pharmacotherapy of gastroparesis: current and future perspectives," *Expert Opinion on Pharmacotherapy*, vol. 14, no. 9, pp. 1171–1186, 2013.

[3] L. K. Phillips, A. M. Deane, K. L. Jones, C. K. Rayner, and M. Horowitz, "Gastric emptying and glycaemia in health and diabetes mellitus," *Nature Reviews Endocrinology*, vol. 11, no. 2, pp. 112–128, 2015.

[4] M. Horowitz and J. Dent, "Disordered gastric emptying: mechanical basis, assessment and treatment," *Baillière's Clinical Gastroenterology*, vol. 5, no. 2, pp. 371–407, 1991.

[5] A. Russo, J. E. Stevens, R. Chen et al., "Insulin-induced hypoglycemia accelerates gastric emptying of solids and liquids in long-standing type 1 diabetes," *The Journal of Clinical Endocrinology & Metabolism*, vol. 90, no. 8, pp. 4489–4495, 2005.

[6] R. Hammersjö, B. Roth, P. Höglund, and B. Ohlsson, "Esophageal and gastric dysmotilities are associated with altered glucose homeostasis and plasma levels of incretins and leptin," *The Review of Diabetic Studies*, vol. 13, no. 1, pp. 79–90, 2016.

[7] S. L. Aronoff, "Rationale for treatment options for mealtime glucose control in patients with type 2 diabetes," *Postgraduate Medicine*, vol. 129, no. 2, pp. 231–241, 2017.

[8] E. J. Stevenson and D. M. Allerton, "The role of whey protein in postprandial glycaemic control," *Proceedings of the Nutrition Society*, vol. 77, no. 1, pp. 42–51, 2018.

[9] K. W. J. Tan, L. J. Sun, K. K. T. Goh, and C. J. Henry, "Lipid droplet size and emulsification on postprandial glycemia, insulinemia and lipidemia," *Food & Function*, vol. 7, no. 10, pp. 4278–4284, 2016.

[10] D. R. Owens, L. Monnier, and M. Hanefeld, "A review of glucagon-like peptide-1 receptor agonists and their effects on lowering postprandial plasma glucose and cardiovascular outcomes in the treatment of type 2 diabetes mellitus," *Diabetes, Obesity & Metabolism*, vol. 19, no. 12, pp. 1645–1654, 2017.

[11] K. L. Tran, Y. I. Park, S. Pandya et al., "Overview of glucagon-like peptide-1 receptor agonists for the treatment of patients with type 2 diabetes," *American Health & Drug Benefits*, vol. 10, no. 4, pp. 178–188, 2017.

[12] K. Laios, M. Karamanou, Z. Saridaki, and G. Androutsos, "Aretaeus of Cappadocia and the first description of diabetes," *Hormones*, vol. 11, no. 1, pp. 109–113, 2012.

[13] A. E. Bharucha, Y. Kudva, A. Basu et al., "Relationship between glycemic control and gastric emptying in poorly controlled type 2 diabetes," *Clinical Gastroenterology and Hepatology*, vol. 13, no. 3, pp. 466–476.e1, 2015.

[14] M. P. Plummer, K. L. Jones, C. E. Cousins et al., "Hyperglycemia potentiates the slowing of gastric emptying induced by exogenous GLP-1," *Diabetes Care*, vol. 38, no. 6, pp. 1123–1129, 2015.

[15] K. A. Tappenden, "Intake: digestion, absorption, transport, and excretion of nutrients," in *Krause's Food & the Nutrition Care Process*, L. K. Mahan and J. L. Raymond, Eds., pp. 2–16, Elsevier, St. Louis, 14th edition, 2017.

[16] T. Okabe, H. Terashima, and A. Sakamoto, "Determinants of liquid gastric emptying: comparisons between milk and isocalorically adjusted clear fluids," *British Journal of Anaesthesia*, vol. 114, no. 1, pp. 77–82, 2015.

[17] T. Okabe, H. Terashima, and A. Sakamoto, "What is the manner of gastric emptying after ingestion of liquids with differences in the volume under uniform glucose-based energy content?," *Clinical Nutrition*, vol. 36, no. 5, pp. 1283–1287, 2017.

[18] T. Okabe, H. Terashima, and A. Sakamoto, "A comparison of gastric emptying of soluble solid meals and clear fluids matched for volume and energy content: a pilot crossover study," *Anaesthesia*, vol. 72, no. 11, pp. 1344–1350, 2017.

[19] C. H. Malbert and Y. Ruckebusch, "Duodenal bulb control of the flow rate of digesta in the fasted and fed dog," *The Journal of Physiology*, vol. 409, no. 1, pp. 371–384, 1989.

[20] H. M. Tasyurek, H. A. Altunbas, M. K. Balci, and S. Sanlioglu, "Incretins: their physiology and application in the treatment of diabetes mellitus," *Diabetes/Metabolism Research and Reviews*, vol. 30, no. 5, pp. 354–371, 2014.

[21] J. Tong and D. D'Alessio, "Give the receptor a brake: slowing gastric emptying by GLP-1," *Diabetes*, vol. 63, no. 2, pp. 407–409, 2014.

[22] T. Edholm, M. Degerblad, P. Grybäck et al., "Differential incretin effects of GIP and GLP-1 on gastric emptying, appetite, and

insulin-glucose homeostasis," *Neurogastroenterology and Motility*, vol. 22, no. 11, pp. 1191–e315, 2010.

[23] T. Wu, C. K. Rayner, and M. Horowitz, "Inter-regulation of gastric emptying and incretin hormone secretion: implications for postprandial glycemic control," *Biomarkers in Medicine*, vol. 10, no. 11, pp. 1167–1179, 2016.

[24] P. Kar, K. L. Jones, M. P. Plummer et al., "Antecedent hypoglycemia does not attenuate the acceleration of gastric emptying by hypoglycemia," *The Journal of Clinical Endocrinology and Metabolism*, vol. 102, no. 11, pp. 3953–3960, 2017.

[25] S. F. A. Caputo, "The Court of Frederick II Hohenstaufen," 2013, November 10, http://www.nobility-association.com/PDF%20Files/2%20TEST%20%20THE%20COURT%20OF%20%20FREDERICK%20II%20HOHENSTAUFEN%20BOOK-1.pdf.

[26] A. A. Lee and W. L. Hasler, "Diabetes and the stomach," *Current Treatment Options in Gastroenterology*, vol. 15, no. 4, pp. 441–459, 2017.

[27] R. J. Fraser, M. Horowitz, A. F. Maddox, P. E. Harding, B. E. Chatterton, and J. Dent, "Hyperglycaemia slows gastric emptying in type 1 (insulin-dependent) diabetes mellitus," *Diabetologia*, vol. 33, no. 11, pp. 675–680, 1990.

[28] A. H. Maurer, "Gastrointestinal motility, part 1: esophageal transit and gastric emptying," *Journal of Nuclear Medicine Technology*, vol. 44, no. 1, pp. 1–11, 2016.

[29] T. L. Abell, M. Camilleri, K. Donohoe et al., "Consensus recommendations for gastric emptying scintigraphy: a joint report of the American Neurogastroenterology and Motility Society and the Society of Nuclear Medicine," *Journal of Nuclear Medicine Technology*, vol. 36, no. 1, pp. 44–54, 2008.

[30] G. Tougas, E. Y. Eaker, T. L. Abell et al., "Assessment of gastric emptying using a low fat meal: establishment of international control values," *The American Journal of Gastroenterology*, vol. 95, no. 6, pp. 1456–1462, 2000.

[31] I. Siddiqui, S. Ahmed, and S. Abid, "Update on diagnostic value of breath test in gastrointestinal and liver diseases," *World Journal of Gastrointestinal Pathophysiology*, vol. 7, no. 3, pp. 256–265, 2016.

[32] L. K. Phillips, C. K. Rayner, K. L. Jones, and M. Horowitz, "Measurement of gastric emptying in diabetes," *Journal of Diabetes and its Complications*, vol. 28, no. 6, pp. 894–903, 2014.

[33] C. Muresan, T. Surdea Blaga, L. Muresan, and D. L. Dumitrascu, "Abdominal ultrasound for the evaluation of gastric emptying revisited," *Journal of Gastrointestinal and Liver Diseases*, vol. 24, no. 3, pp. 329–338, 2015.

[34] R. J. Saad and W. L. Hasler, "A technical review and clinical assessment of the wireless motility capsule," *Gastroenterology & Hepatology*, vol. 7, no. 12, pp. 795–804, 2011.

[35] M. Camilleri and S. F. Phillips, "Disorders of small intestinal motility," *Gastroenterology Clinics of North America*, vol. 18, no. 2, pp. 405–424, 1989.

[36] Y. C. Chiu, M. C. Kuo, C. K. Rayner et al., "Decreased gastric motility in type II diabetic patients," *BioMed Research International*, vol. 2014, Article ID 894087, 6 pages, 2014.

[37] M. Camilleri, "Diabetic gastroparesis," *New England Journal of Medicine*, vol. 356, no. 8, pp. 820–829, 2007.

[38] J. Chang, C. K. Rayner, K. L. Jones, and M. Horowitz, "Diabetic gastroparesis and its impact on glycemia," *Endocrinology and Metabolism Clinics of North America*, vol. 39, no. 4, pp. 745–762, 2010.

[39] S. Yang, B. Wu, H. Sun et al., "Impaired insulin/IGF-1 is responsible for diabetic gastroparesis by damaging myenteric cholinergic neurones and interstitial cells of Cajal," *Bioscience Reports*, vol. 37, no. 5, 2017.

[40] P. Kassander, "Asymptomatic gastric retention in diabetics (gastroparesis diabeticorum)," *Annals of Internal Medicine*, vol. 48, no. 4, pp. 797–812, 1958.

[41] M. Horowitz, D. O'Donovan, K. L. Jones, C. Feinle, C. K. Rayner, and M. Samsom, "Gastric emptying in diabetes: clinical significance and treatment," *Diabetic Medicine*, vol. 19, no. 3, pp. 177–194, 2002.

[42] J. Chang, A. Russo, M. Bound, C. K. Rayner, K. L. Jones, and M. Horowitz, "A 25-year longitudinal evaluation of gastric emptying in diabetes," *Diabetes Care*, vol. 35, no. 12, pp. 2594–2596, 2012.

[43] M. Horowitz, A. F. Maddox, J. M. Wishart, P. E. Harding, B. E. Chatterton, and D. J. C. Shearman, "Relationships between oesophageal transit and solid and liquid gastric emptying in diabetes mellitus," *European Journal of Nuclear Medicine*, vol. 18, no. 4, pp. 229–234, 1991.

[44] A. J. Stunkard, H. G. Wolff, and A. Plescia, "Studies on the physiology of hunger. I. The effect of intravenous administration of glucose on gastric hunger contractions in man," *Journal of Clinical Investigation*, vol. 35, no. 9, pp. 954–963, 1956.

[45] B. A. Laway, T. S. Malik, S. H. Khan, and T. A. Rather, "Prevalence of abnormal gastric emptying in asymptomatic women with newly detected diabetes and its reversibility after glycemic control-a prospective case control study," *Journal of Diabetes and its Complications*, vol. 27, no. 1, pp. 78–81, 2013.

[46] International Diabetes Federation Guideline Development Group, "Guideline for management of postmeal glucose in diabetes," *Diabetes Research and Clinical Practice*, vol. 103, no. 2, pp. 256–268, 2014.

[47] L. Monnier, H. Lapinski, and C. Colette, "Contributions of fasting and postprandial plasma glucose increments to the overall diurnal hyperglycemia of type 2 diabetic patients: variations with increasing levels of HbA (1c)," *Diabetes Care*, vol. 26, no. 3, pp. 881–885, 2003.

[48] M. Horowitz, M. A. L. Edelbroek, J. M. Wishart, and J. W. Straathof, "Relationship between oral glucose tolerance and gastric emptying in normal healthy subjects," *Diabetologia*, vol. 36, no. 9, pp. 857–862, 1993.

[49] K. L. Jones, M. Horowitz, B. I. Carney, J. M. Wishart, S. Guha, and L. Green, "Gastric emptying in early noninsulin-dependent diabetes mellitus," *Journal of Nuclear Medicine*, vol. 37, no. 10, pp. 1643–1648, 1996.

[50] I. A. Macdonald, M. A. Nauck, and M.-F. Kong, "Impact of gastrointestinal function on glycaemic control," in *Gastrointestinal Function in Diabetes Mellitus*, M. Horowitz and M. Samsom, Eds., pp. 285–321, John Wiley & Sons, Chichester, 2004.

[51] J. Lysy, E. Israeli, N. Strauss-Liviatan, and E. Goldin, "Relationships between hypoglycaemia and gastric emptying abnormalities in insulin-treated diabetic patients," *Neurogastroenterology and Motility*, vol. 18, no. 6, pp. 433–440, 2006.

[52] J. Khoo, C. K. Rayner, C. Feinle-Bisset, K. L. Jones, and M. Horowitz, "Gastrointestinal hormonal dysfunction in gastroparesis and functional dyspepsia," *Neurogastroenterology and Motility*, vol. 22, no. 12, pp. 1270–1278, 2010.

[53] G. Parthasarathy, Y. C. Kudva, P. A. Low, M. Camilleri, A. Basu, and A. E. Bharucha, "Relationship between gastric

emptying and diurnal glycemic control in type 1 diabetes mellitus: a randomized trial," *The Journal of Clinical Endocrinology & Metabolism*, vol. 102, pp. jc.2016–jc.2809, 2016.

[54] J. J. Holst, J. Pedersen, N. J. Wewer Albrechtsen, and F. K. Knop, "The gut: a key to the pathogenesis of type 2 diabetes?," *Metabolic Syndrome and Related Disorders*, vol. 15, no. 6, pp. 259–262, 2017.

[55] A. Gastaldelli, M. Gaggini, and R. DeFronzo, "Glucose kinetics: an update and novel insights into its regulation by glucagon and GLP-1," *Current Opinion in Clinical Nutrition and Metabolic Care*, vol. 20, no. 4, pp. 300–309, 2017.

[56] L. G. Trahair, C. S. Marathe, S. Standfield et al., "Effects of small intestinal glucose on glycaemia, insulinaemia and incretin hormone release are load-dependent in obese subjects," *International Journal of Obesity*, vol. 41, no. 2, pp. 225–232, 2017.

[57] X. C. Wang, H. Liu, J. Chen, Y. Li, and S. Qu, "Multiple factors related to the secretion of glucagon-like peptide-1," *International Journal of Endocrinology*, vol. 2015, 11 pages, 2015.

[58] J. J. Meier, G. Kemmeries, J. J. Holst, and M. A. Nauck, "Erythromycin antagonizes the deceleration of gastric emptying by glucagon-like peptide 1 and unmasks its insulinotropic effect in healthy subjects," *Diabetes*, vol. 54, no. 7, pp. 2212–2218, 2005.

[59] M. M. Umapathysivam, M. Y. Lee, K. L. Jones et al., "Comparative effects of prolonged and intermittent stimulation of the glucagon-like peptide 1 receptor on gastric emptying and glycemia," *Diabetes*, vol. 63, no. 2, pp. 785–790, 2014.

[60] M. A. Nauck, G. Kemmeries, J. J. Holst, and J. J. Meier, "Rapid tachyphylaxis of the glucagon-like peptide 1-induced deceleration of gastric emptying in humans," *Diabetes*, vol. 60, no. 5, pp. 1561–1565, 2011.

[61] M. C. Gannon and F. Q. Nuttall, "Amino acid ingestion and glucose metabolism – a review," *IUBMB Life*, vol. 62, no. 9, pp. 660–668, 2010.

[62] J. Tay, C. H. Thompson, and G. D. Brinkworth, "Glycemic variability: assessing glycemia differently and the implications for dietary management of diabetes," *Annual Review of Nutrition*, vol. 35, no. 1, pp. 389–424, 2015.

[63] L. Sun, K. W. J. Tan, C. M. S. Han, M. K.-S. Leow, and C. J. Henry, "Impact of preloading either dairy or soy milk on postprandial glycemia, insulinemia and gastric emptying in healthy adults," *European Journal of Nutrition*, vol. 56, no. 1, pp. 77–87, 2017.

[64] S. Y. Tan, P. C. Siow, E. Peh, and C. J. Henry, "Influence of rice, pea and oat proteins in attenuating glycemic response of sugar-sweetened beverages," *European Journal of Nutrition*, pp. 1–9, 2017.

[65] C. Giezenaar, L. G. Trahair, N. D. Luscombe-Marsh et al., "Effects of randomized whey-protein loads on energy intake, appetite, gastric emptying, and plasma gut-hormone concentrations in older men and women," *The American Journal of Clinical Nutrition*, vol. 106, no. 3, pp. 865–877, 2017.

[66] L. E. Mignone, T. Wu, M. Horowitz, and C. K. Rayner, "Whey protein: the "whey" forward for treatment of type 2 diabetes?," *World Journal of Diabetes*, vol. 6, no. 14, pp. 1274–1284, 2015.

[67] J. Ma, J. E. Stevens, K. Cukier et al., "Effects of a protein preload on gastric emptying, glycemia, and gut hormones after a carbohydrate meal in diet-controlled type 2 diabetes," *Diabetes Care*, vol. 32, no. 9, pp. 1600–1602, 2009.

[68] D. Jakubowicz, O. Froy, B. Ahrén et al., "Incretin, insulinotropic and glucose-lowering effects of whey protein pre-load in type 2 diabetes: a randomised clinical trial," *Diabetologia*, vol. 57, no. 9, pp. 1807–1811, 2014.

[69] S. S. Ullrich, P. C. E. Fitzgerald, I. Nkamba, R. E. Steinert, M. Horowitz, and C. Feinle-Bisset, "Intragastric lysine lowers the circulating glucose and insulin responses to a mixed-nutrient drink without slowing gastric emptying in healthy adults," *The Journal of Nutrition*, vol. 147, no. 7, pp. 1275–1281, 2017.

[70] S. S. Ullrich, P. C. E. Fitzgerald, G. Schober, R. E. Steinert, M. Horowitz, and C. Feinle-Bisset, "Intragastric administration of leucine or isoleucine lowers the blood glucose response to a mixed-nutrient drink by different mechanisms in healthy, lean volunteers," *The American Journal of Clinical Nutrition*, vol. 104, no. 5, pp. 1274–1284, 2016.

[71] F. Mano, K. Ikeda, E. Joo, S. Yamane, N. Harada, and N. Inagaki, "Effects of three major amino acids found in Japanese broth on glucose metabolism and gastric emptying," *Nutrition*, vol. 46, pp. 153–158.e1, 2018.

[72] A. C. Meyer-Gerspach, S. Häfliger, J. Meili et al., "Effect of L-tryptophan and L-leucine on gut hormone secretion, appetite feelings and gastric emptying rates in lean and non-diabetic obese participants: a randomized, double-blind, parallel-group trial," *PLoS One*, vol. 11, no. 11, article e0166758, 2016.

[73] C. J. Homko, F. Duffy, F. K. Friedenberg, G. Boden, and H. P. Parkman, "Effect of dietary fat and food consistency on gastroparesis symptoms in patients with gastroparesis," *Neurogastroenterology and Motility*, vol. 27, no. 4, pp. 501–508, 2015.

[74] K. Yu, M. Y. Ke, W. H. Li, S. Q. Zhang, and X. C. Fang, "The impact of soluble dietary fibre on gastric emptying, postprandial blood glucose and insulin in patients with type 2 diabetes," *Asia Pacific Journal of Clinical Nutrition*, vol. 23, no. 2, pp. 210–218, 2014.

[75] N. Repin, B. A. Kay, S. W. Cui, A. J. Wright, A. M. Duncan, and H. Douglas Goff, "Investigation of mechanisms involved in postprandial glycemia and insulinemia attenuation with dietary fibre consumption," *Food & Function*, vol. 8, no. 6, pp. 2142–2154, 2017.

[76] R. E. Steinert, D. Raederstorff, and T. M. Wolever, "Effect of consuming oat bran mixed in water before a meal on glycemic responses in healthy humans-a pilot study," *Nutrients*, vol. 8, no. 9, 2016.

[77] A. R. Mackie, B. H. Bajka, N. M. Rigby et al., "Oatmeal particle size alters glycemic index but not as a function of gastric emptying rate," *American Journal of Physiology. Gastrointestinal and Liver Physiology*, vol. 313, no. 3, pp. G239–G246, 2017.

[78] A. Ibarra, K. Olli, W. Pasman et al., "Effects of polydextrose with breakfast or with a midmorning preload on food intake and other appetite-related parameters in healthy normal-weight and overweight females: an acute, randomized, double-blind, placebo-controlled, and crossover study," *Appetite*, vol. 110, pp. 15–24, 2017.

[79] M. Voukali, I. Kastrinelli, S. Stragalinou et al., "Study of postprandial lipaemia in type 2 diabetes mellitus: exenatide versus liraglutide," *Journal of Diabetes Research*, vol. 2014, Article ID 304032, 7 pages, 2014.

[80] J. J. Meier, J. Rosenstock, A. Hincelin-Méry et al., "Contrasting effects of lixisenatide and liraglutide on postprandial glycemic control, gastric emptying, and safety parameters in patients with type 2 diabetes on optimized insulin glargine with or

without metformin: a randomized, open-label trial," *Diabetes Care*, vol. 38, no. 7, pp. 1263–1273, 2015.

[81] C. Amouyal and F. Andreelli, "Increasing GLP-1 circulating levels by bariatric surgery or by GLP-1 receptor agonists therapy: why are the clinical consequences so different?," *Journal of Diabetes Research*, vol. 2016, Article ID 5908656, 10 pages, 2016.

[82] M. Lorenz, C. Pfeiffer, A. Steinsträßer et al., "Effects of lixisenatide once daily on gastric emptying in type 2 diabetes – relationship to postprandial glycemia," *Regulatory Peptides*, vol. 185, pp. 1–8, 2013.

[83] J. Jelsing, N. Vrang, G. Hansen, K. Raun, M. Tang-Christensen, and L. Bjerre Knudsen, "Liraglutide: short-lived effect on gastric emptying – long lasting effects on body weight," *Diabetes, Obesity & Metabolism*, vol. 14, no. 6, pp. 531–538, 2012.

[84] Y. Nakatani, M. Maeda, M. Matsumura et al., "Effect of GLP-1 receptor agonist on gastrointestinal tract motility and residue rates as evaluated by capsule endoscopy," *Diabetes & Metabolism*, vol. 43, no. 5, pp. 430–437, 2017.

[85] J. B. Hjerpsted, A. Flint, A. Brooks, M. B. Axelsen, T. Kvist, and J. Blundell, "Semaglutide improves postprandial glucose and lipid metabolism, and delays first-hour gastric emptying in subjects with obesity," *Diabetes, Obesity & Metabolism*, vol. 20, no. 3, pp. 610–619, 2018.

[86] B. Ahrén, "Physiological aspects of the combination of insulin and GLP-1 in the regulation of blood glucose control," *Diabetes & Metabolism*, vol. 41, no. 6, pp. 6S3–6S8, 2015.

[87] A. Albèr, A. Brønden, and F. K. Knop, "Short-acting glucagon-like peptide-1 receptor agonists as add-on to insulin therapy in type 1 diabetes: a review," *Diabetes, Obesity & Metabolism*, vol. 19, no. 7, pp. 915–925, 2017.

[88] American Diabetes Association, "8. Pharmacologic approaches to glycemic treatment," *Diabetes Care*, vol. 40, Supplement 1, pp. S64–S74, 2017.

[89] A. J. Garber, M. J. Abrahamson, J. I. Barzilay et al., "Consensus statement by the American Association of Clinical Endocrinologists and American College of Endocrinology on the comprehensive type 2 diabetes management algorithm – 2017 executive summary," *Endocrine Practice*, vol. 23, no. 2, pp. 207–238, 2017.

[90] C. S. Frandsen, T. F. Dejgaard, H. U. Andersen et al., "Liraglutide as adjunct to insulin treatment in type 1 diabetes does not interfere with glycaemic recovery or gastric emptying rate during hypoglycaemia: a randomized, placebo-controlled, double-blind, parallel-group study," *Diabetes, Obesity & Metabolism*, vol. 19, no. 6, pp. 773–782, 2017.

2

Markers of Local Inflammation and Bone Resorption in the Acute Diabetic Charcot Foot

Rasmus Bo Jansen[1,2] **Tomas Møller Christensen,**[2] **Jens Bülow,**[3] **Lene Rørdam,**[3] **Niklas Rye Jørgensen,**[4,5] **and Ole Lander Svendsen**[1,2]

[1]*Copenhagen Diabetes Foot Center (CODIF), Bispebjerg Hospital, University of Copenhagen, 2400 Copenhagen NV, Denmark*
[2]*Department of Endocrinology, Bispebjerg Hospital, University of Copenhagen, 2400 Copenhagen NV, Denmark*
[3]*Department of Clinical Physiology and Nuclear Medicine, Bispebjerg Hospital, University of Copenhagen, 2400 Copenhagen NV, Denmark*
[4]*Department of Clinical Biochemistry, Rigshospitalet, University of Copenhagen, 2600 Glostrup, Denmark*
[5]*Odense Patient data Explorative Network (OPEN), Odense University Hospital/Institute of Clinical Research, University of Southern Denmark, Odense, Denmark*

Correspondence should be addressed to Rasmus Bo Jansen; rasmus.bo.jansen@regionh.dk

Academic Editor: Mark Yorek

Objective. Due to the localized nature of Charcot foot, systemically altered levels of inflammation markers can be difficult to measure. The aim of this study was to investigate whether it is possible to detect an arteriovenous (A-V) flux in any locally produced inflammatory biomarkers from an acute Charcot foot by comparing local and systemic measurements. *Methods.* We included patients with acute diabetic Charcot foot. Blood was sampled from the vena saphena magna on the distal part of the crus bilaterally as well as from the arteria radialis. To minimize the A-V shunting effect, the feet were externally cooled with ice water prior to resampling. *Results.* Both before and after cooling, the A-V flux of interleukin-6 (IL-6) between the Charcot feet and the arterial level was significantly higher than the flux between the healthy feet and the arterial level ($\Delta\text{value}_{\text{before}}$: 7.25 versus 0.41 pg/mL, resp., $p = 0.008$; $\Delta\text{value}_{\text{after}}$: 10.04 versus 1.68 pg/mL, resp., $p = 0.032$). There were no differences in the fluxes for other markers of inflammation. *Conclusion.* We have found an increased A-V flux of IL-6 in the acute diabetic Charcot foot compared to the healthy foot in the same patients.

1. Introduction

Charcot osteoarthropathy is a rare disorder manifesting with aseptic inflammation and hyperemia in and around load-bearing bones and tissues. The process is normally unilateral and leads to progressive, uncontrolled resorption and degeneration of bone mass, resulting in spontaneous fatigue bone fractures [1–4]. While different locations have been described, the most common is in the feet (Charcot foot (CF)) [5, 6], where the process can cause deformity, ulcerations, and amputations. The Charcot inflammation can be located at different sites in the affected foot, most prominently in the midfoot [2, 7].

The precise pathological mechanisms underlying Charcot foot are still not fully understood. However, it is dependent on relatively unimpaired lower limb blood flow and established peripheral neuropathy [8–11]. It can be triggered by a number of diseases, although today most cases occur in individuals with diabetes mellitus [1, 2, 12].

Recent evidence suggests that the initial inflammation is provoked by repeated local microtrauma and dysregulated bone resorption [13–16], which in turn initiates the inflammatory process.

Several studies have reported changes in biomarkers of bone resorption and inflammation in individuals with

Charcot foot [17–24], and it seems that the inflammation leads to microstructural changes in the affected bones [25, 26].

Related to this, studies have explored the possible relationship between interleukin levels and acute Charcot foot [17, 27–29] and found increased levels of interleukin-1 receptor antagonist (IL-1RA), tumor necrosis factor α (TNF-α), interleukin-6 (IL-6), and interleukin-17 subtypes A, E, and F (IL-17A/E/F), as well as decreased levels of interleukin-1β (IL-1β) and interleukin-8 (IL-8).

In addition, many individuals with Charcot foot also seem to have a degree of vascular calcification and inflammation [30, 31]. This is of particular interest due to the connection between vascular calcification, neuropathy, and the nuclear factor-κB (NF-κB) system, as described by Petrova and Shanahan [32]. A possible way to assess this could be through the system of advanced glycation end products (AGEs) and their soluble receptors (sRAGE) [33–35].

However, the biomarkers in question might only be produced locally around the inflamed bones in the foot, which means that the signal on a systemic level can be difficult to register. Furthermore, a general systemic release of these biomarkers might happen in response to a number of inflammatory processes unrelated to the Charcot foot.

Therefore, it is plausible that a stronger and more specific signal from an acute Charcot foot might be achieved by measuring the flux of a specific marker between the local venous concentration in the foot and the arterial concentration. Local sampling from the dorsal venous arch of the foot in acute Charcot feet has previously been done by Gough et al. and Pearson et al. [21, 23], although neither measured all the markers discussed here. To our knowledge, local fluxes of inflammatory biomarkers across an acute Charcot foot have not been measured previously.

The aim of this study was to investigate whether it is possible to detect a flux in any locally produced biomarkers from an acute Charcot foot by measuring the arteriovenous (A-V) difference.

2. Materials and Methods

2.1. Participants. We included participants with acute Charcot foot, recruited at the Copenhagen Wound Healing Center at Bispebjerg Hospital, Denmark, and at the Steno Diabetes Center, Gentofte, Denmark. The participants were referred by specialists after thorough physical examination, full blood panel, X-ray, bone scintigraphy, and/or MRI. All participants were examined as close as possible to the reported outbreak of the acute Charcot symptom (<3 months).

Exclusion criteria included no diabetes mellitus, temperature difference < 2°C between the feet, duration > 3 months, foot ulcers, prior foot surgery, new objective foot deformities, bilateral Charcot foot, infection in the foot, antiosteoporotic medication, arterial insufficiency, or foot or toe amputation on either side.

To confirm that the Charcot foot still had a high activity on the day of examination as assessed by a locally elevated blood flow, this was measured in the feet with venous occlusion plethysmography [36]. Foot temperature and foot somatosensoric neuropathy as assessed by biothesiometry were measured on the study day as well.

The study was approved by the Regional Ethical Committee for Copenhagen.

2.2. Arteriovenous Flux. To measure the fluxes in biomarker production in the acute Charcot foot, blood was sampled from the vena saphena magna on the distal part of the crus above the ankle. This was done on both the affected (Charcot) side and the healthy side. Arterial blood was sampled from the a. radialis (or from the a. brachialis if the a. radialis was inaccessible).

The venous drainage of the foot happens primarily through the veins saphena magna and parva, while the deep veins only play a minor role. The saphena veins connect through the dorsal venous arch on the dorsal side of the foot. The dorsal venous arch collects blood from both superficial and deep veins in the foot, as well as from the networks rete venosus plantare and rete venosus dorsale pedis. The superficial and deep veins of the foot are linked by communicating perforant veins. The few valves present in these perforants are turned so that blood can only run from the deep to the superficial veins, thus helping with thermoregulation and pressure absorption. This means that parts of the drainage of the deep foot happen through the superficial veins, which can thus be sampled from a superficial vein on the lower leg [37–39].

A portion of the blood flow in the feet bypasses normal microcirculatory exchange by shunting directly through A-V anastomoses. This is in part a thermoregulatory effect and is thus more prevalent at higher skin temperatures [40]. As the shunted blood will not be exposed to any biomarkers produced in the deep foot tissue, this A-V shunting in effect dilutes the signal of any inflammatory biomarkers in a mixed venous sample. To minimize this shunting effect in our setup, we cooled down the feet externally with cold water prior to the final sampling (t_{ice}).

2.3. Experimental Setup. All three sites were sampled simultaneously (t_{start}) (Figure 1). Fluxes between the arterial and venous concentrations were calculated as vein − artery to get a positive gradient if the Charcot foot produced the biomarker in question. After sampling, both feet were cooled down for approximately 10 minutes in an icy water bath, while foot temperature was measured. The three sites were then sampled again while the participants kept their feet in the water (t_{ice}).

In the following, venous samples from the acute Charcot foot are denoted as CF(v) and venous samples from the non-Charcot foot are denoted as non-CF(v).

The blood samples were centrifuged at 4°C and stored at −80°C. All samples were analyzed together at the end of the study.

2.4. Biomarkers. To estimate the existing interleukin profile and the highest relative concentrations, t_{start} samples were analyzed on a Bio-Plex System multiplex immunoassay screening panel (Bio-Rad Laboratories Inc., 4000 Alfred Nobel Drive, Hercules, California 94547, USA). The panel

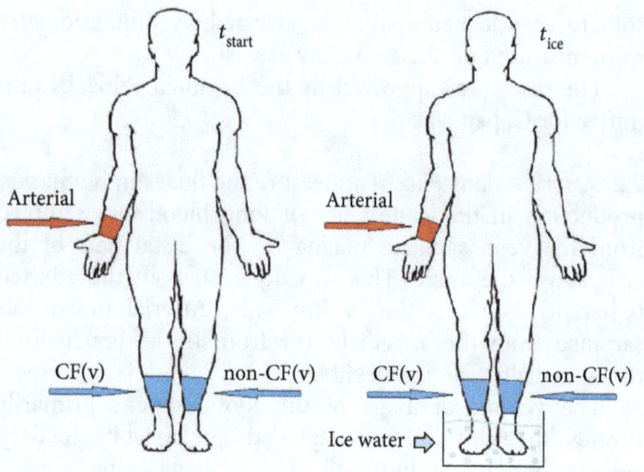

FIGURE 1: Sites of arterial (red) or venous (blue) blood samples before (t_{start}) and after (t_{ice}) external cooling of the feet. Arterial samples were taken from the a. radialis, or from the a. brachialis if the a. radialis was inaccessible. Venous samples were taken from a large superficial vein at the third distal part of the crus both on the side with a Charcot foot (CF(v)) and on the side without a Charcot foot (non-CF(v)).

used screened for IL-1β, IL-1RA, IL-6, IL-8, IL-17A, and TNF-α, with the best signals detected for IL-6 and IL-8.

All analyses were performed by Biolab, Department of Clinical Biochemistry, Rigshospitalet, University of Copenhagen, Denmark. Special ELISA setups were used for IL-6, IL-8, free soluble receptor activator of nuclear factor kappa-*B* ligand (fsRANK-L), osteoprotegerin (OPG), IL-17F, sRAGE, and AGEs. The remaining samples were analyzed as part of the daily hospital sample routines. The accepted intraindividual sample CV for all assays was 20%.

(i) AGEs were measured with a Human sandwich ELISA AGE kit (Nordic BioSite AB, Propellervägen 4A, 183 62 Täby, Sweden) (kit serial number LS-F10641-1; range 0.78–50 ng/mL).

(ii) IL-6 was measured with an IL-6 Quantikine HS ELISA kit (Bio-Techne Ltd., 614 McKinley Place NE, Minneapolis, MN 55413, USA) (kit serial number HS600B).

(iii) IL-8 was measured with a Human CXCL8 Quantikine kit (Bio-Techne Ltd., 614 McKinley Place NE, Minneapolis, MN 55413, USA) (kit serial number D8000C).

(iv) IL-17F was measured with a Human IL-17F Platinum ELISA kit (AH-Diagnostics A/S, Runetoften 18, DK-8210 Aarhus V, Denmark) (kit serial number BMS2037/2).

(v) Assays for fsRANK-L, osteoprotegerin, and sRAGE were performed as previously described [41].

2.5. Statistical Analysis. Data are presented as mean ± 1 SD or range unless otherwise noted. An α-level of <0.05 was considered significant. Normal distribution in data was tested using Shapiro-Wilks tests. No transformations were used. *t*-tests or paired *t*-tests were used for variance analysis between groups in normally distributed data sets. For data sets not normally distributed, nonparametric tests in the form of the Mann-Whitney rank-sum test were used, while Wilcoxon signed-rank tests were used for comparing paired samples.

Statistics and general data handling were done using IBM SPSS Statistics v. 23 by IBM Corporation, SIGMAPLOT v. 11.0.0.77 by Systat Software Inc., Microsoft Excel 2000 v. 9.0.2812 by Microsoft Corporation, and Apache OpenOffice 4.0.1 by the Apache Software Foundation.

3. Results

3.1. Participants. We included 5 patients with acute Charcot foot. In total, 22 patients were screened for inclusion. Of these, 7 patients were excluded due to having foot ulcers or receiving foot surgery and/or ulcer debridement before the examinations. Another 7 did not want to participate or were unable to participate due to personal reasons, while 3 patients had had their Charcot foot for too long to be considered acute (duration > 3 months).

The average time from the reported onset of symptoms to examination was 7.2 weeks. The Charcot feet were on average 2.6°C warmer than the contralateral and had a 3 times increased blood flow. All 5 patients had recently started off-loading treatment with an AirCast® removable walker boot before measurements. All 5 patients were diagnosed with stage 0 Charcot foot.

Anthropometric data for the participants are listed in Table 1, along with the results for biothesiometry, venous occlusion plethysmography, and arterial samples of markers of bone health taken prior to the cooling of the feet (t_{start}). There were a significant higher temperature and blood flow in the acute Charcot feet compared to the healthy feet.

3.2. Multiplex Data. For IL-1β, IL-1RA, IL-17A, and TNF-α, almost all measured values were below the multiplex limit of detection in all samples. This was tested with both serum and plasma. The detection limits were 1.32 pg/mL for IL-1, 29.64 pg/mL for IL-1RA, 7.99 pg/mL for IL-17A, and 12.72 pg/mL for TNF-α. There was a single signal in one patient in IL-1RA and IL-17A (not the same patient for both markers).

The average level of IL-6 detected was 10.6 pg/mL, and for IL-8, it was 12.5 pg/mL.

3.3. Measurements before Cooling. Measurements from all three sites (arterial, CF(v), and non-CF(v)) before and after cooling are listed in Table 2. At t_{start}, there were no differences in the levels of fsRANK-L, OPG, IL-6, IL-8, sRAGE, or AGEs—neither between arterial and CF(v) nor between CF(v) and non-CF(v) samples. The highest relative numerical difference was for IL-6 in arterial versus CF(v) levels (7.31 versus 14.56) ($p = 0.109$). It was not possible to measure IL-17F as it was below the assay detection limit of 7.8 pg/mL for all samples at t_{start} and t_{ice}.

The venous-arterial flux of IL-6 between the Charcot feet and the arterial level was significantly higher than the flux

Table 1: Anthropomorphic data for diabetes patients with acute Charcot foot (CF). Test results are from arterial sampling.

(a)

	Data listed as mean; range or n
Age (years)	48.6; 26.0
Sex (m/f)	3/2
Affected foot (left/right)	1/4
Diabetes type (I/II)	2/3
Diabetes duration (years)	19.2; 31.0
HbA1c (mmol/mol) (31–44 mmol/mol)	73; 53
Ca^{2+}(free, ionized) (mmol/L) (1.18–1.32 mmol/L)	1.24; 0.14
PTH (pmol/L) (1.6–6.9 pmol/L)	4.5; 4.3
CRP (mg/L) (<10 mg/L)	9.8; 15.0
25-OH-vitamin D (nmol/L) (50–160 nmol/L)	36.7; 52.6
Alkaline phosphatase (bone specific) (μg/L) (<20 μg/L)$^{\$}$	20.3; 7.3
CTX (ng/L) (<630 ng/L)$^{\$}$	240; 0.5
P1NP (μg/L) (22–87 μg/L)$^{\$}$	48.3; 53.8
Osteocalcin (μg/L) (9–42 μg/L)	25.3; 42.1

(b)

	Charcot foot	Contralateral foot	Difference, p value
Foot temperature (CF/non-CF) (°C)	33.7	31.1	$\Delta 2.6$, $p = 0.004^{*}$
Biothesiometry (CF/non-CF) (V)	42	39	$\Delta 3$, $p = 0.648$
Plethysmography (CF/non-CF) (mL/(100 g·min))	6.9	1.8	$\Delta 5.1$, $p = 0.045^{*}$

*Significant at the chosen α-level of 0.05. $^{\$}$Reference range listed for 50 y.o. male where ranges differ with age and/or sex.

Table 2: Levels of inflammation markers in local venous samples in the acute Charcot foot (CF(v)), the healthy foot (non-CF(v)), and arterial samples from the a. radialis. Measurements listed before (t_{start}) and after (t_{ice}) external cooling of both feet with ice water.

	Sampling site	t_{start}	t_{ice}
	Arterial	0.14 ± 0.12	0.13 ± 0.11
fsRANK-L (pmol/L)	CF(v)	0.13 ± 0.11	0.14 ± 0.11
	non-CF(v)	0.13 ± 0.11	0.14 ± 0.13
	Arterial	6.5 ± 5.4	6.6 ± 5.1
OPG (pmol/L)	CF(v)	6.4 ± 5.8	7.3 ± 5.9
	non-CF(v)	6.3 ± 5.5	7.5 ± 6.1
	Arterial	7.31 ± 6.88	6.25 ± 5.21
IL-6 (pg/mL)	CF(v)	14.56 ± 14.27	16.29 ± 11.45
	non-CF(v)	7.71 ± 7.07	7.93 ± 5.70
	Arterial	15.6 ± 7.9	13.1 ± 6.3
IL-8 (pg/mL)	CF(v)	13.4 ± 4.4	12.1 ± 6.3
	non-CF(v)	14.5 ± 9.6	11.5 ± 4.7
	Arterial	845 ± 266	860 ± 247
sRAGE (ng/L)	CF(v)	833 ± 292	878 ± 298
	non-CF(v)	827 ± 252	911 ± 293
	Arterial	6.2 ± 7.7	5.4 ± 7.4
AGEs (ng/mL)	CF(v)	5.7 ± 6.8	7.9 ± 7.1
	non-CF(v)	5.9 ± 7.2	8.4 ± 8.4

Data listed as mean ± 1 SD. fsRANKL = free soluble receptor activator of nuclear factor-κB; OPG = osteoprotegerin; IL-6/IL-8 = interleukin 6/interleukin 8; sRAGE = soluble receptor for advanced glycation end products; AGEs = advanced glycation end products.

between the healthy feet and the arterial level (Δvalues: 7.25 versus 0.41 pg/mL, resp.) ($p = 0.008$). There were no differences in fsRANK-L, OPG, IL-8, sRAGE, or AGEs.

3.4. Measurements after External Cooling. The ice bath used for cooling maintained an average temperature of 7.7°C, and it was used for cooling for an average of 11.6 min. The ice bath cooled the Charcot feet at an average of 11.0°C (from 33.7 to 22.7°C), and the non-Charcot feet were cooled at an average of 12.9°C (from 31.1 to 18.2°C). Temperatures in each foot before and after cooling are listed in Table 3.

At t_{ice}, there was a significantly elevated level of IL-6 (Δvalue: 10.04 pg/mL) in the Charcot feet compared to the arterial value ($p = 0.049$) (Figure 2). There was also a significantly elevated level of AGEs (Δvalue: 2.5 ng/mL) ($p = 0.002$) (Table 2). There were no differences in fsRANK-L, OPG, IL-8, or sRAGE.

The venous-arterial flux for IL-6 at t_{ice} was still significantly increased in the Charcot feet (CF(v)-arterial) compared to the healthy feet (non-CF(v)-arterial) (Δvalues: 10.04 versus 1.68 pg/mL) ($p = 0.032$). There were no differences in the fluxes for fsRANK-L, OPG, IL-8, sRAGE, or AGEs.

The fsRANK-L/OPG ratio at t_{ice} was 3.7 in the arterial sample, 4.0 in the CF(v) sample, and 3.8 in the non-CF(v) sample and did not differ in a one-way ANOVA on ranks ($p = 0.970$).

TABLE 3: Temperature measurements on the feet of each individual patient during the study day.

Patient number	Charcot foot temperature (°C) Before cooling (t_{start})	Charcot foot temperature (°C) After cooling (t_{ice})	Non-Charcot foot temperature (°C) Before cooling (t_{start})	Non-Charcot foot temperature (°C) After cooling (t_{ice})
1	32.0	20.0	29.7	18.0
2	33.8	25.9	31.7	18.6
3	33.7	20.2	32.3	20.6
4	34.8	21.8	31.0	17.0
5	34.4	25.7	30.7	17.0

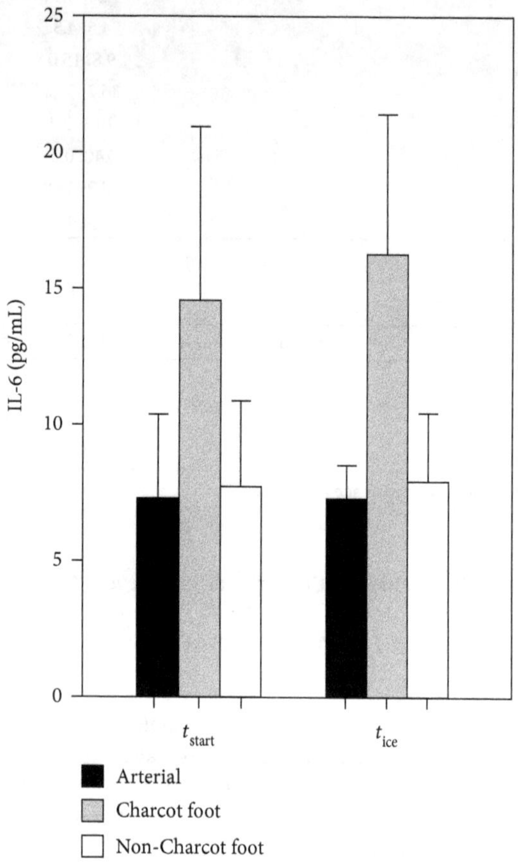

FIGURE 2: Levels of interleukin 6 (IL-6) in arterial and local venous samples in both feet (CF(v) and non-CF(v)) before (t_{start}) and after (t_{ice}) external cooling with ice water. Bars = mean; error bars = SEM.

4. Discussion

In this study, we have tested a novel approach to evaluating the local inflammatory activity in an acute Charcot foot by measuring the venous-arterial flux across the Charcot foot while lowering the possible dilution from A-V shunting by externally cooling the foot.

The data show a difference in the venous-arterial flux of IL-6 both before and after external cooling. We also saw a two-fold elevated level of IL-6 in the Charcot foot compared to the arterial level after cooling, indicating a local production of IL-6. It is interesting that both IL-6 and AGEs only show a significant difference between the Charcot foot and arterial level after cooling, thus possibly indicating an effect of limiting A-V shunting in the feet before sampling.

The results are mostly in line with what other groups have found. Divyateja et al. indicated an increased median IL-6 level in the Charcot foot [24], while both Petrova et al. [17] and Folestad et al. [29] have suggested increased levels of IL-6 systemically (although Folestad et al. did not find an initially increased level of IL-6).

Unlike Folestad et al., we have been unable to demonstrate high levels of IL-17F systemically in acute Charcot patients [27]. However, they did show an initial low level of IL-17F (corresponding to the time where we performed our sampling), and additionally, they used high-sensitivity ECL as opposed to the ELISA that we used.

A finding of locally increased levels of IL-6 is of particular interest for several reasons. As a proinflammatory cytokine, its presence supports the theory regarding the pathogenesis of acute Charcot foot as put forth by, for instance, Jeffcoate et al. [13]. Furthermore, IL-6 is involved in bone resorption through osteoclastic differentiation and activation [42–45]. Thus, the finding further supports local osteoclastic hyperactivation as a central element in the Charcot foot bone metabolism and confirms the findings of IL-6 in osteoclasts in bone samples from Charcot feet as seen by Baumhauer et al. [46]. The source of this local production of IL-6 remains unknown.

Recently, Petrova et al. reported that OPG was elevated in patients with Charcot foot without a corresponding elevation in RANK-L [17] and that osteoclasts from patients with Charcot foot can be modulated by TNF-α through RANK-L [47]. It is important to note however that elevated OPG levels could be associated with neuropathy in itself [48].

Ndip et al. have indicated that individuals with Charcot foot have an increased RANK-L/OPG ratio and suggest that this could play a role in medial vascular calcification [22]. We have also previously shown a higher RANK-L/OPG ratio in patients with acute Charcot foot than non-Charcot diabetic controls [41]. In the current setup, we did not find a difference in the venous-arterial flux or a locally elevated RANK-L/OPG ratio. However, this was not to be expected either as both markers only circulate in very small quantities and furthermore have half-lives sufficient to recirculate the vascular system many times, making it difficult to detect a local difference.

Regarding the increased level of AGEs after cooling, it is unclear whether this is an expression of a local increase in production of AGEs due to cooling, a by-product of the Charcot inflammation, or merely a random sampling variation.

The presence of tissue-bound receptors for AGEs (RAGE) has been associated with impaired bone matrix mineralization and enhanced osteoclast formation [49]. AGEs have been linked to a negative modification of collagen integrity and fragile bones in general [50–52]. Thus, if there is indeed an increased level of AGEs present in Charcot feet, this might account for a further weakening of the bones. Furthermore, there is a link between increased levels of RAGE and activation of the NF-κB system and several associated cytokines [53, 54]. As such, it shares a common pathway of influence of osteoclastic activation with RANK-L/OPG and by extension IL-6.

4.1. Strengths and Limitations. To our knowledge, this is the first time that the local venous-arterial flux across an acute Charcot foot has been studied. Furthermore, we are unaware of other studies that have limited the local A-V shunting effect prior to measuring a Charcot foot.

The study was limited by the number of available participants. In total, we screened 22 patients and most of these were excluded due to foot ulcers or extended time from the symptom onset to diagnosis. Thus, part of the recruitment issue was the rigorous exclusion criteria needed to ensure that any possible findings were not clouded by infections, surgery, or prolonged Charcot inflammation.

Furthermore, most of the assays we have used have a limited accuracy and substantial intraindividual variations, and thus it was difficult to register any possible differences. These variations might be the reason why we saw an increase in AGEs after cooling in the Charcot foot compared to the arterial level. Unless more accurate assays are developed, future tests in a similar setup could be performed with multiple samples from each site and each time point to help alleviate this issue.

5. Conclusion

In conclusion, we have found an increased venous-arterial flux of IL-6 in the acute diabetic Charcot foot compared to the healthy foot. We also found an increased level of IL-6 and AGEs in the acute Charcot foot compared to the arterial level after, but not before, externally cooling the feet.

Disclosure

The foundations had no influence on the design, execution, results, or conclusions of the study.

Conflicts of Interest

The authors declare that they have no conflicts of interest.

Acknowledgments

This study was funded in part by donations from the private Danish foundations: "Toyota-Fonden" and "Brødrene Hartmanns Fond."

References

[1] A. Hartemann-Heurtier, G. H. van, and A. Grimaldi, "The Charcot foot," *The Lancet*, vol. 360, no. 9347, pp. 1776–1779, 2002.

[2] J. Fabrin, K. Larsen, and P. E. Holstein, "Long-term follow-up in diabetic Charcot feet with spontaneous onset," *Diabetes Care*, vol. 23, no. 6, pp. 796–800, 2000.

[3] L. Lee, P. A. Blume, and B. Sumpio, "Charcot joint disease in diabetes mellitus," *Annals of Vascular Surgery*, vol. 17, no. 5, pp. 571–580, 2003.

[4] L. C. Rogers and R. G. Frykberg, "The Charcot foot," *The Medical Clinics of North America*, vol. 97, no. 5, pp. 847–856, 2013.

[5] B. J. Grear, A. Rabinovich, and J. W. Brodsky, "Charcot arthropathy of the foot and ankle associated with rheumatoid arthritis," *Foot & Ankle International*, vol. 34, no. 11, pp. 1541–1547, 2013.

[6] M. E. Munson, J. S. Wrobel, C. M. Holmes, and D. A. Hanauer, "Data mining for identifying novel associations and temporal relationships with Charcot foot," *Journal of Diabetes Research*, vol. 2014, Article ID 214353, 13 pages, 2014.

[7] J. T. Bariteau, S. Tenenbaum, A. Rabinovich, and J. W. Brodsky, "Charcot arthropathy of the foot and ankle in patients with idiopathic neuropathy," *Foot & Ankle International*, vol. 35, no. 10, pp. 996–1001, 2014.

[8] N. L. Petrova and M. E. Edmonds, "Charcot neuro-osteoarthropathy-current standards," *Diabetes/Metabolism Research and Reviews*, vol. 24, Supplement 1, pp. S58–S61, 2008.

[9] J. D. Ward, "The diabetic leg," *Diabetologia*, vol. 22, no. 3, pp. 141–147, 1982.

[10] L. C. Rogers, R. G. Frykberg, D. G. Armstrong et al., "The Charcot foot in diabetes," *Journal of the American Podiatric Medical Association*, vol. 101, no. 5, pp. 437–446, 2011.

[11] A. J. M. Boulton, "Diabetic neuropathy and foot complications," *Handbook of Clinical Neurology*, vol. 126, pp. 97–107, 2014.

[12] S. M. Rajbhandari, R. C. Jenkins, C. Davies, and S. Tesfaye, "Charcot neuroarthropathy in diabetes mellitus," *Diabetologia*, vol. 45, no. 8, pp. 1085–1096, 2002.

[13] W. J. Jeffcoate, F. Game, and P. R. Cavanagh, "The role of proinflammatory cytokines in the cause of neuropathic osteoarthropathy (acute Charcot foot) in diabetes," *The Lancet*, vol. 366, no. 9502, pp. 2058–2061, 2005.

[14] W. J. Jeffcoate, "Charcot neuro-osteoarthropathy," *Diabetes/Metabolism Research and Reviews*, vol. 24, Supplement 1, pp. S62–S65, 2008.

[15] G. Mabilleau and M. E. Edmonds, "Role of neuropathy on fracture healing in Charcot neuro-osteoarthropathy," *Journal of Musculoskeletal & Neuronal Interactions*, vol. 10, no. 1, pp. 84–91, 2010.

[16] E. Chantelau and G. J. Onvlee, "Charcot foot in diabetes: farewell to the neurotrophic theory," *Hormone and Metabolic Research*, vol. 38, no. 6, pp. 361–367, 2006.

[17] N. L. Petrova, T. K. Dew, R. L. Musto et al., "Inflammatory and bone turnover markers in a cross-sectional and prospective

study of acute Charcot osteoarthropathy," *Diabetic Medicine*, vol. 32, no. 2, pp. 267–273, 2015.

[18] L. Uccioli, A. Sinistro, C. Almerighi et al., "Proinflammatory modulation of the surface and cytokine phenotype of monocytes in patients with acute Charcot foot," *Diabetes Care*, vol. 33, no. 2, pp. 350–355, 2010.

[19] A. Piaggesi, L. Rizzo, F. Golia et al., "Biochemical and ultrasound tests for early diagnosis of active neuro-osteoarthropathy (NOA) of the diabetic foot," *Diabetes Research and Clinical Practice*, vol. 58, no. 1, pp. 1–9, 2002.

[20] G. Mabilleau, N. L. Petrova, M. E. Edmonds, and A. Sabokbar, "Increased osteoclastic activity in acute Charcot's osteoarthopathy: the role of receptor activator of nuclear factor-kappaB ligand," *Diabetologia*, vol. 51, no. 6, pp. 1035–1040, 2008.

[21] A. Gough, H. Abraha, F. Li et al., "Measurement of markers of osteoclast and osteoblast activity in patients with acute and chronic diabetic Charcot neuroarthropathy," *Diabetic Medicine*, vol. 14, no. 7, pp. 527–531, 1997.

[22] A. Ndip, A. Williams, E. B. Jude et al., "The RANKL/RANK/OPG signaling pathway mediates medial arterial calcification in diabetic Charcot neuroarthropathy," *Diabetes*, vol. 60, no. 8, pp. 2187–2196, 2011.

[23] R. G. Pearson, K. S. Shu, H. Divyateja et al., "Charcot neuropathic osteoarthropathy, pro-inflammatory cytokines and bone turnover markers," *Orthopaedic Proceedings*, vol. 94-B, Supplement XXXVI, p. 101, 2012.

[24] H. Divyateja, K. S. S. Shu, R. G. Pearson, B. E. Scammell, F. L. Game, and W. J. Jeffcoate, "Local and systemic concentration of pro-inflammatory cytokines, osteoprotegerin, sRANKL and bone turnover markers in acute Charcot foot and in controls," *Diabetologia*, vol. 54, Supplement 1, pp. S11–S12, 2011.

[25] N. L. Petrova, P. K. Petrov, M. E. Edmonds, and C. M. Shanahan, "Novel use of a Dektak 150 surface profiler unmasks differences in resorption pit profiles between control and Charcot patient osteoclasts," *Calcified Tissue International*, vol. 94, no. 4, pp. 403–411, 2014.

[26] J. La Fontaine, N. Shibuya, H. W. Sampson, and P. Valderrama, "Trabecular quality and cellular characteristics of normal, diabetic, and Charcot bone," *The Journal of Foot & Ankle Surgery*, vol. 50, no. 6, pp. 648–653, 2011.

[27] A. Folestad, M. Ålund, S. Asteberg et al., "IL-17 cytokines in bone healing of diabetic Charcot arthropathy patients: a prospective 2 year follow-up study," *Journal of Foot and Ankle Research*, vol. 8, no. 1, p. 39, 2015.

[28] A. Folestad, M. Ålund, S. Asteberg et al., "Role of Wnt/β-catenin and RANKL/OPG in bone healing of diabetic Charcot arthropathy patients," *Acta Orthopaedica*, vol. 86, no. 4, pp. 415–425, 2015.

[29] A. Folestad, M. Ålund, S. Asteberg et al., "Offloading treatment is linked to activation of proinflammatory cytokines and start of bone repair and remodeling in Charcot arthropathy patients," *Journal of Foot and Ankle Research*, vol. 8, no. 1, p. 72, 2015.

[30] S. Sinha, C. S. Munichoodappa, and G. P. Kozak, "Neuroarthropathy (Charcot joints) in diabetes mellitus (clinical study of 101 cases)," *Medicine*, vol. 51, no. 3, pp. 191–210, 1972.

[31] D. G. Armstrong, W. F. Todd, L. A. Lavery, L. B. Harkless, and T. R. Bushman, "The natural history of acute Charcot's arthropathy in a diabetic foot specialty clinic," *Diabetic Medicine*, vol. 14, no. 5, pp. 357–363, 1997.

[32] N. L. Petrova and C. M. Shanahan, "Neuropathy and the vascular-bone axis in diabetes: lessons from Charcot osteoarthropathy," *Osteoporosis International*, vol. 25, no. 4, pp. 1197–1207, 2014.

[33] A. M. Sattler, M. Schoppet, J. R. Schaefer, and L. C. Hofbauer, "Novel aspects on RANK ligand and osteoprotegerin in osteoporosis and vascular disease," *Calcified Tissue International*, vol. 74, no. 1, pp. 103–106, 2004.

[34] L. C. Hofbauer and M. Schoppet, "Clinical implications of the osteoprotegerin/RANKL/RANK system for bone and vascular diseases," *JAMA*, vol. 292, no. 4, pp. 490–495, 2004.

[35] K. A. Witzke, A. I. Vinik, L. M. Grant et al., "Loss of RAGE defense: a cause of Charcot neuroarthropathy?," *Diabetes Care*, vol. 34, no. 7, pp. 1617–1621, 2011.

[36] T. M. Christensen, L. Simonsen, P. E. Holstein, O. L. Svendsen, and J. Bülow, "Sympathetic neuropathy in diabetes mellitus patients does not elicit Charcot osteoarthropathy," *Journal of Diabetes and its Complications*, vol. 25, no. 5, pp. 320–324, 2011.

[37] M. Guillot, G. Vanneuville, G. Escande, J. Chazal, and A. Tanguy, "Anatomical study and systematization of veins in the foot," *Bulletin de l'Association des anatomistes*, vol. 63, no. 183, pp. 425–433, 1979.

[38] J. J. Bergan and N. Bunke, *The Vein Book*, Oxford University Press, 2013.

[39] G. Kuster, E. P. Lofgren, and W. H. Hollinshead, "Anatomy of the veins of the foot," *Surgery, Gynecology & Obstetrics*, vol. 127, no. 4, pp. 817–823, 1968.

[40] L. Walløe, "Arterio-venous anastomoses in the human skin and their role in temperature control," *Temperature*, vol. 3, no. 1, pp. 92–103, 2016.

[41] R. B. Jansen, T. M. Christensen, J. Bülow et al., "Bone mineral density and markers of bone turnover and inflammation in diabetes patients with or without a Charcot foot: an 8.5-year prospective case-control study," *Journal of Diabetes and its Complications*, vol. 32, no. 2, pp. 164–170, 2018.

[42] S. C. Manolagas, "Role of cytokines in bone resorption," *Bone*, vol. 17, no. 2, pp. S63–S67, 1995.

[43] R. Nishimura, K. Moriyama, K. Yasukawa, G. R. Mundy, and T. Yoneda, "Combination of interleukin-6 and soluble interleukin-6 receptors induces differentiation and activation of JAK-STAT and MAP kinase pathways in MG-63 human osteoblastic cells," *Journal of Bone and Mineral Research*, vol. 13, no. 5, pp. 777–785, 1998.

[44] K. Yokota, K. Sato, T. Miyazaki et al., "Combination of tumor necrosis factor α and interleukin-6 induces mouse osteoclast-like cells with bone resorption activity both in vitro and in vivo," *Arthritis & Rheumatology*, vol. 66, no. 1, pp. 121–129, 2014.

[45] C. A. O'Brien, I. Gubrij, S.-C. Lin, R. L. Saylors, and S. C. Manolagas, "STAT3 activation in stromal/osteoblastic cells is required for induction of the receptor activator of NF-κB ligand and stimulation of osteoclastogenesis by gp130-utilizing cytokines or interleukin-1 but not 1,25-dihydroxyvitamin D3or parathyroid hormone," *Journal of Biological Chemistry*, vol. 274, no. 27, pp. 19301–19308, 1999.

[46] J. F. Baumhauer, R. J. O'Keefe, L. C. Schon, and M. S. Pinzur, "Cytokine-induced osteoclastic bone resorption in Charcot arthropathy: an immunohistochemical study," *Foot & Ankle International*, vol. 27, no. 10, pp. 797–800, 2006.

[47] N. L. Petrova, P. K. Petrov, M. E. Edmonds, and C. M. Shanahan, "Inhibition of TNF-α reverses the pathological resorption pit profile of osteoclasts from patients with acute Charcot osteoarthropathy," *Journal of Diabetes Research*, vol. 2015, Article ID 917945, 10 pages, 2015.

[48] M. Nybo, M. K. Poulsen, J. Grauslund, J. E. Henriksen, and L. M. Rasmussen, "Plasma osteoprotegerin concentrations in peripheral sensory neuropathy in type 1 and type 2 diabetic patients," *Diabetic Medicine*, vol. 27, no. 3, pp. 289–294, 2010.

[49] S. Yaturu, "Diabetes and skeletal health," *Journal of Diabetes*, vol. 1, no. 4, pp. 246–254, 2009.

[50] N. C. Chilelli, S. Burlina, and A. Lapolla, "AGEs, rather than hyperglycemia, are responsible for microvascular complications in diabetes: a "glycoxidation-centric" point of view," *Nutrition, Metabolism and Cardiovascular Diseases*, vol. 23, no. 10, pp. 913–919, 2013.

[51] R. G. Paul and A. J. Bailey, "Glycation of collagen: the basis of its central role in the late complications of ageing and diabetes," *The International Journal of Biochemistry & Cell Biology*, vol. 28, no. 12, pp. 1297–1310, 1996.

[52] A. A. Poundarik, P.-C. Wu, Z. Evis et al., "A direct role of collagen glycation in bone fracture," *Journal of the Mechanical Behavior of Biomedical Materials*, vol. 52, pp. 120–130, 2015.

[53] A. Bierhaus, S. Schiekofer, M. Schwaninger et al., "Diabetes-associated sustained activation of the transcription factor nuclear factor-κB," *Diabetes*, vol. 50, no. 12, pp. 2792–2808, 2001.

[54] K.-M. Haslbeck, E. Schleicher, A. Bierhaus et al., "The AGE/RAGE/NF-κB pathway may contribute to the pathogenesis of polyneuropathy in impaired glucose tolerance (IGT)," *Experimental and Clinical Endocrinology & Diabetes*, vol. 113, no. 5, pp. 288–291, 2005.

3

Characterization of the Cicatrization Process in Diabetic Foot Ulcers based on the Production of Reactive Oxygen Species

Alberto López-Delis,[1,2] Suélia de S. Rodrigues Fleury Rosa,[2] Paulo Eduardo Narcizo de Souza,[3] Marcella Lemos Brettas Carneiro,[4] Mário Fabrício Fleury Rosa,[2,5] Yasmin Carneiro Lobo Macedo,[2] Fabiane Hiratsuka Veiga-Souza,[6,7] and Adson Ferreira da Rocha[2]

[1]*Medical Biophysics Center, University of Oriente, Santiago de Cuba, Cuba*
[2]*Biomedical Engineering Program, University of Brasilia, Brasilia, DF, Brazil*
[3]*Laboratory of Electron Paramagnetic Resonance, Institute of Physics, University of Brasilia, Brasilia, DF, Brazil*
[4]*Faculty of Planaltina, University of Brasilia, Planaltina, GO, Brazil*
[5]*Policy-Making in Collective Health, Faculty of Ceilândia, University of Brasilia, Ceilândia, DF, Brazil*
[6]*Laboratory of Biochemistry and Protein Chemistry, Institute of Biological Sciences, University of Brasilia, Brasilia, DF, Brazil*
[7]*Faculty of Ceilândia, University of Brasilia, Ceilândia, DF, Brazil*

Correspondence should be addressed to Alberto López-Delis; alberto.lopez@cbiomed.cu

Academic Editor: Pedro M. Geraldes

The present study aims at evaluating the correlation between the free radical formation and the healing action of lower limbs' ulcers in a randomized controlled trial with the use of an adhesive derived from natural latex associated with a light-emitting diode (LED) circuit. The sample consists of 15 participants with lower limb lesions divided into three groups: group 1 case (5 participants) received the proposed dressing system adhesive of the natural latex associated with the LED circuit; group 2 control (5 participants) received the dressings at home performed by nurses according to and established by the clinic of wounds (treated with calcium alginate or silver foam); and group 3 (5 participants) also received the dressing in their homes with the use of the dressing adhesive derived from the natural latex associated with the LED circuit. The collected data were analyzed qualitatively and quantitatively by electron paramagnetic resonance for determination of free radical formation. Kruskal-Wallis statistical test was used to evaluate the effect of treatment on the lower limb's ulcer cicatrization process and its correlation with free radical. The results obtained corroborated the hypothesis about the reduction of the quantity of these molecules in the end of treatment related to the healing wound.

1. Introduction

The number of people with diabetes has increased from 108 million in 1980 to 422 million in 2014. The global prevalence of diabetes in adults (over 18 years) has increased from 4.7 percent in 1980 to 8.5 percent in 2014. The incidence of diabetes has increased more rapidly in low- and middle-income countries [1]. This pathology is of silent evolution and develops complications such as retinopathy, nephropathy, neuropathy, and cardiovascular and vascular diseases [1]. Among the difficulties, it is concerned with vascular and neuropathic complications that contribute to the formation of lower limb wounds [2].

In this regard, these vascular and neuropathic complications often evolve into lower limb wounds that are a severe problem in public health. Among the comorbidities, the etiology of the diabetic foot is a multifaceted pathophysiological condition characterized by ulcers, infection, or destruction of the deep tissues of the feet in people with diabetes mellitus (DM). The above occurs because of neuropathy, peripheral vascular disease, or deformities in the lower limbs [3]. The diabetic foot is one of the most devastating complications of DM since it may lead to ulcerations that potentially end up in minor to major amputations. The healing process of wounds has different stages, starting from the bedsores to the restoration of the damaged tissue. These stages are hemostasis, inflammation, proliferation, epithelialization, and scar maturation (repair) [4, 5].

In this respect, it is fundamental to choose the correct methods to treat the wound better and to assess healing effectiveness. One example is the use of new coatings, among them the latex derived from *Hevea brasiliensis* in animals [6–8] and humans [9–12]. In a study, Quege [13] analyzed the wound healing efficacy of an essential fatty acid dressing in 11 participants and of a treatment based on a natural latex (Biocure) coating in 8 participants. We noticed that, in both procedures, there was a decrease in the size of the wound with slightly better improvement in the individuals treated with Biocure. Brandão et al. [14] reported the development of a new microperforated vascular graft model made of tissue and covered with a natural latex compound that showed good structural qualities as a vascular substitute, which stimulated endothelial growth and provided adequate tissue integration in dogs.

The LED circuit, associated with latex, was also investigated by Reis [15, 16], who compared the treatment of four participants with silver foam dressing with a treatment of six other participants with latex in association with the LED light for 30 minutes. The clinical findings were analyzed qualitatively and quantitatively, demonstrating that the results obtained by the experimental group were better than those obtained by the control group; the results suggested that the system proposed is a promising treatment option for diabetic foot ulcers, due to its healing properties. The use of LED circuit was also tested with other healing products introduced by Caetano [11], who evaluated the treatment of venous ulcer with silver sulfadiazine, by using the dressing in association with the LED circuit in 7 participants of the research, on a daily basis. Another group (14 participants) used silver sulfadiazine twice a week, also associated with the LED light. Both groups obtained satisfying results; however, the participants of the study that received light emitted at 891 nm showed a better evolution in the healing of the ulcers.

The recent growth in the awareness of free radicals and reactive oxygen species (ROS) in biological studies is bringing about a medical revolution that promises a new age of health and disease management [15]. Most of the potentially harmful effects of oxygen are due to the formation and activity of several chemical compounds, known as ROS, which tend to donate electrons to other substances. Free radicals and antioxidants have become commonly used terms in modern discussions of disease mechanisms [15]. Free radicals and other ROS are derived either from standard essential metabolic processes in the human body or from external sources such as exposure to X-rays, ozone, cigarette smoking, air pollutants, and industrial chemicals [15]. Free radical formation occurs continuously in the cells as a consequence of both enzymatic and nonenzymatic reactions.

Hence, the use of new coatings such as latex biomembrane and other dressings associated with LED, has been shown to be an option for wound healing in the lower limbs. The healing method used in this study is based on the device named RAPHA, and it consists in light-emitting equipment that has a cluster of 30 high-brightness LEDs in red color, aiming at promoting wound healing by stimulating the patient's tissues, regardless of the underlying cause of the ulcer. The treatment protocol with the equipment has a 35-minute duration. The LED phototherapy method in association with the latex biomaterial is noninvasive and nondestructive. The exposition of the light generated by LEDs accelerates cell growth. A set of LEDs that emits light in the visible spectrum increases the energy of the cells, which speeds up the healing process of patients. LED therapy is based on the fact that light can alter cellular metabolism as a result of its absorption by mitochondria.

This survey aims at examining the correlation between the free radical formation and the healing action of lower limb ulcers in a randomized controlled trial by using a natural latex-derived adhesive associated to a LED-based circuit. The main goal of this study is to demonstrate the advantage of the use of LED and latex biomembrane in the healing of ulcers. Additionally, the results may pave the way for a change in the current treatment, by decreasing treatment and healing duration in ulcers.

2. Materials and Methods

2.1. RAPHA Equipment. It is a mobile tissue neoformation system based on the phototherapy principles to assist in the healing of wounds. Its LED light-emitting circuit consists of two modules, a control module and a LED module. The tissue neoformation induction system aims at treating patients who suffer from ulcers caused by various diseases and do not respond well to conventional treatments. This system may be seen as a new form of phototherapy, with reduced costs, due to the use of high-brightness LEDs instead of a laser.

The latex sheet has been made with centrifuged 60% latex biomaterial [15, 16]. In the manufacturing process, the latex was placed in a glass or an acrylic Petri dish, previously cleaned and dried, where the latex biomaterial was spread to form a thin layer, covering the dish surface. The Petri dish was not left horizontally in the oven—it was entirely rested in a vertical position so that any latex excess would be drained [15, 16]. This procedure led to a more transparent sheet. We repeated the process six times, and the resulting final sheet thickness was 0.5 mm.

The latex sheets were cut in rectangular shapes and then sterilized with ethylene oxide. We made layers with different sizes to match different ulcer sizes [15]. Purposely, we made the sheets slightly larger than the extent of the wound, to ensure the total covering of the ulcerated area. The latex sheets were tested at the Optical Spectroscopy Laboratory of the Institute of Physics at the University of Brasilia, to verify if it does not cause excessive attenuation or significant changes in the spectral characteristics of the light irradiated by the LED matrix [15]. The results showed that the sheet causes a reduction of approximately half in the intensity of the light but did not affect its spectrum [15, 16].

2.2. Subjects. The survey was conducted on the premises of the Ceilândia Regional Hospital's ambulatory clinic (Brasilia, Brazil) and at the residence of the participants of the experimental groups. The subjects of the survey previously provide the written consent, give the permission for publication, and share their photographs for scientific and educational purposes. The study has been approved by the Human Research Ethics Committee of the Health Science Teaching and Research Foundation (process number 52305715.6.0000.5553/2018), Brasilia, Brazil.

We chose as a reference site the ambulatory clinic in Ceilândia, at the clinic for treating chronic wounds. At first, we selected the participants of the survey at the ambulatory clinic; then, they were visited in their houses to carry out the other phases of the research (according to the three specific groups). All the participants received the proper information and signed the free and informed consent form.

The sample group consisted of 15 individuals, divided into three groups of 5 participants of the study, regardless of their gender. The sample group presents individuals with lower limb ischemia and neuropathic ulcers. The fifteen participants with lower limb lesions were divided into three groups (the data are presented in the mean ± standard deviation format):

(i) Group 1 (GI) case: 5 participants treated by qualified nurses with the dressings at the ambulatory clinic using the application of latex in association with the LED circuit (age: 61.8 ± 11 yrs; height: 1.65 ± 0.09 m; weight: 90.7 ± 39.5 kg)

(ii) Group 2 (GII) control: 5 participants treated at home by nurses, following the standard wound care recommendations (with silver alginate dressing) (age: 62.6 ± 8.54 yrs; height: 1.54 ± 0.05 m; weight: 70.86 ± 14.4 kg)

(iii) Group 3 (GIII): 5 participants self-treated at home with the dressing in association with the natural latex adhesive and the LED circuit (age 55.4 ± 10.3 yrs; height: 1.67 ± 0.08 m; weight: 81.4 ± 11.6 kg).

To participate in the survey, the participant should meet the following criteria:

(1) Received the treatment on the premises of the Ceilândia Regional Hospital

(2) Participated in the treatment adherence group and sign the informed consent form (TCLE)

(3) Participated in a previous survey on the healing of lower limb ulcers

(4) Had a lower limb ulcer caused by neuropathic or vascular diseases with or without clinical signs of infection

The participant of the research should not

(1) refuse to be part of the research group;

(2) be pregnant, underage, or over 75 years old;

(3) consume alcoholic drinks or illicit drugs;

(4) have evidence of osteomyelitis or gangrene on the affected extremity;

(5) topically apply any medication at the wound site not adopted in this protocol after the start of the trial;

(6) miss the treatment program (for three consecutive times).

2.3. Devices Used. The method proposed for this prospective research is the simultaneous action of the natural latex adhesive and the LED circuit. Both agents have characteristics and properties capable of inducing tissue regeneration and neoformation. Figure 1 presents the flowchart for the application of the randomized clinical trial research with wounds: natural latex and LED circuit.

The latex extracted from the Brazilian rubber tree is a polydisperse system, in which negatively charged particles of various types are suspended in serum due to its neovascularization- and tissue regeneration-inducing properties. Natural latex is healing, for it is a natural defense of the plant. It is of natural origin and presents a low cost, without risk of transmitting pathogens and with great clinical-social applicability.

The process of making the adhesives is done by mixing the bicentrifuged latex with doubly distilled water, placing the mixture in a previously sterilized mold, selected with the approximate dimensions of the wound. This mixture is then accommodated in the mold without leaving extra material or creating air bubbles. After the abovementioned processes, the material undergoes a vulcanization process inside a greenhouse. The adhesive is then removed from the mold and undergoes a sterilization and packaging process before being used by a participant of research.

The LED circuit consists of two modules, a control module and a LED module. The control module has a timer to indicate the duration of light emission that beeps at the end of the procedure. It is directly connected to the module of LEDs that has 30 monochromatic LED lights. The system assists the wound healing process.

2.4. Sample Collection Protocol. All sample solutions were prepared immediately before the experiments in Krebs HEPES buffer (KHB), pH 7.4, dissolved in a bidistilled and deionized water. Ten mM stock solution of CMH was freshly made and dissolved in KHB containing 25 μM deferoxamine methanesulfonate salt (DF) and 5 μM sodium diethyldithiocarbamate trihydrate (DETC). The solutions were kept cooled throughout all the measurements.

Two samples of the wound and venous blood, respectively, and one collection of injured tissues were taken from the subjects to evaluate the healing process (Figure 2). For venous blood collection (1.5 mL), we used a syringe or a

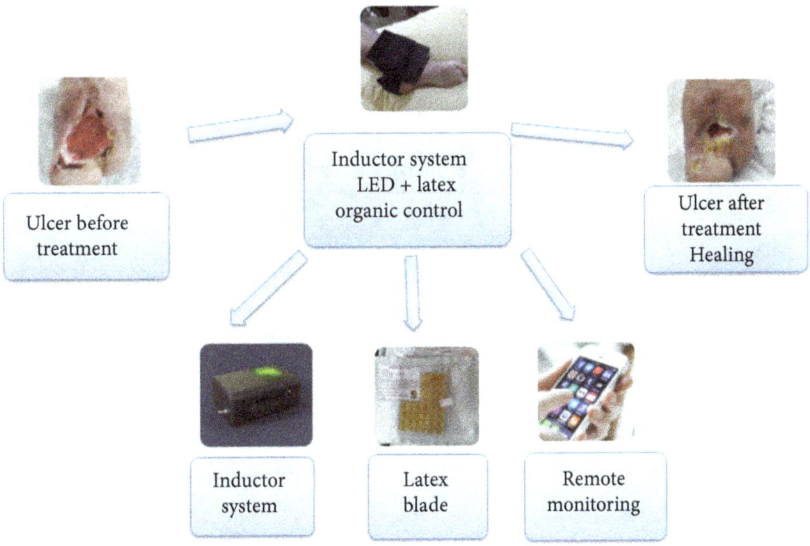

Figure 1: Flowchart for the application of the randomized clinical trial of research participants with wounds: natural latex and light-emitting circuit of LEDs.

heparinized tube. The site of preference for venipunctures is the antecubital fossa, in the anterior area of the forearm and below the elbow, where there are many veins, relatively close to the surface of the skin. First, the patient's arm was set up, by tilting it down from shoulder height. The blood was collected slowly, with a maximum of 40 mmHg of compression in the arm. After removal, the material was frozen in liquid nitrogen.

For the blood collection (2 to 3 drops), we collected a sample from the edges from small holes, where there was forming tissue. We used a syringe or heparinized tube with a special needle (as of insulin, smaller caliber) and deposited the blood in heparinized microtubes. After removal, the material was frozen in liquid nitrogen.

Finally, the collection of wound tissues was accomplished (tissue samples before treatment and granulation tissue formed during healing). The material was collected by scraping (close to the edges) with a sterile wooden spatula. Then, the wooden spatula was hermetically sealed in a tube and frozen in liquid nitrogen.

We established three stages for sample collection: on the first day before the beginning of the treatment, on the second day after two weeks of treatment, and at the end of treatment, around 30 days after the start of the treatment (or sooner, if the wound is healed).

2.5. Detection of ROS in Human Blood. The wound and venous blood were thawed, and 50 μL samples were treated with a solution containing 400 μM 1-hydroxy-3-methoxycarbonyl-2,2,5,5-tetramethylpyrrolidine (CMH) and heparin sodium (100 IU/mL) in 1 : 1 proportion. The tube was incubated under gentle shaking at 37°C for 30 min. After that, 50 μL of the obtained solution was placed between two ice blocks (200 μL each) in a one-mL decapped syringe and snap frozen in liquid nitrogen. All samples were stored at −80°C until the electron paramagnetic resonance measurements were performed. The principle of the method is based upon the ROS interaction with CMH to form a stable radical 3-methoxycarbonyl-2,2,5,5-tetramethylpyrrolidine-1-oxyl ($CM^{\cdot}$), detectable by EPR, which is a signature of ROS generation.

2.6. Electron Paramagnetic Resonance (EPR). EPR measurements were performed in an EPR spectrometer EMX plus (Bruker, Germany), by using X-band (9 GHz) and a high-resolution cavity (ER 4119HS, Bruker, Germany), as illustrated in Figure 3. For ROS detection, the samples were transferred to a liquid nitrogen Dewar (Noxygen, Germany), and the spectra were recorded at 77 K. The instrumental settings were two-mW microwave power, 5G modulation amplitude, 100 kHz of modulation frequency, and 200G sweep width.

We used peak height for detecting the signal. The peak height is the arbitrary distance between lowest and highest point in the first derivative spectrum. The calibration curve was made by using the nitroxide radical $CP^{\cdot}$ diluted in KHB at a dose range of 0, 5, 10, 50, and 100 μM. In this concentration range, a linear calibration curve was obtained, and all the recorded data were within this calibration range.

2.7. Chemicals. The spin probe 1-hydroxy-3-methoxycarbonyl-2.2.5.5-tetramethylpyrrolidine (CMH); the metal chelators deferoxamine (DF) and diethyldithiocarbamate (DETC); Krebs–HEPES buffer (KHB); and the stable radical $CP^{\cdot}$ (3-carboxy-2,2,5,5-tetramethyl-1-pyrrolidinyloxy) were obtained from Noxygen Science Transfer & Diagnostics.

2.8. Statistical Analysis. Statistical analysis was performed by Matlab (Mathworks Inc., Natick, MA). The micromolar concentration metric related to $CM^{\cdot}$ was used to evaluate the real effect of the treatment. The methodology applied for this verification was the Kruskal-Wallis test. This test is a nonparametric version of the classical one-way ANOVA and an extension of the Wilcoxon rank-sum test to more than two

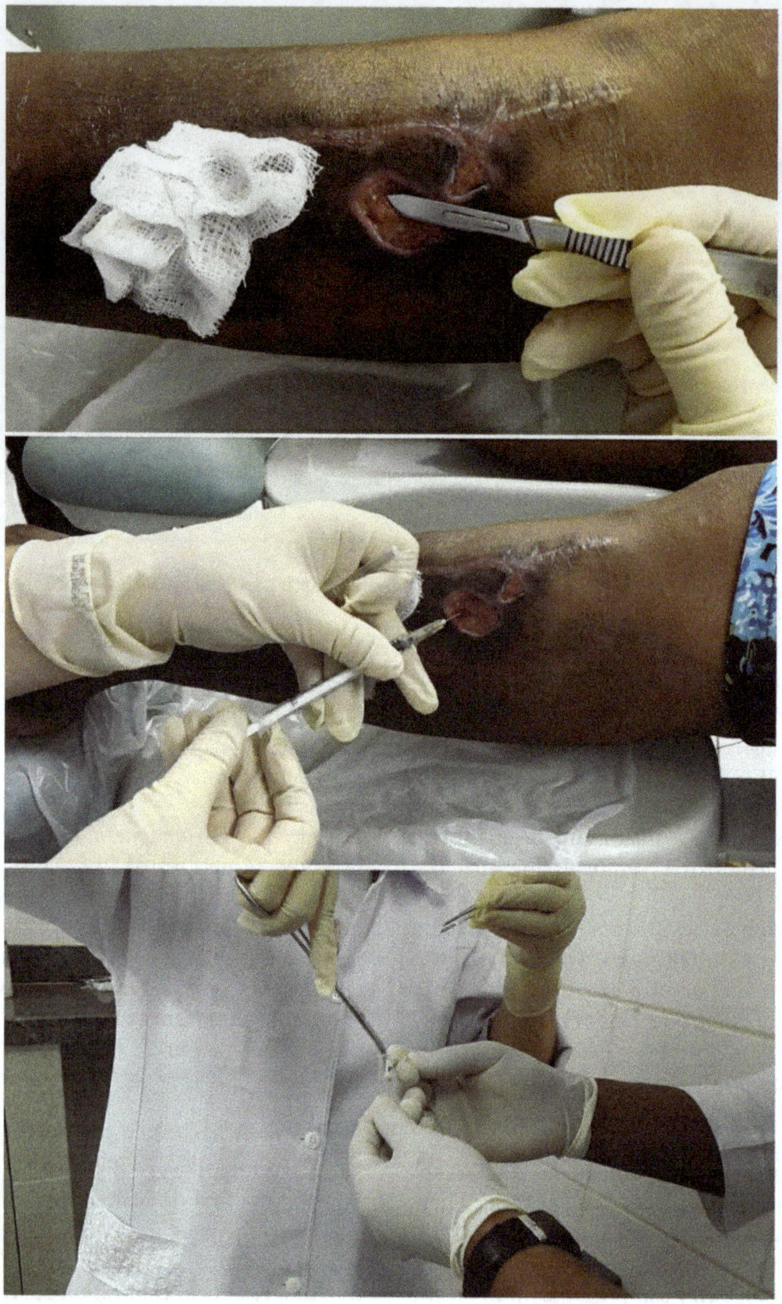

FIGURE 2: Collection of wound tissues on tissue samples before treatment and collection of blood in the wound bed (50 μL).

groups [17]. It compares the medians of the groups of data to determine if the samples come from the same population (or, equivalently, from different populations with the same distribution). The F-statistic used in classical one-way ANOVA is replaced by a chi-square statistic. The p value measures the significance of the chi-square statistic, for this case with a significance of 1% [17].

3. Results

3.1. EPR Measurements. Figure 4 presents the EPR result of ROS quantification from CM˙ in venous (a) and wound (b) blood from the lesions of diabetic patients and wound tissues (c).

In general, the results showed that all experimental groups (G1, G2, and G3) presented similar amounts of ROS in the wound blood considering the same period of analysis (days 01, 15, or 30). Nevertheless, when comparing each experimental stage (days 01, 15, and 30), the results showed a pronounced reduction of CM˙ between days 01 and 30, which correspond to the beginning and the end of the treatment (Figure 4(a)).

Regarding CM˙ data in the venous blood, it was also noticed that G1, G2, and G3 groups presented similar amounts of ROS when comparing each isolated analysis period. However, it was also observed that the ROS concentration was different between days 1 and 15 and between days 15 and 30, considering the same experimental group. Thus,

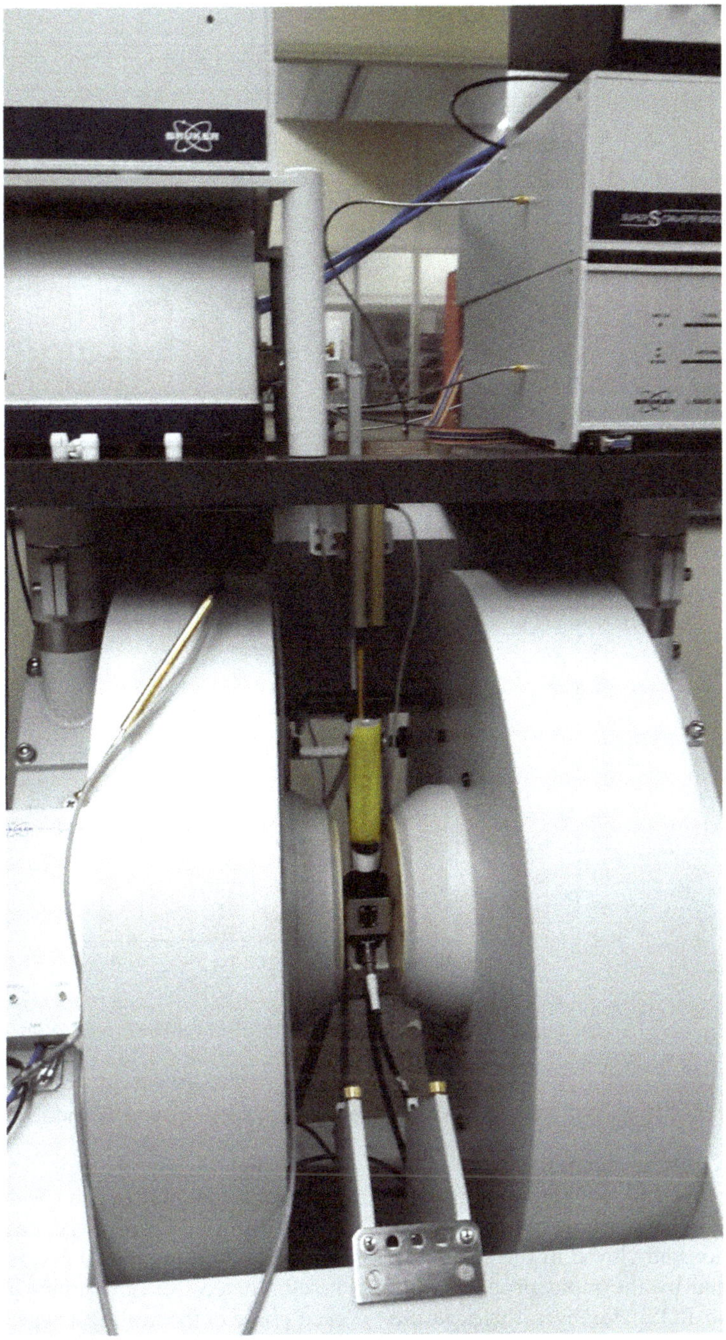

FIGURE 3: Electron paramagnetic resonance spectrometer EMXplus (Bruker, Germany).

we verified the increase of venous blood ROS formation in the middle of the treatment (day 15) in comparison to the beginning (day 01) and the end (day 30) of the treatment period (Figure 4(b)).

According to the analysis of $CM^{\cdot}$ content in wound tissues, there was a statistical difference among the three experimental groups at all times evaluated. Therefore, there was a variation in the generation of ROS in the wound tissues between the beginning and end of treatment (Figure 4(c)).

3.2. Statistical Performance. Figures 5(a)–5(c) present the statistical dispersion obtained along the sample collection stages in the three sample groups with statistical representation in the wound and venous blood as well as in the wound tissues.

4. Discussion

We identified high concentration of $CM^{\cdot}$ in the wound blood at the start and at the middle of the treatment (Figure 4(a)), which is evidence closely related to the inflammation process. The significant reduction in ROS formation at the end of the treatment (Figure 4(b)) is associated with the wound healing process since the decreasing of ROS levels is related to the reduction of the inflammatory process (see statistical

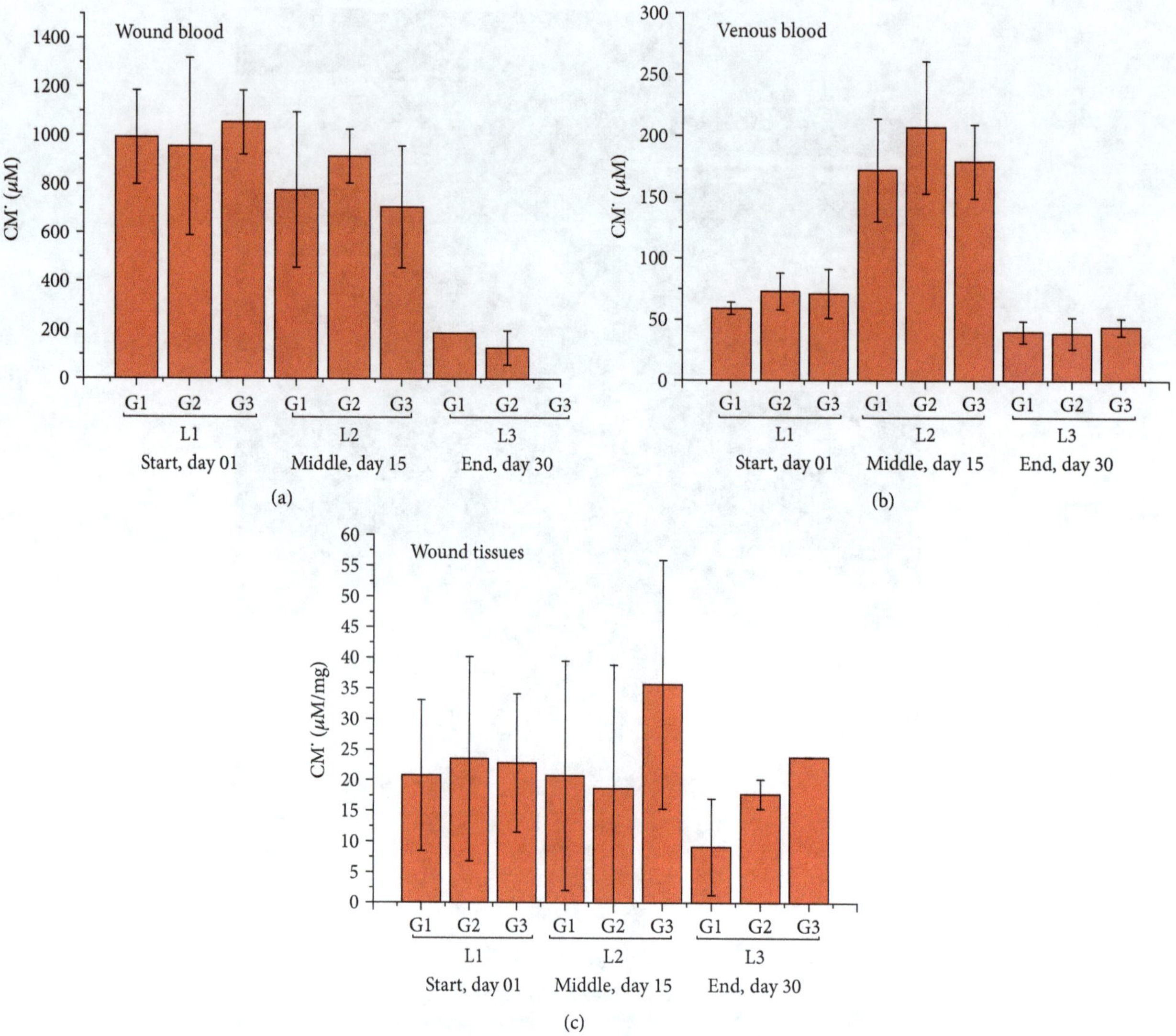

FIGURE 4: CM˙ quantification in the wound (a), venous blood (b), and wound tissues (c).

dispersion in Figure 5(a)). ROS act as inflammation signaling molecules, and they are involved in the host-defense response [18–20]. Neutrophils, macrophages, and immune cells mediate immune reactions employed in the "oxidative burst," which is characterized by the rapid production of large amounts of intracellular ROS. Moreover, the exposure of these cells to proinflammatory cytokines, during the inflammatory process, induces a significant increase of the ROS levels into the immune cells, boosting the ROS production [18, 19]. During the first 15 days of the treatment, a high generation of ROS was identified in the wound blood (Figure 4(a)), corresponding to the inflammatory process which precedes the wound healing.

By the end of treatment, at about the 30th day, we noticed a significant reduction of ROS generation in the wound blood (Figure 4(b)), which is related not only to the decline of the inflammation but also to the induction of the apoptosis in wound cell remnants.

Apoptosis, or programmed cell death, is closely related to the control of the swelling, and it has an essential role in the advancing epithelial edge toward the center of the wound, evidencing healing progress. The wound healing involves a series of rapid increases in specific cell populations that prepare the wound for repair, deposit new matrices, and, finally, mature the wound. For this reason, these types of cells must be eliminated from the injury before the progression to the next phase of the healing, triggered through apoptosis, which allows the eliminations of entire populations without an inflammatory response or tissue damage [18–20].

It is widely reported that ROS behave as signaling molecules for inflammation in the endothelial dysfunction. Under the inflammatory conditions, oxidative stress, produced by immune cells, leads to the opening of interendothelial junctions and promotes the migration of inflammatory/immune cells across the endothelial barrier. The immune cell emigration elicits the acute inflammatory response essential to repair injury tissue [18, 19]. Thus, the increase of ROS formation, observed in the patient venous blood in the middle of the treatment period (day 15, Figure 4(b)) could be related to the endothelial dysfunction and to mobilization of immune cells to the wound area. The mechanism described results in higher ROS formation in the venous blood in the 15th day (see statistical

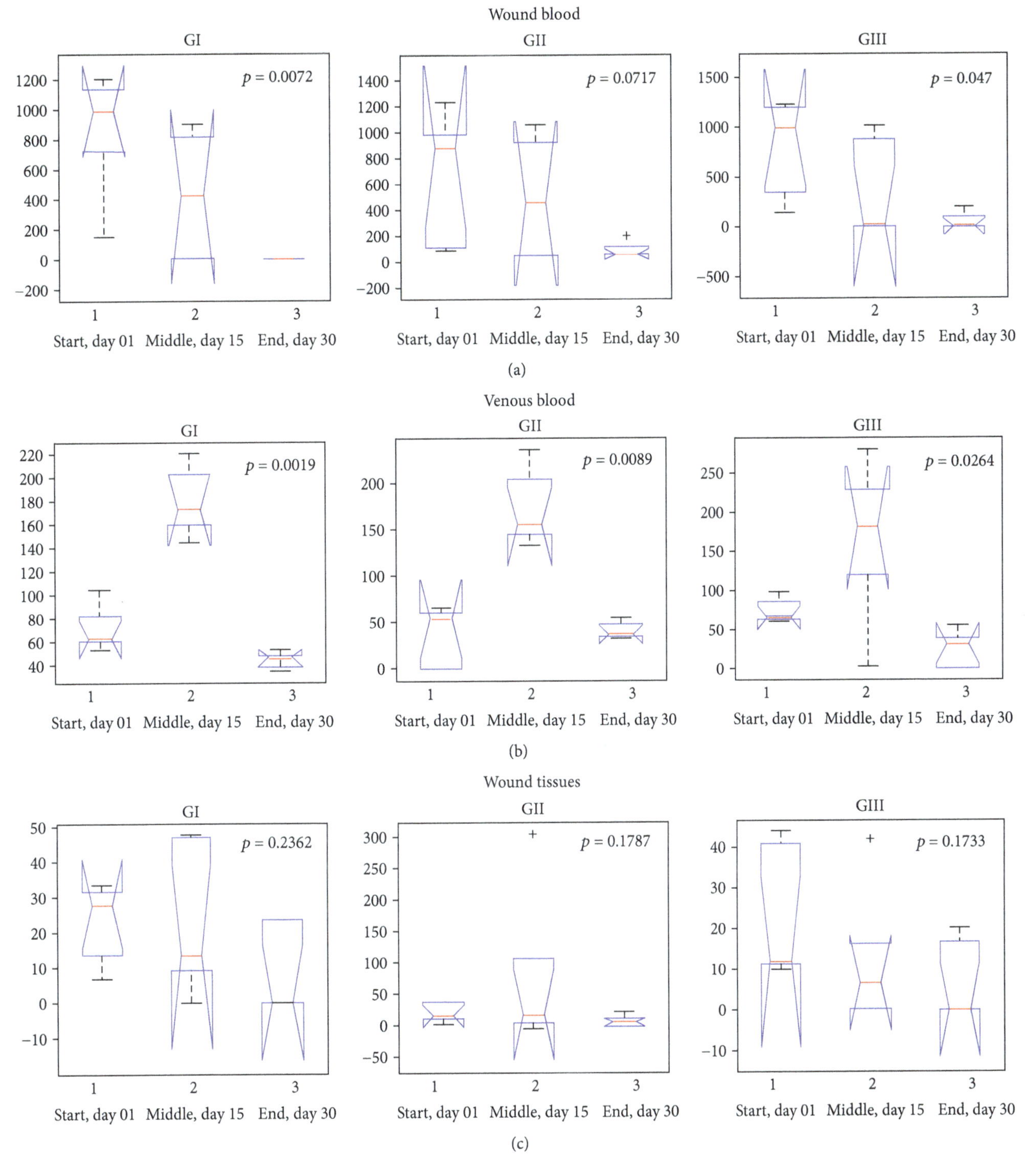

FIGURE 5: The statistical dispersion obtained along the sample collection stages in the three sample groups with statistical signification in the wound (a), venous blood (b), and wound tissues (c).

dispersion from Figure 5(b)). Similarly, there was a variation in the amount of ROS in the wound tissues between the beginning and end of treatment (Figure 4(c), see statistical dispersion in Figure 5(c)). In particular, in groups G1 and G3 (patients that are receiving latex and LED treatment), a reduction in wound ROS concentration at the end of the treatment (30th day, Figure 4) was observed, which corresponds to a decrease of the inflammation. It is related to the roles of ROS antioxidants in skin wound healing, their possible involvement in chronic wounds, and the potential value of ROS-induced biomarkers in wound healing prognosis [21].

Together, these results suggest the existence of modulation of environmental oxidative stress in chronic wounds and their contribution to healing in these scars. It is known that the ROS generation is critical for the inflammatory modulation response and plays a significant role in the impact on several functions in the cells. There are multiple sources of ROS, both inside and outside the cell, and diverse ROS species that are generated in different zones within a cell, at different times and at different concentrations. All these factors significantly influence the effectiveness of ROS and present distinct results [19]. Thus, the understanding of the effect of ROS generation in the wound blood, venous blood, and wound tissues, conducted in this survey, was essential to elucidate its biological effects as a target molecule in the healing wound.

Moreover, the participation of the nurses was fundamental to the evaluation of the wound. For this process, elements such as the degree of healing and the sample collection site can affect the sample data (ROS equal to zero) and the nurse evaluation in avoiding injuring the newly formed area. In this analysis, we noticed that the reduction of the pH of bedsore stimulated the production of cytokines and the reproduction of these cells, thereby reducing the growth of pathogenic microorganisms. We also concluded that the system acted as debridement and that it had an anti-inflammatory action, as evidenced in the images obtained in the analysis of the contraction and the junction of borders of the healing wounds.

We concluded that this system could be implemented in various healing stages, with different concentrations, according to the type of the wound tissue (this is the next step of the study). In this context, it is necessary to evaluate the best options for data collection, considering its effectiveness.

We must also take into consideration that, in clinical practice, the evidence presented in this study contributes to the decision making for the treatment approach, suggesting that it can be done by modifying the light intensity, the duration of exposure, and the thickness of the latex adhesive according to the stage of the healing process. The granulation tissue observed for the applied light intensity and the characteristics of the lamina and when there is a presence of necrosis of innovative liquefaction approach of intensity and time of use of the lamina must be incorporated and finally should be performed in coagulation necrosis and escharotomy.

There were no side effects observed in this survey, although the participants reported burning and pain during and after the treatment. Considering that it was a subjective perception, there was no need to specify the concentration and intensity of climbing point for future studies. The system (latex and phototherapy) yielded better good debridement and acceleration of the healing process with the formation of granulated tissue, when compared to the current standard procedures.

We also point out the necessity of training the nursing team on the manipulation of the product, to collect samples and especially to manage the patient's ability to obtain samples of wounds already healed. The use of latex demonstrated a maceration of the wound edges and a granulation tissue susceptible to fragmentation due to its softened feature. The system presented in this study can be applied in different stages of the healing process in diverse etiologies, but it still requires further investigation.

We concluded that high ROS formation in the wound blood, in the beginning and in the middle of the treatment, correspond to the inflammation process and that the reduction of the quantity of these molecules by the end of the treatment is related to the healing process of the wound.

Conflicts of Interest

The authors declare that they have no conflicts of interest.

Acknowledgments

This research is supported by grants from the General Coordination of Equipment and Materials for Health Use (CGEMS), the Department of Industrial Complex and Innovation in Health (DECIIS), the Secretary of Science, Technology and Strategic Inputs (SCTIE), the Ministry of Health, and the CNPq for productivity and postdoctoral fellowships.

References

[1] A. Alwan, *Global status report on noncommunicable diseases 2010*, World Health Organization, Geneva, Switzerland, 2011.

[2] C. E. D. A. Rocha, M. I. Martins, M. H. Foss et al., "Improving quality of life of neuropathic pain patients by continuous outpatient setting monitoring," *Revista Dor*, vol. 12, no. 4, pp. 291–296, 2011.

[3] H. C. Pedrosa, "Diabetic polyneuropathy: new strategies for early diagnosis and therapeutic intervention - guidelines NeurALAD (in Portuguese)," in *The Latin America Congress on Controversies to Consensus in Diabetes, Obesity and Hypertension (CODHy)*, pp. 2–8, Buenos Aires, Argentina, 2010.

[4] C. L. Baum and C. J. Arpey, "Normal cutaneous wound healing: clinical correlation with cellular and molecular events," *Dermatologic Surgery*, vol. 31, no. 6, pp. 674–686, 2005.

[5] M. B. Serra, W. A. Barroso, N. N. da Silva et al., "From inflammation to current and alternative therapies involved in wound healing," *International Journal of Inflammation*, vol. 2017, Article ID 3406215, 17 pages, 2017.

[6] R. J. Mendonça, V. B. Maurício, B. Teixeira Lde, J. J. Lachat, and J. Coutinho-Netto, "Increased vascular permeability, angiogenesis and wound healing induced by the serum of natural latex of the rubber tree *Hevea brasiliensis*," *Phytotherapy Research*, vol. 24, no. 5, pp. 764–768, 2010.

[7] E. C. C. M. Pinho, *The Use of the Natural Latex Biomembrane Compared to the Autologous Conjunctival Transplantation on the Ocular Surface (in Portuguese), [Ph.D. thesis]*, Universidade de São Paulo, Faculdade de Medicina de Ribeirão Preto, Ribeirão Preto, SP, Brazil, 2011.

[8] T. A. M. Andrade, *Tissue Modifications and Mechanisms of Action of the F 1 Fraction of Latex and the Hevea brasiliensis Serinigera in the Healing of Cutaneous Ulcers in Diabetic Rats (in Portuguese), [Ph.D. thesis]*, Universidade de São Paulo, Faculdade de Medicina de Ribeirão Preto, Ribeirão Preto, SP, Brazil, 2012.

[9] C. P. C. M. Siqueira, D. O. T. Filho, F. M. Lima et al., "Biological effects of light: application of low power therapy using LEDs in venous ulcer healing: case report (in Portuguese)," *Seminário: Ciências Biológicas e da Saúde*, vol. 30, no. 1, pp. 37–46, 2009.

[10] M. M. Araujo, E. T. Massuda, and M. A. Hyppolito, "Anatomical and functional evaluation of tympanoplasty using a transitory natural latex biomembrane implant from the rubber tree

Hevea brasiliensis," *Acta Cirurgica Brasileira*, vol. 27, no. 8, pp. 566–571, 2012.

[11] K. S. Caetano, "Evaluation of the treatment of chronic venous ulcers with phototherapy (LEDs) and silver sulfadiazine 1% (in Portuguese)," in *Programa de Pós-graduação em Interunidades Bioengenharia, Escola de Engenharia de São Carlos da universidade São Paulo*, p. 96, São Carlos, SP, Brazil, 2008.

[12] M. A. C. Frade, *Leg Ulcer: Clinical Characterization and Immuno Histotopathological Profile of Cicatrization in the Presence of Natural Latex Biomembrane of Rubber Tree Hevea Brasilienses (in Portuguese), [Ph.D. thesis]*, Universidade de São Paulo, Faculdade de Medicina de Ribeirão Preto, Ribeirão Preto, SP, Brazil, 2003.

[13] G. E. Quege, "Comparative study of the use of a product based on essential fatty acids (AGEs) and a latex biomembrane in the treatment of chronic infected wounds (in Portuguese)," in *Universidade federal de Goiás, Programa de Pósgraduação em Enfermagem*, p. 235, Goiânia, GO, Brazil, 2008.

[14] M. L. Brandão, J. C. Netto, J. A. Thomazini, J. J. Lachat, V. F. Muglia, and C. E. Piccinato, "Latex-derived vascular prosthesis," *Jornal Vascular Brasileiro*, vol. 6, no. 2, pp. 130–141, 2007.

[15] M. D. Reis, *Tissue Neoformation Inducer System for Diabetic Foot with Led Emitting Circuit and Use of Natural Latex (in Portuguese), [Ph.D. thesis]*, Universidade de Brasilia, Faculdade de Tecnologia, Brasilia, DF, Brazil, 2013.

[16] G. A. M. de Almeida Nunes, M. do Carmo dos Reis, M. F. F. Rosa, L. R. T. Peixoto, A. F. da Rocha, and S. de Siqueira Rodrigues Fleury Rosa, "A system for treatment of diabetic foot ulcers using led irradiation and natural latex," *Research on Biomedical Engineering*, vol. 32, no. 1, pp. 3–13, 2016.

[17] J. D. Spurrier, "On the null distribution of the Kruskal–Wallis statistic," *Journal of Nonparametric Statistics*, vol. 15, no. 6, pp. 685–691, 2003.

[18] M. Mittal, M. R. Siddiqui, K. Tran, S. P. Reddy, and A. B. Malik, "Reactive oxygen species in inflammation and tissue injury," *Antioxidants & Redox Signaling*, vol. 20, no. 7, pp. 1126–1167, 2014.

[19] H. Blaser, C. Dostert, T. W. Mak, and D. Brenner, "TNF and ROS crosstalk in inflammation," *Trends in Cell Biology*, vol. 26, no. 4, pp. 249–261, 2016.

[20] D. G. Greenhalgh, "The role of apoptosis in wound healing," *The International Journal of Biochemistry & Cell Biology*, vol. 30, no. 9, pp. 1019–1030, 1998.

[21] R. Moseley, J. R. Hilton, R. J. Waddington, K. G. Harding, P. Stephens, and D. W. Thomas, "Comparison of oxidative stress biomarker profiles between acute and chronic wound environments," *Wound Repair and Regeneration*, vol. 12, no. 4, pp. 419–429, 2004.

4

Changes in Immunoreactivity of Sensory Substances within the Enteric Nervous System of the Porcine Stomach during Experimentally Induced Diabetes

Michał Bulc,[1] Katarzyna Palus,[1] Jarosław Całka,[1] and Łukasz Zielonka[2]

[1]*Department of Clinical Physiology Faculty of Veterinary Medicine, University of Warmia and Mazury in Olsztyn, Oczapowskiego Str. 13, 10-719 Olsztyn, Poland*

[2]*Department of Veterinary Prevention and Feed Hygiene, Faculty of Veterinary Medicine, University of Warmia and Mazury in Olsztyn, 10-718 Olsztyn, Poland*

Correspondence should be addressed to Michał Bulc; michal.bulc@uwm.edu.pl

Academic Editor: Mark Yorek

One of the most frequently reported disorders associated with diabetes is gastrointestinal (GI) disturbance. Although pathogenesis of these complications is multifactorial, the complicity of the enteric nervous system (ENS) in this respect has significant importance. Therefore, this paper analysed changes in substance P- (SP-), calcitonin gene-related peptide- (CGRP-), and leu5-enkephalin (L ENK-) like immunoreactivity (LI) in enteric stomach neurons caused by chemically induced diabetes in a porcine model. Using double immunofluorescent labelling, it was found that acute hyperglycaemia led to significant changes in the chemical coding of stomach enteric neurons. Generally, the response to artificially inducted diabetes depended on the "kind" of enteric plexus as well as the stomach region studied. A clear increase in the percentage of neurons immunoreactive to SP and CGRP was visible in the myenteric plexus (MP) in the antrum, corpus, and pylorus as well as in the submucosal plexus (SmP) in the corpus. For L-ENK, an increase in the number of L-ENK-LI neurons was observed in the MP of the antrum and SmP in the corpus, while in the MP of the corpus and pylorus, a decrease in the percentage of L-ENK-LI neurons was noted.

1. Introduction

Diabetes mellitus is actually considered an epidemic in the 21st century. The diabetic population has systematically increased worldwide, and it is expected to rise to 592 million patients/cases by the year 2035 [1]. Improper treatment of diabetes leads to long-term increased blood glucose level, which is considered to be a major pathophysiological factor in the development of severe diabetic complications [2, 3]. It has been evaluated that up to 75% of patients with type 1 or type 2 diabetes will have the complication of neuropathy. One of the clinical signs of neuropathy is gastrointestinal (GI) disorder [4–6]. Regardless of their etiology, it is possible that the molecular mechanisms of pathological changes within the GI tract are partly due to changes within the enteric nervous system (ENS) [4].

The enteric nervous system regulates gastrointestinal functions, which is independent of the central nervous system and is embedded in the wall of the gastrointestinal tract [7]. The ENS is comprised approximately of millions of sensory, motor, and interneurons formed in intramural ganglionated plexuses interconnected with a very dense network of nerves [8]. In the porcine stomach, it is formed by the myenteric plexus (MP) located between the longitudinal and circular muscle layers, which mainly regulates the proper gastric motility, both after and between the meals, and the submucosal plexus (SmP) is situated in the inner side of the circular muscle layer, primarily regulating fluid secretion and resorption [9, 10].

Gastrointestinal complications in the course of diabetes mellitus appear to be multifactorial [11]. Several possibilities have been suggested, such as diabetic autonomic neuropathy altering the parasympathetic and sympathetic nerve functions. Moreover, other possibilities have been proposed. Namely, enteric neurons may undergo changes caused by adaptive and/or neuroprotective processes during many gastrointestinal and extraintestinal diseases, and these changes are mainly manifested in the modification of neuronal chemical phenotyping [12, 13]. Proper sensory perception is conditioned by a functional balance between nociceptive substances such as substance P (SP) or calcitonin gene-related peptide (CGRP) and, on the other hand, an appropriate level of antinociceptive factors, particularly the opioid family, for example, leu5-enkephalin (L-ENK) [14–17].

SP is an undecapeptide and belongs to the tachykinin/neurokinin family. The neurokinin family consists of (in addition to SP) neurokinin A (NKA) and neurokinin B (NKB) [18]. SP and NKA are encoded by the preprotachykinin I gene, while NKB is encoded by the preprotachykinin II gene [19]. SP is widely distributed in the ENS. Till now, SP-like immunoreactivity has been described in different fragments of the GI tract, like the oesophagus, stomach, duodenum, jejunum, and descending colon [20]. SP in the GI tract is first of all considered to be a neurotransmitter for primary sensory afferent nerve fibres, which are involved in pain signal transmission. Furthermore, SP is engaged in the regulation of blood flow, both by relaxation and by contraction of muscular cells of blood vessels [21–24]. The expression of SP within the enteric nervous system, as well as their changes, has been described in various species under different pathological conditions, including inflammatory bowel disease [22], bisfenol A intoxication [25], parasite infection [26], *Bacteroides fragilis* infection [27], or carcinoma [28].

Calcitonin gene-related peptide (CGRP) is a member of the calcitonin family of peptides [29]. CGRP is one of the most abundant peptides, produced in both the peripheral and central nervous systems [28]. One of the better-known functions of CGRP in the GI tract is its participation in nociception signal transmission. It is also known that CGRP plays a role as a neuromediator and/or neuromodulator, participating in the regulation of motor activity, blood flow, and gastric acid secretion [27]. CGRP is also considered to be a marker of intrinsic primary afferent neurons. This class of neurons plays an essential role in short reflexes in the intestinal wall excluding the central nervous system. This mentioned function corresponds with wide distribution of CGRP in the GI tract. Namely, CGRP-immunoreactive nerve structures were described in the wall of the GI tract from the oesophagus to the rectum [30]. Multiple functions of CGRP in the GI tract were confirmed by numerous studies regarding pathological conditions resulting in changes in expression of CGRP [30].

In turn, met-enkephalin, leu-enkephalin, β-endorphin, α-neo-endorphin, dynorphin, and nociceptin/orphanin are opioid peptides. Leu-enkephalin (L-ENK) was the first time isolated from the porcine brain in 1975. Opioid peptides in the stomach originate from both enteroendocrine cells and ENS neurons. LENK is a factor that most often is present in sensory neurons and its participation in sensory and pain transmission is well known [31, 32].

Therefore, this experiment was designed to determine the possible alterations in expression of sensory substances in the stomach enteric neurons under the influence of acute hyperglycaemia. Streptozotocin-induced hyperglycaemic/diabetic porcine model was used in this study. In many publications on diabetic complications, much attention is paid to issues that affect life-threatening conditions or are threatened with irreversible crippling. As high as 75% of patients with diabetes may experience gastrointestinal symptoms. These complications represent a major cause of morbidity and have a negative impact on healthcare (leads to a significant impairment in the quality of life) and costs in diabetes. Taking this into account, it seems highly important to find an appropriate animal model that allows learning the exact etiology of changes occurring in diabetes in the gastrointestinal tract. Especially in the area of diabetes, the swine in the last time has gained considerable interest [33, 34]. It is due to the fact that biochemical and pathophysiological responses to diabetes remain in part like those observed in people. It has been documented that blood flow of the pig pancreas is similar to that of the human pancreas and the number of insulin producing cells is within a similar number as that observed in humans [35]. Moreover, pigs, in contrast to rodents, are omnivorous and active during the day. It all makes the pig a much better model for studying diabetic complications than rodents. The current study for the first time focused on the examination of SP, CGRP, and leu5-enkephalin expression in stomach neurons during streptozotocin-inducted diabetes. The choice of these neuropeptides was dictated by the fact that these substances are involved in sensory signal modulation. It is well documented that abdominal pain is one of the most serious GI diabetic complications. The current results may help to create the foundation for further, more detailed, and clinically oriented studies, involving these neuropeptides and their roles in gastrointestinal diabetic symptom treatment.

2. Materials and Methods

2.1. Animals. We followed the methods of Bulc et al. [36]. This study was conducted on ten juvenile female pigs of the white large Polish breed, weighing from 17.0 kg to 20 kg. At the beginning of the experiment, the animals were randomly distributed into two groups: the diabetic group (D, $n = 5$) and the control group (C, $n = 5$) and were housed in cages suitable for pigs. The animals were given one week of acclimatization to observe their general health, to minimize physiological stress, and to ensure the proper conduct of the study. The treatment of animals was conducted in compliance with the instructions of the Local Ethical Committee in Olsztyn (Poland) (decision number 13/2015/DTN) with special attention paid to minimizing any stress reaction.

2.2. Chemical Induction of Diabetes. After acclimatization, hyperglycaemia was induced as previously described [36]. Streptozotocin (STZ) (Sigma-Aldrich, St Louis, MO, USA, S0130), 150 mg/kg of body weight, was dissolved in a freshly prepared disodium citrate buffer solution (pH = 4.23, 1 g streptozotocin/10 mL solution). For this purpose, pigs were

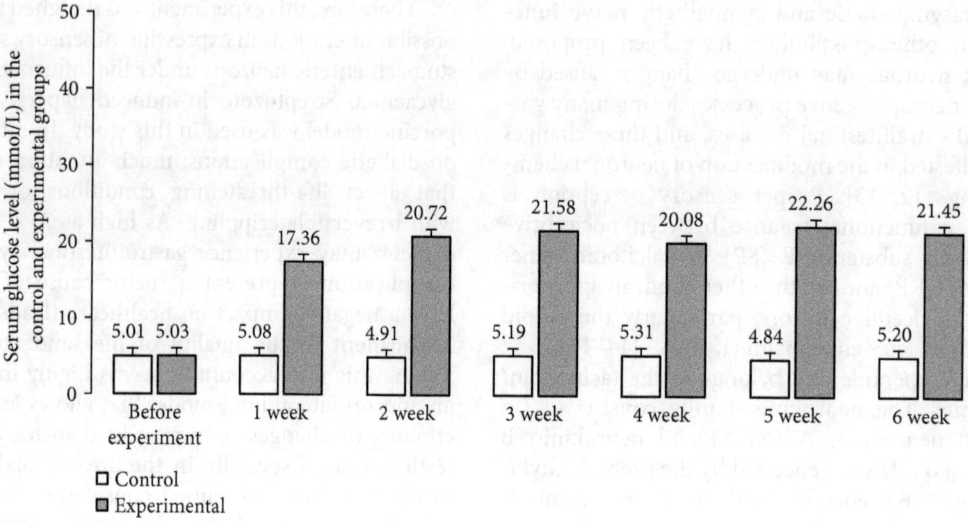

FIGURE 1: Serum glucose levels. Serum glucose levels after induction of diabetes and glucose concentration after streptozotocin administration (1 to 6 weeks).

anesthetized and the solution was administrated via an intravenous needle inserted into an ear with continuous infusion for approximately 5 minutes. To avoid gastrointestinal complications such as nausea and vomiting after streptozotocin injection, animals were fasted for 18 h before the experiment and the control pigs were injected with equal amounts of vehicle (citrate buffer).

The pigs were continuously observed for 24 h after streptozotocin injection. Because streptozotocin often causes temporary hypoglycaemia, 250 mL of 50% glucose solution per animal was administered. The pigs received a normal diet throughout the experiment twice a day and tap water ad libitum. The blood glucose level was measured to confirm hyperglycaemia. The blood glucose concentration was estimated using an Accent-200 (Germany) biochemical analyser, with the colorimetric measurement at a wavelength of 510 nm/670 nm. For this purpose, capillary blood from the ear was collected. The plasma glucose level was measured prior to the experiment initiation in both control and experimental groups. The next measurement was made 48 hours after the induction of diabetes. Subsequent measurements of glucose levels were monitored weekly until the end of the experiment.

2.3. Tissue Collection. Six weeks after streptozotocin injection, pigs were deeply anesthetized via intravenous administration of pentobarbital (Vetbutal, Biowet, Poland) and perfused transcardially via the ascending aorta with 4% paraformaldehyde in a 0.1 M phosphate buffer (PB, pH 7.4). The samples were postfixed by immersion in the same fixative for 1 h, rinsed several times with (PB), and then transferred into a 30% sucrose solution and stored at 4°C until sectioning. The frozen tissue blocks were cut in frontal or sagittal planes using a Microm HM 560 cryostat (Carl Zeiss, Germany) at a thickness of 12 μm and mounted on chrome-coated slides.

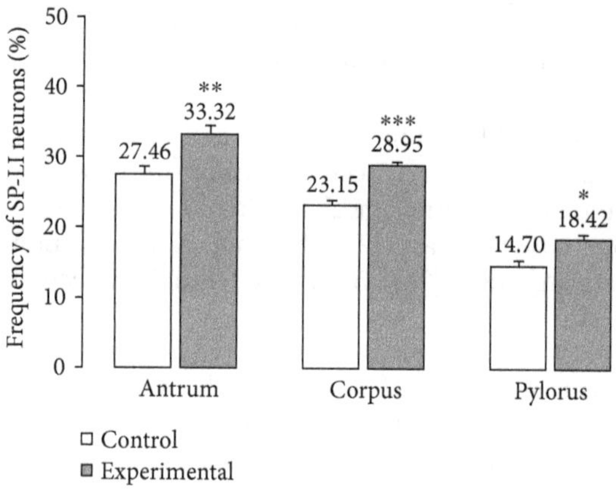

FIGURE 2: The average percentage of MP neurons immunoreactive to SP. The mean of SP-like immunoreactive (SP-LI) neurons in the myenteric plexus (MP) of the stomach antrum, corpus, and pylorus regions in the control and streptozotocin-inducted diabetes groups. Data are presented as mean ± SEM; statistically significant data ($^{*}P < 0.05$, $^{**}P < 0.01$, and $^{***}P < 0.001$).

2.4. Immunofluorescence Procedure. The sections were processed for double immunofluorescence staining. Briefly, after air drying at room temperature for 45 min and rinsing in 0.1 M phosphate-buffered saline (PBS; pH 7.4; 3 × 10 min), the sections were incubated in a blocking buffer containing 10% normal goat serum (MP Biomedicals, USA), in 0.1 M PBS, 0.1% donkey serum (Abcam, UK), 1% Triton X-100 (Sigma-Aldrich, USA), 0.05% Thimerosal (Sigma-Aldrich, USA), and 0.01% NaN_3 for 1 h at room temperature to reduce nonspecific background staining. Subsequently, after another wash in PBS (3 × 10 min), the sections were incubated overnight at 4°C with primary antibodies raised in different species and directed towards general neuronal marker Hu C/D proteins (mouse polyclonal: Invitrogen USA; code A-212711:1.000; working dilution 1 : 1000), anti-

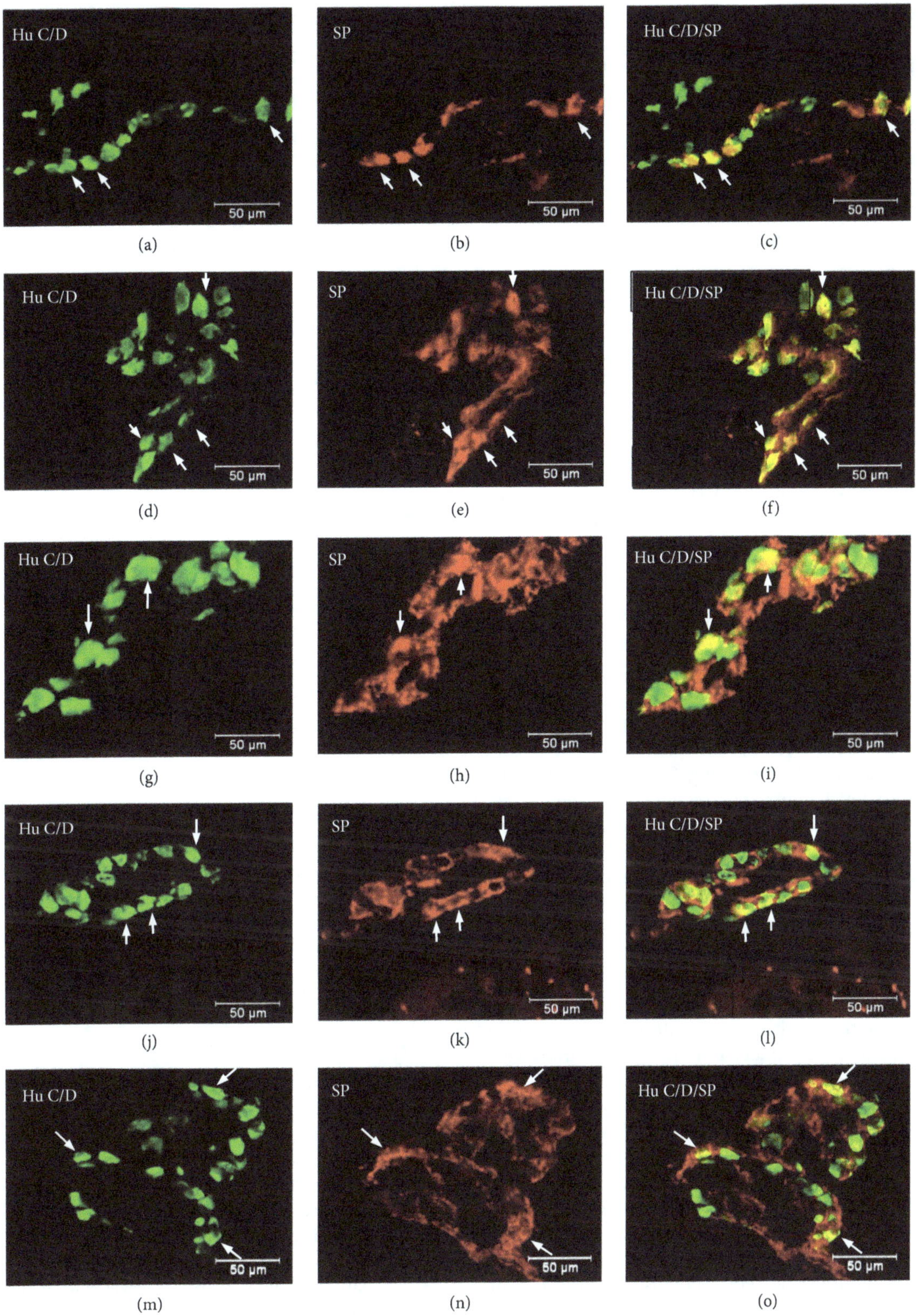

FIGURE 3: Continued.

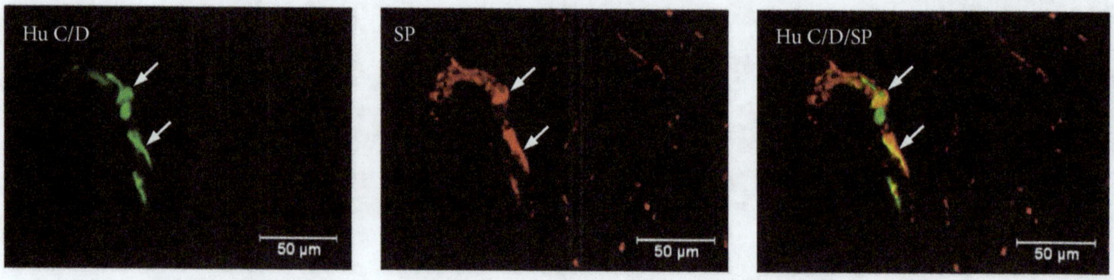

(p) (q) (r)

FIGURE 3: Myenteric ganglion of the porcine stomach immunoreactive to SP. Myenteric ganglion of the porcine antrum under physiological condition (a–c) and during experimentally inducted diabetes (d–f); myenteric ganglion of the porcine corpus under physiological condition (g–i) and during experimentally inducted diabetes (j–l); and myenteric ganglion of the porcine pylorus under physiological condition (m–o) and during experimentally inducted diabetes (p–r), immunostained for Hu C/D (green/arrows) and SP (red/arrows). The right column of the pictures shows the overlap of both stainings. Colocalization of both antigens in the studied cell bodies is indicated with arrows.

nSP antibodies (rat monoclonal: AbD Serotec, cat. number 8450-0505; working dilution 1:150), CGRP (rabbit polyclonal; Millipore, cat. number AB15360; working dilution 1: 4000), and L-ENK (rabbit polyclonal: Abcam, cat. number ab85798; working dilution 1:1000). All antibodies were diluted in PBS containing 0.3% Triton X-100 and 1% BSA. On the following day, the sections were rinsed (PBS, 3×15 min) and incubated with secondary antibodies (donkey anti-mouse Alexa Fluor 488, 1:1000 Invitrogen USA, code A21202; donkey anti-rabbit Alexa Fluor 546 1:1000 Invitrogen, USA, code A10040 diluted in PBS containing 0.25% BSA and 0.1% Triton X-100; and donkey anti-rat Alexa Fluor 546, 1:1000 Invitrogen, USA; code A21208 diluted in PBS containing 0.25% BSA and 0.1% Triton X-100) for 4 hours. The sections were then rinsed three times (PBS, 3×5 min) and mounted in fluorescent mounting medium (DAKO, Carpinteria, CA, USA). The prepared specimens were viewed and photographed using an Olympus BX51 microscope equipped with epifluorescence and appropriate filter sets, coupled with a digital monochromatic camera (Olympus XM 10) connected to a PC, and analysed with Cell Dimension software (Olympus, Tokyo, Japan). Standard controls, that is, preabsorption of the neuropeptide antisera with appropriate antigen, omission, and replacement of the primary antisera by nonimmune sera, were performed to test the antibodies and specificity of the method. The test was performed as follows: sections of the stomach were incubated with a "working" dilution of the primary immunoserum, which had been previously preabsorbed for 18 h at 37°C with 20 μg of appropriate purified protein SP (ab120170, Abcam), CGRP (ab158017, Abcam), and L-ENK (ab159087, Abcam). Additional negative controls, such as the omission and replacement of all primary antisera with nonimmune sera, were also performed. This procedure completely eliminated specific staining.

2.5. Counting of the Nerve Structures and Statistical Evaluation. The number of SP-, CGRP-, and L-ENK-like immunoreactive (LI) enteric neurons was expressed as a percentage of the total number of Hu C/D-positive perikarya. At least 700 Hu C/D-labelled cell bodies of intramural ganglia of each part of the stomach were examined. Only neurons with

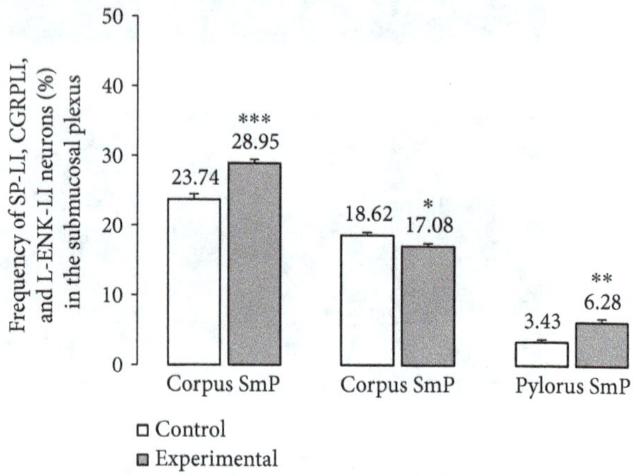

FIGURE 4: The average percentage of SmP neurons immunoreactive to SP, CGRP, and L-ENK. The mean of SP-like immunoreactive (SP-IL), CGRP-like immunoreactive (CGRP-LI), and L-ENK-like immunoreactive (LENK-LI) neurons in the submucosal plexus (SmP) of the stomach corpus in the control and streptozotocin-inducted diabetes groups. Data are presented as mean ± SEM; statistically significant data ($^{*}P < 0.05$, $^{**}P < 0.01$, and $^{***}P < 0.001$).

well-visible nucleus were counted. To prevent the double counting of Hu C/D-immunoreactive neurons, the sections were located at least 100 μm apart. The data pooled from all animal groups were statistically analysed using Statistica 10 software (StatSoft Inc., Tulsa, OK, USA) and expressed as a mean ± standard error (SE) of mean. Significant differences were evaluated using Student's t-test for independent samples ($^{*}P < 0.05$, $^{**}P < 0.001$, and $^{***}P > 0.001$).

Evaluation of the density of nerves within the muscular or mucosal layers was based on counting all the nerve fibres which were immunoreactive to SP, CGRP, and L-ENK per microscopic observation and was assessed under ×40 objective (0.55 mm2) by subjective observation (two independent researchers). Nerve profiles with clearly visible varicosities were counted in four sections per animal (in five fields per section) and the obtained data were pooled and presented as a mean ± SEM.

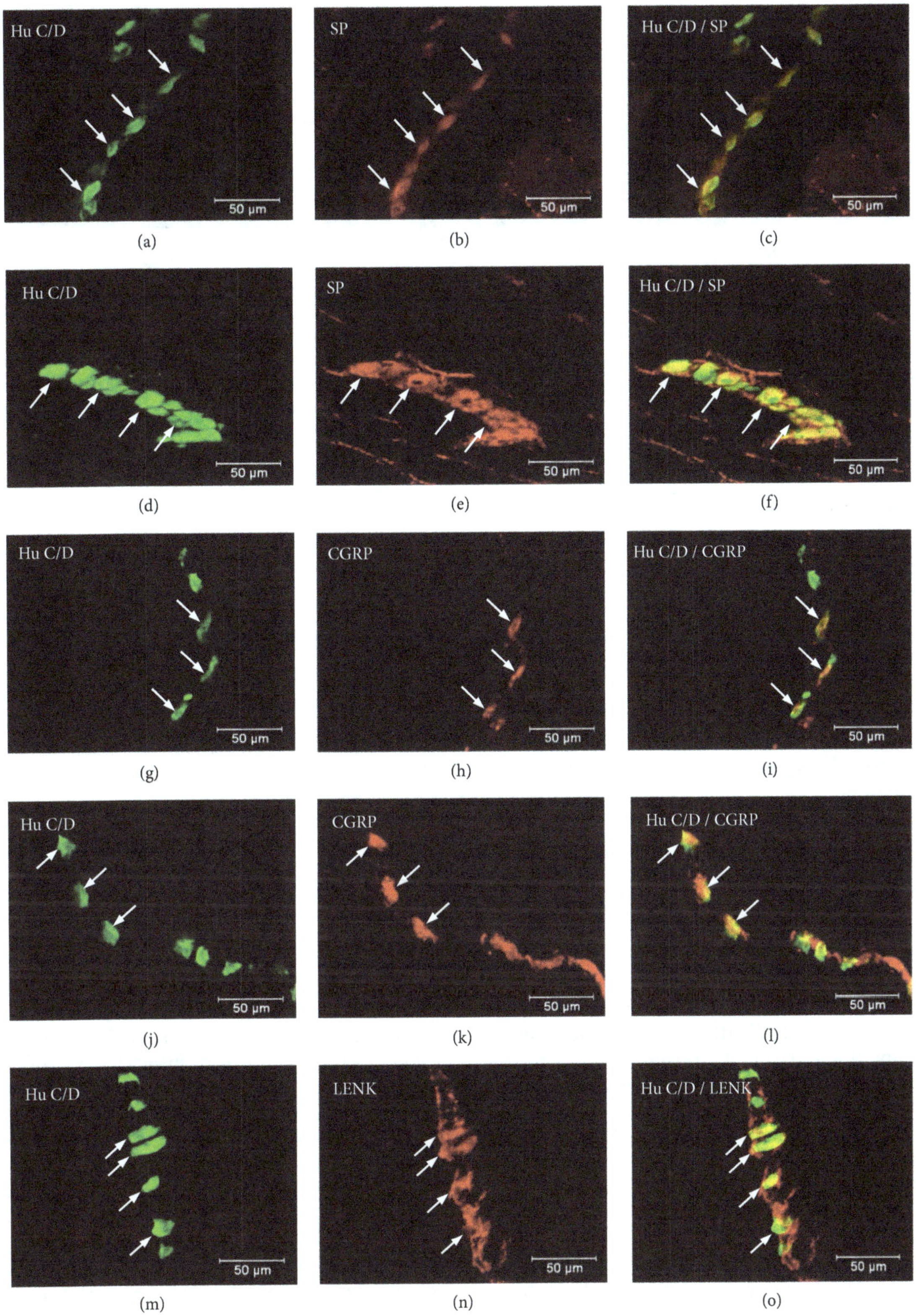

FIGURE 5: Continued.

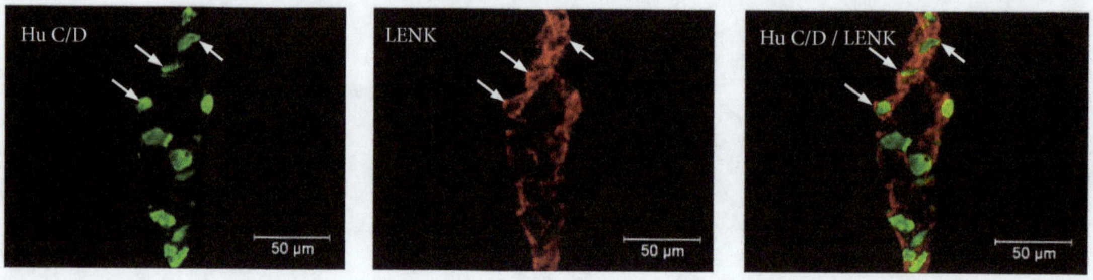

(p) (q) (r)

FIGURE 5: Submucosal ganglion of the porcine stomach immunoreactive to SP, CGRP, and L-ENK. Submucosal ganglion of the porcine corpus under physiological condition (a–c) and during experimentally inducted diabetes (d–f) immunoreactive to SP; submucosal ganglion of the porcine corpus under physiological condition (g–i) and during experimentally inducted diabetes (j–l) immunoreactive to CGRP; and submucosal ganglion of the porcine corpus under physiological condition (m–o) and during experimentally inducted diabetes (p–r) immunoreactive to L-ENK, immunostained for Hu C/D (green/arrows) and SP,CGRP, and L-ENK (red/arrows). The right column of the pictures shows the overlap of both stainings. Colocalization of both antigens in the studied cell bodies is indicated with arrows.

TABLE 1: SP-, CGRP-, and L-ENK-immunoreactive nerve fibres in various parts of the porcine stomach under physiological conditions (control group) and during experimentally induced diabetes (experimental group).

Stomach part	Control group			Experimental group		
	Antrum	Corpus	Pylorus	Antrum	Corpus	Pylorus
SP						
Circular muscle layer[a]	4.82 ± 0.16	3.65 ± 0.16	6.07 ± 0.13	7.42 ± 0.37**	5.63 ± 0.15***	10.75 ± 0.4***
Submucosal/mucosal layer[a]	2.8 ± 0.28	5.19 ± 0.20	2.41 ± 0.18	6.72 ± 0.16***	9.46 ± 0.41***	2.89 ± 0.25
CGRP						
Circular muscle layer[a]	6.10 ± 0.08	6.20 ± 0.18	6.24 ± 0.33	10.44 ± 0.26***	11.38 ± 0.34***	8.85 ± 0.19
Submucosal/mucosal layer[a]	2.58 ± 0.12	2.08 ± 0.14	3.40 ± 0.18	2.88 ± 0.18	2.45 ± 0.09	3.14 ± 0.26
L-ENK						
Circular muscle layer[a]	1.63 ± 0.21	3.11 ± 0.22	1.78 ± 0.15	1.98 ± 0.12	1.47 ± 0.37**	2.10 ± 0.24
Submucosal/mucosal layer[a]	1.81 ± 0.24	1.43 ± 0.09	2.25 ± 0.10	1.62 ± 0.51	1.58 ± 0.11	2.55 ± 0.25

Statistically significant data (**$P > 0.01$ and ***$P > 0.001$). [a]Average number of nerve profiles per area (0.55 μm^2) studied (mean ± SEM).

3. Results

The mean glycaemia level in pigs before streptozotocin injection was within standard reference values for the pig (5.01 mmol/L ± 0.10 mmol/L) (Figure 1) and did not differ between individual animals. Following the STZ induction, a consistent increase in plasma glucose concentration was observed (Figure 1). A significant (17.36 mmol/L ± 0.38 mmol/L) increase in glucose level was observed on the 7th day after STZ injection. The highest increase in blood glucose concentration was detected 4-5 weeks after the STZ injection (22.26 mmol/L ± 1.21 mmol/L) (Figure 1). In the last week of the experiment, the mean serum glucose level increased slightly, reaching 21.24 mmol/L ± 1.11 mmol/L (Figure 1). It should be noted that although chronic glycaemia in experimental animals was significantly higher than that in controls, all pigs which received streptozotocin survived the duration of the experiment in a good general condition and none of the animals required exogenous insulin injection.

Double labelling immunohistochemistry revealed that in the control group, the SP distribution in the ENS neurons was varied and clearly depended on the analysed area of the stomach (Figure 2). In the myenteric ganglia of the antrum, the SP-positive cell bodies constitute 27.46 ± 1.09% of all HuC/D neurons studied (Figure 2, Figures 3(a)–3(c)). In turn, inside the MP of the corpus, the quantity of SP-positive cell bodies was slightly lower (23.15 ± 0.75%) (Figure 2, Figures 3(g)–3(i)). A very similar number of SP-LI neurons were observed in the submucosal plexus (SmP) of the corpus (23.74 ± 0.80%) (Figure 4, Figures 5(a)–5(c)). The smallest number of SP-LI perikarya was found in the MG of the pylorus (14.70 ± 0.80%) (Figure 2, Figures 3(m)–3(o)).

In the diabetic group, a statistically significant increase in the number of SP-positive cell bodies was observed in all investigated area of the stomach. In the MG of the antrum, the population of SP neurons amounted to 33.32 ± 1.21%. (Figure 2, Figures 3(d)–3(f)). The highest increase in SP expression was observed in the MG of the corpus, where the number of SP-LI neurons was 36.58 ± 0.64% (Figure 2, Figures 3(j)–3(l)). A slightly lower increase in SP-positive neurons (to 28.5 ± 0.56%) in the submucosal ganglia of the corpus was noted (Figure 4, Figures 5(d)–5(f)). With regard

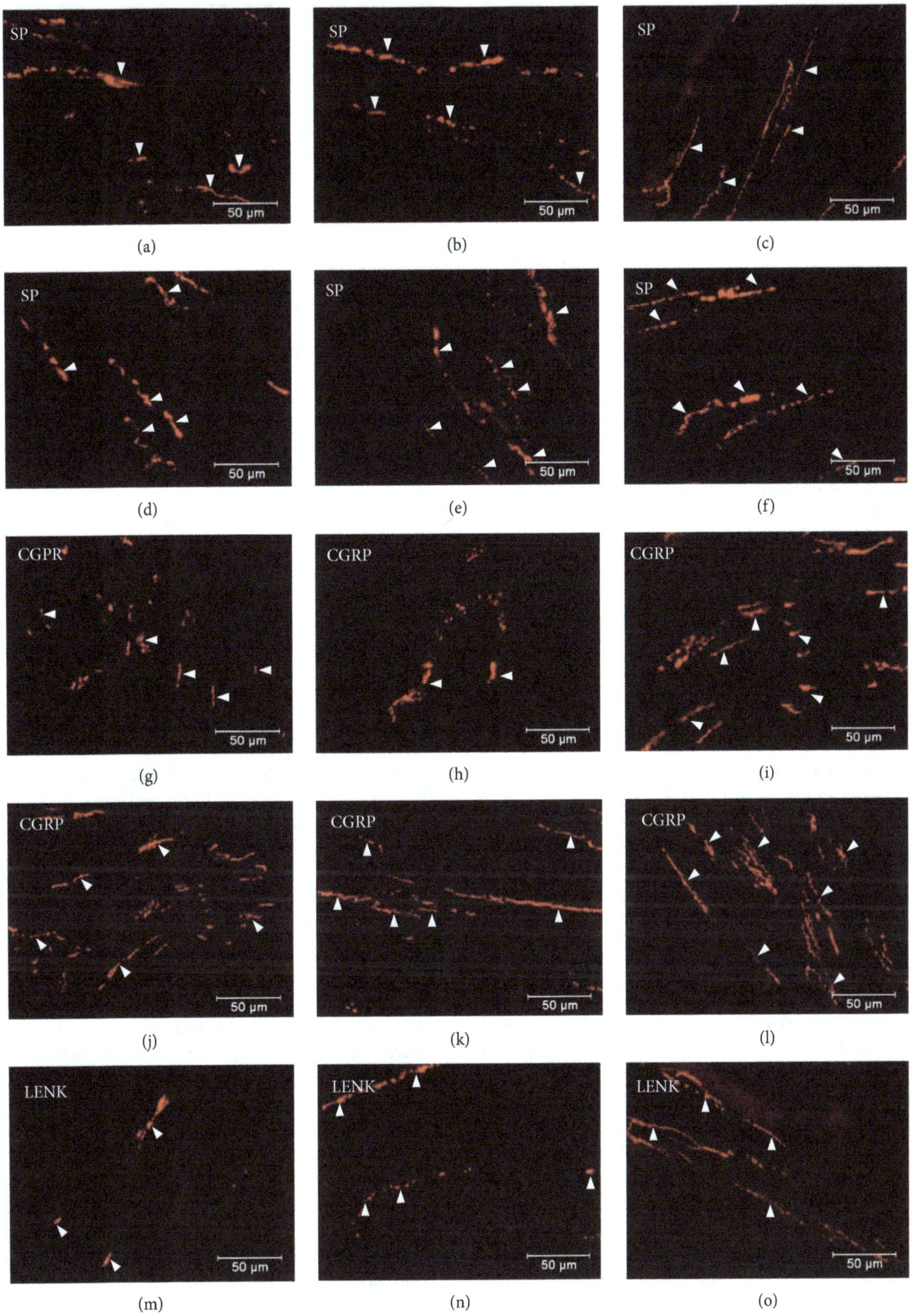

Figure 6: Continued.

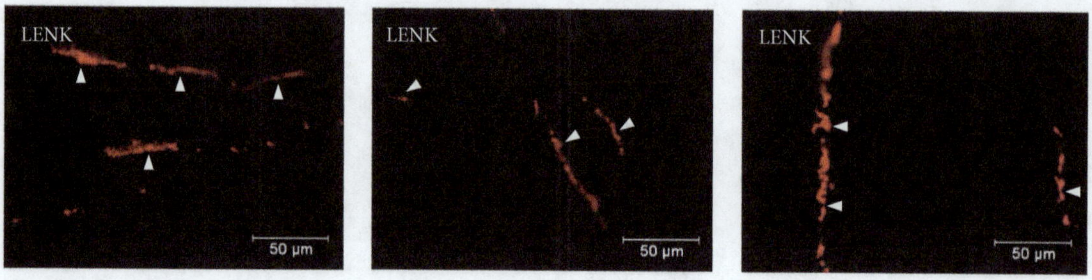

(p) (q) (r)

FIGURE 6: Distribution pattern of nerve fibres (arrow) immunoreactive to SP, CGRP, and L-ENK within the circular muscle layer. Distribution pattern of nerve fibres (arrows) within the circular muscle layer immunoreactive to SP under physiological condition: antrum (a), corpus (b), and pylorus (c) and under experimentally inducted diabetes: antrum (d), corpus (e), and pylorus (f); for CGRP under physiological condition: antrum (g) corpus (e), and pylorus (f) and under experimentally inducted diabetes: antrum (j), corpus (k), and pylorus (l); and for L-ENK under physiological condition: antrum (m), corpus (n), and pylorus (o) and under experimentally inducted diabetes: antrum (p), corpus (q), and pylorus (r).

to the MG in the pylorus, changes in chemical coding were relativity smaller and amounted to 18.42 ± 0.82% (Figure 2, Figures 3(p)–3(r)).

Moreover, in addition to cell bodies, the density of nerve fibres was also investigated. Namely, SP-positive nerve fibres were present in the circular and submucosal muscle layers. In the control group, the SP-immunoreactive nerve fibres were more numerous in the circular muscle layer and they constitute 4.82 ± 0.16 in the antrum, 3.65 ± 0.16 in the corpus, and 6.07 ± 0.13 in the pylorus (Table 1, Figures 6(a)–6(c)). In the diabetic group, a statistically significant increase was observed in the density of SP-LI nerve fibres in the circular muscle layer in all areas of the stomach. In the antrum, SP-positive nerve fibres constituted 7.42 ± 0.37, 5.63 ± 0.16 in the corpus, and 10.75 ± 0.40 in the pylorus (Table 1, Figures 6(d)–6(f)). In the submucosal layer, the SP-positive nerve fibres in the control group were more numerous in the corpus 5.19 ± 0.20, while in the antrum and pylorus, they constituted only 2.8 ± 0.28 and 2.41 ± 0.18, respectively (Table 1, Figures 7(a)–7(c)). Under hyperglycaemia conditions, a statistically significant increase in the density of SP nerve fibres in the antrum and corpus was observed (6.72 ± 0.16 and 9.46 ± 0.41, resp.) (Table 1, Figures 7(d) and 7(e)), while in the pylorus, no statistically significant changes were observed (Table 1, Figure 7(f)).

The other investigated substance was CGRP. Similar to SP, CGRP-positive neurons were presented in all studied areas, but clear differences were noted between various regions of the stomach. In the control group, the highest population of CGRP was noted in the antrum (33.07 ± 1.10%) (Figure 8, Figures 9(a)–9(c)), while in the other regions of the stomach, the number of CGRP-immunoreactive cell bodies was relatively lower and amounted to 23.95 ± 0.64% within the MG in the corpus (Figure 8, Figures 9(g)–9(i)) and 16.15 ± 0.80% in the pylorus (Figure 8, Figures 9(m)–9(o)) and 18.62 ± 0.44% in the submucosal ganglia in the corpus (Figure 4, Figures 5(g)–5(h)). In the diabetic group, statistically significant changes were observed in all investigated areas. The number of CGRP-positive neurons within the MG was estimated at 41.6 ± 0.99% in the antrum (Figure 8, Figures 9(d)–9(f)), 38.61 ± 0.81% in the corpus (Figure 8, Figures 9(j)–9(l)), and 22.33 ± 0.86% in the pylorus (Figure 8, Figures 9(p)–9(r)). In turn, in the submucosal ganglia inside the corpus, the numbers of GGRP-positive neurons were 17.08 ± 0.40% (Figure 4, Figures 5(j)–5(l)). Nerve fibres immunoreactive to CGRP were observed in the circular muscle layer and in the submucosal layer (Table 1). In the control group, the density of CGRP-LI neuronal processes was similar in all investigated areas. In the circular muscle layer, an average of 6.10 ± 0.37 of CGRP-positive fibres were noted in the antrum (Figure 6(g)), 6.20 ± 0.18 in the corpus (Figure 6(h)), and 6.24 ± 0.33 in the pylorus (Figure 6(i), Table 1).

In the diabetic group, a statistically significant increase in the density of CGRP-LI fibres within the circular muscle layer was observed. In the antrum, the density of CGRP-containing nerve fibres was estimated at 10.44 ± 0.23 (Figure 7(j)), whereas in the corpus and pylorus, it was 11.38 ± 0.32 (Figure 7(k)) and 8.85 ± 0.19, respectively (Table 1, Figure 7(l)). Within the submucosal layer, the density of CGRP-positive nerve fibres was scarce. In the antrum of control animals, 2.58 ± 0.12 of CGRP-positive nerve fibres was observed, while in the corpus, it was 2.08 ± 0.14 and it was 3.40 ± 0.18 in the pylorus (Table 1, Figures 7(g)–7(i)). Moreover, in the experimental pigs, no statistically significant changes in the density of CGRP-immunoreactive nerve fibres were observed (Table 1, Figures 7(j)–7(l)).

Another substance studied was L-ENK. The population of neurons containing L-ENK was the least numerous among investigated peptides. In the control group, the population of L-ENK-positive neurons was the highest in the MG of the corpus (15.06 ± 0.47%) (Figure 10, Figures 11(g)–11(i)), a bit lower in the antrum (8.84 ± 0.54%) (Figure 10, Figures 11(a)–11(c)), and the lowest in the pylorus (5.43 ± 0.32%) (Figure 10, Figures 11(m)–11(o)). In turn, in the submucosal ganglia within the corpus, this value was calculated at 3.43 ± 0.40% (Figure 4, Figures 5(m)–5(o)).

Hyperglycaemia triggered the following changes in the chemical phenotyping of L-ENK-positive enteric neurons. In the MG of the antrum, an increase was noted in L-ENK-LI neurons (to 11.45 ± 0.44%) (Figure 10,

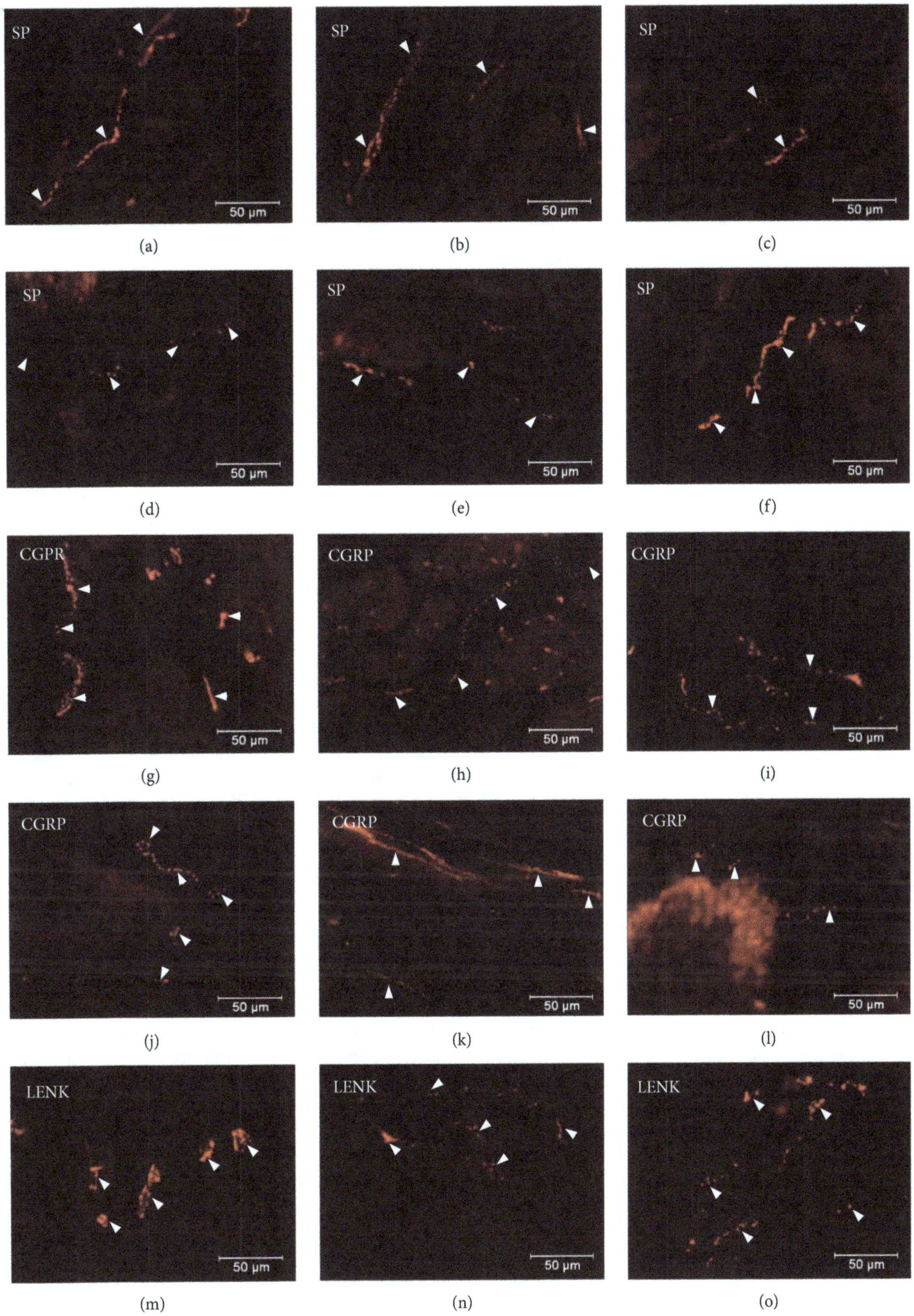

(a) (b) (c) (d) (e) (f) (g) (h) (i) (j) (k) (l) (m) (n) (o)

FIGURE 7: Continued.

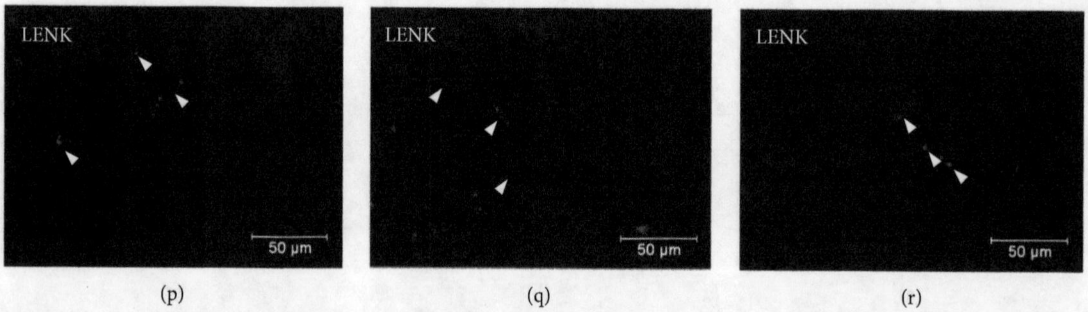

FIGURE 7: Distribution pattern of nerve fibres (arrow) immunoreactive to SP, CGRP, and L-ENK within the submucosal muscle layer. Distribution pattern of nerve fibres (arrows) within the submucosal muscle layer immunoreactive to SP under physiological condition: antrum (a), corpus (b), and pylorus (c) and under experimentally inducted diabetes: antrum (d), corpus (e), and pylorus (f); for CGRP under physiological condition: antrum (g), corpus (e), and pylorus (f) and under experimentally inducted diabetes: antrum (j), corpus (k), and pylorus (l); and for L-ENK under physiological condition: antrum (m), corpus (n), and pylorus (o) and under experimentally inducted diabetes: antrum (p), corpus (q), and pylorus (r).

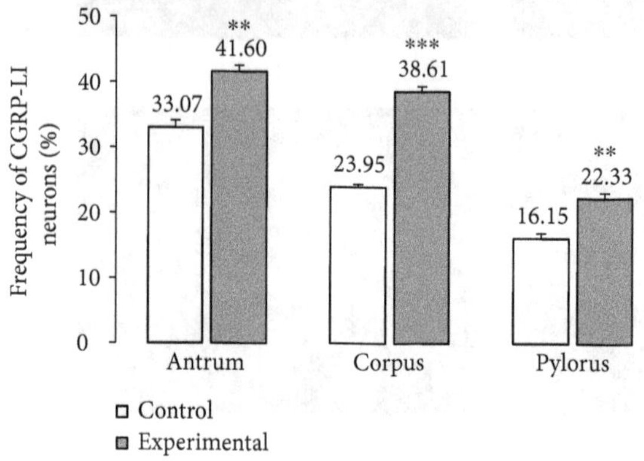

FIGURE 8: The average percentage of MP neurons immunoreactive to CGRP. The mean of CGRP-like immunoreactive (CGRP-LI) neurons in the myenteric plexus (MP) of the antrum, corpus, and pylorus regions of the stomach in the control and streptozotocin-inducted diabetes groups. Data are presented as mean ± SEM; statistically significant data (**$P < 0.01$ and ***$P < 0.001$).

Figures 11(d)–11(f)), while in the corpus, there was a decrease in L-ENK-LI neurons (to 6.94 ± 0.42%) (Figure 10, Figures 11(j)–11(l)), while in the pylorus, the number of L-ENK-immunopositive cell bodies was decreased (1.90 ± 0.16%) (Figure 10, Figures 11(p)–11(r)). In turn, in the submucosal ganglion of the corpus, the population of L-ENK-LI neurons was increased (to 6.28 ± 1.67%) (Figure 4, Figures 5(p)–5(r)).

On the other hand, L-ENK-positive nerve fibres were visible in both the circular and submucosal muscle layers. In the control group, the density of nerve fibres within the circular muscle layer amounted to 1.63 ± 0.21 in the antrum, 3.11 ± 0.22 in the corpus, and 1.78 ± 0.15 in the pylorus (Table 1, Figures 6(m)–6(o)). In a diabetes condition, statistically significant changes were observed only in the corpus, that is, a decrease was noted in L-ENK-positive nerve fibres (to 1.47 ± 0.37) (Table 1, Figures 6(p)–6(r)). In the submucosal layer, the density of nerve fibres in the control group was as follows: 1.81 ± 0.24 in the antrum, 1.43 ± 0.09 in the corpus, and 2.25 ± 0.01 in the pylorus (Table 1, Figures 7(m)–7(o)). In the diabetic group, the density of L-ENK-containing nerves fibres changed only in a statistically insignificant manner compared to that in the control group (Figures 7(p)–7(r)). In the preabsorbtion test positive reaction was not observed (Figure 12).

4. Discussion

The present study showed that the porcine gastric enteric neurons, after six weeks of sustained hyperglycaemia, exhibit alterations in the chemical phenotyping of the ENS neurons situated in the porcine stomach. Hitherto, data describing chemical changes in the intramural enteric neurons in response to hyperglycaemia were limited to studies on small animal models, especially rats [12, 37, 38]. The population of the SP-IR neurons has been described in a different region of the gastrointestinal tract [20, 24, 25]. Previous studies clearly showed that the level of SP expression in the GI tract is dependent on diabetes duration. In the human stomach, after 15 years of diabetes condition, a decreased concentration of SP in Cajal cells was described [39]. However, in rats, 48 weeks after the induction of diabetes, significant changes in SP expression in both the stomach and small intestine were not observed [40]. The results obtained in the present experiment, performed on immature gilts, are different than those presented above. Namely, a statistically significant increase was observed in the number of SP-positive neurons in all investigated areas of the stomach. It is hypothesized that the observed augmentation in SP expression in diabetic pigs may be explained by the time of hyperglycaemia duration. Moreover, throughout the entire time of the experiment, all animals in the diabetic group exhibited an approx. fourfold increase in glucose serum compared to those in the control group. Additionally, none of the pigs in the diabetic group received exogenous insulin. The supplementation of exogenous insulin seems to be an important factor to restore an appropriate level of SP [41]. In turn, with respect to differentiation of SP distribution due to the region of the gastrointestinal tract, previous studies demonstrated differences between the stomach and small and large intestines, as well as among each ganglion [42–44]. For example, in diabetic rats, an increase in SP

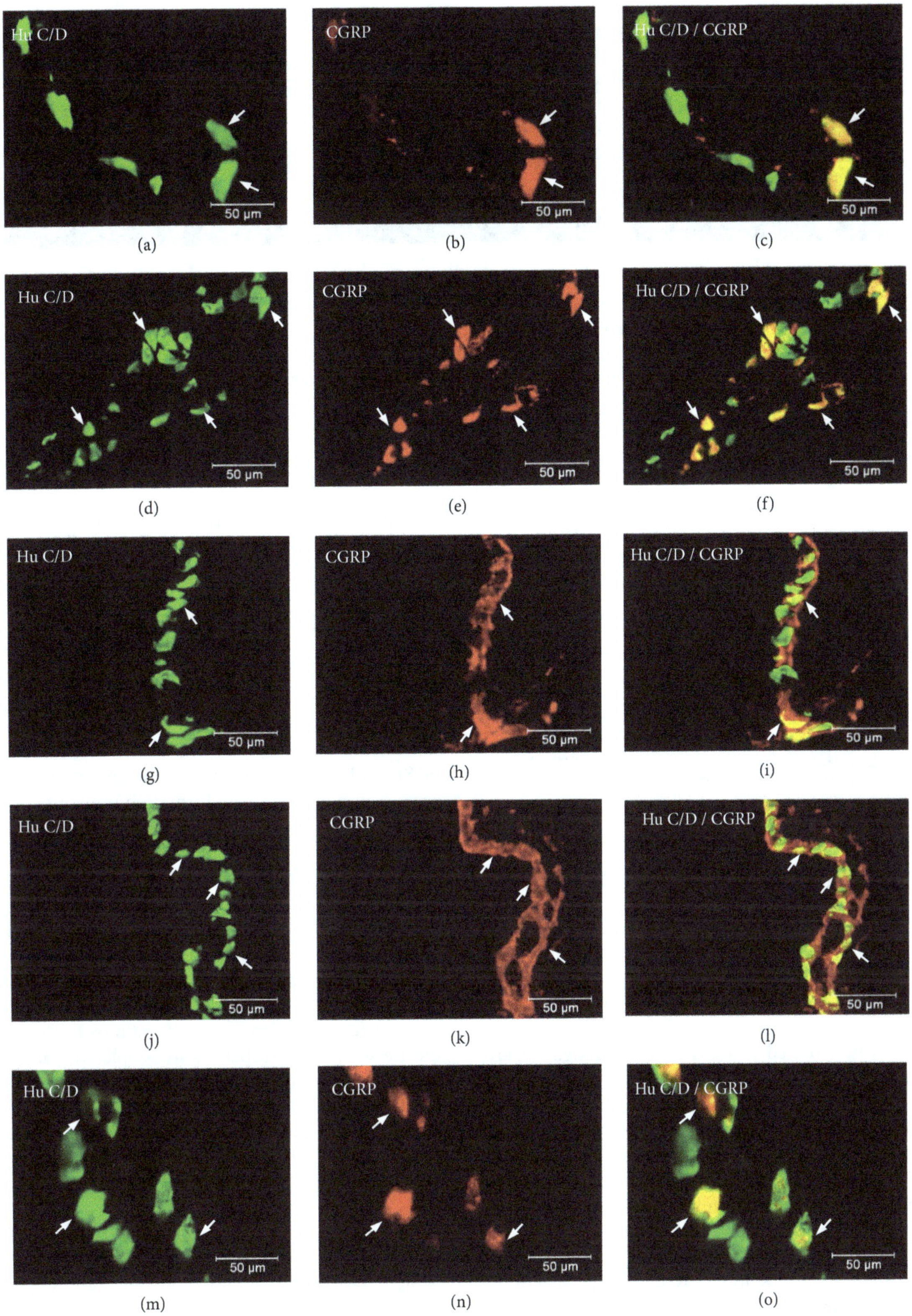

FIGURE 9: Continued.

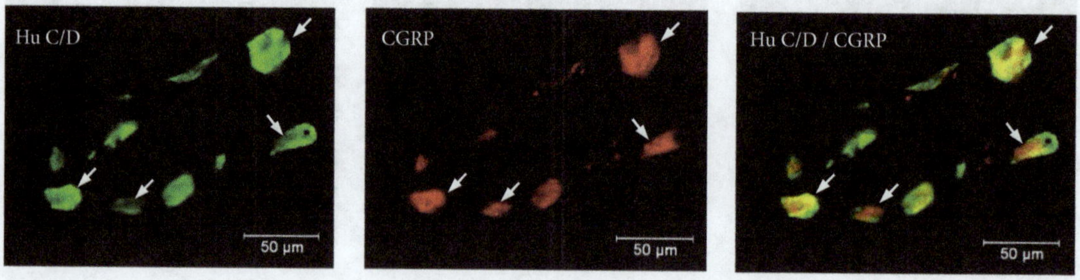

(p) (q) (r)

Figure 9: Myenteric ganglion of the porcine stomach immunoreactive to CGRP. Myenteric ganglion of the porcine antrum under physiological condition (a–c) and during experimentally inducted diabetes (d–f); myenteric ganglion of the porcine corpus under physiological condition (g–i) and during experimentally inducted diabetes (j–l); and myenteric ganglion of the porcine pylorus under physiological condition (m–o) and during experimentally inducted diabetes (p–r), immunostained for Hu C/D (green/arrows) and CGRP (red/arrows). The right column of the pictures shows the overlap of both stainings. Colocalization of both antigens in the studied cell bodies is indicated with arrows.

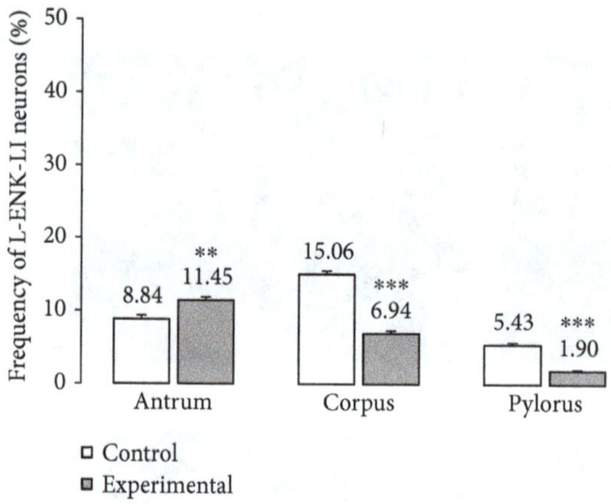

Figure 10: The average percentage of MP neurons immunoreactive to L-ENK. The mean of L-ENK-like immunoreactive (LENK-LI) neurons in the myenteric plexus (MP) of the antrum, corpus, and pylorus regions of the stomach in the control and streptozotocin-inducted diabetes group. Data are presented as mean ± SEM; statistically significant data (**$P < 0.01$ and ***$P < 0.001$).

expression has been noted in the myenteric ganglia of the duodenum and colon, as well as within the ileum [12]. Moreover, we have observed an increase in the number of SP-positive nerve fibres. A similar process was also observed in other pathological conditions [20]. But it should be noted that the exact origin of these fibres (extrinsic/intrinsic) is unclear and its elucidation requires application of retrograde tracing techniques.

Furthermore, CGRP immunoreactivity was found to be significantly reduced after 8 and 12 weeks of diabetes in the myenteric and submucosal plexuses of rat ileum and colon [43, 44]. On the other hand, there is a lack of information about changes in CGRP expression in the stomach. The current study indicates that in the myenteric ganglia of the antrum, corpus, and pylorus in diabetic pigs, the expression level of CGRP was higher than the number of CGRP-LI neurons observed in the healthy group. In the submucosal ganglia in the corpus, statistically significant changes in the CGRP expression were also noted. It should be emphasized that previous studies were performed on rats using the streptozotocin diabetes model, while the current study, for the first time, used pigs as a model to focus studying on a phenotype of stomach enteric neurons. The rate of metabolism in swine is similar to humans [45]. In addition, pigs are increasingly used as experimental models in diseases with metabolic disorders [46].

The role of SP and CGRP in the gastrointestinal tract is well established [15, 16]. One of the best-known functions of SP and CGRP, not only in the gastrointestinal tract, is sensory and nociceptive information transmission [20]. Both SP and CGRP are markers of primary afferent neurons whose main role is to participate in short reflexes within the gastrointestinal wall. These neurons also take part in the transmission of nociceptive stimuli from the lamina mucosa and muscular layer of the gastrointestinal tract [30]. This observation strongly suggests that SP and CGRP may be actively involved in the pathophysiological mechanisms of abdominal pain during diabetes. This function seems to be very important because pain episodes are one of the most often disturbances in people with long-term diabetes [2]. Our studies show that an increase in the number of SP and CGRP neurons can be correlated with pain episodes. In order to fully answer of this question, further research should be carried out using analogues or agonists/antagonists of these substances to confirm the role of SP and CGRP in this process.

It should also be added that in the course of many gastrointestinal symptoms, gastrointestinal motility is impaired. Gastrointestinal symptoms including dysfunction of motor activity appear more commonly in diabetes [47]. The most important manifestation of gastrointestinal autonomic neuropathy is gastroparesis [4, 5]. The molecular mechanism underlying the above symptoms is not fully understood. The receptor for advanced glycation end products (RAGE) has recently gained attention as a potential contributor to neuropathy including autonomic neuropathy [48]. The mechanism triggering RAGE-related neurodegenerative

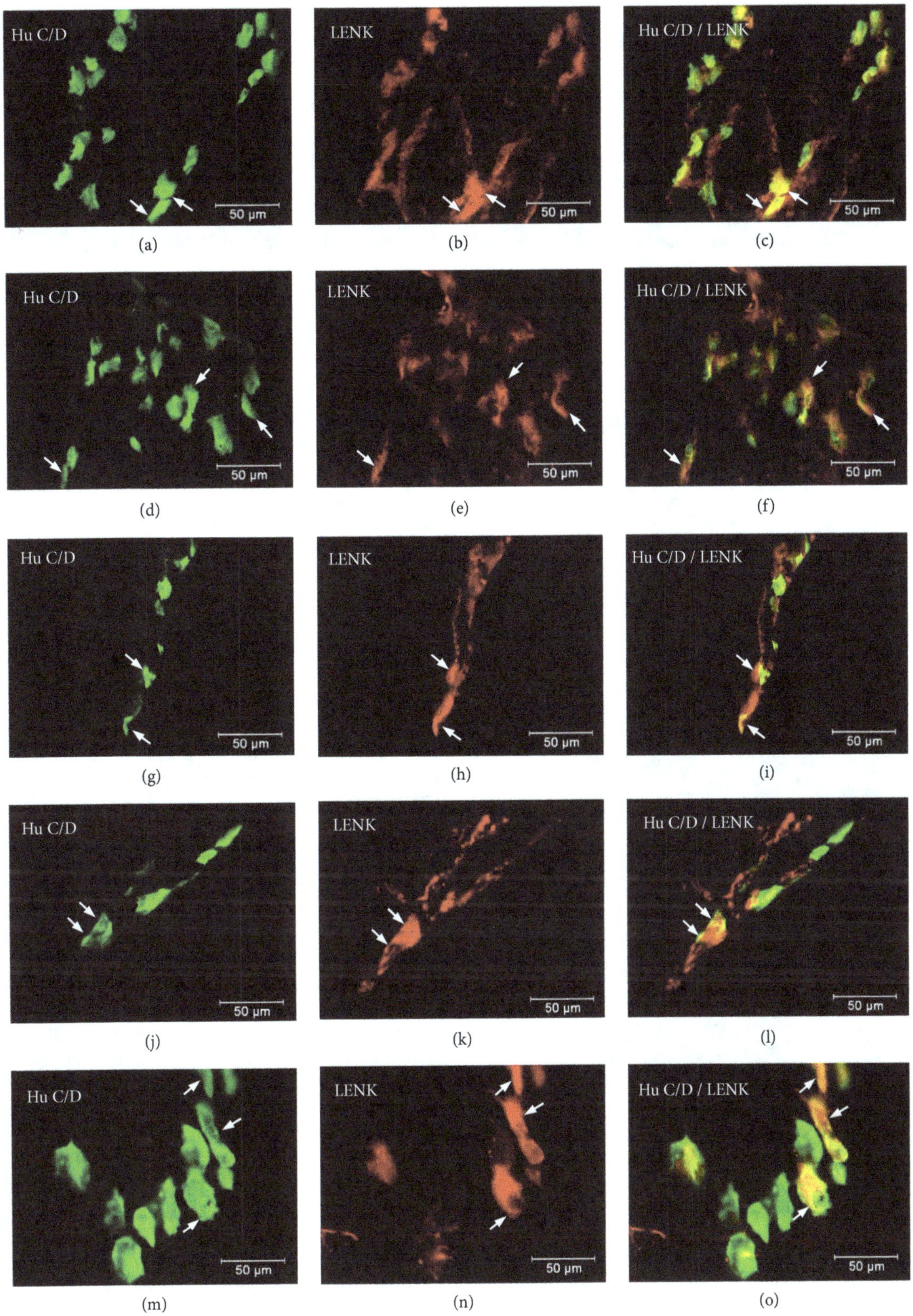

FIGURE 11: Continued.

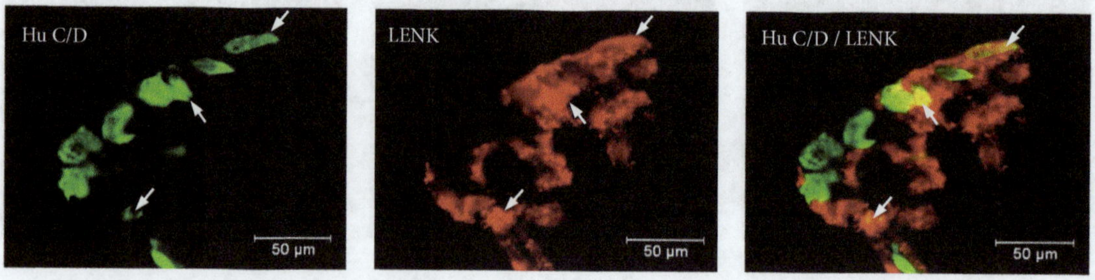

(p) (q) (r)

FIGURE 11: The average percentage of MP neurons immunoreactive to L-ENK. The mean of L-ENK-like immunoreactive (LENK-LI) neurons in the myenteric plexus (MP) of the antrum, corpus, and pylorus regions of the stomach in the control and streptozotocin-inducted diabetes group. Data are presented as mean ± SEM; statistically significant data ($^{**}P < 0.01$ and $^{***}P < 0.001$).

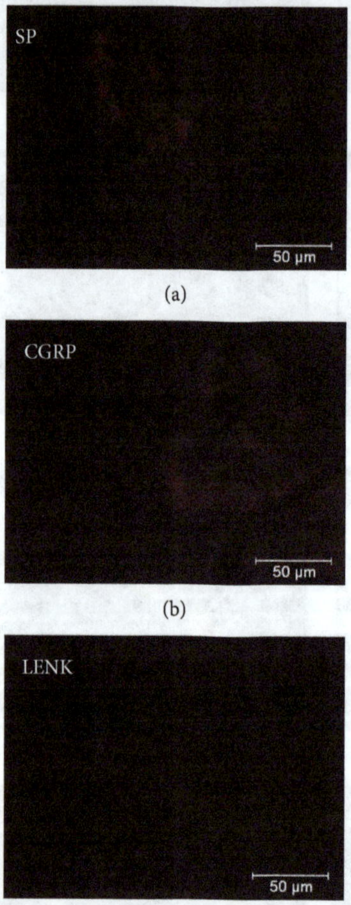

(a) (b) (c)

FIGURE 12: Negative controls for SP (a), CGRP (b), and LENK (c).

processes is likely related to oxidative stress caused by an increase in reactive oxygen species through an NF-κB-activated inflammatory pathway [49]. In the above described processes, SP and CGRP can be at least partially involved. Inflammatory and immune modulatory actions of SP are relatively well known [50]. Namely, SP is considered to be an important proinflammatory factor, which inducts cytokine release [51], as well as an agent sending information between the nervous and immune systems [50].

Leu5-enkephalin, which was also investigated in the present study, belongs to a group of opioid peptides [31]. The sources of opioid peptides in the GI tract include both endocrine cells and enteric neurons. Enkephalins are predominantly located in submucosal and myenteric neurons. They are also present in stomach muscle membranes, as well as in the muscle layer of the small and large intestines. These peptides exhibit various effects on the function of the gastrointestinal tract. Generally, they show a modulatory effect on the secretion of other peptides and are able to enhance or inhibit the contractility of particular parts of the gastrointestinal tract [17, 52, 53].

The current results, for the first time, describe changes in the expression of leu5-enkephalin in stomach enteric neurons under acute hyperglycaemia. In contrast to SP and CGRP, an increase in the number of neurons containing leu5-enkephalin in investigated areas of the stomach was not observed. With regard to myenteric ganglia, in the corpus and pylorus, a decrease in the expression of leu5-enkephalin was observed. To date, changes of leu5-enkephalin in the course of diabetes in enteric neurons have not been investigated. Till now, the expression and distribution of leu5-enkephalin were described in the human large intestine in the course of drug-resistant colitis [30]. Moreover, the distribution of opiate receptors in the gastrointestinal tract were also described [54]. It is well known that endogenous opioids have strong antinociceptive properties. Based on the current results, it can be concluded that changes in the amount of leu5-enkephalin neurons may be at least partially responsible for increasing pain reactions in the course of long-lasting hyperglycaemia in diabetes patients. Also, like in the case of CGRP and SP utilization of agonists or antagonists of opioids, receptors can provide more information concerning engagement of investigated substances in gastrointestinal complications in the course of diabetes.

5. Conclusion

In conclusion, the obtained results proved that hyperglycaemia causes significant changes in the neurochemical profile of the porcine stomach enteric neurons with respect to SP, CGRP, and L-ENK. It also seems that the participation of investigated substances in the development of gastric complications is significant. Undoubtedly, they are involved in the process of transmitting and modulating sensory information and may also influence the immune response, inflammatory processes, and regulate motor activity. It cannot be excluded that, in the future, research on the role of these peptides may result in the development of effective pharmacotherapy of gastrointestinal disorders. In addition, it seems that the pig is an appropriate model for studying the effect of hyperglycaemia on the neurochemical coding of enteric neurons.

Conflicts of Interest

The authors declare no conflict of interest.

Acknowledgments

This study was financed by a statutory Grant no. 15.610.003-300 and KNOW (Leading National Research Center) scientific consortium "Healthy Animal—Safe Food" and decision of the Ministry of Science and Higher Education (no. 05-1/KNOW2/2015).

References

[1] A. T. Kharroubi and H. M. Darwish, "Diabetes mellitus: the epidemic of the century," *World Journal of Diabetes*, vol. 6, no. 6, pp. 850–867, 2015.

[2] A. I. Vinik, R. E. Maser, B. D. Mitchell, and R. Freeman, "Diabetic autonomic neuropathy," *Diabetes Care*, vol. 26, no. 5, pp. 1553–1579, 2003.

[3] O. Vikulova, L. Bolotskaya, E. Bessmertnaya et al., "Frequency of diabetic complications and HbA1C level by active screening and diabetes registry data: comparative study," *Atherosclerosis*, vol. 263, article e171, 2017.

[4] A. Gatopoulou, N. Papanas, and E. Maltezos, "Diabetic gastrointestinal autonomic neuropathy: current status and new achievements for everyday clinical practice," *European Journal of Internal Medicine*, vol. 23, no. 6, pp. 499–505, 2012.

[5] M. Camilleri, A. E. Bharucha, and G. Farrugia, "Epidemiology, mechanisms and management of diabetic gastroparesis," *Clinical Gastroenterology and Hepatology*, vol. 9, no. 1, pp. 5–12, 2011.

[6] M. Horowitz, A. F. Maddox, J. M. Wishart, P. E. Harding, B. E. Chatterton, and D. J. C. Shearman, "Relationships between oesophageal transit and solid and liquid gastric emptying in diabetes mellitus," *European Journal of Nuclear Medicine*, vol. 18, no. 4, pp. 229–234, 1991.

[7] J. B. Furness, B. P. Callaghan, L. R. Rivera, and H. J. Cho, "The enteric nervous system and gastrointestinal innervation: integrated local and central control," *Advances in Experimental Medicine and Biology*, vol. 817, pp. 39–71, 2014.

[8] J. B. Furness, "The enteric nervous system and neurogastroenterology," *Nature Reviews Gastroenterology & Hepatology*, vol. 9, no. 5, pp. 286–294, 2012.

[9] J. Wojtkiewicz, S. Gonkowski, M. Bladowski, and M. Majewski, "Characterisation of cocaine- and amphetamine- regulated transcript-like immunoreactive (CART-LI) enteric neurons in the porcine small intestine," *Acta Veterinaria Hungarica*, vol. 60, no. 3, pp. 371–381, 2012.

[10] S. Gonkowski, P. Burlinski, and J. Calka, "Proliferative enteropathy (PE)-induced changes in galanin—like immunoreactivity in the enteric nervous system of the porcine distal colon," *Acta Veterinaria*, vol. 59, no. 4, pp. 321–330, 2009.

[11] B. Chandrasekharan and S. Srinivasan, "Diabetes and the enteric nervous system," *Neurogastroenterology and Motility*, vol. 19, no. 12, pp. 951–960, 2007.

[12] A. Belai, J. Lincoln, P. Milner, and G. Burnstock, "Progressive changes in adrenergic, serotonergic, and peptidergic nerves in proximal colon of streptozotocin-diabetic rats," *Gastroenterology*, vol. 95, no. 5, pp. 1234–1241, 1988.

[13] T. Ordög, Y. Hayashi, and S. J. Gibbons, "Cellular pathogenesis of diabetic gastroenteropathy," *Minerva Gastroenterologica e Dietologica*, vol. 55, no. 3, pp. 315–343, 2009.

[14] P. Holzer and U. Holzer-Petsche, "Tachykinins in the gut. Part I. Expression, release and motor function," *Pharmacology & Therapeutics*, vol. 73, no. 3, pp. 173–217, 1997.

[15] P. Holzer and U. Holzer-Petsche, "Tachykinins in the gut. Part II. Roles in neural excitation, secretion and inflammation," *Pharmacology & Therapeutics*, vol. 73, no. 3, pp. 219–263, 1997.

[16] P. Holzer and U. Holzer-Petsche, "Tachykinin receptors in the gut: physiological and pathological implications," *Current Opinion in Pharmacology*, vol. 1, no. 6, pp. 583–590, 2001.

[17] J. J. Galligan and H. I. Akbarali, "Molecular physiology of enteric opioid receptors," *American Journal of Gastroenterology Supplements*, vol. 2, no. 1, pp. 17–21, 2014.

[18] P. Datar, S. Srivastava, E. Coutinho, and G. Govil, "Substance P: structure, function, and therapeutics," *Current Topics in Medicinal Chemistry*, vol. 4, no. 1, pp. 75–103, 2004.

[19] N. P. Gerard, L. A. Garraway, R. L. Eddy Jr. et al., "Human substance P receptor (NK-1): organization of the gene, chromosome localization, and functional expression of cDNA clones," *Biochemistry*, vol. 30, no. 44, pp. 10640–10646, 2002.

[20] S. Gonkowski, "Substance P as a neuronal factor in the enteric nervous system of the porcine descending colon in physiological conditions and during selected pathogenic processes," *BioFactors*, vol. 39, no. 5, pp. 542–551, 2013.

[21] C. A. Maggi, "Principles of tachykininergic co-transmission in the peripheral and enteric nervous system," *Regulatory Peptides*, vol. 93, no. 1–3, pp. 53–64, 2000.

[22] C. R. Mantyh, S. R. Vigna, J. E. Maggio, P. W. Mantyh, R. R. Bollinger, and T. N. Pappas, "Substance P binding sites on intestinal lymphoid aggregates and blood vessels in inflammatory bowel disease correspond to authentic NK-1 receptors," *Neuroscience Letters*, vol. 178, no. 2, pp. 255–259, 1994.

[23] P. J. Thor, R. Sendur, and S. J. Konturek, "Influence of substance P on myoelectric activity of the small bowel," *American Journal of Physiology-Gastrointestinal and Liver Physiology*, vol. 243, no. 6, pp. G493–G496, 1982.

[24] M. Lordal, E. Theodorsson, and P. M. Hellstrom, "Tachykinins influence interdigestive rhythm and contractile strength of human small intestine," *Digestive Diseases and Sciences*, vol. 42, no. 9, pp. 1940–1949, 1997.

[25] K. Szymanska, K. Makowska, and S. Gonkowski, "The influence of high and low doses of bisphenol a (BPA) on the enteric

nervous system of the porcine ileum," *International Journal of Molecular Sciences*, vol. 19, no. 3, 2018.

[26] S. D. Masson, D. M. McKay, R. H. Stead, A. Agro, A. Stanisz, and M. H. Perdue, "Nippostrongylus brasiliensis infection evokes neuronal abnormalities and alterations in neurally regulated electrolyte transport in rat jejunum," *Parasitology*, vol. 113, no. 2, pp. 173–182, 1996.

[27] S. Gonkowski, B. Kamińska, A. Bossowska, M. Korzon, P. Landowski, and M. Majewski, "The influence of experimental Bacteroides fragilis infection on substance P and somatostatin-immunoreactive neural elements in the porcine ascending colon - a preliminary report," *Folia Morphologica*, vol. 62, no. 4, pp. 455–457, 2003.

[28] J. Godlewski and J. Kaleczyc, "Somatostatin, substance P and calcitonin gene-related peptide-positive intramural nerve structures of the human large intestine affected by carcinoma," *Folia Histochemica et Cytobiologica*, vol. 48, no. 3, pp. 475–483, 2010.

[29] M. G. Rosenfeld, J. J. Mermod, S. G. Amara et al., "Production of a novel neuropeptide encoded by the calcitonin gene via tissue-specific RNA processing," *Nature*, vol. 304, no. 5922, pp. 129–135, 1983.

[30] K. Makowska and S. Gonkowski, "The influence of inflammation and nerve damage on the neurochemical characterization of calcitonin gene-related peptide-like Immunoreactive (CGRP-LI) neurons in the enteric nervous system of the porcine descending Colon," *International Journal of Molecular Sciences*, vol. 19, no. 2, 2018.

[31] B. Kamińska, S. Gonkowski, M. Korzon, A. Bossowska, P. Landowski, and M. Majewski, "Relations between Leu^5-enkephalin- (LENK) and VIP-immunoreactive nerve fibres during human drug-resistant colitis. A case study," *Folia Morphologica*, vol. 62, no. 4, pp. 509–511, 2003.

[32] K. Nihei and T. Iwanaga, "Localization of Met-enkephalin-Arg6-Gly7-Leu8-like immunoreactivity in the gastrointestinal tract of rat and pig," *The Journal of Histochemistry and Cytochemistry*, vol. 33, no. 10, pp. 1001–1006, 2017.

[33] M. O. Larsen and B. Rolin, "Use of the Gottingen minipig as a model of diabetes, with special focus on type 1 diabetes research," *ILAR Journal*, vol. 45, no. 3, pp. 303–313, 2004.

[34] J. Fricker, "The pig: a new model of diabetic atherosclerosis," *Drug Discovery Today*, vol. 6, no. 18, pp. 921-922, 2001.

[35] R. J. Arner, K. S. Prabhu, V. Krishnan, M. C. Johnson, and C. C. Reddy, "Expression of myo-inositol oxygenase in tissues susceptible to diabetic complications," *Biochemical and Biophysical Research Communications*, vol. 339, no. 3, pp. 816–820, 2006.

[36] M. Bulc, K. Palus, Ł. Zielonka, M. Gajęcka, and J. Całka, "Changes in expression of inhibitory substances in the intramural neurons of the stomach following streptozotocin- induced diabetes in the pig," *World Journal of Gastroenterology*, vol. 23, no. 33, pp. 6088–6099, 2017.

[37] A. Belai, N. A. Calcutt, A. L. Carrington, L. T. Diemel, D. R. Tomlinson, and G. Burnstock, "Enteric neuropeptides in streptozotocin-diabetic rats; effects of insulin and aldose reductase inhibition," *Journal of the Autonomic Nervous System*, vol. 58, no. 3, pp. 163–169, 1996.

[38] P. C. Kniel, U. Junker, I. V. Perrin, G. E. Bestetti, and G. L. Rossi, "Varied effects of experimental diabetes on the autonomic nervous system of the rat," *Laboratory Investigation*, vol. 54, no. 5, pp. 523–530, 1986.

[39] C. L. He, J. H. Szurszewski, G. Farrugia, E. E. Soffer, R. M. Walsh, and C. D. Ferris, "Loss of interstitial cells of Cajal and inhibitory innervation in insulin-dependent diabetes," *Gastroenterology*, vol. 121, no. 2, pp. 427–434, 2001.

[40] R. E. Schmidt, D. A. Plurad, and K. A. Roth, "Effects of chronic experimental streptozotocin-induced diabetes on the nor-adrenergic and peptidergic innervation of the rat alimentary tract," *Brain Research*, vol. 458, no. 2, pp. 353–360, 1988.

[41] M. Ballmann and J. M. Conlon, "Changes in the somatostatin, substance P and vasoactive intestinal polypeptide content of the gastrointestinal tract following streptozotocin-induced diabetes in the rat," *Diabetologia*, vol. 28, no. 6, pp. 355–358, 1985.

[42] E. Fehér, B. Batbayar, A. Vér, and T. Zelles, "Changes of the different neuropeptide-containing nerve fibers and immunocells in the diabetic rat's alimentary tract," *Annals of the New York Academy of Sciences*, vol. 1084, no. 1, pp. 280–295, 2006.

[43] A. Belai and G. Burnstock, "Changes in adrenergic and peptidergic nerves in the submucous plexus of streptozocin-diabetic rat ileum," *Gastroenterology*, vol. 98, no. 6, pp. 1427–1436, 1990.

[44] A. Belai, J. Lincoln, and G. Burnstock, "Lack of release of vasoactive intestinal polypeptide and calcitonin gene-related peptide during electrical stimulation of enteric nerves in streptozotocin-diabetic rats," *Gastroenterology*, vol. 93, no. 5, pp. 1034–1040, 1987.

[45] M. M. Swindle and A. C. Smith, "Comparative anatomy and physiology of the pig," *Scandinavian Journal of Laboratory Animal Science*, vol. 25, pp. 11–21, 1998.

[46] M. O. Larsen, M. Wilken, C. F. Gotfredsen, R. D. Carr, O. Svendsen, and B. Rolin, "Mild streptozotocin diabetes in the Göttingen minipig. A novel model of moderate insulin deficiency and diabetes," *American Journal of Physiology. Endocrinology and Metabolism*, vol. 282, no. 6, pp. E1342–E1351, 2002.

[47] P. Bytzer, N. J. Talley, M. Leemon, L. J. Young, M. P. Jones, and M. Horowitz, "Prevalence of gastrointestinal symptoms associated with diabetes mellitus: a population-based survey of 15000 adults," *Archives of Internal Medicine*, vol. 161, no. 16, pp. 1989–1996, 2001.

[48] J. K. Juranek, G. K. Daffu, J. Wojtkiewicz, D. Lacomis, J. Kofler, and A. M. Schmidt, "Receptor for advanced glycation end products and its inflammatory ligands are upregulated in amyotrophic lateral sclerosis," *Frontiers in Cellular Neuroscience*, vol. 9, pp. 9–485, 2015.

[49] J. K. Juranek, A. Aleshin, E. M. Rattigan et al., "Morphological changes and immunohistochemical expression of RAGE and its ligands in the sciatic nerve of hyperglycemic pig (Sus Scrofa)," *Biochemistry Insights*, vol. 3, no. 3, article BCI.S5340, 2010.

[50] V. Vasina, G. Barbara, L. Talamonti et al., "Enteric neuroplasticity evoked by inflammation," *Autonomic Neuroscience*, vol. 126-127, pp. 264–272, 2006.

[51] D. ZHAO, S. Kuhnt-Moore, H. Zeng et al., "Substance P-stimulated interleukin-8 expression in human colonic epithelial cells involves Rho family small GTPases," *The Biochemical Journal*, vol. 368, no. 2, pp. 665–672, 2002.

[52] J. J. Galligan and C. Sternini, "Insights into the role of opioid receptors in the GI tract: experimental evidence and therapeu-

tic relevance," *Handbook of Experimental Pharmacology*, vol. 239, pp. 363–378, 2017.

[53] K. Palus and J. Całka, "Neurochemical plasticity of the coeliac-superior mesenteric ganglion complex neurons projecting to the prepyloric area of the porcine stomach following hyperacidity," *Neural Plasticity*, vol. 2016, Article ID 8596214, 9 pages, 2016.

[54] P. Holzer, "Opioids and opioid receptors in the enteric nervous system: from a problem in opioid analgesia to a possible new prokinetic therapy in humans," *Neuroscience Letters*, vol. 361, no. 1–3, pp. 192–195, 2004.

5

Insulin Secretion and Risk for Future Diabetes in Subjects with a Nonpositive Insulinogenic Index

Daisuke Aono,[1] Rie Oka,[1,2] Mitsuhiro Kometani,[1] Yoshimichi Takeda,[1] Shigehiro Karashima,[1] Kenichi Yoshimura,[3] Yoshiyu Takeda,[1] and Takashi Yoneda[1]

[1]*Department of Cardiovascular and Internal Medicine, Kanazawa University Graduate School of Medicine, Kanazawa, Japan*
[2]*Department of Internal Medicine, Hokuriku Central Hospital, Oyabe, Japan*
[3]*Department of Biostatistics, Innovative Clinical Research Center (iCREK), Kanazawa University Hospital, Kanazawa, Japan*

Correspondence should be addressed to Rie Oka; ririoka@goo.jp

Academic Editor: Janet H. Southerland

Aim. To characterize subjects with a nonpositive insulinogenic index and longitudinally observe changes in their glucose tolerance. *Subjects and Methods.* A historical cohort study was conducted using data from the medical checkups of public school workers. Indices of insulin secretion and insulin sensitivity derived from oral glucose tolerance test (OGTT) and the incidences of diabetes and impaired glucose tolerance (IGT) were compared among subgroups of subjects with different insulinogenic index (change in insulin/change in glucose over the first 30 min on the OGTT). *Results.* Of the 1464 nondiabetic subjects at baseline, 72 (4.9%) subjects had a nonpositive insulinogenic index: 42 of those subjects had a nonpositive glucose response ($\Delta Glu_{0-30} \leq 0$) and 30 had a nonpositive insulin response ($\Delta Ins_{0-30} \leq 0$). Compared with subjects who had normal glucose tolerance (NGT) with insulinogenic index ≥ 0.4, subjects with a nonpositive glucose response had a higher first-phase Stumvoll and lower incidences of diabetes and IGT based on a log-rank test ($p < 0.05$), whereas subjects with a nonpositive insulin response had lower indices of insulin secretion and a higher incidence of diabetes ($p < 0.05$). *Conclusions.* These results demonstrate that in the first 30 min on the OGTT, subjects with a nonpositive insulinogenic index due to a nonpositive glucose response ($\Delta Glu_{0-30} \leq 0$) had a lower risk for future diabetes and that subjects with nonpositive insulin response ($\Delta Ins_{0-30} \leq 0$) had a higher risk for future one.

1. Introduction

Insulinogenic index (change in insulin/change in glucose over the first 30 min after the load) on the oral glucose tolerance test (OGTT) has been widely used as an index of early phase insulin secretion in clinical studies [1–4]. It is highly correlated with the acute insulin response (AIR) on intravenous glucose tolerance test (IVGTT) and is considered a reasonable surrogate [5, 6]. Measuring insulinogenic index has several advantages; it involves less complex protocols, needs less costs, and utilizes a physiological route of glucose administration [7, 8]. Simpler methods for the assessment of insulin secretion are those based on basal glucose and insulin concentrations, such as HOMA-beta [9], but fasting levels cannot provide insight into the secretory response of beta cells to rising glucose concentrations [8]. Indeed, insulinogenic index or its composite with insulin sensitivity (oral disposition index) has been demonstrated to be predictive of type 2 diabetes, independent of fasting plasma glucose in different populations [4, 10–12].

Sometimes, however, a small number of subjects in general populations exhibit a nonpositive insulinogenic index due to either a decrement in insulin or in glucose value 30 min after glucose ingestion from fasted states [13]. Most studies, including ours, exclude them from the main analysis [14]. Abdul-Ghani et al. have reported a lower risk for future diabetes in individuals whose plasma glucose concentrations returned to equal to or below fasting levels within 30 min compared with those who required longer time to return their plasma glucose to fasting levels [15]. Besides the report by Abdul-Ghani et al., there has been no report on the clinical characteristics and the risk for future diabetes in subjects with a nonpositive insulinogenic index.

The aim of this study, therefore, was to characterize subjects with a nonpositive insulinogenic index and longitudinally observe changes in their glucose tolerance.

2. Methods

2.1. Study Participants. A historical cohort study was conducted using data from the medical checkups of public school employees collected at Hokuriku Central Hospital [14]. During April 2006 and March 2010 (baseline period), 2340 employees underwent an OGTT at a medical checkup [16]. If employees received more than one checkup during the baseline period, the initial checkup data were used. After those who had fasting plasma glucose ≥ 126 mg/dL and/or 2 h plasma glucose ≥ 200 mg/dL ($n = 85$), those who had HbA1c values ≥ 6.9% (52 mmol/mol) ($n = 42$), those who had undergone gastrectomy ($n = 32$), those who were taking steroids ($n = 1$) or anticancer drugs ($n = 1$), those who or had any missing data ($n = 18$) were excluded, 2161 nondiabetic individuals were selected. Of these, 1464 individuals repeated checkups at least once until March 2016 and comprised our study sample. The remaining 697 participants did not have a repeat checkup, yielding a follow-up rate of 67.7%. If the subjects developed diabetes, the follow-up ended at that time. An OGTT was performed at all checkups during the follow-up period; however, within the last two years (April 2014 to March 2016), an OGTT was performed on 1191 participants and the measurement of fasting plasma glucose only was performed in the remaining 273 participants for financial reasons. Information on smoking and drinking habits and a medical history were obtained via a questionnaire. Participants were considered current smokers if they smoked at least one cigarette per day. Alcohol use was defined by the number of days per week it was consumed, regardless of the amount. Informed consent was obtained by an opt-out method, and the institutional review board of the Kanazawa University approved the study protocol on June 21, 2017 (IRB number 2497-1); the study protocol conforms to the provisions of the Declaration of Helsinki. The study was registered on the University Hospital Medical Information Network Clinical Trials Registry (UMIN-CTR, http://www.umin.ac.jp/ctr, UMIN ID: UMIN000017662).

2.2. Blood Sampling and Assay. All evaluations were performed at the Health Check Department of the Hokuriku Central Hospital. Participants were asked to visit the hospital between 8:00 a.m. and 9:00 a.m. after an overnight fast. At the baseline visit, an OGTT (75 g dextrose monohydrate in 250 mL water) with 0, 30, 60, and 120 min sampling to determine plasma glucose and insulin concentrations was performed on all participants [16]. Plasma glucose was assessed using the glucose oxidase method (Automatic Glucose Analyzer ADAMS Glucose GA-1160, Arkray, Kyoto, Japan) at the hospital laboratory. Insulin concentration assays were performed by the chemiluminescence immunoassay method at a commercial laboratory (BML Inc., Tokyo, Japan), with an intra-assay coefficient of variation (CV) of 2.4–3.2% based on 10 replicates of 3 different samples. Height and weight were measured, and body mass index (BMI) was calculated by dividing weight (kg) by height squared (m^2).

2.3. Calculations of Indices of Insulin Secretion and Insulin Sensitivity. The indices of insulin secretion used in this study were as follows: insulinogenic index = $(Ins_{30} - Ins_0)/(Gluc_{30} - Gluc_0)$ or $\Delta Ins_{0-30}/\Delta Glu_{0-30}$, where Ins_y and Glu_y represent values at time (y: min) during the OGTT [5, 6]; the ratio of area under the curve (AUC) for insulin to AUC for glucose for the specific time frame, which was calculated by applying the trapezoid rule; first-phase Stumvoll = $1283 + 1.829 \times Ins_{30} - 138.7 \times Glu_{30} + 3.772 \times Ins_0$; and second-phase Stumvoll = $286 + 0.416 \times Ins_{30} - 25.94 \times Glu_{30} + 0.926 \times Ins_0$ [17]. The indices of insulin sensitivity were as follows: Matsuda insulin sensitivity index (ISI) = $10{,}000/(Glu_0 \times Ins_0 \times Glu_{120} \times Ins_{120})^{0.5}$ [18] and homeostatic model assessment of insulin resistance (HOMA-IR) = $Glu_0 \times Ins_0/405$ [9]. We used different units for glucose concentration and insulin concentration in calculating each index, as described in Table 1.

2.4. Statistical Analysis. The data are presented as the mean ± standard deviation or median with interquartile ranges for continuous variables or as a frequency for categorical variables. Continuous variables were compared using one-way analysis of variance (ANOVA) or Kruskal-Wallis test, and categorical values were compared using a χ^2 test, with a Bonferroni correction for multiple comparisons. The participants were classified by their insulinogenic index at 0.4 because this threshold was adopted by the Japan Diabetes Society to identify individuals at a high risk of progression to diabetes [19]. Participants were further classified by their glucose tolerance using the criteria of the American Diabetes Association (ADA) [20]; subjects were categorized as having NGT (fasting plasma glucose < 100 mg/dL and 2 h plasma glucose < 140 mg/dL), impaired fasting glucose (IFG) (fasting plasma glucose = 100–125 mg/dL), and impaired glucose tolerance (IGT) (2-hour plasma glucose = 140–199 mg/dL). Among groups, indices of insulin sensitivity and insulin secretion were compared using analysis of covariance (ANCOVA) with age, gender, and BMI as covariates. Insulinogenic index and HOMA-IR were log-transformed using the natural log prior to analysis to reduce skewness; the transformed values produced a good fit to normal distribution. Finally, the progression to diabetes defined as fasting plasma glucose ≥ 126 mg/dL, 2-hour plasma glucose ≥ 200 mg/dL, and/or taking treatments for diabetes or to IGT among subjects grouped by insulinogenic index was compared by the Kaplan-Meier method. The analysis of the progression to IGT was performed in 982 out of the 1169 NGT subjects at baseline, because the remaining 187 NGT subjects did not receive an OGTT at follow-up. A p value of < 0.05 was considered statistically significant. All analyses were conducted using SPSS software version 24.0 for Windows (SPSS Inc., Chicago, USA).

Table 1: Indices of insulin secretion and insulin sensitivity among groups by insulinogenic index.

	Positive insulinogenic index				Nonpositive insulinogenic index	
	NGT		IFG and/or IGT			
	Insulinogenic index ≥ 0.4 ($n = 515$)	Insulinogenic index < 0.4 ($n = 221$)	Insulinogenic index ≥ 0.4 ($n = 42$)	Insulinogenic index < 0.4 ($n = 340$)	$\Delta Glu_{0-30} \leq 0$ ($n = 42$)	$\Delta Ins_{0-30} \leq 0$ ($n = 30$)
Insulin secretion						
Insulinogenic index (mU/L/mg/dL)	0.92 (0.87–0.97)†	0.24 (0.22–0.26)*†	0.79 (0.73–0.84)*	0.20 (0.18–0.21)*†	Not calculable	Not calculable
AUC (Ins_{30})/AUC (Glu_{30}) (pmol/mmol)	27.6 (26.6–28.7)	12.7 (11.2–14.2)*†	26.7 (25.4–28.0)	10.9 (9.6–12.1)*†	24.3 (20.8–27.8)	3.8 (−0.4–7.9)*†
AUC (Ins_{120}) (nmol*min)	28.4 (27.3–29.7)†	17.0 (15.2–18.8)*†	34.5 (33.0–36.1)*	19.4 (17.9–20.9)*†	20.0 (15.9–24.1)*†	10.4 (5.6–15.3)*†
AUC (Ins_{120})/AUC (Glu_{120}) ($\times 10^{-2}$ mU/mg)	2.79 (2.69–2.90)	1.41 (1.25–1.57)*†	2.86 (2.72–2.99)	1.37 (1.25–1.50)*†	2.51 (2.16–2.87)	0.85 (0.43–1.27)*†
First-phase Stumvoll (pmol/L, mmol/L)	945 (918–972)†	464 (423–506)*†	853 (818–888)*	276 (243–309)*†	1156 (1062–1251)*†	232 (121–343)*†
Second-phase Stumvoll (pmol/L, mmol/L)	254 (248–260)	150 (141–159)*†	240 (232–248)	115 (107–122)*†	285 (264–306)†	99 (74–124)*†
Insulin sensitivity						
Matsuda insulin sensitivity index (mU/L, mg/dL)	14.0 (13.0–15.1)†	18.4 (16.8–20.0)*†	10.1 (8.7–11.4)*	10.7 (9.4–12.0)*	17.2 (13.6–20.9)†	14.5 (10.1–18.8)
HOMA-IR (mU/L, mmol/L)	0.89 (0.85–0.93)†	0.70 (0.65–0.76)*†	1.13 (1.06–1.20)*	0.92 (0.87–0.98)†	0.87 (0.73–1.03)	0.88 (0.73–1.08)

Data are means (95% confidence intervals) adjusted for body mass index, age, and gender. Insulinogenic index and HOMA-IR were log-transformed before analysis, and calculated values were untransformed after analysis. *$p < 0.05$ compared to NGT with insulinogenic index ≥ 0.4 and †$p < 0.05$ compared to IFG and/or IGT with insulinogenic index ≥ 0.4 with Bonferroni correction for multiple comparisons. AUC(Glu_{time}): area under the curve for glucose by time (min) elapsed; AUC(Ins_{time}): area under the curve for insulin by time (min) elapsed; ΔGlu_{0-30} and ΔIns_{0-30}: change in glucose and in insulin, respectively, over the first 30 min on the oral glucose tolerance test; HOMA-IR: homeostasis model of insulin resistance.

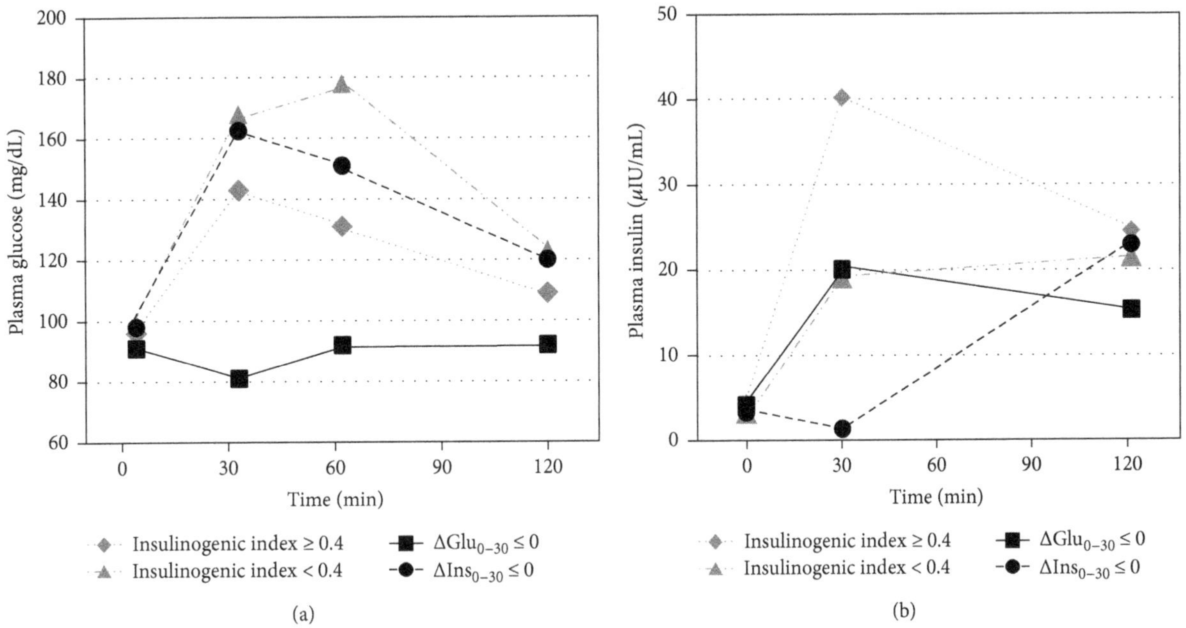

FIGURE 1: Plasma glucose and insulin concentrations on the OGTT among subgroups of subjects with a different insulinogenic index as presented as median values.

3. Results

Study subjects were 1464 nondiabetic individuals with a mean age of 52.0 years and a mean BMI of 23.9 kg/m^2 at baseline. There were 42 (2.9%) subjects whose plasma glucose concentrations fell equal to or below their fasting levels at 30 min ($\Delta Glu_{0-30} \leq 0$) and 30 (2.0%) subjects whose insulin concentrations fell equal to or below the fasting levels at 30 min after the oral glucose load ($\Delta Ins_{0-30} \leq 0$). Three subjects with double nonpositive values, resulting in a positive insulinogenic index, were excluded from the following analysis. As shown in Figure 1, subjects with $\Delta Ins_{0-30} \leq 0$ increased their insulin concentrations at 120 min from 30 min, while those with $\Delta Glu_{0-30} \leq 0$ got to return their insulin concentrations at 120 min. As shown in Table 2, subjects with $\Delta Glu_{0-30} \leq 0$ included a lower proportion of men and had a lower BMI and lower glucose and insulin concentrations during OGTT, compared with subjects with insulinogenic index ≥ 0.4 ($p < 0.05$). Subjects with $\Delta Ins_{0-30} \leq 0$ had a higher BMI and higher glucose and fasting insulin concentrations compared with subjects with $\Delta Glu_{0-30} \leq 0$ ($p < 0.05$). Subjects with $\Delta Glu_{0-30} \leq 0$ had a significantly higher proportion of NGT (92.9%) compared with the other three groups listed in Table 2 ($p < 0.05$).

To evaluate insulin secretion and insulin sensitivity on the basis of the OGTT, we classified subjects with nonpositive insulinogenic index into 2 groups (i.e., $\Delta Glu_{0-30} \leq 0$ and $\Delta Ins_{0-30} \leq 0$) and those with positive insulinogenic index into 2 groups as well [with subgroups] (i.e., NGT [insulinogenic index ≥ 0.4 or <0.4] and IFG and/or IGT [insulinogenic index ≥ 0.4 or <0.4]) (Table 1). In subjects with $\Delta Glu_{0-30} \leq 0$, indices of insulin secretion such as $AUC(Ins_{30})/AUC(Glu_{30})$ and $AUC(Ins_{120})/AUC(Glu_{120})$ were not significantly decreased and first-phase Stumvoll was increased compared with NGT with insulinogenic index ≥ 0.4. In subjects with $\Delta Ins_{0-30} \leq 0$, all indices of insulin secretion examined were significantly decreased compared with IFG and/or IGT as well as NGT with insulinogenic index ≥ 0.4. Matsuda ISI and HOMA-IR were not significantly different in subgroups with nonpositive insulinogenic index compared with NGT with insulinogenic index ≥ 0.4. These indices were estimated after adjustments for gender, age, and BMI; however, the results were essentially the same before the adjustments (data not shown).

The progression to diabetes (Figure 2) or to IGT (Figure 3) was assessed among different subgroups by insulinogenic index. In subjects with $\Delta Glu_{0-30} \leq 0$, there was no progression to diabetes nor to IGT during a mean follow-up period of 5.6 years, which was significantly less than NGT with insulinogenic index ≥ 0.4 by log-rank test ($p < 0.05$). In subjects with $\Delta Ins_{0-30} \leq 0$, the incidence of diabetes was significantly higher compared with NGT with insulinogenic index ≥ 0.4 ($P < 0.05$) while that of IGT was not statistically different by log-rank test. In comparison between subjects with $\Delta Glu_{0-30} \leq 0$ and those with $\Delta Ins_{0-30} \leq 0$, the incidences of diabetes and of IGT were significantly different ($p = 0.016$ and $p < 0.001$, resp.).

4. Discussion

In this study, subjects with a nonpositive insulinogenic index were characterized based on insulin secretion and insulin sensitivity and diabetes and IGT incidences were compared with subjects who had a positive insulinogenic index. Although the prevalence of nonpositive insulinogenic index was low in agreement with prior studies investigating Western cohorts [13], this is the first study in Asian populations that longitudinally observed the future incidence of glucose intolerance in subjects with a nonpositive insulinogenic index. The findings of the current study could be useful for

Table 2: Baseline characteristics by level of the insulinogenic index.

	Positive insulinogenic index		Nonpositive insulinogenic index	
	Insulinogenic index ≥ 0.4 (n = 828)	Insulinogenic index < 0.4 (n = 561)	$\Delta Glu_{0-30} \leq 0$ (n = 42)	$\Delta Ins_{0-30} \leq 0$ (n = 30)
Age (years)	51.6 ± 7.0	52.9 ± 6.7*	50.6 ± 7.1	50.2 ± 8.5
Male gender (%)	65.3	79.5*	42.9*†	63.3
Body mass index (kg/m^2)	24.3 ± 3.3	23.6 ± 2.9*	22.4 ± 2.7*	24.8 ± 4.3‡
Fasting plasma glucose (mg/dL)	92/96/101	94/99/106*	88/91/95*†	92/98/108‡
30 min plasma glucose (mg/dL)	126/143/162	150/168/186*	76/81/88*†	132/163/182‡
1-hour plasma glucose (mg/dL)	106/131/159	146/178/205*	72/92/101*†	112/151/192*‡
2-hour plasma glucose (mg/dL)	96/109/126	105/123/146*	81/92/111*†	90/120/142‡
Fasting insulin (μIU/mL)	3.1/4.3/6.2	2.6/3.3/4.3*	2.8/4.2/4.7	2.4/3.3/6.2
30 min insulin (μIU/mL)	29.2/40.2/58.3	13.7/19.1/24.1*	13.7/20.1/32.9*	0.8/1.4/2.1*†‡
120 min insulin (μIU/mL)	16.3/24.6/39.7	14.5/21.5/34.9*	9.1/15.3/21.9*	10.6/23.0/39.1
HbA1c (%)	5.2 ± 0.3	5.3 ± 0.4*	5.1 ± 0.3†	5.3 ± 0.4
Glucose tolerance				
Normal glucose tolerance (%)	62.2	39.4*	92.9*†	46.7‡
Impaired fasting glucose (%)	32.1	49.8	7.2*†	43.3
Impaired glucose tolerance (%)	13.2	30.9*	2.4	30.0
Current smokers (%)	17.5	25.0*	19.0	20.0
Drinkers (%)	59.9	71.3*	42.9†	63.3
Antihypertensive medications (%)	13.6	14.6	7.1	10.0
Lipid-lowering medications (%)	6.9	7.3	2.4	6.7

Data are expressed as mean ± standard deviation, 25/50/75th percentile values, or %. Characteristics among groups were compared using one-way ANOVA for continuous variables and chi-square tests for categorical variables with Bonferroni correction for multiple comparisons. *$p < 0.05$ compared to insulinogenic index ≥ 0.4, †$p < 0.05$ compared to insulinogenic index < 0.4, ‡$p < 0.05$ compared to $\Delta Glu_{0-30} \leq 0$. ΔGlu_{0-30} and ΔIns_{0-30}, change in glucose and in insulin, respectively, over the first 30 min on the oral glucose tolerance test.

estimating the risk for diabetes when clinicians encounter subjects with a nonpositive insulinogenic index.

The prevalence of a nonpositive insulinogenic index was 4.9% (72/1464) in nondiabetic subjects in this study. The prevalence in other cohorts has been reported as 8.2% in the San Antonio Heart Study, 3.4% in the Genetics of NIDDM Study, and 2.5% in the Japanese American Community Diabetes Study [13]. There were two reasons for a nonpositive insulinogenic index: a nonpositive glucose response ($\Delta Glu_{0-30} \leq 0$) and a nonpositive insulin response ($\Delta Ins_{0-30} \leq 0$) after a glucose load. The former included a higher proportion of NGT than the latter in this study (92.9% versus 46.7%), which is in agreement with the results from the San Antonio Heart Study (81.4% versus 11.8%). We confirmed and extended the observation that a nonpositive insulinogenic index occurs at a given frequency in Japanese populations.

Subjects with a nonpositive glucose response 30 min after a glucose load had similar or even higher insulin secretion compared with NGT with insulinogenic index ≥ 0.4 and a lower risk for future deterioration of glucose tolerance. Abdul-Ghani et al. have reported that individuals whose plasma glucose concentrations return to equal to or below the fasting levels by 30 min after a glucose load showed the highest insulin sensitivity, the highest insulin secretion, and the lowest risk for future diabetes, compared with those who required >30 min for their plasma glucose to return to fasting levels in Mexican Americans [15] and Caucasians [21]. Of note, the insulinogenic index could not be calculated due to nonpositive glucose response in their study, so they assessed insulin secretion by AUC (Ins_{30})/AUC(Glu_{30}), which was also applied in this study. The subjects with a nonpositive glucose response are likely to be highly efficient in disposing glucose and in maintaining normal glucose homeostasis following a glucose load.

Subjects with a nonpositive insulin response 30 min after the glucose load had the lowest insulin secretion among different groups of the insulinogenic index. This group comprised of more IFG and/or IGT and showed a higher BMI compared with the abovementioned subjects with a nonpositive glucose response. In the study examining the acute (first-phase) insulin response to intravenous glucose, a paradoxically nonpositive insulin response had also been observed in subjects with fasting hyperglycemia [22]. A nonpositive insulin response at 30 min on the OGTT may reflect an impairment of early insulin response, which is one of the primary pathophysiologic changes of type 2 diabetes.

Of note, insulin levels at 120 min in subjects with a nonpositive insulin response were similar to other groups,

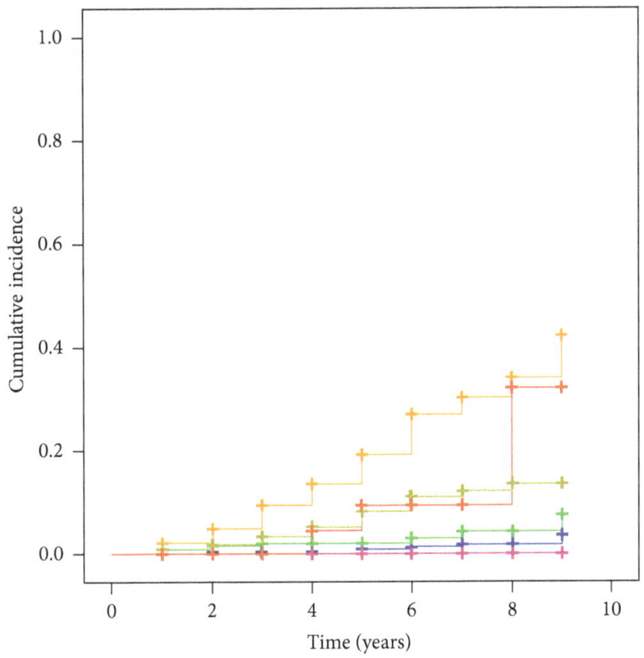

	Positive insulinogenic index				Nonpositive insulinogenic index	
	NGT		IFG and/or IGT			
	Insulinogenic index ≥ 0.4 ($n = 515$)	Insulinogenic index < 0.4 ($n = 221$)	Insulinogenic index ≥ 0.4 ($n = 313$)	Insulinogenic index < 0.4 ($n = 340$)	$\Delta Glu_{0-30} \leq 0$ ($n = 42$)	$\Delta Ins_{0-30} \leq 0$ ($n = 30$)
Incidence (%)	6 (1.2)	7 (3.2)	25 (8.0)*	69 (20.3)*	0*	4 (13.3)*#
Mean follow-up time (years)	5.4	5.2	4.9	4.6	5.6	4.7
Incidence rate (per 100 person-years)	0.2	0.6	1.6	4.4*	0.0*	2.8*#

*Significantly different from NGT with insulinogenic index ≥ 0.4 by log-rank test ($p < 0.001$). #Significantly different between $\Delta Glu_{0-30} \leq 0$ and $\Delta Ins_{0-30} \leq 0$ ($P = 0.016$).

FIGURE 2: Cumulative incidence of diabetes by the Kaplan-Meier method among groups by insulinogenic index.

indicating that insulin secretion was delayed but preserved (Figure 1). Recently, Lorenzo et al. have reported that indices of insulin secretion derived from the late OGTT period as well as the early period (e.g., insulinogenic index) independently predict the incidence of diabetes from the San Antonio Study [23]. Although the late insulin secretion may keep the subjects with a nonpositive insulin response from the development of diabetes, they are likely to have a higher risk of diabetes compared with the IFG and/or IGT with insulinogenic index ≥ 0.4.

We evaluated several OGTT-based indices of insulin secretion. When glucose is administered intravenously, the insulin response to a hyperglycemic stimulation is biphasic [24]; plasma insulin concentrations increase rapidly to a peak at 2 to 4 min, decrease within 10 to 15 min (first-phase insulin release), and gradually increase over 120 min (second-phase insulin release) [25]. First-phase Stumvoll has been validated against this first-phase insulin release on hyperglycemic clamp test [26]. Although measurements of plasma insulin are ordinarily performed at 30 min on the OGTT, this time point may be too late to capture the early insulin response in some subjects with a prompt secretory response to glucose stimulation. In these subjects, the first burst of insulin secreted into the portal vein would suppress hepatic glucose production and decrease their plasma glucose equal to or below the fasting levels by 30 min after the glucose load.

The strength of our study is the longitudinal design, which allows for a comparison of future risk for diabetes among groups by insulinogenic index. However, several limitations of this study should be considered. First, the

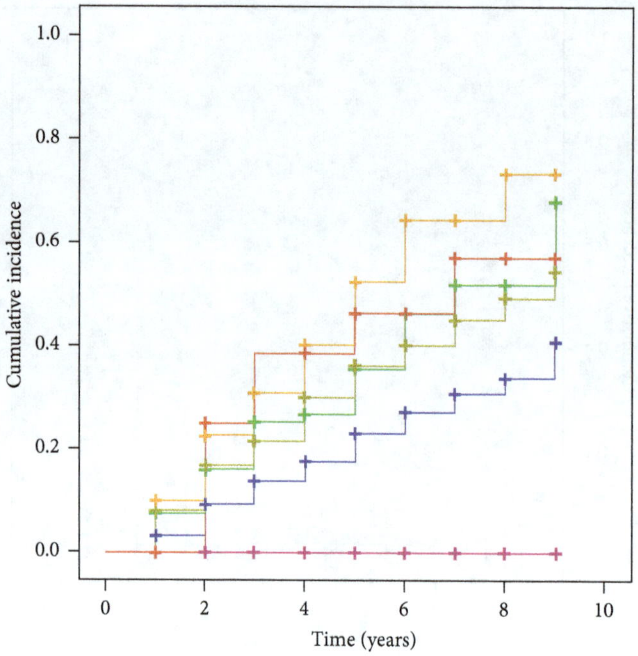

	Positive insulinogenic index				Nonpositive insulinogenic index	
	NFG		IFG			
	Insulinogenic index ≥ 0.4 ($n = 441$)	Insulinogenic index < 0.4 ($n = 194$)	Insulinogenic index ≥ 0.4 ($n = 160$)	Insulinogenic index < 0.4 ($n = 131$)	$\Delta Glu_{0-30} \leq 0$ ($n = 38$)	$\Delta Ins_{0-30} \leq 0$ ($n = 18$)
Incidence (%)	107 (24.3)	75 (38.7)*	56 (35.0)*	65 (49.6)*	0 (0.0)*	8 (44.4)#
Mean follow-up time (years)	4.9	4.2	4.2	3.8	5.6	4.2
Incidence rate (per 100 person-years)	5.0	9.2*	8.3*	13.1*	0.0*	10.6#

*Significantly different from NGT with insulinogenic index ≥ 0.4 by log-rank test ($p < 0.001$). #Significantly different between $\Delta Glu_{0-30} \leq 0$ and $\Delta Ins_{0-30} \leq 0$ ($p < 0.001$).

FIGURE 3: Cumulative incidence of impaired glucose tolerance or type 2 diabetes (2-hour PG ≥ 140 mg/dL) by the Kaplan-Meier method among groups by insulinogenic index.

follow-up rate of the subjects was 67.7%. Subjects who missed checkups during the follow-up period might be less conscious about their health, which biased the study subjects toward metabolically healthy people. However, baseline characteristics including BMI, glucose, and insulin concentrations between the subjects who were and were not followed were not significantly different. Second, measurements of C-peptide were not performed. C-peptide has been utilized to assess the insulin secretory function of beta cells because it is not degraded by the liver and thus represents prehepatic insulin secretion [27]. However, in estimation of the prehepatic insulin secretion, the calculation from insulin and that from C-peptide has been shown to be highly correlated ($R^2 = 0.75$, $p < 0.001$) [28]. Third, the measurement of plasma glucose concentrations relied on a single OGTT, which is known to have within-subject variability [29].

In conclusion, a nonpositive insulinogenic index occurs at a given frequency in Japanese populations, due to a nonpositive glucose response or due to a nonpositive insulin response 30 min after the load. The former is efficient in disposing glucose and has a lower risk for future diabetes, while the latter showed a lower early insulin response and has a higher risk for future diabetes.

Conflicts of Interest

The authors declare that there are no conflicts of interest associated with this manuscript.

Acknowledgments

The authors thank the study participants and the staff at the Health Check Department of Hokuriku Central Hospital and

Dr. Masaru Sakurai at Kanazawa Medical University for advice on the study design. This study was supported in part by Grants-in-Aid for Scientific Research from the Ministry of Education, Science, Sports, and Culture of Japan (17K09199).

References

[1] M. Hanefeld, C. Koehler, K. Fuecker et al., "Insulin secretion and insulin sensitivity pattern is different in isolated impaired glucose tolerance and impaired fasting glucose: the risk factor in impaired glucose tolerance for atherosclerosis and diabetes study," *Diabetes Care*, vol. 26, no. 3, pp. 868–874, 2003.

[2] Y. Nishi, M. Fukushima, H. Suzuki et al., "Insulin secretion and insulin sensitivity in Japanese subjects with impaired fasting glucose and isolated fasting hyperglycemia," *Diabetes Research and Clinical Practice*, vol. 70, no. 1, pp. 46–52, 2005.

[3] D. Tripathy, M. Carlsson, P. Almgren et al., "Insulin secretion and insulin sensitivity in relation to glucose tolerance: lessons from the Botnia study," *Diabetes*, vol. 49, no. 6, pp. 975–980, 2000.

[4] K. Kosaka, T. Kuzuya, H. Yoshinaga, and R. Hagura, "A prospective study of health check examinees for the development of non-insulin-dependent diabetes mellitus: relationship of the incidence of diabetes with the initial insulinogenic index and degree of obesity," *Diabetic Medicine*, vol. 13, no. 9, Supplement 6, pp. S120–S126, 1996.

[5] R. E. Pratley and C. Weyer, "The role of impaired early insulin secretion in the pathogenesis of type II diabetes mellitus," *Diabetologia*, vol. 44, no. 8, pp. 929–945, 2001.

[6] K. Kosaka, T. Kuzuya, R. Hagura, and H. Yoshinaga, "Insulin response to oral glucose load is consistently decreased in established non-insulin-dependent diabetes mellitus: the usefulness of decreased early insulin response as a predictor of insulin-dependent diabetes mellitus," *Diabetic Medicine*, vol. 13, no. 9, Supplement 6, pp. S109–S119, 1996.

[7] G. Pacini and A. Mari, "Methods for clinical assessment of insulin sensitivity and β-cell function," *Best Practice & Research Clinical Endocrinology & Metabolism*, vol. 17, no. 3, pp. 305–322, 2003.

[8] E. Cersosimo, C. Solis-Herrera, M. E. Trautmann, J. Malloy, and C. Triplitt, "Assessment of pancreatic β-cell function: review of methods and clinical applications," *Current Diabetes Reviews*, vol. 10, no. 1, pp. 2–42, 2014.

[9] D. R. Matthews, J. P. Hosker, A. S. Rudenski, B. A. Naylor, D. F. Treacher, and R. C. Turner, "Homeostasis model assessment: insulin resistance and β-cell function from fasting plasma glucose and insulin concentrations in man," *Diabetologia*, vol. 28, no. 7, pp. 412–419, 1985.

[10] L. J. C. J. den Biggelaar, S. J. S. Sep, S. J. P. M. Eussen et al., "Discriminatory ability of simple OGTT-based beta cell function indices for prediction of prediabetes and type 2 diabetes: the CODAM study," *Diabetologia*, vol. 60, no. 3, pp. 432–441, 2017.

[11] K. M. Utzschneider, R. L. Prigeon, M. V. Faulenbach et al., "Oral disposition index predicts the development of future diabetes above and beyond fasting and 2-h glucose levels," *Diabetes Care*, vol. 32, no. 2, pp. 335–341, 2009.

[12] M. A. Abdul-Ghani, K. Williams, R. A. DeFronzo, and M. Stern, "What is the best predictor of future type 2 diabetes?," *Diabetes Care*, vol. 30, no. 6, pp. 1544–1548, 2007.

[13] M. V. Faulenbach, L. A. Wright, C. Lorenzo et al., "Impact of differences in glucose tolerance on the prevalence of a negative insulinogenic index," *Journal of Diabetes and Its Complications*, vol. 27, no. 2, pp. 158–161, 2013.

[14] R. Oka, T. Aizawa, S. Miyamoto, T. Yoneda, and M. Yamagishi, "One-hour plasma glucose as a predictor of the development of type 2 diabetes in Japanese adults," *Diabetic Medicine*, vol. 33, no. 10, pp. 1399–1405, 2016.

[15] M. A. Abdul-Ghani, C. P. Jenkinson, D. K. Richardson, D. Tripathy, and R. A. DeFronzo, "Insulin secretion and action in subjects with impaired fasting glucose and impaired glucose tolerance: results from the Veterans Administration Genetic Epidemiology Study," *Diabetes*, vol. 55, no. 5, pp. 1430–1435, 2006.

[16] R. Oka, K. Yagi, M. Sakurai et al., "Insulin secretion and insulin sensitivity on the oral glucose tolerance test (OGTT) in middle-aged Japanese," *Endocrine Journal*, vol. 59, no. 1, pp. 55–64, 2012.

[17] M. Stumvoll, T. van Haeften, A. Fritsche, and J. Gerich, "Oral glucose tolerance test indexes for insulin sensitivity and secretion based on various availabilities of sampling times," *Diabetes Care*, vol. 24, no. 4, pp. 796-797, 2001.

[18] R. A. DeFronzo and M. Matsuda, "Reduced time points to calculate the composite index," *Diabetes Care*, vol. 33, no. 7, article e93, 2010.

[19] The Committee of the Japan Diabetes Society on the Diagnostic Criteria of Diabetes Mellitus, Y. Seino, K. Nanjo et al., "Report of the committee on the classification and diagnostic criteria of diabetes mellitus," *Journal of Diabetes Investigation*, vol. 1, no. 5, pp. 212–228, 2010.

[20] S. Genuth, K. G. Alberti, P. Bennett et al., "Follow-up report on the diagnosis of diabetes mellitus," *Diabetes Care*, vol. 26, no. 11, pp. 3160–3167, 2003.

[21] M. A. Abdul-Ghani, V. Lyssenko, T. Tuomi, R. A. DeFronzo, and L. Groop, "The shape of plasma glucose concentration curve during OGTT predicts future risk of type 2 diabetes," *Diabetes/Metabolism Research and Reviews*, vol. 26, no. 4, pp. 280–286, 2010.

[22] S. A. Metz, J. B. Halter, D. Porte Jr., and R. P. Robertson, "Suppression of plasma catecholamines and flushing by clonidine in man," *The Journal of Clinical Endocrinology & Metabolism*, vol. 46, no. 1, pp. 83–90, 1978.

[23] C. Lorenzo, K. Williams, and S. M. Haffner, "Insulin secretion based on the late oral glucose tolerance test period and incident diabetes: the San Antonio Heart Study," *Diabetic Medicine*, vol. 29, no. 8, pp. e151–e158, 2012.

[24] D. L. Curry, L. L. Bennett, and G. M. Grodsky, "Dynamics of insulin secretion by the perfused rat pancreas," *Endocrinology*, vol. 83, no. 3, pp. 572–584, 1968.

[25] J. E. Gerich, "Is reduced first-phase insulin release the earliest detectable abnormality in individuals destined to develop type 2 diabetes?," *Diabetes*, vol. 51, Supplement 1, pp. S117–S121, 2002.

[26] M. Stumvoll, A. Mitrakou, W. Pimenta et al., "Use of the oral glucose tolerance test to assess insulin release and insulin sensitivity," *Diabetes Care*, vol. 23, no. 3, pp. 295–301, 2000.

[27] S. H. Kim and G. M. Reaven, "Insulin clearance: an underappreciated modulator of plasma insulin concentration," *Journal of Investigative Medicine*, vol. 64, no. 7, pp. 1162–1165, 2016.

6

Insulin Adherence in Type 2 Diabetes in Mexico: Behaviors and Barriers

Janneth Bermeo-Cabrera,[1] Paloma Almeda-Valdes,[1,2] Josefa Riofrios-Palacios,[1] Carlos A. Aguilar-Salinas,[1,2] and Roopa Mehta[1,2]

[1]*Departamento de Endocrinología y Metabolismo, Instituto Nacional de Ciencias Médicas y Nutrición Salvador Zubirán, Mexico City, Mexico*

[2]*Unidad de Investigación de Enfermedades Metabólicas, Instituto Nacional de Ciencias Médicas y Nutrición Salvador Zubirán, Mexico City, Mexico*

Correspondence should be addressed to Roopa Mehta; roopamehta@yahoo.com

Academic Editor: Andrea Flex

Objective. To investigate factors associated with insulin adherence in subjects with type 2 diabetes mellitus (T2D) attending a tertiary care centre in Mexico City. *Material and Methods.* Cross-sectional study, including 200 patients. Adherence to insulin therapy was measured with a medication adherence questionnaire. Sociodemographic data and factors related to insulin omission were collected and compared between the nonadherent and adherent groups. *Results.* We categorized 117 (58.5%) patients as nonadherent and 83 (41.5%) as adherent. Among the adherent, only 22 patients (11%) had excellent adherence to insulin therapy. The following factors were associated with nonadherence: lack of planning of daily activities (46.1%), fear of hypoglycemia (41%), economic factors (15.4%), and number of insulin applications (2.31 versus 1.76 applications per day). *Conclusions.* In this study, patients with type 2 diabetes attending a tertiary care referral centre showed inadequate adherence to insulin therapy. The principal factors associated with insulin omission were low socioeconomic status, fear of hypoglycemia, and a greater number of insulin applications per day.

1. Introduction

In their treatment guidelines, both the American Diabetes Association and the American Association of Clinical Endocrinologists confirm that insulin (either for initiation in patients with severe hyperglycemia or for treatment intensification) is the most efficient glucose-lowering agent [1, 2]. Despite this, insulin use remains relatively low. In the United States, the National Health and Nutrition Examination Survey (2005–2012) reported that the proportion of patients with diabetes on any insulin (includes insulin only and insulin plus oral diabetes medications) was 29.1% (95% CI 26.7–31.5) [3]. Rebolledo and Arellano comment that the usage rate of oral diabetes medications among adults with type 2 diabetes has remained almost three times higher than that of insulin (50.3 versus 17.8%) [4]. In Mexico, the most recent National Health Survey showed that even though insulin use has increased, it is still inadequate; between 2012 and 2016, the prevalence of insulin plus oral medication increased from 6.6% to 8.8%, while that of insulin only regimens increased from 6.5% to 11.1% [5]. Among the barriers associated with insulin use (including patients' perceptions regarding insulin safety, cultural beliefs, social factors, health literacy, medication costs, and physician-related attitudes), patient noncompliance is commonly encountered [6]. Insulin nonadherence may be considered in terms of primary nonadherence (failure to fill pharmacy prescriptions) or poor persistence due to insulin dose omissions, either deliberate or accidental [7]. Peyrot et al. have explored factors related to insulin omission/nonadherence. In the Global Attitudes of Patients and Physicians in Insulin Therapy for Diabetes Mellitus (GAPP) Survey, 8.6% of subjects omitted insulin doses because of pain associated with the injection [8]. Almost half of the participants (43.3%) omitted injections because they felt that insulin interfered or was intrusive in their daily activities. The perception of insulin injections as painful or embarrassing was also associated with dose omission, as were a large number of daily injections. Unsurprisingly, in those reporting insulin omission, glycemic control was inadequate with elevated glycated hemoglobin (A1c) levels.

The diabetes attitudes, wishes, and needs (DAWN) study also evaluated patient attitudes towards insulin therapy [7]. Patients rated the efficacy of insulin as low, and about a quarter believed that insulin would not help them. Many blamed themselves for having to initiate insulin therapy and reported high degrees of diabetes distress.

In the Hispanic-Latino population, patients with diabetes often show reluctance to start insulin therapy, frequently due to myths and misconceptions about its use [9]. In a systematic review, Rodríguez-Gutiérrez et al. reported that the main concerns regarding insulin use included the following: that it is associated with blindness, indicated more advanced disease, a punishment, difficult to administer, expensive, and more time-consuming to manage [10]. Herrero and Caballero found that those patients with such beliefs had a poorer perception of their health, were more likely to have insulin omission, had greater emotional distress, and generally showed lower treatment adherence [11].

In Mexico, Lerman et al. reported that insulin therapy was delayed; the mean duration of type 2 diabetes (T2D) at insulin initiation was 14 years [9]. In addition, 41% of patients were nonadherent to insulin therapy. This was more common in women and was associated with depression and a negative attitude about insulin. Patients felt that insulin therapy was required because their disease had worsened due to their failure in treatment adherence. Patients also mentioned a fear of injections and felt that insulin would restrict their lifestyle. Others believed that insulin was associated with the development of diabetic complications. These attitudes were most common in lower income subjects and those with less diabetes-related knowledge. To our knowledge, there are no studies evaluating adherence to insulin therapy in Mexico.

The aim of this study is to evaluate the adherence to insulin therapy in patients with T2D treated at a large tertiary care centre and to identify the factors associated with omission or nonadherence to the insulin regimen.

2. Methods

We performed a cross-sectional study in patients with T2D attending the diabetes clinic of a tertiary care centre in Mexico City. In the diabetes clinic, there are approximately 2800 patients with type 2 diabetes, 878 of which have been prescribed insulin treatment. Between March and December 2017, 200 patients were recruited utilizing convenience sampling. All participants were adult subjects under treatment with at least one insulin dose per day over the last 3 months (i.e., a stable dose of insulin). Patients were recruited the day of their appointment and underwent a personal interview. Sample size was estimated considering an alpha error of 0.05 and a precision of 0.05 to detect a 15% prevalence of nonadherence. This study was approved by the Comité de Ética del Instituto Nacional de Ciencias Médicas y Nutrición Salvador Zubirán (study reference number 1967). Informed consent was obtained from all participants. Patients were excluded if they had type 1 diabetes mellitus, a secondary cause of diabetes, or had been admitted to hospital for an acute illness a month prior to commencing the study. In all patients, a brief medical history and current laboratory results were obtained. The questionnaires for evaluating adherence and related factors were self-administered with supervision from one of the study investigators. Participants completed the questionnaires in a quiet room and were given sufficient time to do so.

The main outcome was adherence or nonadherence to insulin therapy, evaluated using the 8 item Morisky-Green Questionnaire [12, 13]. A score of 8 indicated excellent adherence; 6 to <8, moderately good adherence; and <6 was indicative of poor adherence.

Factors associated with omission were sought using a questionnaire formulated using evidence from previous publications [7, 9] and a pilot study carried out at our centre. A double-interview method was used. Consecutive patients were recruited to complete the 23-item questionnaire ($n = 10$). Participants were asked to explain what each item meant and why they chose a particular response. The questionnaire was adapted taking into account the discrepancies, namely, what was intended and what was understood. In a second step, the revised questionnaire was tested in a further 10 patients whose results suggested good acceptability of this instrument.

The following three aspects associated with insulin adherence were evaluated: interference with daily activities, experience with insulin injections, and economic factors. The instrument contained 23 questions with answers captured on a 5-point Likert scale. The responses were analyzed in a dichotomized fashion (using chi-squared test). The extremes of the scale, that is, the percentage of patients answering totally agree + agree, were considered as one group, while, completely unsatisfied + unsatisfied all of the time + a lot of the time constituted the comparison group.

In the statistical analysis, patients who had excellent adherence or moderately good adherence to insulin therapy (≥6 in the Morisky-Green Questionnaire) were compared to those who had poor adherence (<6 in the Morisky-Green Questionnaire). The distribution of continuous variables was assessed by the Kolmogorov-Smirnov test. Continuous variables were compared between adherence groups using the Student t-test (parametric) or the Mann–Whitney U test (nonparametric). The chi-squared test was used to analyze categorical variables. A multivariate regression model was generated with adherence as the dependent variable (Morisky score) and the factors identified in bivariate analysis as independent variables. A p value of <0.05 was considered as statistically significant. All analyses were performed using SPSS version 21.

3. Results

Of the T2D patients under insulin treatment, 200 consecutive subjects fulfilled the selection criteria and were included in this study. The majority of participants were women (65%), the mean age was 61.5 ± 12.0 years, the mean duration of diabetes was 19.6 ± 8.7 years, and the median time since insulin initiation was 6 (3.25–10) years. Excellent adherence (Morisky score of 8) was found in only 11% ($n = 22$), moderate adherence in 30.5% ($n = 61$), and low adherence in 58.5% ($n = 117$).

Table 1 shows the characteristics of the population according to 2 adherence categories (adherent versus nonadherent). The "adherent" group was formed by combining those subjects with excellent adherence with those showing moderate adherence ($n = 83$ subjects); this was compared with the "nonadherent" group (Morisky score ≤ 5) ($n = 117$). There was no gender difference between these groups ($p = 0.359$). The age of participants in the adherent group was significantly greater than the age those in the adherent group (64 versus 59 years, respectively, $p = 0.037$). The age at diagnosis of diabetes was similar between groups (41.8 versus 42.1 years, $p = 0.502$). Regarding the duration of diabetes, this was significantly longer in the adherent group (20 versus 17.5 years, $p = 0.022$). With respect to the median time since insulin initiation, no differences were found between the groups (5 versus 6 years, $p = 0.685$). There was no difference in the education level between groups ($p = 0.536$), approximately 30% of participants had less than middle school education.

The characteristics of both groups with respect to insulin treatment are shown in Table 2. A simple insulin regimen (only basal insulin) was present in 62.5% of the population. There was no difference between groups with respect to the use of only basal insulin (NPH and basal analogues, $p = 0.136$). The commonest basal insulin was NPH (NPH 65.3%, glargine U100 28.6%, and degludec U100 6.1%). However, when comparing adherence groups, basal insulin analogues were more frequently used in the adherent group (42.7 versus 28.9%, adherent versus nonadherent group, resp., $p = 0.046$). Insulin intensification regimens were present in the remaining subjects. The use of premixed insulin was rare (2%). No subject utilized GLP-1 agonists. Basal-bolus and basal-plus regimens were predominant, recorded in 35.5%. Regular insulin was the most prevalent preprandial agent (90.1%). In the nonadherent group, a significantly higher number of patients were on such complex regimens (25.3 versus 42.7%, adherent versus nonadherent groups, resp., $p = 0.011$). Insulin dose was significantly higher in the nonadherent subjects (0.40 [0.28–0.54] versus 0.54 [0.37–0.73], $p < 0.0001$). As one would anticipate, the number of insulin applications was also higher in the nonadherent group (1.76 ± 0.79 versus 2.31 ± 0.96, $p < 0.0001$). The use of prefilled insulin pen devices was significantly higher in the adherent group (31.3 versus 17.9%, $p = 0.028$).

The biochemical characteristics according to adherence category are shown in Table 3. The nonadherent group had a significantly higher A1c compared to the adherent group (8.4 versus 8.9%, $p = 0.024$). The levels of fasting plasma glucose, triglycerides, and LDL cholesterol did not show differences between groups.

3.1. Interference with Daily Activities. The adherent group reported that they planned their daily activities around the application of insulin (58.7% versus 53.9%, adherent versus nonadherent, resp., $p = 0.012$) (Table 4). This group also reported greater interference with meals ($p = 0.001$) and exercise ($p = 0.003$). There was no difference between groups regarding interference with social and recreational activities, sexual activity or work, and professional development.

3.2. Experience with Insulin Injections. The second factor evaluated was subject experience with regard to the application of insulin (Table 5). Persons who were nonadherent felt that injecting was the most difficult part of their treatment (19.0% versus 21.4%, adherent versus nonadherent, resp., $p = 0.044$). This group reported pain and bruising more frequently than the adherent group (33.7% versus 59.8%, $p = 0.002$ and 32.5% versus 55.5%, $p = 0.002$). The nonadherent group also felt greater embarrassment with insulin application (8.4% versus 25.7%, $p = 0.033$). Finally, the most significant difference between adherence groups was fear of hypoglycemia; here again, the nonadherent subjects more frequently reported fear (28.9% versus 41.0%, $p < 0.0001$).

3.3. Economic Aspects. The final aspect examined was economic reasons for insulin omission (Table 6). The nonadherent group reported that this was an important factor all the time or almost all the time (9.6% versus 15.4%, adherent versus nonadherent, resp., $p < 0.0001$). Health insurance or access to social security was significantly less prevalent in the nonadherent group (51.8% versus 35.9%, $p = 0.025$). Economic support from relatives was also more commonly cited in the nonadherent subjects (26.5% versus 37.6%, $p = 0.012$). Finally, inadequate beliefs surrounding insulin application were equally present in both adherence categories ($p = 0.116$).

A linear regression model was constructed to determine factors independently associated with adherence. The dependent variable was the adherence score. The independent variables were age, use of needle and syringe, planning of activities around the application of insulin, fear of hypoglycemia, and economic factors. The factors significantly associated with better adherence were adequate economic resources, planning of daily activities around insulin application, lack of fear of hypoglycemia, and fewer insulin applications per day. This model is shown in Table 7.

4. Discussion

In this study, we describe the characteristics of insulin-treated patients in a tertiary care centre in Mexico City. We evaluated the level of insulin adherence and explored the factors related to nonadherence. About a third (30.5%) of subjects showed moderate adherence to insulin therapy and excellent adherence was infrequent (11%).

In our population, one important characteristic was that the average duration of diabetes was almost twenty years; however, the mean number of years on insulin therapy was only six, suggesting a significant delay for commencing insulin. Lerman et al. have shown similar findings in a Mexican population; at the time of insulin initiation, the mean duration of type 2 diabetes was 14 ± 9 years and the mean A1c

Table 1: Characteristics of study participants, classified by adherence category.

Variable	Nonadherent $n = 117$	Adherent $n = 83$	p
Gender			0.359
Women	73 (62.4)	57 (68.7)	
Men	44 (37.6)	26 (31.3)	
Age, years	59 [53–69]	64 [54–73]	0.037
Weight, kg	71.7 ± 14.9	70.5 ± 10.9	0.551
Age at diagnosis of diabetes, years	42.1 ± 11.2	41.8 ± 11.6	0.502
Duration of diabetes, years	17.5 [12–25]	20 [15–26]	0.022
Time since insulin initiation, months	72 [42–120]	60 [36–120]	0.685
Education level			0.536
Incomplete primary	19 (16.2)	9 (10.8)	
Primary/elementary	17 (14.5)	13 (15.7)	
Secondary/middle school	39 (33.3)	32 (38.6)	
High school	13 (11.1)	12 (14.5)	
College	24 (20.5)	11 (13.3)	
Postgraduate	5 (4.3)	6 (7.2)	

Data are expressed as means ± standard deviation, median [interquartile range], or number (%).

Table 2: Insulin regimen characteristics according to adherence category.

Variable	Nonadherent $n = 117$	Adherent $n = 83$	p
Insulin applications/day, number	2.31 ± 0.96	1.76 ± 0.79	<0.0001
Insulin dose, units/kg	0.54 [0.37–0.73]	0.40 [0.28–0.54]	<0.0001
Form of insulin application			0.028
Pen	21 (17.9)	26 (31.3)	
Syringe	96 (82.1)	57 (68.7)	
Basal insulin			0.046
NPH	81 (71.1)	47 (57.3)	
Basal insulin analogue (glargine U100 and degludec U100)	33 (28.9)	35 (42.7)	
Preprandial insulin			0.611
Regular	44 (88.0)	20 (95.2)	
Rapid acting insulin analogue (lispro and aspart)	6 (12.0)	1 (4.8)	
Basal-bolus or basal-plus regimen	50 (42.7)	21 (25.3)	0.011

Data are expressed as means ± standard deviation or number (%).

Table 3: Biochemical parameters of the participants according to adherence category.

Variable	Nonadherent $n = 117$	Adherent $n = 83$	p
Glucose, mg/dl	134 [96–181.5]	123.5 [88–170]	0.303
A1c, %	8.9 [7.9–10.4]	8.4 [7.5–9.6]	0.024
Triglycerides, mg/dl	136.5 [100–198]	131 [100–185]	0.771
Total cholesterol, mg/dl	171 [145–193]	166 [144–196]	0.711
HDL cholesterol, mg/dl	46 [38–55]	46 [41–54.5]	0.727
LDL cholesterol, mg/dl	98 [79.5–114.5]	98 [79–114]	0.938

Data are expressed as means ± standard deviation or median [interquartile range].

concentration was 10.8 ± 1.4% [9]. Rodríguez-Gutiérrez et al. reported that inappropriate beliefs (negative attitudes towards insulin therapy, psychosocial barriers, and myths regarding insulin use) are an important barrier for physicians when trying to initiate and sustain insulin treatment (persistence of treatment) in this region [10]. Available information regarding insulin adherence in Latin American countries is scarce, and Lerman et al. reported that 41% of Mexican patients did not adhere to insulin treatment [9]. In our population, 58.5% were nonadherent (when this was considered as a dichotomous variable).

Regarding factors associated with nonadherence, both age (64 versus 59 years, adherent versus non adherent, resp., $p = 0.037$) and mean duration of diabetes (20 versus 17 years, $p = 0.02$) were significantly lower in the nonadherent group

TABLE 4: Interference with daily activities according to adherence category.

	Nonadherent $n = 117$	Adherent $n = 83$	p
Do you plan your activities around insulin application?	63 (53.9)	57 (58.7)	0.012
Applying insulin interferes with your meals?	39 (33.3)	41 (49.4)	0.001
Applying insulin interferes with doing exercise?	34 (29)	37 (44.6)	0.003
Applying insulin has a negative impact in your social and recreational activities?	19 (16.3)	9 (10.8)	0.336
Applying insulin has a negative impact in your sexual activity?	15 (12.8)	6 (7.2)	0.487
Applying insulin has a negative impact in your work and professional development?	20 (17.1)	6 (7.2)	0.225

Data are expressed as number (%).

TABLE 5: Experience with insulin application according to adherence groups.

	Nonadherent $n = 117$	Adherent $n = 83$	p
Injecting is the most difficult part of the treatment	25 (21.4)	38 (19)	0.044
Injecting insulin causes pain	70 (59.8)	28 (33.7)	0.002
Injecting insulin causes bruising	65 (55.5)	27 (32.5)	0.002
Injecting insulin is embarrassing	30 (25.7)	7 (8.4)	0.033
Worry of having a hypoglycemia episode	48 (41)	24 (28.9)	<0.0001

TABLE 6: Economic factors and inadequate beliefs associated with the omission of insulin according to adherence groups.

	Nonadherent $n = 117$	Adherent $n = 83$	p
Do you omit your insulin for economic reasons?	18 (15.4)	8 (9.6)	<0.0001
Do you have social security or private health insurance?	42 (35.9)	43 (51.8)	0.025
Do you receive economic support from family to buy insulin?	44 (37.6)	22 (26.5)	0.012
Do you believe insulin causes health problems (blindness, amputation, kidney damage)?	13 (11.1)	7 (8.4)	0.116

TABLE 7: Linear regression model showing the factors associated with adherence (as quantified using the Morisky adherence score).

Variables	Coefficient beta (95% CI)	p
Planning of daily activities around the application of insulin	0.218 (0.122 to 0.449)	0.001
Number of insulin applications per day	−0.151 (−0.012 to −0.028)	0.023
Lack of fear of hypoglycemia	−0.128 (−0.492 to −0.139)	0.001
Lack of economic resources	−0.249 (−0.598 to −0.198)	<0.0001

Dependent variable: Morisky score. Included variables: age, use of syringe and needle, $R^2 = 0.234$, $p < 0.0001$.

compared to the adherent group. There is no clear explanation for this finding. We can speculate that older patients and patients with a longer disease duration may have better adherence because they have learnt to accept the disease to a greater extent than younger patients or patients with recent diagnosis. In the Global Attitudes of Patients and Physicians in Insulin Therapy (GAPP) study, 34.6% of the study population admitted to omitting their insulin dose at least once in the previous month. Insulin omission was more frequent among women (50.8%), and age and duration of diabetes were lower in the low adherence group (50 and 6 years, resp.) [8]. Peyrot et al. found similar results in an internet survey in 502 diabetic individuals, 388 of which had T2D [14]. Intentional insulin omission was identified in 20% of participants. Sociodemographic factors associated with insulin omission were younger age, lower income, and higher education level. In our study, we did not find differences in adherence associated with educational level ($p = 0.536$).

In the nonadherent group, the number of insulin applications per day was significantly higher ($p < 0.0001$). In addition, a higher proportion of nonadherent individuals applied insulin using needle and syringe compared to the adherent group (68.7% versus 82.1%, adherent versus nonadherent, resp., $p = 0.028$). Slabaugh et al. in a retrospective analysis of Medicare data reported that adherence-adjusted probability (proportion of covered days ≥ 80%) was positively associated with pen device use (OR 2.19; 95% CI 1.86–2.59) [15]. The nonpersistence-adjusted risk was significantly lower (58%) in the cohort using pen devices compared to those using syringes (HR 0.42; 95% CI 0.38–0.45). The simplicity of use and lower pain associated with pen devices probably promotes improved compliance [16].

In our study, the nonadherent subjects did not plan their activities around insulin application. They also believed that insulin did not interfere with meals or exercise. In the GAPP study subjects who omitted insulin reported interference with daily activities (43.3%), this difference suggests that subjects who omit insulin in our centre do not consider insulin treatment as an integral part of their daily lives [8].

With respect to the experience associated with insulin injection, the nonadherent group reported that fear of hypoglycemia, pain, bruising, embarrassment, and injecting insulin were considered the most difficult parts of treatment. Ross et al. identified anxiety related to disease progression, fear of hypoglycemia, embarrassment, panic of injections, regimen complexity, and fear of weight gain as the factors most strongly associated with insulin omission in Canada [17]. In the GAPP study, 28.9% omitted insulin because of pain related to injections [8]. Peyrot et al. reported that the most important factors were a greater number of injections per day, interference with daily activities, pain, and embarrassment related to insulin injection [14]. Farsaei et al. reported the following factors associated with insulin noncompliance: time-consuming application of insulin, injection site pain, embarrassment, forgetfulness, feeling worse after insulin injection, difficulties in injecting, concurrent illness, insulin shortage, cost, and weight gain associated with insulin [18].

Finally, with respect to economic factors, a lower proportion of nonadherent subjects had health coverage or economic support from their families. In Mexico, diabetes treatment is often an out of pocket expense and insulin treatment is perceived as costly [19]. Farsaei et al. reported that medication cost had a significant relationship with low compliance in a similar population [18].

Although there is extensive worldwide literature regarding patient barriers to insulin therapy and nonadherence, there is little information on interventions to improve adherence to insulin [20]. Possible actions to address the principle factors include the use of newer therapies, in particular insulin analogues, and pen devices instead of needle and syringe for insulin administration. Insulin analogues are associated with a lower risk of hypoglycemia, in particular nocturnal hypoglycemia [21, 22]. In a systematic review investigating real-world factors affecting adherence to insulin, Davies et al. found that switching or initiating insulin administered by a pen device improved adherence in four of five studies investigating this factor. They also suggested that a more flexible insulin regimen (e.g., use of newer insulin analogues) would impact the perceptions of interference with daily activities and may result in fewer applications per day. Finally, these authors comment that adherence is improved when the financial burden to the patient is reduced [23]. Education regarding the prevention and treatment of hypoglycemia is also necessary to allay patient fears. Lerman et al. showed that a support from a diabetic nurse specialist was a positive predictor for adherence [9]. Improving access to health care services is also necessary.

The results of this study may help to establish actions to confront and improve the lack of adherence to insulin treatment in patients with T2D. Health care providers should be encouraged to address the factors identified in this study in the consultation. Doggrell and Chan found that the best strategy was to involve patients in all aspects of the decision-making process around insulin therapy [20]. Finally, the implementation of education programs, patient empowerment, and specific interventions targeting young and recently diagnosed individuals (possibly utilizing newer technologies or social media) may be worth considering for improving insulin adherence [19].

Some limitations of the present study should be acknowledged. Only the most important factors reported in other studies were evaluated; this was not a totally inclusive search. Insulin omission was evaluated through questionnaires and not directly. Patient self-reporting has previously been shown to either underestimate or overestimate adherence [24]. The impact of participating in a study with researchers present at the time of questionnaire completion may have influenced the way participants responded. To minimize this limitation, questionnaires were completed anonymously and patients were encouraged to be honest knowing that the answers would not affect subsequent patient care. Factors related to health care providers were not evaluated, and the study was performed in a referral centre; thus, results might not be generalizable. Finally, insulin treatment is only one component of the integral treatment in patients with T2D. This study did not evaluate other components of the treatment (e.g., number of concomitant medications).

5. Conclusions

In this study, excellent adherence to insulin was identified in only a minority of patients with T2D. The principal factors associated with insulin nonadherence were fear of hypoglycemia, interference with daily activities, a greater number of applications per day, and economic factors. In order to address these findings, education programs designed to tackle these issues in a multidisciplinary team setting should be considered.

Conflicts of Interest

There are no potential conflicts of interest relevant to this article.

Acknowledgments

This study was carried out and supported by the INCMNSZ.

References

[1] American Diabetes Association, "8. Pharmacologic approaches to glycemic treatment: *Standards of Medical Care in Diabetes—2018*," *Diabetes Care*, vol. 41, Supplement 1, pp. S73–S85, 2018.

[2] A. J. Garber, M. J. Abrahamson, J. I. Barzilay et al., "Consensus statement by the American Association of Clinical Endocrinologists and American College of Endocrinology on the comprehensive type 2 diabetes management algorithm – *2018 executive summary*," *Endocrine Practice*, vol. 24, no. 1, pp. 91–120, 2018.

[3] E. Selvin, C. M. Parrinello, N. Daya, and R. M. Bergenstal, "Trends in insulin use and diabetes control in the U.S.: 1988–1994 and 1999–2012," *Diabetes Care*, vol. 39, no. 3, pp. e33–e35, 2016.

[4] J. A. Rebolledo and R. Arellano, "Cultural differences and considerations when initiating insulin," *Diabetes Spectrum*, vol. 29, no. 3, pp. 185–190, 2016.

[5] Instituto Nacional de Salud Pública and Secretaría de Salud, "Encuesta Nacional de Salud y Nutrición de Medio Camino 2016," April 2018, http://promocion.salud.gob.mx.

[6] K. Khunti, M. L. Wolden, B. L. Thorsted, M. Andersen, and M. J. Davies, "Clinical inertia in people with type 2 diabetes: a retrospective cohort study of more than 80,000 people," *Diabetes Care*, vol. 36, no. 11, pp. 3411–3417, 2013.

[7] M. Peyrot, R. R. Rubin, T. Lauritzen et al., "Resistance to insulin therapy among patients and providers: results of the cross-national diabetes attitudes, wishes, and needs (DAWN) study," *Diabetes Care*, vol. 28, no. 11, pp. 2673–2679, 2005.

[8] M. Peyrot, A. H. Barnett, L. F. Meneghini, and P. M. Schumm-Draeger, "Factors associated with injection omission/non-adherence in the Global Attitudes of Patients and Physicians in Insulin Therapy study," *Diabetes, Obesity and Metabolism*, vol. 14, no. 12, pp. 1081–1087, 2012.

[9] I. Lerman, J. Díaz, M. Ibarguengoitia et al., "Nonadherence to insulin therapy in low-income, type 2 diabetic patients," *Endocrine Practice*, vol. 15, no. 1, pp. 41–46, 2009.

[10] R. Rodríguez-Gutiérrez, A. Millan-Ferro, and E. A. Caballero, "Myths and misconceptions about insulin therapy among Latinos/ Hispanics with diabetes: a fresh look at an old problem," *Journal of Diabetes & Metabolism*, vol. 6, 2015.

[11] M. M. Herrero and A. E. Caballero, "The presence of the blindness myth in Latino patients with type 2 diabetes," *Presented in the International Diabetes Federation Meeting*, 2006.

[12] D. E. Morisky, A. Ang, M. Krousel-Wood, and H. J. Ward, "Predictive validity of a medication adherence measure in an outpatient setting," *The Journal of Clinical Hypertension*, vol. 10, no. 5, pp. 348–354, 2008.

[13] C. Y. Osborn and J. S. Gonzalez, "Measuring insulin adherence among adults with type 2 diabetes," *Journal of Behavioral Medicine*, vol. 39, no. 4, pp. 633–641, 2016.

[14] M. Peyrot, R. R. Rubin, D. F. Kruger, and L. B. Travis, "Correlates of insulin injection omission," *Diabetes Care*, vol. 33, no. 2, pp. 240–245, 2010.

[15] S. L. Slabaugh, J. R. Bouchard, Y. Li, J. C. Baltz, Y. A. Meah, and D. C. Moretz, "Characteristics relating to adherence and persistence to basal insulin regimens among elderly insulin-naïve patients with type 2 diabetes: pre-filled pens versus vials/syringes," *Advances in Therapy*, vol. 32, no. 12, pp. 1206–1221, 2015.

[16] S. L. Slabaugh, B. H. Curtis, G. Clore, H. Fu, and D. P. Schuster, "Factors associated with increased healthcare costs in Medicare advantage patients with type 2 diabetes enrolled in a large representative health insurance plan in the US," *Journal of Medical Economics*, vol. 18, no. 2, pp. 106–112, 2015.

[17] S. A. Ross, H. D. Tildesley, and J. Ashkenas, "Barriers to effective insulin treatment: the persistence of poor glycemic control in type 2 diabetes," *Current Medical Research and Opinion*, vol. 27, Supplemet 3, pp. 13–20, 2011.

[18] S. Farsaei, M. Radfar, Z. Heydari, F. Abbasi, and M. Qorbani, "Insulin adherence in patients with diabetes: risk factors for injection omission," *Primary Care Diabetes*, vol. 8, no. 4, pp. 338–345, 2014.

[19] I. Lerman, "Barreras que dificultan la aplicación temprana de insulina en el paciente con diabetes tipo 2," *Asociación Latinoamericana de Diabetes*, vol. 12, no. 2, pp. 66–68, 2009.

[20] S. A. Doggrell and V. Chan, "Adherence to insulin treatment in diabetes: can it be improved?," *Journal of Diabetes*, vol. 7, no. 3, pp. 315–321, 2015.

[21] A. Cahn, R. Miccoli, A. Dardano, and S. Del Prato, "New forms of insulin and insulin therapies for the treatment of type 2 diabetes," *The Lancet Diabetes & Endocrinology*, vol. 3, no. 8, pp. 638–652, 2015.

[22] K. Horvath, K. Jeitler, A. Berghold et al., "Long-acting insulin analogues versus NPH insulin (human isophane insulin) for type 2 diabetes mellitus," *Cochrane Database of Systematic Reviews*, no. 2, article CD005613, 2007.

[23] M. J. Davies, J. J. Gagliardino, L. J. Gray, K. Khunti, V. Mohan, and R. Hughes, "Real-world factors affecting adherence to insulin therapy in patients with type 1 or type 2 diabetes mellitus: a systematic review," *Diabetic Medicine*, vol. 30, no. 5, pp. 512–524, 2013.

[24] G. B. Sarbacker and E. M. Urteaga, "Adherence to insulin therapy," *Diabetes Spectrum*, vol. 29, no. 3, pp. 166–170, 2016.

7

The Antidiabetic Agent Sodium Tungstate Induces Abnormal Glycogen Accumulation in Renal Proximal Tubules from Diabetic IRS2-Knockout Mice

Romina Bertinat,[1] Francisco Westermeier,[2,3] Pamela Silva,[4] Rodrigo Gatica,[5] Joana Moitinho Oliveira,[6,7] Francisco Nualart,[1] Ramón Gomis,[6,7,8,9] and Alejandro J. Yáñez[10]

[1]*Centro de Microscopía Avanzada (CMA BIO-BIO), Universidad de Concepción, Concepción, Chile*
[2]*Institute of Biomedical Science, FH Joanneum Gesellschaft mbH University of Applied Sciences, Eggenberger Allee 13, 8020 Graz, Austria*
[3]*Facultad de Ciencia, Universidad San Sebastián, Santiago, Chile*
[4]*Facultad de Salud, Universidad Santo Tomás, Osorno, Chile*
[5]*Escuela de Veterinaria, Facultad de Ciencias, Universidad Mayor, Santiago, Chile*
[6]*CIBER de Diabetes y Enfermedades Metabólicas Asociadas (CIBERDEM), Barcelona, Spain*
[7]*Diabetes and Obesity Research Laboratory, IDIBAPS, Barcelona, Spain*
[8]*Department of Endocrinology and Nutrition, Hospital Clinic, Barcelona, Spain*
[9]*Faculty of Medicine, University of Barcelona, Barcelona, Spain*
[10]*Facultad de Ciencias, Universidad Austral de Chile, Valdivia, Chile*

Correspondence should be addressed to Romina Bertinat; romibert@gmail.com and Alejandro J. Yáñez; ayanez@uach.cl

Academic Editor: Sergiu Catrina

The kidney is an insulin-sensitive organ involved in glucose homeostasis. One major effect of insulin is to induce glycogen storage in the liver and muscle. However, no significant glycogen stores are detected in normal kidneys, but diabetic subjects present a characteristic renal histopathological feature resulting from extensive glycogen deposition mostly in nonproximal tubules. The mechanism of renal glycogen accumulation is yet poorly understood. Here, we studied in situ glycogen accumulation in the kidney from diabetic IRS2-knockout mice and the effect of the insulin-mimetic agent sodium tungstate (NaW). IRS2-knockout mice displayed hyperglycemia and hyperinsulinemia. NaW only normalized glycemia. There was no evident morphological difference between kidneys from untreated wild-type (WT), NaW-treated WT, and untreated IRS2-knockout mice. However, NaW-treated IRS2-knockout mice showed tubular alterations resembling clear cells in the cortex, but not in the outer medulla, that were correlated with glycogen accumulation. Immunohistochemical detection of the gluconeogenic enzyme phosphoenolpyruvate carboxykinase, mostly expressed by renal proximal tubules, showed that altered tubules were of proximal origin. Our preliminary study suggests that IRS2 differentially regulates glycogen accumulation in renal tubules and that NaW treatment in the context of IRS2 ablation induces abnormal glycogen accumulation in cortical proximal tubules.

1. Introduction

Insulin participates in a wide spectrum of growth and metabolic responses by binding to the insulin receptor (IR) and inducing IR tyrosine kinase activity to phosphorylate IR itself and several other proteins, among them IR substrates (IRS) [1]. Knockout (KO) studies have been critical to understand IRS relevance in insulin signaling in different tissues, indicating that IRS1 plays a major role in adipose tissue and skeletal muscle metabolism [1–3], whereas IRS2 is critical for liver metabolism and pancreatic β-cell development and survival [1–4]. Moreover, IRS1 and IRS2 show differential relevance in mitogenic and metabolic insulin effects, respectively, as IRS1-KO mice are 50% smaller in size and insulin resistant but maintain normal glucose tolerance due to compensatory β-cell hyperplasia [3], whereas IRS2-KO mice develop type 2 diabetes due to β-cell failure [4] and decreased suppression of endogenous glucose production and hepatic glycogen synthesis [2].

Two key effects of insulin are its ability to induce glycogen synthesis in the liver and muscle and to suppress gluconeogenesis in the liver [1]. Indeed, insulin inhibits the expression of rate-limiting enzymes of gluconeogenesis, that is, phosphoenolpyruvate carboxykinase (PEPCK), fructose 1,6-bisphosphatase (FBPase), and glucose 6-phosphatase (G6Pase), whereas it activates the key enzyme of glycogen synthesis, that is, glycogen synthase (GS) [1]. The kidney is also an insulin-sensitive organ involved in normal glucose homeostasis and enhanced gluconeogenesis during diabetes [1, 5, 6]. However, contrary to the liver and muscle, no significant glycogen stores are detected in the kidney under normal conditions, but diabetes induces abnormal glycogen deposition especially in nonproximal tubular epithelial cells [7–10]. This pathological feature has long been recognized, but the triggering mechanisms are not fully understood, albeit overexpression and activation of GS may be involved [8, 9].

Sodium tungstate (NaW) is an inorganic salt that exerts potent insulin-mimetic and antidiabetic actions in animal models of diabetes by normalizing hepatic glycogen metabolism and blood glucose levels [11]. NaW is a phosphatase inhibitor [11–13], but this property cannot account for all its antidiabetic effects [13]. Notably, NaW stimulates hepatic glycogen synthesis bypassing IR [13, 14], with the common intracellular target of all NaW insulin-mimetic effects reported to date being the mitogen-activated protein kinase (MAPK) pathway, through phosphorylation/activation of extracellular signal-regulated kinase (ERK) 1/2, both *in vitro* and *in vivo* [11]. NaW has been shown to reverse the pathological accumulation of glycogen in the diabetic kidney [15], but it remains to be established whether NaW requires an intact insulin signaling pathway to exert its renal effects. In parallel, the adverse effects of NaW treatment are poorly defined, which has hampered further clinical study of this antidiabetic agent [11, 16].

The molecular pathways involved in the opposite response between the liver/muscle and kidney in glycogen accumulation during diabetes are poorly understood. On the basis that IRS2 is critical for the proper regulation of glycogen metabolism in the liver [2, 4], we hypothesized that it also has a pivotal role in the kidney, especially because IRS2 mRNA expression is higher in mouse kidney than in the liver [17]. Therefore, in this preliminary work, we examined the effect of IRS2 ablation and the impact of NaW treatment on glycogen accumulation in the kidney in situ. To this end, we used a total IRS2-KO mouse model that exhibits a diabetic phenotype [2, 4]. Our data suggest that IRS2 plays an important role in renal glycogen metabolism and that NaW treatment in the context of IRS2 ablation is harmful for the kidney.

2. Materials and Methods

2.1. Animals. Wild-type (WT) and whole-body IRS2-KO mice were generated by intercrossing Irs2$^{+/-}$ mice (C57Bl/6 genetic background) [4]. The principles of laboratory animal care were followed (European and local government guidelines), and protocols were approved by the Animal Research Committee of Barcelona University. 10-week-old male WT and IRS2-KO mice with glycemia inferior to 16 mM were randomly divided into two groups. For 3 weeks, one WT group received distilled water as drinking water (untreated group), whereas the other received ad libitum a solution of 2 mg/ml NaW (Sigma-Aldrich, St. Louis, MO) in distilled water (treated group). The same is true for the two IRS2-KO groups. Glycemia was measured with a clinical glucometer. Insulinemia was analyzed with an ELISA kit (Mercodia, Uppsala, Sweden). Animals were euthanized by cervical dislocation.

2.2. Antibodies. Rabbit anti-cytosolic PEPCK was prepared in our laboratory [18]. Goat anti-muscle pyruvate kinase (PK-M) was from Rockland Immunochemicals Inc. (Gilbertsville, PA). An HRP-conjugated β-actin antibody was from Santa Cruz Biotechnology (sc-47778-HRP; Santa Cruz, CA). Rabbit monoclonal anti-phospho-p44/42 MAPK (Erk1/2) (Thr202/Tyr204) was from Cell Signaling Technology Inc. (#4370, Beverly, MA). Secondary antibodies were goat anti-rabbit IgG-HRP, rabbit anti-goat IgG-HRP (Jackson ImmunoResearch, West Grove, PA), and Alexa Fluor 488-conjugated donkey anti-rabbit IgG (Molecular Probes, Eugene, OR).

2.3. Histochemical Analysis. Pieces of the kidney were fixed in formalin and embedded in paraffin. Immunohistochemical studies were conducted as previously described [18]. Briefly, tissue was deparaffinized in xylene, rehydrated in graded ethanol, blocked with 3% BSA, and permeabilized with 0.05% Triton X-100 for 20 min. For immunoperoxidase and immunofluorescence analyses, primary antibodies were incubated overnight at 4°C and secondary antibodies were incubated for 1 h at room temperature. For periodic acid-Schiff (PAS) staining, we used the PAS Staining Kit from Merck Millipore (Billerica, MA), following the manufacturer's instructions. In situ digestion of glycogen was performed with α-amylase (Sigma-Aldrich, St. Louis, MO; 0.2% *w/v* α-amylase in 0.1 M Na_2HPO_4 and 0.05 M sodium citrate, pH 5.0) for 30 min at 37°C in a humidified chamber. Serial sections of the kidney were mounted on separate slides: one was digested and the other was not, but both were stained with PAS reagents. For semiquantitation of PAS staining, images were smoothed by applying a 3-pixel Gaussian filter. Areas of interest with higher PAS signal, before and after α-amylase treatment, were manually selected using the Wand tracing tool from ImageJ v1.48 software (NIH, USA), and the total area was calculated. Calculation of the total tissue area was based on the selection of all pixels with saturation higher than 30. For combined PAS staining and immunofluorescence, we applied a previously described protocol where tandem detection was standardized [19], using DAPI for nuclear counter staining. ImageJ v1.48 software (NIH,

Table 1: Blood glucose and insulin levels and body weight in groups of mice.

	WT	NaW-WT	IRS2-KO	NaW-IRS2-KO
Glycemia (mM)	7.6 ± 0.3	7.1 ± 0.2	13.0 ± 0.9^a	7.0 ± 0.5^b
Insulinemia (μg/l)	1.5 ± 0.6	1.5 ± 0.7	2.1 ± 0.5^a	2.0 ± 0.5
Body weight (g)	24.8 ± 3.5	25.5 ± 2.7	27.2 ± 1.3	24.0 ± 4.1

Values are means ± SD. $n = 5$ mice per group. $^aP < 0.01$ compared to WT. $^bP < 0.001$ compared to IRS2-KO.

USA) was used to digitally combine images from immunofluorescence and bright-field PAS staining.

2.4. Western Blot. Proteins were prepared in lysis buffer (50 mM Tris pH 7.5, 5 mM EDTA, 150 mM NaCl, 1% Triton X-100, 10 mM sodium phosphate, 10 mM sodium fluoride, 10 mM sodium orthovanadate, and protease inhibitors), resolved by 10–12% SDS-PAGE, transferred onto PVDF membranes, and probed overnight with a primary antibody. β-Actin was used as a loading control. Reaction was developed using the Pierce ECL Western Blotting Substrate (Pierce Biotechnology, Rockford, IL).

2.5. Statistical Analysis. Data are expressed as mean ± SD. Statistical comparison between groups was performed with 2-way ANOVA (followed by Tukey's post hoc test) using GraphPad Prism software, version 6.01. Data were considered statistically significant for $P < 0.05$.

3. Results

Ten-week-old IRS2-KO mice displayed fasting hyperglycemia and hyperinsulinemia. Three weeks of NaW treatment had no effect on control WT mice and was able to only normalize glycemia but not insulinemia in IRS2-KO mice. Body weight was not significantly affected by the treatment (Table 1). Noteworthy, IRS2-KO mice did not display polydipsia at this stage yet; therefore, both control and IRS2-KO mice ingested almost the same amount of water and consumed almost the same amount of NaW, which was approximately 120 mg per kg body weight per day. In order to complement the morphological data and extend the study of IRS2 and NaW participation in renal insulin signaling from IRS2-KO mice, we conducted PAS staining with or without α-amylase digestion to asses for glycogen deposition in situ. Unexpectedly, no differences were detected between untreated WT (WT), treated WT (NaW-WT), and untreated IRS2-KO (IRS2-KO) kidneys with or without α-amylase digestion (Figures 1(a)–1(f), resp.), indicating that no significant glycogen stores were present in these conditions, despite hyperglycemia in IRS2-KO mice. In contrast, the same analysis in kidneys from NaW-treated IRS2-KO (NaW-IRS2-KO) mice showed a significant increase in PAS staining (Figure 1(g)) that was α-amylase-sensitive (Figure 1(h)). Hematoxylin/eosin staining confirmed that no significant differences in kidney morphology were evident between WT, NaW-WT, and IRS2-KO mice (Figures 1(i)–1(k), resp.), but kidneys from NaW-IRS2-KO mice showed a distinctive pattern of tubular morphology (Figure 1(l)). A more detailed comparison of kidneys from IRS2-KO (Figures 1(m) and 1(n)) and NaW-IRS2-KO (Figures 1(o)–1(r)) mice at higher magnification showed that increased α-amylase-sensitive PAS-positive tubules were mainly localized to the renal cortex and not to the outer medulla from NaW-IRS2-KO mice (Figures 1(o) and 1(p)). Semiquantitation of those renal areas that were positive for PAS staining and sensitive to α-amylase revealed that approximately 20% of the renal cortex presented an increased signal in NaW-IRS2-KO mice that was the result of glycogen accumulation (Figure 1(s)).

To define which renal tubules were affected by glycogen accumulation in NaW-IRS2-KO mice, we analyzed the cellular expression of different metabolic enzymes that display a characteristic pattern of zonation along the nephron, which may help to understand the segment specificity (if any) of the glycogenic alteration. We studied the gluconeogenic enzyme PEPCK, which is specifically expressed in proximal tubules, and the muscle isoform of the glycolytic enzyme pyruvate kinase (PK-M) that is mostly expressed downstream of the proximal tubules. Given that tubular structures downstream of the proximal tubule have different functions and names, hereafter, we will refer to them just as nonproximal tubules for simplification. As expected, PEPCK was exclusively detected in the renal cortex and outer medulla from WT, NaW-WT, IRS2-KO, and NaW-IRS2-KO mice, where proximal tubules are organized (Figures 2(a)–2(d), resp.). Instead, PK-M was detected in the cortex and outer medulla and all tubule segments from the inner medulla in the same groups (Figures 2(e)–2(h)), in agreement with the distribution of nonproximal tubules throughout the tissue. However, in the particular case of NaW-IRS2-KO mice, PEPCK showed a different immunoreactivity in the renal cortex but not in the outer medulla (Figure 2(d)), whereas PK-M immunostaining remains virtually the same among the groups (Figures 2(e)–2(h)). Although PEPCK detection was limited to proximal tubules (Figures 2(i)–2(l)), its immunoreactivity was reduced in those tubules that show a different morphology in NaW-IRS2-KO kidneys, in comparison to tubules not affected in the same samples (Figure 2(l)) and to those in WT, NaW-WT, and IRS2-KO mice (Figures 2(i)–2(k), resp.). A similar pattern of immunoreactivity as for PEPCK was detected with an antibody against FBPase, another gluconeogenic enzyme expressed in proximal tubules (data not shown). Again, no significant changes in the immunostaining of PK-M were detected in any group (Figures 2(m)–2(p)). We provide more evidence supporting the fact that neither NaW treatment nor IRS2 ablation per se produced an evident impact on renal morphology, but instead we observed that NaW treatment in

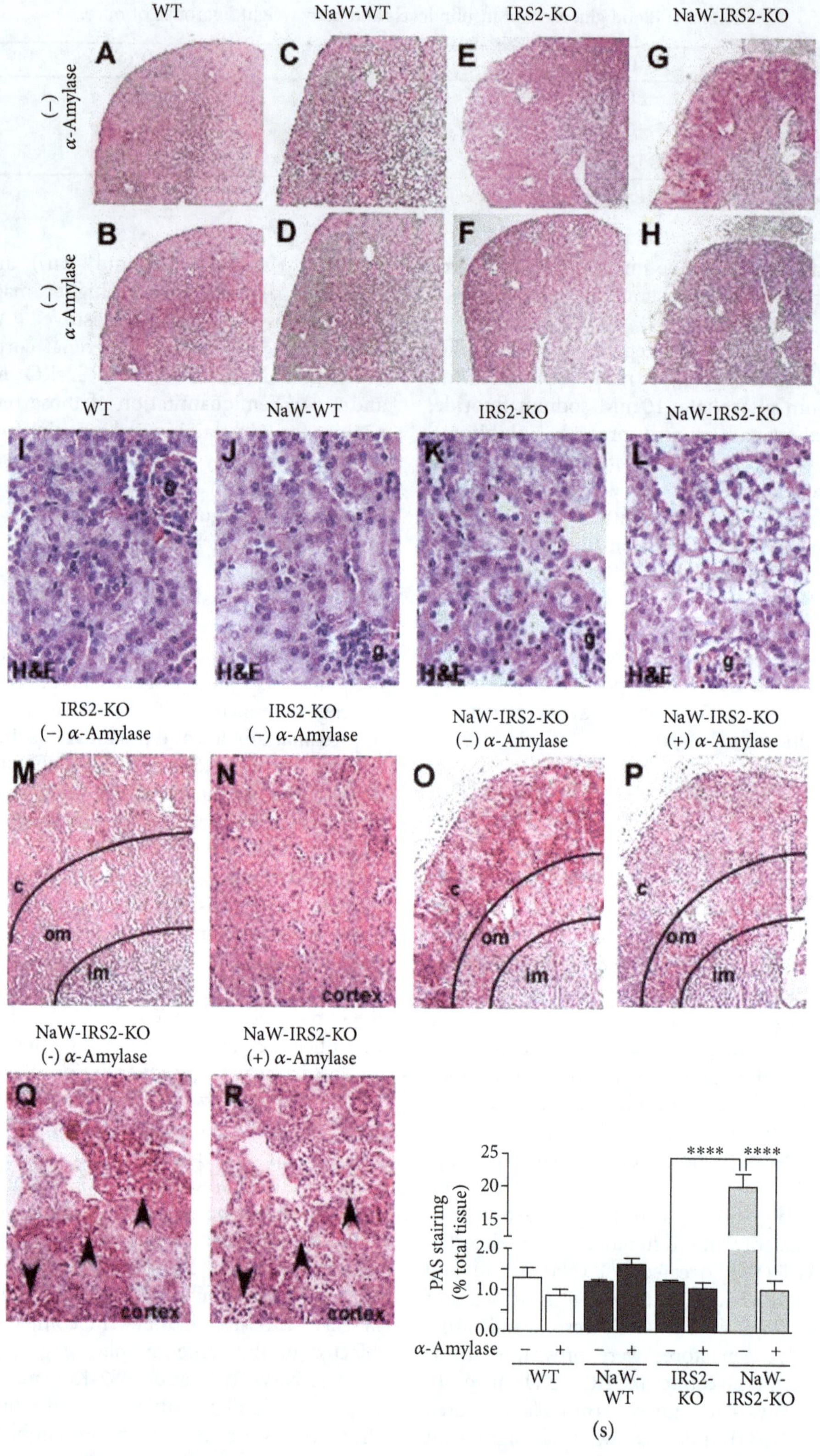

Figure 1: NaW induces glycogen accumulation in renal cortical tubules from IRS2-KO mice. Serial sections of the kidney from untreated WT (WT; a, b), treated WT (NaW-WT; c, d), untreated IRS2-KO (IRS2-KO; e, f), and treated IRS2-KO (NaW-IRS2-KO; g, h) mice were processed for PAS staining with (+) or without (−) α-amylase digestion. (i–l) Hematoxylin/eosin (H&E) staining to compare renal morphology. (m) Magnification of (e). (n) Magnification of (m). (o) Magnification of (g). (p) Magnification of (h). (q) Magnification of (g) and (o). (r) Magnification of (h) and (p). Areas of positive PAS staining were semiquantified and normalized against total tissues. c: cortex; om: outer medulla; im: inner medulla. Arrowheads show the same tubules in serial renal sections before and after α-amylase digestion. Representative images of $n = 5$ each group. $^{****}P < 0.0001$.

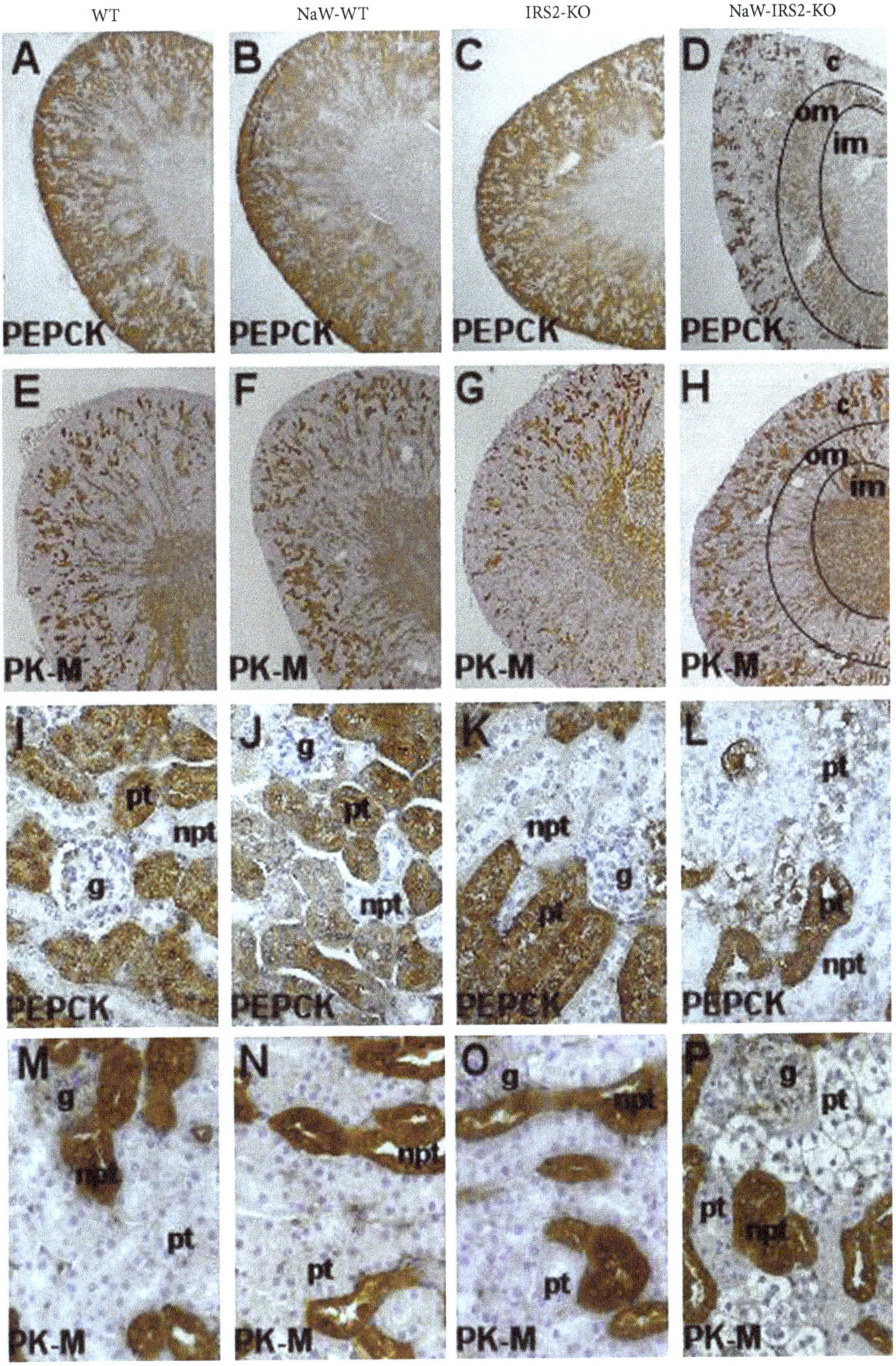

FIGURE 2: Zonation of metabolic enzymes in the kidney from NaW-IRS2-KO mice. The gluconeogenic enzyme PEPCK (a–d) and the glycolytic enzyme PK-M (e–h) were immunodetected in formalin-fixed paraffin-embedded kidneys from untreated WT (WT), treated WT (NaW-WT), untreated IRS2-KO (IRS2-KO), and treated IRS2-KO (NaW-IRS2-KO) mice. (i–l) Magnifications of the renal cortex from (a)–(d), respectively. (m–p) Magnifications of the renal cortex from (e)–(h), respectively. c: cortex; om: outer medulla; im: inner medulla, pt: proximal tubule; npt: nonproximal tubule; g: glomerulus. Representative images of $n = 5$ each group.

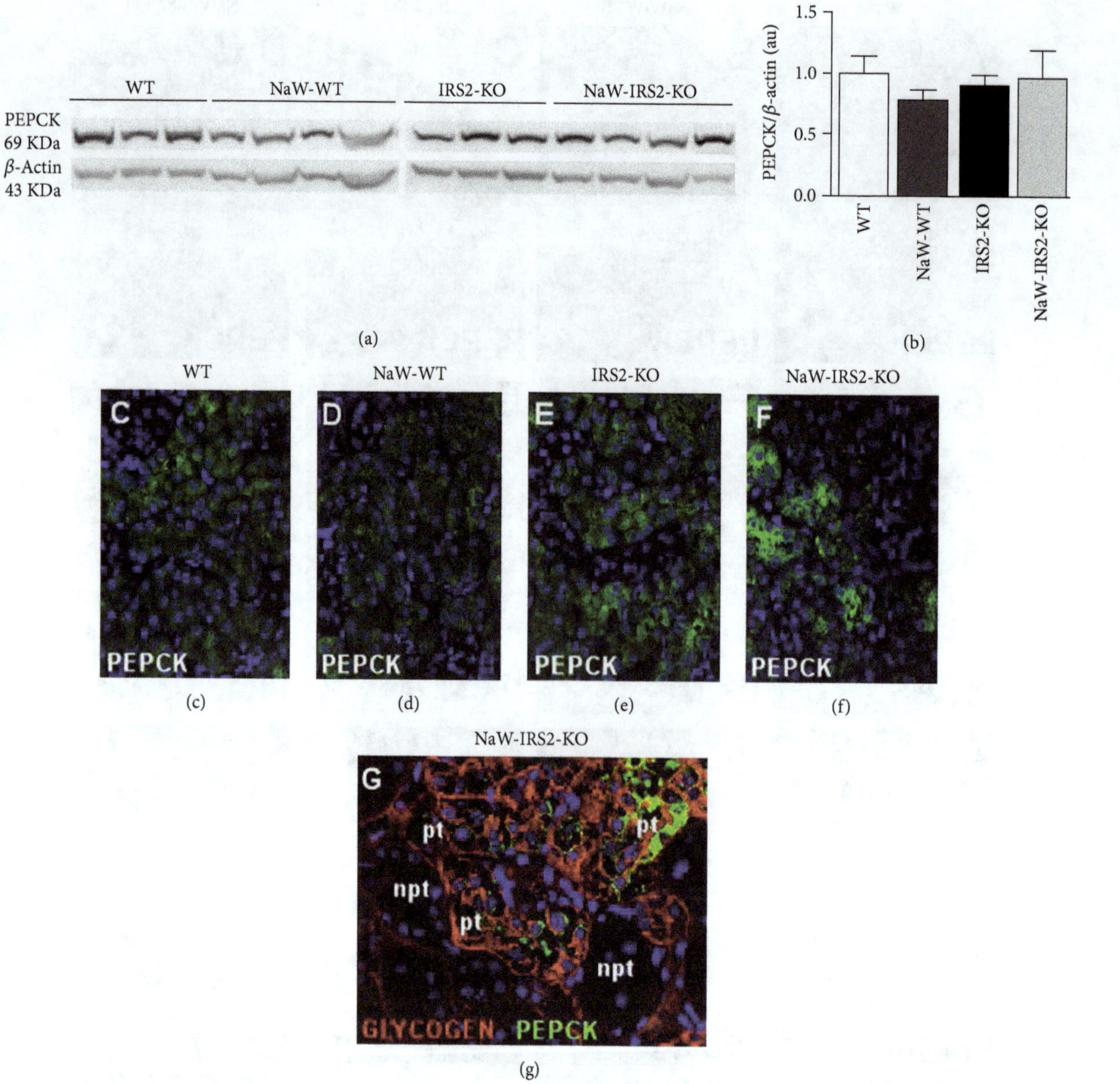

FIGURE 3: Protein expression of the gluconeogenic enzyme PEPCK in the kidney from NaW-IRS2-KO mice. Western blot analysis of PEPCK in the total kidney from untreated WT (WT), treated WT (NaW-WT), untreated IRS2-KO (IRS2-KO), and treated IRS2-KO (NaW-IRS2-KO) mice (a, b). (c–f) Immunofluorescence analysis of PEPCK in the cortex from WT, NaW-WT, IRS2-KO, and NaW-IRS2-KO kidneys. (g) Combined glycogen (red) and PEPCK (green) detection in kidneys from NaW-IRS2-KO mice without α-amylase treatment. DAPI was used for nuclear staining. pt: proximal tubule, npt: nonproximal tubule. Representative images of $n = 5$ each group.

the context of IRS2 ablation generated a disarrangement of cortical glycogen metabolism, which was concentrated in proximal tubules.

Interestingly, despite that the immunohistochemical data showed an apparent reduction in the intensity of PEPCK immunostaining in the kidney cortex between NaW-IRS2-KO and the other groups (Figures 2(a)–2(d) and 2(i)–2(l)), Western blot analysis revealed no significant differences in the level of expression of PEPCK in whole kidney samples (Figures 3(a) and 3(b)). Given that immunoperoxidase analysis produced strong signal amplification, we performed immunofluorescence analysis to study PEPCK expression and distribution with more detail. Confocal analysis showed no significant differences among samples from WT, NaW-WT, and IRS2-KO mice (Figures 3(c)–3(e), resp.), but a great variability in PEPCK signal among proximal tubules from NaW-IRS2-KO mice was observed, with some proximal tubules showing enhanced reaction and others showing very poor levels (Figure 3(f)), which was further confirmed by a combination of PAS staining and PEPCK immunofluorescence (Figure 3(g)).

Given that one main intracellular target of NaW is ERK1/2, which has been shown to mediate NaW-dependent glycogen production in hepatocytes [13], we studied in situ phosphorylation of this signaling molecule to assess its role in renal glycogen accumulation in the IRS2-KO model.

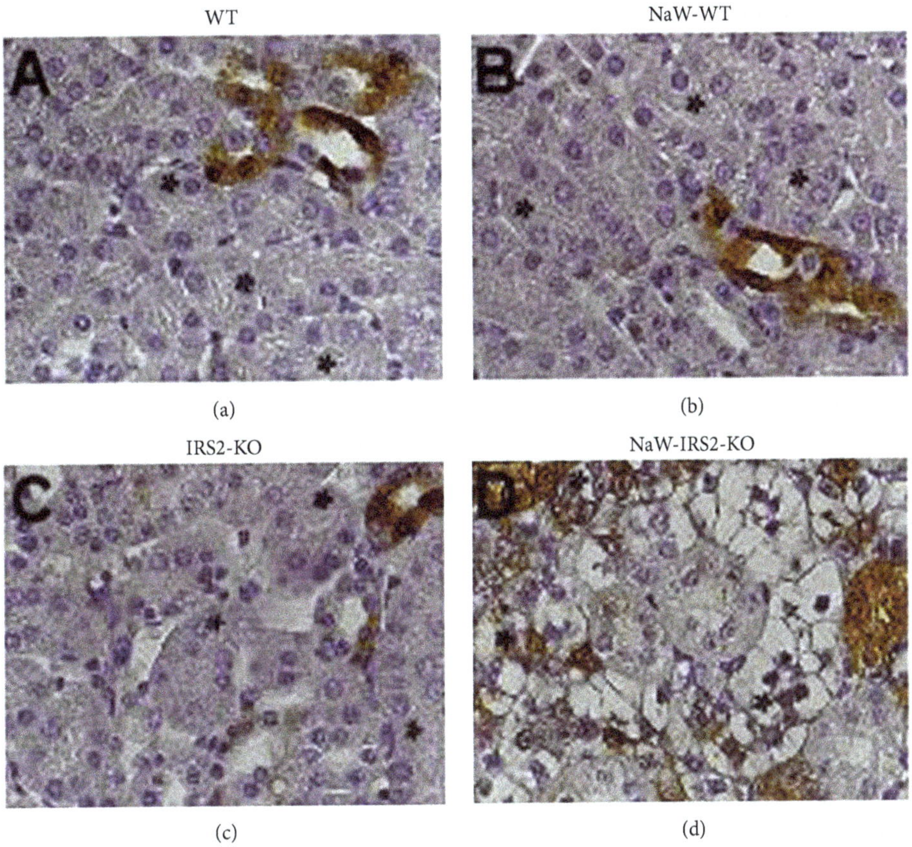

FIGURE 4: NaW-induced ERK1/2 activation in proximal tubules from the IRS2-KO kidney. Activation of ERK1/2 was analyzed in situ by immunodetection of phosphorylated residues Thr202/Tyr204 in formalin-fixed paraffin-embedded kidneys from (a) untreated WT (WT), (b) treated WT (NaW-WT), (c) untreated IRS2-KO (IRS2-KO), and (d) treated IRS2-KO (NaW-IRS2-KO) mice. Asterisks: proximal tubule. Representative images of $n = 4$ each group.

Interestingly, phosphorylation of ERK1/2 was detected in the kidney from both untreated WT and IRS2-KO mice, but only in nonproximal tubules (Figures 4(a) and 4(c), resp.). NaW treatment had no evident effect on further activation of ERK1/2 in the kidney from WT mice (Figure 4(b)), but instead it stimulated ERK1/2 phosphorylation in proximal tubules from IRS2-KO mice (Figure 4(d)).

4. Discussion

Despite the relevance of the kidney in glucose homeostasis and the well-known antidiabetic properties of NaW, only one study has addressed its effect on renal tissue, showing that glycogen accumulation in renal tubules, which is the most characteristic histopathological lesion related to the diabetic kidney, was absent in NaW-treated WT diabetic rats compared with the untreated diabetic group [15]. Given that NaW mimics most of insulin effects but acts through different downstream effectors, in the present work, we aimed to extend our understanding regarding its effects on renal glucose metabolism by using the diabetic IRS2-KO mouse model that shows reduced hepatic glycogen metabolism [2, 4]. On this basis, we hypothesized that this diabetic model is characterized by decreased glycogen accumulation in the liver and increased glycogen accumulation in the kidney. Interestingly, a previous report showed that IRS2 mRNA expression was higher in the mouse kidney than in the liver [17]. However, despite these differences, no significant morphological alterations were detected between kidneys from WT and IRS2-KO mice [4, 17, present study].

NaW treatment normalized glycemia but not insulinemia in IRS2-KO mice, in agreement with a previous work where improved glucose tolerance was not associated with enhanced peripheral insulin sensitivity, but rather with increased β-cell mass and replication and a reduction in β-cell apoptosis [4]. Indeed, IRS2-KO mice showed altered hepatic glucose metabolism, with lower glycogen levels and a marked decrease in the ability of insulin to suppress hepatic glucose production [2, 4], a phenotype that was not improved by NaW treatment [4]. Conversely, NaW has been previously shown to restore hepatic glycogen metabolism in other diabetic animal models with an intact insulin pathway [11], strongly suggesting that IRS2 is associated with hepatic insulin-mimetic effects of NaW.

Insulin signaling negatively modulates hepatic and renal gluconeogenesis by inhibiting expression of gluconeogenic enzymes [1, 5, 6], although renal regulation seems to differ from that of the liver [5]. The metabolic zonation of gluconeogenic enzymes in proximal tubules and glycolytic enzymes in nonproximal tubules is in agreement with the differential ability of each nephron portion to handle glucose [20, 21]. In the present work, we observed that PEPCK immunostaining was severely reduced only in those cortical proximal tubules affected by glycogenic alteration in NaW-IRS2-KO mice. It has been reported that NaW, as an insulin-mimetic agent, downregulates PEPCK expression in the liver from WT diabetic rats [22] and in human proximal tubules *in vitro* [23]. However, previous findings described an inconsistent effect of NaW in downregulating PEPCK in the liver from IRS2-KO mice [4], suggesting that IRS2 expression is required. Although further analysis is needed, we show that NaW is also unable to downregulate renal PEPCK expression in the context of IRS2 ablation, and therefore the preservation of PEPCK total protein levels in the kidney from NaW-IRS2-KO compared to IRS2-KO mice might be explained by overexpression in proximal tubules not affected, together with downregulation in proximal tubules affected by glycogen accumulation, which in combination may not be reflected in Western blot from the total kidney. Thus, the reduced expression of PEPCK may be the consequence of cell death after extensive glycogen accumulation [7, 9] rather than a direct downregulating effect exerted by NaW on the expression of gluconeogenic enzymes, as reduced immunodetection is only observed in proximal tubules that show severe glycogenic alterations.

One main and unexpected finding of our preliminary work is the absence of tubular alterations related to abnormal glycogen accumulation in diabetic IRS2-KO mice. We expected some level of glycogen deposition due to the diabetic phenotype. It has been shown that expression and/or activation of GS may be involved in abnormal glycogen accumulation of diabetic kidney [8, 9, 24]. GS is regulated by glucose 6-phosphate (G6P) allosteric activation and by inactivating phosphorylation [1, 8, 25]. Fully phosphorylated GS is considered to be inactive. Noteworthy, it has been described that glycogen-storing cells are mainly originated by nonproximal tubules in kidneys from WT diabetic rats [7–10] and that NaW treatment reverses this phenotype [15]. However, no glycogen-storing cells were detected in the kidney from diabetic IRS2-KO mice, indicating that hyperglycemia itself is not enough to promote renal glycogen synthesis. At this regard, it has been reported that adiponectin activates AMP-activated protein kinase (AMPK) in distal tubules and thick ascending limb to phosphorylate and inhibit GS, inhibiting in turn glycogen accumulation [8]. Although the involvement of IRS2 in the renal adiponectin-AMPK-GS axis remains to be elucidated, we detected activation of ERK1/2 in renal proximal tubules from IRS2-KO but not from WT mice after NaW treatment, strongly suggesting that this signaling molecule participates in NaW-induced glycogen production in IRS2-KO kidney. In agreement, ERK1/2 is pivotal for most insulin-mimetic effects of NaW, especially glycogen production in hepatocytes [11, 13]. Overstimulation of ERK1/2 by NaW in the absence of IRS2 may aberrantly activate glycogen synthesis, suggesting that insulin signaling through IRS2 keeps ERK1/2 activity restrained in proximal tubules to avoid glycogen production in WT mice.

Then, what is happening in the kidney from IRS2-KO mice after NaW treatment? Our preliminary data show that when IRS2 is absent and mice are treated with NaW, glycogen synthesis is activated in cortical proximal tubules, suggesting that IRS2 somehow inhibits glycogen accumulation in this particular tubular structure, possibly by keeping ERK1/2 inactive or at a low rate. During hyperglycemia, proximal tubules reabsorb more glucose from the glomerular ultrafiltrate [26]. However, it has been proposed that they just participate in transepithelial glucose movement but are not able to phosphorylate it into G6P, because proximal tubules virtually lack hexokinase activity [20, 21]. Then, reabsorbed luminal glucose cannot be directly phosphorylated into G6P, the actual precursor/activator of glycogen synthesis [1, 25]. Other possibility is indirect glycogen synthesis from G6P provided by gluconeogenesis, which is an important pathway in hepatic glycogen synthesis [27]. Moreover, NaW has been shown to inhibit G6Pase activity [12], the gluconeogenic enzyme that converts G6P into free glucose, but has no direct effect on FBPase activity [28]. Hence, during normal or enhanced gluconeogenesis in combination with reduced G6Pase activity, accumulation of G6P might be the triggering mechanism for glycogen accumulation, despite that GS is phosphorylated. Indeed, although phosphorylation leads to inactivation of GS, the activity can be restored in the presence of the allosteric activator G6P [25]. Thus, we speculate that NaW cannot inhibit gluconeogenesis in renal cortical proximal tubules in the absence of IRS2 that, together with NaW-induced G6Pase inhibition, favors G6P accumulation. This idea is sustained by the fact that gluconeogenic enzymes are not uniformly expressed along the proximal tubule, with higher levels in cortical proximal tubules [20] where we observed the glycogenic effect. Indeed, a recent report showed that targeted deletion of G6Pase in the kidney induces glycogen accumulation specifically in cortical proximal tubules [29], producing a pattern of tubular alteration similar to that observed in NaW-IRS2-KO mice. Accumulation of renal glycogen in the animal model studied by Clar et al. [29] confirmed its nephrotoxicity in the long term. While the effect of NaW on renal function in KO-IRS2 mice remains to be established, our histological data suggest that NaW-KO-IRS2 mice have nephropathy, although maybe incipient because of the short treatment compared with the 6 months of the experiment by Clar et al. [29].

NaW has been widely studied as an insulin-mimetic and antidiabetic drug because of its low hypoglycemic action, but other undesirable effects remain to be established [11]. The fact that NaW treatment affects glycogen metabolism in renal proximal tubules in IRS2-KO mice, similar to glycogen storage disease type 1a [29], turns on a red light on its potential use as a drug for type 2 diabetes treatment. Although IRS2 mutations are unusual and have not been associated with human type 2 diabetes, enhanced phosphorylation on serine/threonine residues, many of which negatively regulate IRS2 function [30], may affect the proper IRS2 downstream signals, which in turn would affect NaW renal effects. Indeed, only one study on human subjects has reached the clinical trial phase with inconclusive results [16], and a study with an organovanadium compound for the treatment of diabetes mellitus (with activity analogous to that of NaW) reached preclinical phase II but was terminated after 3 months because of renal complications (http://www.biospace.com/

news/akesispharmaceuticalsdiscontinuessoleclinical/123583), indicating that the use of this kind of drugs might be specifically related to renal alterations *in vivo*. However, understanding the reasons behind clinical failure is essential for clinical development. Thus, a kidney-specific IRS2 deletion model would be critical to further understand the complex and particular roles of IRS2 in renal insulin signaling, glycogen metabolism, and NaW effects and also the participation of renal IRS2 in whole-body glucose homeostasis. In this sense, whole-body IRS2-KO mice showed impaired suppression of gluconeogenesis and reduced glycogen synthesis in the liver, but a liver-specific IRS2 deletion model showed that IRS2 is not required for glucose homeostasis, and rather extrahepatic IRS2-dependent mechanisms regulate this process [31].

5. Conclusions

In conclusion, our preliminary study showed two interesting and totally unexpected facts: (1) young diabetic IRS2-KO mice are protected against glycogen accumulation in renal tubules despite hyperglycemia and (2) NaW treatment normalized glycemia in IRS2-KO mice but induced glycogen accumulation in the kidney, specifically in proximal tubules from the cortex. Although more studies are needed, we propose that IRS2 is involved in pathological glycogen accumulation in the diabetic kidney and that the use of NaW in the context of altered IRS2 signaling induces abnormal renal glycogen accumulation that should be considered a new undesirable effect.

Conflicts of Interest

The authors declare that there is no conflict of interest regarding the publication of this article.

Acknowledgments

The authors thank Joanna Tereszczuk and Germán Osorio for the technical support. Microscopic images were obtained at Centro de Microscopía Avanzada (CMA BIO-BIO), Universidad de Concepción, Chile. The work was supported by Dirección de Investigación y Desarrollo de la Universidad Austral de Chile (DID-UACh) to Alejandro J. Yáñez, Fondo Nacional de Desarrollo Científico y Tecnológico (FONDECYT) (11160854) from the Chilean State to Romina Bertinat, and Proyecto PIA-CONICYT ECM-12 (CMA BIO-BIO) to Francisco Nualart.

References

[1] A. R. Saltiel, "Insulin signaling in the control of glucose and lipid homeostasis," *Handbook of Experimental Pharmacology*, vol. 233, pp. 51–71, 2016.

[2] S. F. Previs, D. J. Withers, J. M. Ren, M. F. White, and G. I. Shulman, "Contrasting effects of IRS-1 versus IRS-2 gene disruption on carbohydrate and lipid metabolism *in vivo*," *Journal of Biological Chemistry*, vol. 275, no. 50, pp. 38990–38994, 2000.

[3] A. C. P. Thirone, C. Huang, and A. Klip, "Tissue-specific roles of IRS proteins in insulin signaling and glucose transport," *Trends in Endocrinology & Metabolism*, vol. 17, no. 2, pp. 72–78, 2006.

[4] J. M. Oliveira, S. A. Rebuffat, R. Gasa et al., "Tungstate promotes β-cell survival in $Irs2^{-/-}$ mice," *American Journal of Physiology-Endocrinology and Metabolism*, vol. 306, no. 1, pp. E36–E47, 2014.

[5] L. J. Hale and R. J. M. Coward, "Insulin signalling to the kidney in health and disease," *Clinical Science*, vol. 124, no. 6, pp. 351–370, 2013.

[6] G. Pandey, K. Shankar, E. Makhija et al., "Reduced insulin receptor expression enhances proximal tubule gluconeogenesis," *Journal of Cellular Biochemistry*, vol. 118, no. 2, pp. 276–285, 2017.

[7] S. Bamri-Ezzine, Z. J. Ao, I. Londoño, D. Gingras, and M. Bendayan, "Apoptosis of tubular epithelial cells in glycogen nephrosis during diabetes," *Laboratory Investigation*, vol. 83, no. 7, pp. 1069–1080, 2003.

[8] P. G. Cammisotto, I. Londono, D. Gingras, and M. Bendayan, "Control of glycogen synthase through ADIPOR1-AMPK pathway in renal distal tubules of normal and diabetic rats," *American Journal of Physiology-Renal Physiology*, vol. 294, no. 4, pp. F881–F889, 2008.

[9] R. Gatica, R. Bertinat, P. Silva et al., "Over-expression of muscle glycogen synthase in human diabetic nephropathy," *Histochemistry and Cell Biology*, vol. 143, no. 3, pp. 313–324, 2015.

[10] J. Kang, X. S. Dai, T. B. Yu, B. Wen, and Z. W. Yang, "Glycogen accumulation in renal tubules, a key morphological change in the diabetic rat kidney," *Acta Diabetologica*, vol. 42, no. 2, pp. 110–116, 2005.

[11] R. Bertinat, F. Nualart, X. Li, A. J. Yáñez, and R. Gomis, "Preclinical and clinical studies for sodium tungstate: application in humans," *Journal of Clinical & Cellular Immunology*, vol. 6, no. 1, 2015.

[12] J. D. Foster, S. E. Young, T. D. Brandt, and R. C. Nordlie, "Tungstate: a potent inhibitor of multifunctional glucose-6-phosphatase," *Archives of Biochemistry and Biophysics*, vol. 354, no. 1, pp. 125–132, 1998.

[13] J. E. Domínguez, M. C. Muñoz, D. Zafra et al., "The antidiabetic agent sodium tungstate activates glycogen synthesis through an insulin receptor-independent pathway," *Journal of Biological Chemistry*, vol. 278, no. 44, pp. 42785–42794, 2003.

[14] D. Zafra, L. Nocito, J. Domínguez, and J. J. Guinovart, "Sodium tungstate activates glycogen synthesis through a non-canonical mechanism involving G-proteins," *FEBS Letters*, vol. 587, no. 3, pp. 291–296, 2013.

[15] A. Barberà, R. R. Gomis, N. Prats et al., "Tungstate is an effective antidiabetic agent in streptozotocin-induced diabetic rats: a long-term study," *Diabetologia*, vol. 44, no. 4, pp. 507–513, 2001.

[16] F. Hanzu, R. Gomis, M. J. Coves et al., "Proof-of-concept trial on the efficacy of sodium tungstate in human obesity," *Diabetes, Obesity and Metabolism*, vol. 12, no. 11, pp. 1013–1018, 2010.

[17] R. M. Carew, M. Sadagurski, R. Goldschmeding, F. Martin, M. F. White, and D. P. Brazil, "Deletion of Irs2 causes reduced kidney size in mice: role for inhibition of GSK3β?," *BMC Developmental Biology*, vol. 10, no. 1, p. 73, 2010.

[18] R. Gatica, R. Bertinat, P. Silva et al., "Altered expression and localization of insulin receptor in proximal tubule cells from human and rat diabetic kidney," *Journal of Cellular Biochemistry*, vol. 114, no. 3, pp. 639–649, 2013.

[19] G. Schaart, R. P. Hesselink, H. A. Keizer, G. van Kranenburg, M. R. Drost, and M. K. Hesselink, "A modified PAS stain combined with immunofluorescence for quantitative analyses of glycogen in muscle sections," *Histochemistry and Cell Biology*, vol. 122, no. 2, pp. 161–169, 2004.

[20] J. W. Lee, C. L. Chou, and M. A. Knepper, "Deep sequencing in microdissected renal tubules identifies nephron segment-specific transcriptomes," *Journal of the American Society of Nephrology*, vol. 26, no. 11, pp. 2669–2677, 2015.

[21] A. J. Yañez, H. C. Ludwig, R. Bertinat et al., "Different involvement for aldolase isoenzymes in kidney glucose metabolism: aldolase B but not aldolase A colocalizes and forms a complex with FBPase," *Journal of Cellular Physiology*, vol. 202, no. 3, pp. 743–753, 2005.

[22] L. Nocito, D. Zafra, J. Calbó, J. Domínguez, and J. J. Guinovart, "Tungstate reduces the expression of gluconeogenic enzymes in STZ rats," *PLoS One*, vol. 7, no. 8, article e42305, 2012.

[23] R. Bertinat, F. Westermeier, P. Silva et al., "Anti-diabetic agent sodium tungstate induces the secretion of pro- and anti-inflammatory cytokines by human kidney cells," *Journal of Cellular Physiology*, vol. 232, no. 2, pp. 355–362, 2017.

[24] X. Lau, Y. Zhang, D. J. Kelly, and D. I. Stapleton, "Attenuation of Armanni–Ebstein lesions in a rat model of diabetes by a new anti-fibrotic, anti-inflammatory agent, FT011," *Diabetologia*, vol. 56, no. 3, pp. 675–679, 2013.

[25] M. Bouskila, R. W. Hunter, A. F. M. Ibrahim et al., "Allosteric regulation of glycogen synthase controls glycogen synthesis in muscle," *Cell Metabolism*, vol. 12, no. 5, pp. 456–466, 2010.

[26] V. Vallon, "The proximal tubule in the pathophysiology of the diabetic kidney," *American Journal of Physiology-Regulatory, Integrative and Comparative Physiology*, vol. 300, no. 5, pp. R1009–R1022, 2011.

[27] T. H. van Dijk, F. H. van der Sluijs, C. H. Wiegman et al., "Acute inhibition of hepatic glucose-6-phosphatase does not affect gluconeogenesis but directs gluconeogenic flux toward glycogen in fasted rats. A pharmacological study with the chlorogenic acid derivative S4048," *The Journal of Biological Chemistry*, vol. 276, no. 28, pp. 25727–25735, 2001.

[28] R. Bertinat, F. Nualart, J. C. Slebe, and A. J. Yáñez, "Sodium tungstate mimics insulin effect on nuclear translocation of FBPase in rat liver," *Postdoc Journal*, vol. 5, no. 3, 2017.

[29] J. Clar, B. Gri, J. Calderaro et al., "Targeted deletion of kidney glucose-6 phosphatase leads to nephropathy," *Kidney International*, vol. 86, no. 4, pp. 747–756, 2014.

[30] K. D. Copps and M. F. White, "Regulation of insulin sensitivity by serine/threonine phosphorylation of insulin receptor substrate proteins IRS1 and IRS2," *Diabetologia*, vol. 55, no. 10, pp. 2565–2582, 2012.

[31] M. Simmgen, C. Knauf, M. Lopez et al., "Liver-specific deletion of insulin receptor substrate 2 does not impair hepatic glucose and lipid metabolism in mice," *Diabetologia*, vol. 49, no. 3, pp. 552–561, 2006.

8

The Humanistic and Economic Burden Associated with Anxiety and Depression among Adults with Comorbid Diabetes and Hypertension

Kimberly Wallace,[1] **Xiaohui Zhao**,[2] **Ranjita Misra**,[3] **and Usha Sambamoorthi**[2]

[1]*School of Nursing, West Virginia University, Morgantown 26506, USA*
[2]*School of Pharmacy, West Virginia University, Morgantown, 26506 WV, USA*
[3]*School of Public Health, West Virginia University, Morgantown, 26506 WV, USA*

Correspondence should be addressed to Xiaohui Zhao; xozhao@mix.wvu.edu

Academic Editor: Ilaria Campesi

We conducted a retrospective cross-sectional study to estimate the humanistic and economic burden associated with depression and anxiety among adults with comorbid diabetes and hypertension. Pooled data from the 2013 and 2015 Medical Expenditure Panel Survey were used to include adults (≥18 years old) who were alive and diagnosed with both diabetes and hypertension during the observation period. We assessed the humanistic burden with health-related quality of life (HRQoL) and economic burden with the total annual healthcare expenditures. Depending on the presence/absence of depression and anxiety, the study sample was divided into four groups (i.e., no depression/anxiety, depression only, anxiety only, and depression and anxiety). Multivariable regression analyses were used to evaluate the associations between the depression/anxiety categories and disease burden measures. The incremental burden associated with depression and/or anxiety was estimated with the counterfactual recycled prediction. Of the 4560 adults with comorbid diabetes and hypertension, 13.2% reported depression only, 8.7% reported anxiety only, and 7.7% reported both. Results from adjusted analyses indicated that the presence/absence of depression and anxiety was associated with significantly poorer HRQoL, especially on the mental component. Having either depression or anxiety corresponded to reduced mental component summary scores by more than four points. The reduction was as high as 10.35 points when both conditions occurred. Comparing to adults without depression or anxiety, the per-capital incremental annual healthcare expenditures were $4607 for the depression group, $2481 for the anxiety group, and $8709 for adults with both conditions. Furthermore, adults with depression and anxiety were 58% more likely to spend at least 10% of annual household income on healthcare as compared to those with neither the conditions. Our results highlight the needs for integrating cost-effective mental health services into diabetes management to improve the HRQoL and reduce healthcare costs for adults with comorbid diabetes and hypertension.

1. Introduction

Comorbid chronic conditions can post an enormous challenge in diabetes care. Hypertension is one of the most common comorbid conditions due to a considerable overlap of risk factors [1]. Approximately 75% of individuals diagnosed with diabetes have concomitant hypertension, representing nearly 23 million adults in the United States (US) [1, 2]. Individuals with multiple chronic conditions usually have impaired mental health [3]. Like many other chronic conditions, diabetes and hypertension are independently associated with a higher prevalence of mental conditions, particularly depression and anxiety [4]. The prevalence of depression and anxiety ranges from 15% to 35% among individuals with diabetes [5, 6] and 22% to 56% among those with hypertension [7, 8].

The presence of depression and/or anxiety can impose substantial disease burdens on adults with comorbid diabetes and hypertension as they ranked amongst the top ten causes of disease burden in the 2013 Global Burden of Disease Study [9]. The presence of either the condition can complicate the course of diabetes and hypertension by causing increased inflammation, unhealthy lifestyles, and poor adherence to treatments [10]. Furthermore, depression and anxiety can lead to significant functional impairments, resulting in poor quality of life [11, 12]. Results from several observational studies have indicated that depression and anxiety manifest themselves in multiple facets of the quality of life for individuals with diabetes, including functional, cognitive, and emotional domains [13–15].

The impairment in quality of life also represents a considerable economic burden on patients, their family members, and the whole healthcare system due to high use of healthcare services. Diabetes is one of the most expensive chronic conditions in the US, with an estimated medical expenditure of $237 billion in 2017 [16]. Based on the finding of a recent study, the national burden of comorbid diabetes and hypertension could exceed $350 billion [17]. Depression and anxiety have been indicated with higher risks of diabetes complications and heart diseases, leading to excess costs from more physician office visits, emergency room or inpatient admissions, and prescription consumption [18, 19].

Depression, anxiety, diabetes, and hypertension are closely linked and affect a substantial proportion of the US population. Individuals that carry more than one, or even all four conditions, face unique challenges regarding access to the healthcare resources and the emotional state to achieve optimal treatment goals. Evaluating the burden of mental comorbidities has indispensable roles in achieving these goals because it helps direct resource allocation for policymakers. Like diabetes and hypertension, depression and anxiety also have substantial overlap in occurrence [20]. Although previous studies have evaluated the impact of depression and anxiety on individuals with diabetes or hypertension separately, no study has comprehensively quantified the effect of either of the condition alone. Furthermore, researchers have reported that treating comorbid depression and anxiety could be more challenging than managing each condition alone [21]. Research attention on comorbid depression and anxiety is therefore warranted to help understand the unmet needs in providing care to patients with such complex conditions. Therefore, the objective of this study is to estimate the humanistic and economic burden of depression and/or anxiety among adults with comorbid diabetes and hypertension.

2. Materials and Methods

2.1. Study Design. This study utilized a retrospective cross-sectional design.

2.2. Data Source. We pooled data from the 2013 and 2015 Medical Expenditure Panel Survey (MEPS). The MEPS is a nationally representative survey of noninstitutionalized adults. It collects information on demographics and various facets of healthcare, including medical conditions, access to care, health-related quality of life (HRQoL), and medical expenditures. The MEPS employs a panel design, in which participants were followed for two years. As recommended by MEPS, we utilized alternate years to avoid duplicate observations of the same participant [22].

2.3. Study Sample. Our descriptive sample consisted of 4560 adults (aged 18 or older) who were alive and diagnosed with both diabetes and hypertension during the study period (2013 and 2015). Diabetes and hypertension were identified from the full-year consolidated file based on queries regarding the diagnosis of specific conditions or medical condition files using the clinical classification codes (49–50 for diabetes, 98–99 for hypertension). These conditions were reported by households, recorded by professional coders, and then converted into clinical classification codes by MEPS researchers. Because the MEPS only collects data on HRQoL through self-administered questionnaires (SAQ), we further restricted our sample to adults who were eligible for SAQ to analyze humanistic outcomes. For economic outcomes, the analytic cohort only included adults with positive expenditures.

2.4. Dependent Variables

2.4.1. Humanistic Outcome: Health-Related Quality of Life (HRQoL). MEPS measures HRQoL with the 12-item short-form health survey version 2 (SF-12v2). The SF-12v2 is a widely used generic measure for HRQoL in health services research. MEPS researchers combined, scored, and weighted the responses to create physical component summary (PCS) and mental component summary (MCS) scores. The scores range from 0 to 100, with higher scores indicating better HRQoL related to physical and/or mental health [23].

2.4.2. Economic Outcomes: Total Annual Healthcare Expenditures. The MEPS is considered as the most complete source of data on healthcare expenditures. Healthcare expenditures are measured as any payment to healthcare providers (i.e., hospitals, outpatient facilities, private practices, and long-term care facilities) for healthcare services (i.e., inpatient, outpatient, prescription, dental, vision, and home health services). Payers include patients or their families paying for a service out-of-pocket as well as third-party payers (Medicare, Medicaid, private insurance, Veterans Administration, Tricare, HMOs, etc.). Total annual per-person healthcare expenditures were calculated as the sum of all medical payments from all payers. We conducted separate analyses on total expenditures, those paid by third parties and out-of-pocket (OOP) spending from patients. Third-party expenditures were calculated as the difference between total expenditures and OOP spending. All expenditures were adjusted to 2015 US dollars using the consumer price index for medical services from the Bureau of Labor Statistics.

2.4.3. Economic Outcomes: OOP Spending Burden. The economic burden from OOP spending was measured as the percentage of annual household income spent on healthcare as OOP payments [24]. We used a conventional cut-off of 10% to define high burden [25].

2.5. Key Independent Variable

2.5.1. Depression/Anxiety Categories. We identified depression and anxiety from the medical condition files using the clinical classification code of "657" and "651." A variable with four categories (depression and anxiety, depression only, anxiety only, and no depression/anxiety) was created based on the presence/absence of depression and anxiety.

2.6. Other Independent Variables. We selected other independent variables under the guidance of the Andersen's behavioral model [26], in which an individual's use of healthcare services and associated outcomes is considered as a function of predisposing factors, enabling factors, need factors, personal health practices, and external environment. We included sex (male/female), race/ethnicity (Whites/African-American/Latino/other racial minorities), and age (18–39/40–54/55–64/65–74/75+) as predisposing factors. Enabling factors were comprised of marital status (married/not married), education (less than high school/high school/more than high school), family poverty status (poor/near poor/middle income/high income), health insurance (private/public/uninsured), and prescription insurance status (yes/no). Need factors included having a chronic condition (yes/no) other than diabetes and hypertension from a list of eight conditions (asthma, arthritis, cancer, chronic obstructive pulmonary disease, heart disease, and stroke), perceived physical and mental health status (excellent/very good, good, and fair/poor), and pain interference (mild/no, moderate, and a lot/extreme). Personal health practice factors included obesity (yes/no), smoking status (current smoker/others), and physical activities (five times or more/week, less than five times/week). We also used geographic region (northeast/midwest/south/west) of residency to account for variations due to the external environment.

2.7. Statistical Analyses. We used chi-square tests to determine statistically significant differences across study groups for categorical variables and Student's independent *t*-tests for continuous variables. Multivariable regression analyses were used to examine the association between the depression/anxiety categories and disease burden measures. Ordinary least square regressions were employed to analyze MCS and PCS scores. Logistic regressions were used for binary outcomes such as OOP spending burden. To overcome common challenges associated with modeling expenditures (e.g., high positive skewness and heteroscedasticity), we used generalized linear models with a log link function and gamma family distribution for expenditure outcomes [27].

To estimate excess healthcare expenditures contributed by depression and/or anxiety, we utilized counterfactual recycled prediction. This technique is preferable because, by creating counterfactual scenarios, it allows for adjustment for differences in characteristics across all groups (i.e., depression and anxiety, depression only, anxiety only, and neither depression nor anxiety) [28]. To account for the complex survey design of the MEPS, we utilized the survey procedures in the statistical analysis software (SAS) version 9.4 (Cary, NC, USA) and STATA 14. As recommended by MEPS researchers, we computed annualized weights by dividing personal weights by the number of years pooled (two, in our study) [29]. Annualized SAQ weights were used for analyzing MCS and PCS.

3. Results

3.1. Description of Study Sample. The study sample was almost evenly female (50.1%) and male (49.9%). The majority were white (62%), aged greater than 55 (76%), with multimorbidity (73%), and adults who had at least a high school education (80%). Twenty-seven percent of individuals considered themselves as having excellent or very good physical health while 48% reported having excellent or very good mental health (Table 1).

Within our sample, approximately one-fifth had either depression (13.2%) or anxiety (8.7%), and 7.7% had both conditions. We observed significant differences in the prevalence of depression and/or anxiety across all predisposing factors, enabling factors, need factors, personal health practices, and external environment with the exception for education. For example, females with comorbid diabetes and hypertension reported a significantly higher rate of depression and anxiety, either alone or together, as compared to their male counterparts. Similar patterns were observed for adults with public insurances relative to private insurances or no insurance, adults reporting multimorbidity in addition to diabetes and hypertension versus those without additional chronic conditions, and adults with severe pain interference as compared to those with mild or no pain interference (Table 1).

3.2. Humanistic Outcomes: Physical and Mental Component Summary Scores (PCS and MCS). Adults with depression and/or anxiety reported significant lower health scores, both physically and mentally, as compared to those with neither the condition. Across the four groups, adults with both depression and anxiety reported the lowest MCS scores while those with depression had the lowest PCS scores (Table 1). However, after adjusting for all other covariates, we only observed significant differences in MCS scores. Results from adjusted analyses indicated that, compared to adults with neither depression nor anxiety, the MCS scores were 10.35 points lower for those with depression and anxiety and 7.67 and 4.88 points lower for those with either depression or anxiety, respectively (Table 2).

3.3. Economic Outcomes: Total Annual Healthcare Expenditures. Adults with depression and/or anxiety also had significantly higher annual healthcare expenditures than those with neither the condition (Table 3). Adults with depression and anxiety had the highest expenditures at $28,832 per person per year, followed by those with either depression ($19,648) or anxiety ($16,990). After adjusting for all other factors that may influence healthcare expenditures, results from recycled predictions showed that the annual per-person mean healthcare expenditures were $20,963 (95% confidence interval (CI): $20,581–$21,329) for those with both depression and anxiety and $16,861

Table 1: Description of study sample by depression and anxiety categories among adults with comorbid diabetes and hypertension, using pooled data from the 2013 and 2015 Medical Expenditure Panel Survey.

	All		Depression and anxiety		Depression only		Anxiety only		No depression/ anxiety			
	N	Wt%	*N*	Wt row%	*N*	Wt row%	*N*	Wt row%	*N*	Wt row%	*p* value	sig
All	4560	100.0	309	7.7	561	13.2	366	8.7	3324	70.4		
Predisposing factors												
Sex											<0.001	***
Female	2477	50.1	227	10.9	368	16.5	227	10.3	1655	62.3		
Male	2083	49.9	82	4.4	193	10.0	139	7.0	1669	78.6		
Race/ethnicity											<0.001	***
White	1658	61.6	163	9.2	237	14.6	173	10.4	1085	65.8		
African-American	1267	16.1	51	4.0	140	11.1	90	6.3	986	78.6		
Latino	1210	14.4	80	6.8	156	13.2	87	6.4	887	73.6		
Others	425	7.9	15	4.5	28	6.9	16	4.2	366	84.4		
Age groups											<0.001	***
18–39 years	224	4.4	21	10.5	30	15.5	23	8.7	150	65.3		
40–54 years	1016	19.9	96	10.3	121	13.2	77	8.3	722	68.1		
55–64 years	1304	26.8	98	8.6	191	16.0	98	8.8	917	66.6		
65–74 years	1165	28.6	65	7.3	152	13.8	92	8.2	856	70.8		
75 years or older	851	20.3	29	3.7	67	8.4	76	9.4	679	78.5		
Enabling factors												
Marital status											<0.001	***
Married	2352	57.5	110	5.7	265	12.9	170	8.0	1807	73.3		
Not married	2208	42.5	199	10.3	296	13.6	196	9.5	1517	66.6		
Education level[†]											0.186	
<High school	1301	19.1	74	6.0	158	11.4	106	9.3	963	73.3		
High school	1447	34.2	110	8.9	174	12.9	126	9.2	1037	69.0		
>HS	1751	46.7	121	7.5	223	14.2	131	8.1	1276	70.2		
Poverty status[‡]											<0.001	***
Poor	1014	13.5	100	11.5	165	15.6	95	9.6	654	63.2		
Near poor	1174	22.7	88	9.4	138	13.2	105	10.3	843	67.1		
Middle income	1321	30.5	77	7.6	152	13.7	92	7.0	1000	71.6		
High income	1051	33.3	44	5.0	106	11.8	74	8.6	827	74.6		
Insurance coverage											<0.001	***
Private	2119	57.0	100	5.8	230	13.2	161	8.3	1628	72.7		
Public	2067	37.3	193	10.8	294	14.0	190	9.8	1390	65.4		
Uninsured	374	5.7	16	6.1	37	9.1	15	4.6	306	80.1		
Prescription insurance											0.020	*
Yes	1670	44.7	79	5.9	182	13.8	128	8.6	1281	71.7		
No	2890	55.3	230	9.1	379	12.8	238	8.7	2043	69.4		
Need factors												
Perceived physical health											<0.001	***
Excellent/very good	1037	26.7	36	4.3	85	9.2	69	8.0	847	78.5		
Good	1642	38.2	81	6.1	160	11.3	117	8.1	1284	74.6		
Fair/poor	1881	35.1	192	11.9	316	18.4	180	9.8	1193	59.8		
Perceived mental health											<0.001	***
Excellent/very good	1979	48.2	56	3.8	135	8.0	124	7.6	1664	80.6		
Good	1702	35.8	103	7.3	228	15.3	134	8.7	1237	68.6		
Fair/poor	879	16.0	150	20.1	198	24.5	108	11.6	423	43.8		

Table 1: Continued.

	All		Depression and anxiety		Depression only		Anxiety only		No depression/ anxiety			
	N	Wt%	*N*	Wt row%	*N*	Wt row%	*N*	Wt row%	*N*	Wt row%	*p* value	sig
Multimorbidity											<0.001	***
Yes	3179	72.6	198	8.6	369	15.3	212	8.8	1729	67.3		
No	1381	27.4	104	6.3	180	10.4	146	8.3	1525	75.0		
Pain interference											<0.001	***
None/little	2240	50.5	95	5.5	191	9.7	143	7.6	1811	77.3		
Moderate	757	17.5	58	8.4	103	14.4	64	8.6	532	68.6		
A lot/extreme	1204	25.0	136	12.1	228	20.2	132	11.2	708	56.6		
Not reported	359	7.1	20	5.9	39	11.3	27	7.5	273	75.3		
Personal health practice												
Obesity[†], [¶]											<0.001	***
Yes	2508	57.3	198	8.6	369	15.3	212	8.8	1729	67.3		
No	1955	42.7	104	6.3	180	10.4	146	8.3	1525	75.0		
Current smoker											<0.001	***
Yes	578	12.2	77	12.8	103	21.0	49	7.7	349	58.5		
No	3553	79.2	214	7.1	415	12.4	281	8.7	2643	71.7		
Not reported	429	8.6	18	5.5	43	9.7	36	9.1	332	75.7		
Exercise ≥ 5 times/week[†]											<0.001	***
Yes	1584	34.7	77	6.1	154	10.1	99	6.6	1254	77.2		
No	2938	65.3	229	8.5	402	14.9	266	9.8	2041	66.8		
External environment												
Region											0.027	*
Northeast	740	17.2	76	11.1	99	12.7	56	8.1	509	68.0		
Midwest	800	22.0	69	8.9	106	13.0	80	10.2	545	67.9		
South	2011	42.6	109	5.7	250	13.9	166	8.7	1486	71.7		
West	1009	18.3	55	7.6	106	12.4	64	7.2	784	72.8		

Note: study sample included adults (≥18 years old) with comorbid diabetes and hypertension who were alive in the observation year (2013/2015). Wt%: weighted percentages; Wt row%: weighted row percentages; Sig.: statistical significance level. [†]Some groups with missing data were not reported here due to small cell size (<10). [‡]Poverty status was calculated from the annual family income and family composition using the federal poverty line (FPL). Poor was defined as <100% FPL; near poor was defined as >100% FPL and <199% FPL; middle income was defined as >200% FPL and <399% FPL; high income was defined as >400% FPL. [¶]Obesity was defined as body mass index ≥ 30.0. $^{*}p < 0.05$; $^{**}0.001 < p < 0.01$; $^{***}p < 0.001$.

(95% CI: $16,533–$17,155) and $14,735 (95% CI: $14,466–$14,992) for those with either depression or anxiety. The expenditures in these three groups were all significantly higher than the group with neither condition, with an incremental expenditure of $8709 (95% CI: $8550–$8861), $4607 (95% CI: $4523–$4687), and $2481 (95% CI: $2436–$2525), respectively (Table 3).

Similar results were found for analyses on third-party expenditures and out-of-pocket (OOP) spending (Table 3). For instance, third-party payers spent an excess of $9132 (95% CI: $8956–$9304) annually among adults with both depression and anxiety than those with neither condition. Furthermore, the former group also had $399 (95% CI: $393–$406) more OOP spending than the latter group.

3.4. Economic Outcomes: OOP Spending Burden. We found significantly higher percentages of adults with depression and/or anxiety bearing a high OOP spending burden (i.e., spending 10% or more of income on healthcare) than those without these two conditions (Table 4). Specifically, approximately one-third (34.0%) of those with both depression and anxiety had high OOP burden versus 18.3% of those with neither the conditions. Results from unadjusted and adjusted logistic regressions consistently indicated that adults having depression and anxiety were more likely to suffer from high OOP burden as compared to those with neither the conditions. However, we did not observe any significant association between either condition alone (depression or anxiety) and high OOP burden after adjusting for all the predisposing factors, enabling factors, need factors, personal health practices, and external environment (Table 4).

4. Discussion

This study comprehensively evaluated the humanistic and economic burden associated with depression and anxiety, alone and together, among a nationally representative sample of adults with comorbid diabetes and hypertension. Our

Table 2: Unadjusted and adjusted coefficients for depression and anxiety categories from ordinary least square (OLS) regressions on physical component summary (PCS) and mental component summary (MCS) scores among adults with comorbid diabetes and hypertension, using pooled data from the 2013 and 2015 Medical Expenditure Panel Survey (MEPS).

	Unadjusted means and SE			
	PCS		MCS	
	Mean (SE)	p value	Mean (SE)	p value
Depression and anxiety	37.27 (0.96) ***	<0.001	40.45 (0.94) ***	<0.001
Depression only	37.02 (0.97) ***	<0.001	43.76 (0.71) ***	<0.001
Anxiety only	38.38 (1.04) *	0.016	46.96 (0.78) ***	<0.001
No depression/anxiety (reference group)	40.92 (0.34)		52.8 (0.23)	
	Parameter estimates and SE from multivariable OLS regressions†			
	PCS		MCS	
	Beta (SE)	p value	Beta (SE)	p value
Depression and anxiety	−0.68 (0.87)	0.432	−10.35 (0.91) ***	<0.001
Depression only	−1.37 (0.83)	0.098	−7.67 (0.66) ***	<0.001
Anxiety only	0.01 (0.80)	0.987	−4.88 (0.74) ***	<0.001
No depression/anxiety (reference group)				

Note: the analytic sample consisted of adults (>18 years) with comorbid diabetes and hypertension who were alive and eligible for the self-administered questionnaires of MEPS in the observation year (2013/2015). SE: standard error of the mean; Beta: parameter estimates from multivariable OLS regressions. †Covariates included in the multivariable OLS regressions included predisposing factors (sex, age groups, and race/ethnicity), enabling factors (marital status, education level, poverty status, health insurance coverage, and prescription drug insurance coverage), enabling factor (presence/absence of other chronic conditions, pain interference), personal health practice (obesity, smoking status, and exercise level), and external environment (region). Pain interference was not included in the regression on PCS scores because it was used in the computation of PCS scores with heavy weights. $^{*}p < 0.05$; $^{**}p < 0.01$; $^{***}p < 0.001$.

results revealed that a substantial proportion of adults with comorbid diabetes and hypertension suffered from depression and/or anxiety. Some subgroups such as females, individuals with low socioeconomic status, current smokers, and those with severe pain were more vulnerable than others to be affected. Adding regular check-ups for mental health to diabetes management for these subgroups may help prevent the development of depression or anxiety.

Our study findings showed that depression and anxiety, either alone or together, were associated with poorer quality of life relative to mental health, but not physical health, among adults with comorbid diabetes and hypertension. It is expected that individuals with mental health diagnoses perceived poorer mental health. Although previous literature suggested that depression could impact physical health [30], we did not observe such association after adjusting for all the predisposing factors, enabling factors, need factors, personal health practice, and the external environment. We speculated that adults with diabetes and hypertension perceived the role limitations and impaired functional status affected by emotional problems rather than physical sufferings. It is also possible that they received more medical attention to physical symptoms than mental problems from healthcare providers. Results from the National Comorbidity Survey Replication indicated that 60% of adults with a recent mental health condition did not receive care from healthcare professional [31]. Removing barriers to seeking mental healthcare (i.e., mental health stigma) and increasing access to mental health services are pivotal to improve the quality of life for patients with comorbid diabetes and hypertension.

In addition to impairments in quality of life, adults with comorbid diabetes and hypertension also born excess economic burden from depression and anxiety, especially when both conditions occurred. Li and colleagues reported that almost one-fourth of adults with diabetes spent considerable proportion (>10%) of family income for healthcare [32]. The presence of comorbid depression and anxiety may expose more diabetes patients and their families to financial difficulties. Such excess spending burden may come from paying for behavioral health interventions, which have relatively low reimbursement rates. Lifting restrictions and increasing reimbursement rates for behavioral health services can enable more diabetes patients to afford the care needed for their overall well-being. Not only patients but also healthcare payers such as Medicare, Medicaid, and private insurance companies have significantly higher costs due to depression, anxiety, and the combination of these two. We estimated that depression and anxiety together accounted for an excess of $14.3 billion medical expenditures (2015 USD) for third-party payers annually. The new payment model for behavioral health services implemented by the Centers for Medicare and Medicaid Services may be promising in reducing costs for both patients and payers [33].

Like any other research study, our findings should be interpreted along with the study strengths and limitations. We believe this to be the first study that comprehensively examined the humanistic and economic burden of depression and anxiety among adults with comorbid diabetes and hypertension in a nationally representative sample. Also, our study utilized data that allows for adjustment of a comprehensive list of confounders. The recycled predictions

TABLE 3: Unadjusted and adjusted annual per-person mean healthcare expenditures (2015 US$) by depression and anxiety categories among adults with comorbid diabetes and hypertension, using pooled data from the 2013 and 2015 Medical Expenditure Panel Survey.

	N	Unadjusted mean Mean (SE), $	Adjusted mean[†] Mean (95% CI)[‡], $	Adjusted incremental[†] Mean (95% CI)[‡], $
		All payers		
Depression and anxiety	309	28,832.15 (5963.66) **	20,962.68 (20,580.69–21,328.80)	8708.81 (8550.11–8860.90)
Depression only	559	19,648.34 (1,542.8) ***	16,860.66 (16,553.42–17,155.13)	4606.78 (4522.84–4687.24)
Anxiety only	366	16,990.31 (2008.43) **	14,735.14 (14,466.63–14,992.49)	2481.26 (2436.05–2524.60)
No depression/anxiety	3256	11,543.4 (448.52)	12,253.88 (12,030.58–12,467.89)	(reference group)
		Third-party payers		
Depression and anxiety	309	27,009.6 (5928.43) **	20,396.77 (20,003.49–20,782.35)	9132.19 (8956.11–9304.83)
Depression only	559	17,844.71 (1436.02) ***	15,659.59 (15,357.65–15,955.62)	4395.01 (4310.27–4478.09)
Anxiety only	366	15,236.58 (1996.7) *	13,273.26 (13,017.34–13,524.18)	2008.69 (1969.96–2046.66)
No depression/anxiety	3256	10,420.07 (445.14)	11,264.58 (11,047.38–11,477.53)	(reference group)
		Out-of-pocket		
Depression and anxiety	309	1822.54 (207.53) ***	1382.75 (1361.19–1405.12)	399.31 (393.08–405.77)
Depression only	559	1803.64 (236.02) **	1364.25 (1342.98–1386.32)	380.81 (374.88–386.98)
Anxiety only	366	1753.73 (231.31) **	1312.70 (1292.23–1333.94)	329.26 (324.12–334.59)
No depression/anxiety	3256	1123.33 (41.17)	983.44 (968.10–999.35)	(reference group)

Note: the analytic sample consisted of adults (>18 years) with comorbid diabetes and hypertension who were alive and had positive expenditures in the observation year (2013/2015). All the expenditures were converted to 2015 US dollars using the consumer product index from the US Bureau of Labor Statistics. SE: standard error of the mean. [†]The adjusted annual per-person mean/incremental healthcare expenditures were obtained from recycled predictions based on the estimates of generalized linear model (GLM) with log link function and gamma distribution. Covariates adjusted in the GLM included predisposing factors (sex, age groups, and race/ethnicity), enabling factors (marital status, education level, poverty status, health insurance coverage, and prescription drug insurance coverage), enabling factor (presence/absence of other chronic conditions, pain interference), personal health practice (obesity, smoking status, and exercise level), and external environment (region). [‡]Confidence intervals are based on 2000 bootstrap replications using the percentile method. $^{*}p < 0.05$; $^{**}p < 0.01$; $^{***}p < 0.001$.

TABLE 4: Unadjusted and adjusted association between depression and anxiety categories and high out-of-pocket (OOP) spending burden among adults with comorbid diabetes and hypertension, using pooled data from the 2013 and 2015 Medical Expenditure Panel Survey.

	Bivariate association between depression and anxiety categories and high OOP spending burden					
	High burden[†]		Not high burden			
	N	Wt row%	*N*	Wt row%	*p* value	Sig.
Depression and anxiety	90	34.0	219	66.0	<0.001	***
Depression only	158	28.2	403	71.8		
Anxiety only	96	23.5	270	76.5		
No depression/anxiety	650	18.3	2674	81.7		
	Logistic regressions on high OOP spending burden[†]					
	Unadjusted model			Adjusted model[‡]		
	OR	95% CI	Sig.	AOR	95% CI	Sig.
Depression and anxiety	2.26	(1.66–3.07)	***	1.55	(1.06–2.25)	*
Depression only	1.72	(1.28–2.32)	***	1.25	(0.91–1.70)	
Anxiety only	1.34	(1.04–1.74)	*	1.03	(0.77–1.38)	
No depression/anxiety			(reference group)			

Note: the analytic sample consisted of adults (>18 years) with comorbid diabetes and hypertension who were alive and had positive expenditures in the observation year (2013/2015). Wt row%: weighted row percentages; Sig.: statistical significance level; OR: odds ratio; AOR: adjusted odds ratio; 95% CI: 95% confidence interval. [†]OOP spending burden was measured by the percentage of household income spent on healthcare. It was calculated by dividing OOP spending by household income. High OOP spending burden was defined as 10% or more. [‡]Covariates adjusted in the logistic regression included predisposing factors (sex, age groups, and race/ethnicity), enabling factors (marital status, education level, poverty status, health insurance coverage, and prescription drug insurance coverage), enabling factor (presence/absence of other chronic conditions, pain interference), personal health practice (obesity, smoking status, and exercise level), and external environment (region). $^{*}p < 0.05$; $^{**}p < 0.01$; $^{***}p < 0.001$.

provide realistic estimates of healthcare expenditures for a typical diabetes patient. Such estimates can be better comprehended by policymakers than parameter estimates from conventional regression analyses. However, there are limitations as well. First, the study results may subject to recall and social desirability bias due to the self-reported nature of the MEPS data. Second, there might be misclassification bias from undiagnosed depression/anxiety, leading to underestimation of the disease burdens. Third, the diagnostic codes and clinical classification codes provided by the MPES do not allow us to further examine the burden of anxiety and depression on different types of diabetes and/or hypertension. Also, we could not evaluate the duration and severity of diabetes and hypertension from MEPS data. Future studies considering these factors are warranted to confirm our findings. Finally, the cross-sectional design of our study may limit the ability to demonstrate causality.

5. Conclusions

In summary, the present study indicated that depression and anxiety, especially the combination of these two conditions, are associated with significant impairments in quality of life and excess economic burden for patients with comorbid diabetes and hypertension. The burden estimates can be used as benchmarks to evaluate future diabetes management programs. Our findings highlight the needs for timely screening and early interventions that could help prevent anxiety and/or depression among adults with comorbid diabetes and hypertension to reduce their clinical, humanistic, and economic burden. Furthermore, it is necessary to integrate mental healthcare into diabetes management to improve the quality of life for adults with comorbid diabetes and hypertension. Innovative payment models that encourage collaboration among primary care providers, diabetes specialists, and mental health professionals are needed to reduce healthcare costs for both patients and healthcare payers.

Disclosure

A portion of the information presented in this manuscript was presented as a poster at the International Society for Pharmacoeconomics and Outcome Research 2018 meeting in Baltimore, Maryland. The abstract of the poster presentation was published in *Value in Health*, 2018, volume 21, supplement 1, page S228.

Conflicts of Interest

The authors declare that there is no conflict of interest regarding the publication of this paper.

References

[1] A. N. Long and S. Dagogo-Jack, "Comorbidities of diabetes and hypertension: mechanisms and approach to target organ protection," *Journal of Clinical Hypertension (Greenwich, Conn.)*, vol. 13, no. 4, pp. 244–251, 2011.

[2] Centers for Disease Control Prevention (CDC), *National Diabetes Statistics Report, 2017*, Centers for Disease Control and Prevention, US Dept of Health and Human Services, Atlanta, GA, 2017.

[3] J. R. Read, L. Sharpe, M. Modini, and B. F. Dear, "Multimorbidity and depression: a systematic review and meta-analysis," *Journal of Affective Disorders*, vol. 221, pp. 36–46, 2017.

[4] N. Taneja, M. Adhikary, S. Chandramouleeswaan, and S. K. Kapoor, "Prevalence of common mental disorders among patients with diabetes mellitus and hypertension in an urban east delhi slum–a cross sectional study," *Hindu*, vol. 44, pp. 43–46, 2015.

[5] E. Andreoulakis, T. Hyphantis, D. Kandylis, and A. Iacovides, "Depression in diabetes mellitus: a comprehensive review," *Hippokratia*, vol. 16, no. 3, pp. 205–214, 2012.

[6] M. M. Collins, P. Corcoran, and I. J. Perry, "Anxiety and depression symptoms in patients with diabetes," *Diabetic Medicine*, vol. 26, no. 2, pp. 153–161, 2009.

[7] Z. Li, Y. Li, L. Chen, P. Chen, and Y. Hu, "Prevalence of depression in patients with hypertension: a systematic review and meta-analysis," *Medicine*, vol. 94, no. 31, article e1317, 2015.

[8] I. A. Kretchy, F. T. Owusu-Daaku, and S. A. Danquah, "Mental health in hypertension: assessing symptoms of anxiety, depression and stress on anti-hypertensive medication adherence," *International Journal of Mental Health Systems*, vol. 8, no. 1, p. 25, 2014.

[9] T. Vos, R. M. Barber, B. Bell et al., "Global, regional, and national incidence, prevalence, and years lived with disability for 301 acute and chronic diseases and injuries in 188 countries, 1990–2013: a systematic analysis for the Global Burden of Disease Study 2013," *The Lancet*, vol. 386, no. 9995, pp. 743–800, 2015.

[10] E. H. B. Lin, W. Katon, M. von Korff et al., "Relationship of depression and diabetes self-care, medication adherence, and preventive care," *Diabetes Care*, vol. 27, no. 9, pp. 2154–2160, 2004.

[11] M. V. Mendlowicz and M. B. Stein, "Quality of life in individuals with anxiety disorders," *American Journal of Psychiatry*, vol. 157, no. 5, pp. 669–682, 2000.

[12] K. B. Wells, A. Stewart, R. D. Hays et al., "The functioning and well-being of depressed patients. Results from the Medical Outcomes Study," *Journal of the American Medical Association*, vol. 262, no. 7, pp. 914–919, 1989.

[13] L. E. Egede, "Diabetes, major depression, and functional disability among U.S. adults," *Diabetes Care*, vol. 27, no. 2, pp. 421–428, 2004.

[14] M. A. B. dos Santos, L. B. Ceretta, G. Z. Réus et al., "Anxiety disorders are associated with quality of life impairment in patients with insulin-dependent type 2 diabetes: a case-control study," *Revista Brasileira de Psiquiatria*, vol. 36, no. 4, pp. 298–304, 2014.

[15] K. Mosaku, B. Kolawole, C. Mume, and R. Ikem, "Depression, anxiety and quality of life among diabetic patients: a comparative study," *Journal of the National Medical Association*, vol. 100, no. 1, pp. 73–78, 2008.

[16] American Diabetes Association, "Economic costs of diabetes in the U.S. in 2017," *Diabetes Care*, vol. 41, no. 5, pp. 917–928, 2018.

[17] G. Wang, X. Zhou, X. Zhuo, and P. Zhang, "Annual total medical expenditures associated with hypertension by diabetes status in U.S. adults," *American Journal of Preventive Medicine*, vol. 53, no. 6, Supplement 2, pp. S182–S189, 2017.

[18] A. Alzoubi, R. Abunaser, A. Khassawneh, M. Alfaqih, A. Khasawneh, and N. Abdo, "The bidirectional relationship between diabetes and depression: a literature review," *Korean Journal of Family Medicine*, vol. 39, no. 3, pp. 137–146, 2018.

[19] A. M. Roest, E. J. Martens, P. de Jonge, and J. Denollet, "Anxiety and risk of incident coronary heart disease: a meta-analysis," *Journal of the American College of Cardiology*, vol. 56, no. 1, pp. 38–46, 2010.

[20] R. C. Kessler, C. B. Nelson, K. A. McGonagle, J. Liu, M. Swartz, and D. G. Blazer, "Comorbidity of DSM-III-R major depressive disorder in the general population: results from the US National Comorbidity Survey," *British Journal of Psychiatry*, vol. 168, no. S30, pp. 17–30, 1996.

[21] J. D. Coplan, C. J. Aaronson, V. Panthangi, and Y. Kim, "Treating comorbid anxiety and depression: psychosocial and pharmacological approaches," *World Journal of Psychiatry*, vol. 5, no. 4, pp. 366–378, 2015.

[22] J. P. Sommers, *An Examination of State Estimates Using Multiple Years of Data from the Medical Expenditure Panel Survey, Household Component*, Agency for Healthcare Research and Quality, 2006.

[23] J. E. Ware Jr, M. Kosinski, and S. D. Keller, "A 12-item short-form health survey: construction of scales and preliminary tests of reliability and validity," *Medical Care*, vol. 34, no. 3, pp. 220–233, 1996.

[24] S. Crystal, R. W. Johnson, J. Harman, U. Sambamoorthi, and R. Kumar, "Out-of-pocket health care costs among older Americans," *The Journals of Gerontology Series B: Psychological Sciences and Social Sciences*, vol. 55, no. 1, pp. S51–S62, 2000.

[25] K. A. Paez, L. Zhao, and W. Hwang, "Rising out-of-pocket spending for chronic conditions: a ten-year trend," *Health Affairs*, vol. 28, no. 1, pp. 15–25, 2009.

[26] R. M. Andersen, "Revisiting the behavioral model and access to medical care: does it matter?," *Journal of Health and Social Behavior*, vol. 36, no. 1, pp. 1–10, 1995.

[27] B. Mihaylova, A. Briggs, A. O'hagan, and S. G. Thompson, "Review of statistical methods for analysing healthcare resources and costs," *Health Economics*, vol. 20, no. 8, pp. 897–916, 2011.

[28] A. Basu and P. J. Rathouz, "Estimating marginal and incremental effects on health outcomes using flexible link and variance function models," *Biostatistics*, vol. 6, no. 1, pp. 93–109, 2005.

[29] Agency for Healthcare Research and Quality (AHRQ), "MEPS HC-036: 1996–2007 Pooled Estimation File," 2009, June 2018 https://meps.ahrq.gov/data_stats/download_data/pufs/h36/h36u07doc.shtml#40Other.

[30] M. H. Trivedi, "The link between depression and physical symptoms," *Primary care companion to the Journal of clinical psychiatry*, vol. 6, suppl 1, pp. 12–16, 2004.

[31] P. S. Wang, M. Lane, M. Olfson, H. A. Pincus, K. B. Wells, and R. C. Kessler, "Twelve-month use of mental health services in the United States: results from the National Comorbidity Survey Replication," *Archives of General Psychiatry*, vol. 62, no. 6, pp. 629–640, 2005.

[32] R. Li, L. E. Barker, S. Shrestha et al., "Changes over time in high out-of-pocket health care burden in U.S. adults with diabetes, 2001–2011," *Diabetes Care*, vol. 37, no. 6, pp. 1629–1635, 2014.

[33] M. J. Press, R. Howe, M. Schoenbaum et al., "Medicare payment for behavioral health integration," *New England Journal of Medicine*, vol. 376, no. 5, pp. 405–407, 2017.

9

Determinants of Change in Glycemic Status in Individuals with Prediabetes: Results from a Nationwide Cohort Study in Germany

Rebecca Paprott, Christa Scheidt-Nave, and Christin Heidemann

Department of Epidemiology and Health Monitoring, Robert Koch Institute, 12101 Berlin, Germany

Correspondence should be addressed to Christin Heidemann; heidemannc@rki.de

Academic Editor: Paolo Fiorina

Previous studies investigating determinants of changes in glycemic status among individuals with prediabetes mainly focused on glucose-defined prediabetes. In this study, we examined determinants of a regression to normoglycemia or a progression to diabetes among individuals with HbA1c-defined prediabetes. The study included 817 participants (18–79 years) with prediabetes (HbA1c 5.7–6.4% (39–47 mmol/mol)) at baseline. Glycemic status at follow-up was categorized as diagnosed diabetes (self-reported physician diagnosis or antidiabetic medication), undiagnosed diabetes (HbA1c ≥ 6.5% (≥48 mmol/mol)), prediabetes (as defined at baseline), and normoglycemia (HbA1c < 5.7% (<39 mmol/mol)). Determinants of glycemic changes were identified by multinomial logistic regression (OR (95% CI)), with those remaining in the prediabetic state as reference. During a mean follow-up time of 12.0 years, 33.8% of the participants reverted to normoglycemia, 7.2% progressed to undiagnosed diabetes, 12.8% progressed to diagnosed diabetes, and 46.2% remained prediabetic. Determinants of a regression to normoglycemia were female sex (male vs. female: 0.67 (0.46; 0.98)) and higher HDL cholesterol levels (1.17 (1.02; 1.35) per 10 mg/dl). Determinants of a progression to undiagnosed or diagnosed diabetes were higher values of BMI (1.10 (1.02; 1.18); 1.13 (1.06; 1.21) per kg/m^2), waist circumference (1.04 (1.01; 1.07); 1.06 (1.03; 1.09) per cm), alanine aminotransferase (1.06 (1.03; 1.09); 1.07 (1.03; 1.10) per U/l), and gamma-glutamyl transferase (1.02 (1.00; 1.03); 1.03 (1.01; 1.04) per U/l). Higher age (1.04 (1.02; 1.06) per year), female sex (male vs. female: 0.56 (0.33; 0.97)), and parental history of diabetes (yes vs. no: 1.82 (1.05; 3.15)) were further associated with a progression to diagnosed diabetes, whereas higher triglyceride levels (1.03 (1.01; 1.06) per 10 mg/dl) were associated with a progression to undiagnosed diabetes. In conclusion, among the investigated determinants, potentially modifiable anthropometric and metabolic markers were associated with glycemic changes in individuals with HbA1c-defined prediabetes. The findings of this study demonstrate the need for more refined case finding strategies for diabetes prevention.

1. Introduction

Type 2 diabetes is a chronic metabolic disease characterized by elevated blood glucose levels that increase the risk for severe micro- and macrovascular complications [1]. Prediabetes is considered a prestage of manifest diabetes and is associated with an increased risk of developing type 2 diabetes [2–5]. Approximately 5% to 10% of individuals with prediabetes progress to diabetes yearly [2]. However, progression can be prevented by lifestyle and pharmacological interventions and prediabetes may even revert to normoglycemia [2, 3].

Prediabetes can be defined by impaired fasting glucose (IFG) (5.6–6.9 mmol/l), impaired glucose tolerance (IGT) (7.8–11.0 mmol/l), or elevated HbA1c levels (5.7–6.4% (39–47 mmol/mol)) [5]. Previous studies on determinants of progression or regression from prediabetes were mostly based on prediabetes defined by IFG or IGT, whereas studies using elevated HbA1c levels for definition are sparse.

In these studies, among individuals with IFG or IGT, measures of lipid metabolism [6–10] and anthropometry [4, 8, 11–14] were associated with changes in glycemic status. Moreover, several previous studies among persons with IFG or IGT examined the effect of modifiable lifestyle factors (mostly physical activity, smoking, and alcohol intake) on glycemic changes but the majority did not find an association [4, 6–10, 15–17]. In addition, a recent study that included individuals with HbA1c-defined prediabetes found no association between physical activity and a regression to normoglycemia [17].

Since the characteristics of individuals with prediabetes who are diagnosed by different criteria may vary due to differences in the underlying pathophysiological pathways [2, 18], determinants of changes in glycemic status may also differ according to the applied diagnostic criterion.

In the present study, we therefore aimed to identify determinants of a regression to normoglycemia or a progression to undiagnosed or diagnosed diabetes in a nationwide sample of German adults with HbA1c-defined prediabetes who were followed for 12 years. In addition to sociodemographic characteristics, we investigated potentially modifiable risk factors such as anthropometric, metabolic, and lifestyle factors as determinants of change in glycemic status.

2. Materials and Methods

2.1. National Health Examination Surveys. The "German National Health Interview and Examination Survey 1998" (GNHIES98) was conducted from 1997 to 1999 and targeted the residential German population aged 18 to 79 years (response: 61%). A two-stage cluster sampling procedure was applied. First, sample points were selected, and then, age- and sex-stratified random samples from local population registries were drawn [19]. Out of all GNHIES98 participants, 3959 participants (response: 62%) also took part in the subsequent "German Health Interview and Examination Survey for Adults" (DEGS1), conducted from 2008 to 2011 (Figure 1) [20]. Both surveys were conducted in accordance with the Declaration of Helsinki and approved by the Federal and State Commissioners for Data Protection. DEGS1 was approved by the ethics committee of the Charité-Universitätsmedizin Berlin (No. EA2/047/08). Participants provided written informed consent before participation [20].

2.2. Study Population. Figure 1 depicts a flow chart reflecting the composition of the study population. After applying different exclusion criteria among those who participated in both GNHIES98 (baseline) and DEGS1 (follow-up), a cohort consisting of 2900 participants remained. The final study sample comprised 817 participants with prediabetes at baseline.

2.3. Assessment of Glycemic Status. Diagnosed diabetes was determined by a self-reported history of diagnosed diabetes assessed in physician-administered standardized interviews or by the intake of antidiabetic agents within the 7 days prior to the interview documented through a detailed medication review. Among participants without diagnosed diabetes, normoglycemia (HbA1c < 5.7% (<39 mmol/mol)), prediabetes (HbA1c 5.7–6.4% (39–47 mmol/mol)), and undiagnosed diabetes (HbA1c ≥ 6.5% (≥48 mmol/mol)) were defined according to recent ADA recommendations [5]. In GNHIES98, HbA1c was measured using a Diamat high-performance liquid chromatography (HPLC) analyzer (Bio-Rad Laboratories, Munich, Germany) and RECIPE reagents (RECIPE Chemicals and Instruments, Munich, Germany). In DEGS1, HbA1c was measured using an immunoturbidimetric method (ARCHITECT ci8200; Abbott, Wiesbaden, Germany). Both methods were traceable to the National Glycohemoglobin Standardization Program [21], and no systematic deviation of HbA1c measurements between the surveys was evident [22].

2.4. Assessment of Risk Factors for Type 2 Diabetes. The assessment of several health-related risk factors in GNHIES98 has been previously described in detail [20, 22–25]. Briefly, information about educational level, sport activity, smoking status, residential traffic intensity, and mental distress was obtained through a standardized self-administered questionnaire. For the current analyses, middle and high educational levels were combined. Sport activity was ascertained as regular sport activity over the past three months and categorized as either no sport or any sport. Smoking status was categorized into never, former, and current smoker. Residential traffic intensity was dichotomized into rare to considerable traffic versus heavy to extreme traffic. Psychosocial distress was measured by the Mental Health Inventory (MHI-5) on a scale ranging from 0 to 100 points, with lower values indicating mental distress and higher values indicating mental well-being. A parental history of diabetes was assessed in DEGS1 through a standardized physician-administered personal interview. In GNHIES98, measures of body height, weight, and waist circumference were obtained while participants wore light clothing. BMI was calculated as the ratio of body weight (kg) and height squared (m^2).

The intake of coffee, red meat, and whole grains (including whole grain bread, buns, and muesli) (as components of the German Diabetes Risk Score (GDRS) that is described below) was assessed through a questionnaire on frequency of consumption of these food groups. The average amount consumed per day was estimated by further considering information on dietary intake assessed through a diet history method in a GNHIES98 subsample ($n = 4030$) as previously described [23].

As a summary measure of overall risk for type 2 diabetes, we calculated the GDRS including age, height, waist circumference, history of hypertension, physical activity, smoking, family history of diabetes, and intake of coffee, red meat, and whole grains as score components [26]. The GDRS has been shown to be a valid tool for prediction of diagnosed diabetes in the general adult population [23].

Venous blood samples were taken, processed within an hour, and stored at −40°C in the central laboratory unit at the Robert Koch Institute until further analyses. HDL cholesterol was determined based on the cholesterol oxidase-peroxidase 4-aminophenazone method (MEGA, Merck, Darmstadt, Germany) (intra-assay CV: 1.2–2.5%). Triglycerides were determined by the glycerol-3-phosphate oxidase-peroxidase 4-aminophenazone method using the MEGA measurement device (Merck, Darmstadt, Germany) (intra-assay CV: 1.6–2.2%). Both gamma-glutamyl transferase

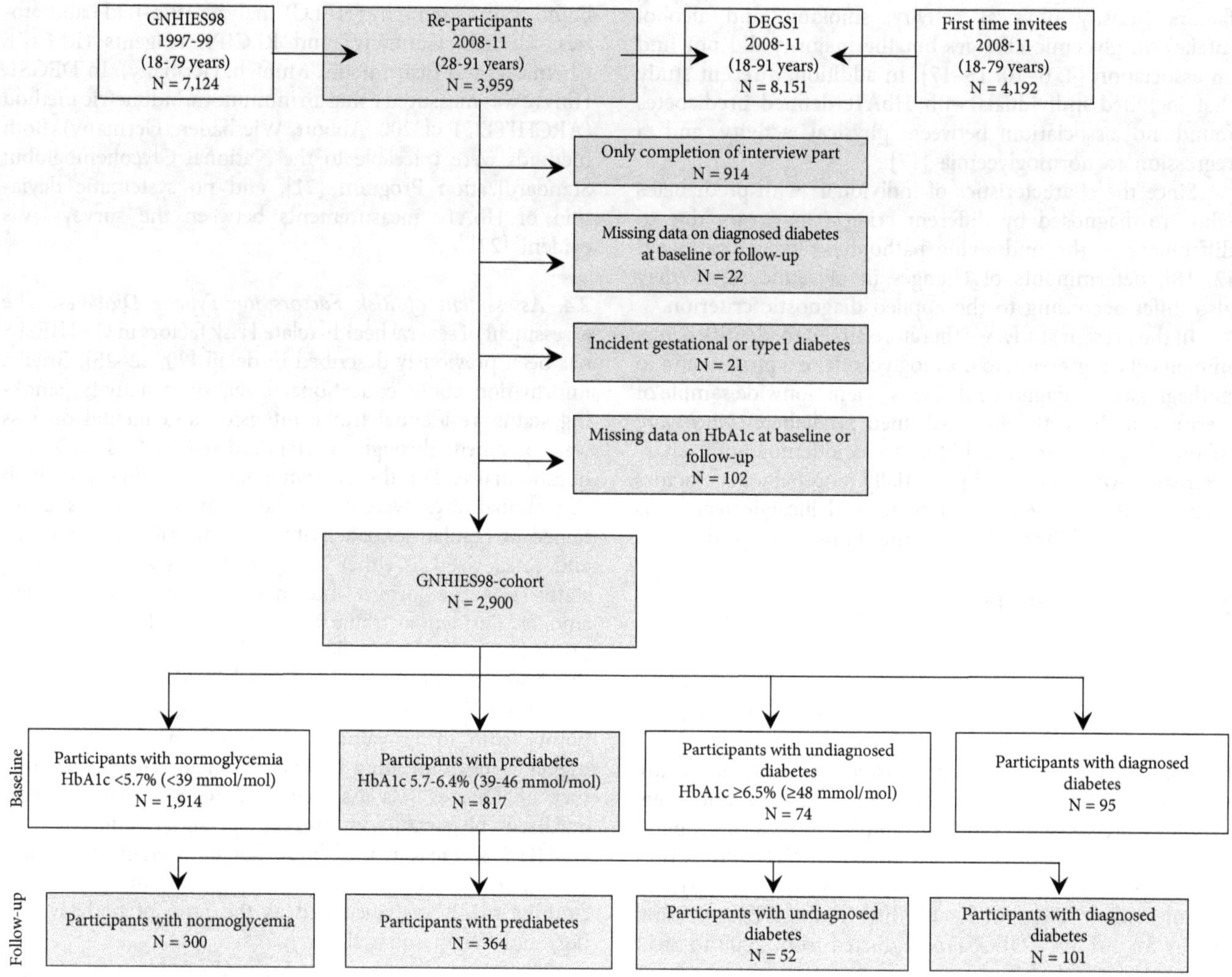

FIGURE 1: Flow chart showing the definition and distribution of participants within categories of glycemic status. Definitions applied for glycemic status were the same at baseline and follow-up. The numbers shown were drawn from the unimputed data set.

(GGT) and alanine aminotransferase (ALT) were measured according to standards of the DGKC (German Association of Clinical Chemistry) (EPOS, Eppendorf, Wesseling, Germany) (intra-assay CV for GGT: 1.3–2.7%; for ALT: 1.1–4.8%). High-sensitivity C-reactive protein (hs-CRP) was measured in serum by an immunoturbidimetric method (ARCHITECT ci8200, Abbott, Munich, Germany) (intra-assay CV: 4.0).

Additionally, diagnosed hypertension, hyperlipidemia, myocardial infarction, and stroke were considered as comorbidities and assessed through a physician-administered personal interview. The use of statins and thiazide diuretics was considered as concomitant therapy known to favor the progression from prediabetes to diabetes and was ascertained through a detailed medication review. However, we found that the number of participants taking thiazide diuretics ($n = 20$) or statins ($n = 32$) at the time of baseline examination (1997–99) was too low to enable further analyses.

2.5. Statistical Analysis. The SAS software 9.4 (SAS Institute Inc., Cary, NC) was used for all statistical analyses. A weighting factor was applied that corrects for deviations of the DEGS1 sample from population figures from the Federal Statistical Office (as of 31 December 2010) and accounts for the incomplete follow-up [27]. For the current analyses, the probability of GNHIES98 participants with prediabetes participating in DEGS1 was derived from a generalized linear mixed model with age at the time of GNHIES98 (4 categories) and age at the time of DEGS1 (8 categories), as well as smoking (yes or no), education (3 categories), income (3 categories), and migration background (yes or no) at the time of GNHIES98, as independent variables.

Multinomial logistic regression was performed to calculate the odds ratios (OR) and 95% confidence intervals (CI) for considered risk factors. For the dependent variable, three categories were defined according to a participant's glycemic status at follow-up, with those who remained in the prediabetic state as the reference group. In the case of a regression to normoglycemia, an OR > 1.00 indicates a higher chance for a regression (i.e., favorable). In the case of a progression to diabetes, an OR > 1.00 indicates a higher chance of a progression (i.e., unfavorable).

TABLE 1: Baseline characteristics of individuals with prediabetes at baseline ($n = 817$) according to HbA1c-defined glycemic status at follow-up.

	Regression to normoglycemia	Remained prediabetic	Progression to Undiagnosed diabetes	Progression to Diagnosed diabetes
n (%)	300 (33.8%)	364 (46.2%)	52 (7.2%)	101 (12.8%)
Unmodifiable risk factors				
Sociodemographic factors				
Age (years)	48.5 (45.9; 51.1)	49.6 (47.6; 51.7)	**53.8 (50.5; 57.2)**	**57.0 (54.8; 59.2)**
Male sex	53.3 (46.5; 60.1)	61.5 (54.8; 67.8)	48.1 (30.4; 66.2)	**41.6 (31.1; 52.9)**
Educational level				
Low	52.2 (45.0; 59.4)	52.6 (45.6; 59.6)	52.4 (34.2; 70.2)	**71.8 (61.6; 82.0)**
Medium/high	47.8 (40.6; 55.0)	47.4 (40.4; 54.4)	47.3 (29.8; 65.8)	28.2 (18.0; 38.4)
Family history of diabetes				
At least one parent with diabetes	27.1 (19.6; 34.5)	35.4 (29.9; 40.8)	31.1 (10.6; 51.6)	46.7 (34.6; 58.8)
Modifiable risk factors				
Anthropometric markers				
BMI (kg/m^2)	**26.6 (25.8; 27.3)**	27.5 (27.0; 28.1)	**29.6 (28.5; 30.6)**	**30.4 (29.3; 31.6)**
Waist circumference (cm)	**91.1 (89.1; 93.1)**	94.3 (92.8; 95.7)	**98.6 (94.7; 102.5)**	**101.3 (98.0; 104.5)**
Lifestyle factors				
Any sport activity per week	44.9 (37.5; 52.4)	51.2 (44.3; 58.1)	43.8 (29.1; 59.9)	39.6 (29.8; 49.4)
Smoker at baseline				
Never	36.9 (30.4; 43.4)	38.2 (31.4; 45.0)	51.2 (36.5; 65.9)	43.9 (33.1; 54.7)
Former	16.7 (11.7; 21.7)	24.7 (19.7; 29.7)	26.7 (15.6; 42.1)	25.2 (15.7; 34.8)
Current	46.4 (39.1; 53.8)	37.1 (30.9; 43.3)	**21.8 (11.9; 36.7)**	30.9 (20.7; 41.1)
Intake of whole grains (portions/day)	1.3 (1.2; 1.5)	1.2 (1.1; 1.4)	**1.0 (0.8; 1.2)**	1.1 (1.0–1.3)
Intake of red meat (portions/day)	0.58 (0.55; 0.60)	0.59 (0.57; 0.61)	0.54 (0.50; 0.58)	**0.52 (0.47–0.57)**
Intake of coffee (cups/day)	3.2 (2.9; 3.4)	3.1 (2.8; 3.3)	2.8 (2.4; 3.1)	2.8 (2.4; 3.2)
Residential traffic intensity				
Heavy/extreme residential traffic intensity	25.5 (18.3; 32.7)	23.5 (17.7; 29.4)	28.1 (13.5; 49.6)	**33.5 (22.8; 44.2)**
Mental distress (points)	73.9 (71.6; 76.1)	75.4 (73.3; 77.4)	79.0 (74.2; 83.7)	70.9 (67.0; 74.8)
GDRS (points)	**538 (514; 563)**	575 (557; 592)	**633 (599; 666)**	**690 (661; 720)**
Metabolic markers				
HDL cholesterol (mg/dl)	**56.4 (53.5; 59.4)**	52.4 (50.4; 54.6)	51.3 (47.9; 54.9)	50.3 (47.5; 53.2)
Triglycerides (mg/dl)	**121.9 (111.0; 133.8)**	144.1 (134.2; 154.7)	**187.0 (150.2; 232.9)**	**175.2 (155.0; 198.0)**
GGT (U/l)	**13.9 (12.7; 15.1)**	15.6 (14.6; 16.7)	**18.9 (16.2; 22.1)**	**20.1 (17.2; 23.5)**
ALT (U/l)	12.3 (11.4; 13.2)	12.7 (12.0; 13.5)	**16.0 (13.3; 19.2)**	**15.0 (13.5; 16.5)**
hs-CRP (mg/l)	1.4 (1.1; 1.7)	1.3 (1.2; 1.5)	1.4 (0.9; 2.3)	**2.3 (1.7; 3.1)**

Information is given as weighted proportions (95% CI) for categorical variables, as weighted arithmetic mean (95% CI) for continuous variables, and in case of metabolic markers and predicted 5-year diabetes risk as weighted geometric mean (95% CI). Differences in proportions and means between groups of glycemic status (reference group: remained prediabetic) were assessed by logistic regression and ANOVA. Bold numbers indicate $p < 0.05$.

We classified a total of 19 potential determinants (Table 1) into the following categories and subcategories: (1) *unmodifiable diabetes risk factors* comprising sociodemographic factors and family history of diabetes and (2) *potentially modifiable risk factors*, including anthropometric markers, lifestyle factors, residential traffic intensity, mental distress, the diabetes risk score (as a summary measure of predominantly modifiable factors), and metabolic markers. Risk factors were examined in separate multinomial regression models, adjusting for age and sex (model 1). For potentially modifiable risk factors, a second model (model 2) was fitted that additionally adjusted for educational level and other potential confounders that were selected by applying directed acyclic graphs [28].

Among individuals with prediabetes at baseline, 22% had missing data in at least one of the considered determinants. To account for the missing values, multiple imputation was applied that included all potential determinants, glycemic status at follow-up, the weighting factor, and the cluster variable. The SAS procedure "PROC MI" with the fully conditional specification method for an arbitrary pattern of missingness was used, and 25 complete data sets were imputed [29, 30]. The fraction of missing information ranged from <0.001 for height to 0.08 for hs-CRP. The relative efficiency was >0.99 for all risk factors imputed. SAS survey procedures were also applied to the individual imputed data sets again using the weighting factor and the cluster variable [29]. Results from the individual imputed data sets were then combined using the SAS procedure "PROC MIANALYZE," which accounts for the variability between the results of imputed data sets [31].

A considerable proportion of participants had an HbA1c level of 5.7% (39 mmol/mol; equivalent to 26.1%) or of 6.4% (47 mmol/mol; equivalent to 2.4%), i.e., an HbA1c level that was borderline for the definition of normoglycemia or diabetes, respectively. Therefore, *relevant* changes in glycemic status were defined for a sensitivity analysis as a change in the category of glycemic status combined with a change of at least ±0.3 percentage points in HbA1c. This definition of a *relevant* glycemic change was adapted from Kowall et al., who defined relevant changes in glycemic status based on fasting or 2 h glucose [12].

In additional analyses, the associations between changes in modifiable risk factors during follow-up and changes in glycemic status were examined. A change in a modifiable risk factor was defined as the measurement at follow-up minus the measurement at baseline. In addition to models 1 and 2 described above, a third model (model 3) was analyzed additionally including the baseline value of the respective risk factor.

3. Results

During a mean follow-up time of 12.0 years, 7.2% of the 817 participants with prediabetes at baseline progressed to undiagnosed diabetes and 12.8% progressed to diagnosed diabetes. During the same period, 33.8% reverted to normoglycemia and 46.2% remained prediabetic (Table 1). When considering *relevant* changes in glycemic status, the proportion of participants who reverted to normoglycemia was 28.1% (95% CI: 22.5–34.4%), while 51.9% (46.2–57.6%) remained in the prediabetic stage. The proportion of participants with a progression to undiagnosed or diagnosed diabetes remained unchanged (data not shown).

Baseline characteristics of participants according to changes in glycemic status during follow-up are shown in Table 1. Compared to those who remained in the prediabetic state, participants who regressed to normoglycemia had lower values for BMI, waist circumference, triglycerides, GGT, and the diabetes risk score. Additionally, they showed higher levels of HDL cholesterol. On the other hand, participants who progressed to diagnosed or undiagnosed diabetes were older and had higher values for BMI, waist circumference, triglycerides, GGT, ALT, and the diabetes risk score. Those who progressed to diagnosed diabetes were also more often female, living in streets with heavy or extreme residential traffic intensity, of a low educational level, and characterized by a lower intake of red meat and a higher level of hs-CRP. Those who progressed to undiagnosed diabetes were less likely to be current smokers and had a lower intake of whole grains compared to those who remained prediabetic.

Additional descriptive analyses considering diagnosed comorbidities at baseline (hypertension, hyperlipidemia, myocardial infarction, and stroke) showed that, as expected, participants with a progression to diagnosed diabetes were more likely and those with a regression to normoglycemia were less likely to have been diagnosed with hypertension or hyperlipidemia than those who remained prediabetic. No significant differences across categories of glycemic changes were observed with respect to myocardial infarction and stroke (data not shown).

Table 2 depicts the association between the investigated baseline determinants and changes in glycemic status as determined from multivariate analyses. Among the unmodifiable risk factors, female sex was associated with a regression to normoglycemia and a progression to diagnosed diabetes. Higher age and a parental history of diabetes were associated with a progression to diagnosed diabetes. Among the potentially modifiable risk factors, higher levels of HDL cholesterol and lower values of the diabetes risk score were associated with a regression to normoglycemia. Higher values of BMI, waist circumference, GGT, ALT, and the diabetes risk score were associated with a progression to both undiagnosed diabetes and diagnosed diabetes. In addition, a higher triglyceride level was associated with a progression to undiagnosed diabetes. The lifestyle factors considered, residential traffic intensity, and mental distress were not individually associated with a change in glycemic status. The results persisted when analyses were repeated considering only *relevant* glycemic changes (data not shown).

Further analyses of changes in potentially modifiable risk factors between baseline and follow-up (Supplementary Table 1) revealed that decreases in the levels of BMI (OR: 0.86 (95% CI: 0.77–0.95)), waist circumference (0.96 (0.93–0.99)), and triglycerides (0.94 (0.89–1.00)) during follow-up were associated with a regression to normoglycemia. However, an increased waist circumference (1.04 (1.00–1.08)) was associated with a progression to undiagnosed diabetes whereas an increased triglyceride level (1.05 (1.02–1.09)) was related to a progression to diagnosed diabetes. An increase in the diabetes risk score during follow-up was associated with a progression to undiagnosed diabetes (1.04 (1.01–1.08)) and to diagnosed diabetes (1.06 (1.01–1.10)).

4. Discussion

After 12.0 years of follow-up, 20% of HbA1c-defined prediabetic adults from a nationwide German study had progressed to diagnosed or undiagnosed diabetes, whereas 46% had remained prediabetic and 34% had reverted to normoglycemia. Figure 2 provides an overview of the hypothesized determinants of the study and its findings. Among the unmodifiable risk factors, female sex was related to a higher chance of a regression to normoglycemia and a progression to diagnosed diabetes. Additionally, older age and a parental diabetes history were related to a higher chance of a progression to

TABLE 2: Multivariable adjusted odds ratios (95% CI) for associations between risk factors of type 2 diabetes and change in glycemic status during follow-up among individuals with prediabetes at baseline ($n = 817$).

Risk factor at baseline		Regression to normoglycemia	Remained prediabetic	Progression to Undiagnosed diabetes	Progression to Diagnosed diabetes
n (%)		300 (33.8%)	364 (46.2%)	52 (7.2%)	101 (12.8%)
Unmodifiable risk factors					
Sociodemographic factors					
Age (per year)	Model 1	0.99 (0.97; 1.01)	1.00 (ref)	1.02 (1.00; 1.04)	**1.04 (1.02; 1.06)**
Sex (male vs. female)	Model 1	**0.67 (0.46; 0.98)**	1.00 (ref)	0.66 (0.30; 1.44)	**0.56 (0.33; 0.97)**
Educational level (low vs. middle/high)	Model 1	1.03 (0.69; 1.54)	1.00 (ref)	0.82 (0.38; 1.77)	1.72 (0.90; 3.30)
Family history of diabetes					
At least one parent with diabetes (yes vs. no)	Model 1	0.65 (0.41; 1.03)	1.00 (ref)	0.85 (0.31; 2.35)	**1.82 (1.05; 3.15)**
Modifiable risk factors					
Anthropometric markers					
BMI (per 1 kg/m^2)	Model 1	0.95 (0.90; 1.01)	1.00 (ref)	**1.09 (1.03; 1.16)**	**1.12 (1.05; 1.19)**
	Model 2	0.95 (0.90; 1.00)	1.00 (ref)	**1.10 (1.02; 1.18)**	**1.13 (1.06; 1.21)**
Waist circumference (per 1 cm)	Model 1	0.98 (0.96; 1.00)	1.00 (ref)	**1.04 (1.01; 1.07)**	**1.06 (1.03; 1.09)**
	Model 2	0.98 (0.96; 1.00)	1.00 (ref)	**1.04 (1.01; 1.07)**	**1.06 (1.03; 1.09)**
Lifestyle factors					
Sport (no sport vs. any sport)	Model 1	1.29 (0.89; 1.88)	1.00 (ref)	1.28 (0.64; 2.55)	1.48 (0.88; 2.50)
	Model 2	1.39 (0.96; 2.01)	1.00 (ref)	1.04 (0.47; 2.27)	0.93 (0.52; 1.65)
Smoker (former vs. never)	Model 1	0.81 (0.49; 1.33)	1.00 (ref)	0.94 (0.37; 2.47)	1.22 (0.62; 2.42)
	Model 2	0.79 (0.48; 1.30)	1.00 (ref)	0.96 (0.39; 2.36)	1.21 (0.59; 2.48)
Smoker (current vs. never)	Model 1	1.40 (0.87; 2.27)	1.00 (ref)	0.57 (0.24; 1.33)	1.42 (0.75; 2.66)
	Model 2	1.29 (0.79; 2.13)	1.00 (ref)	0.59 (0.23; 1.52)	1.58 (0.78; 3.20)
Intake of whole grains (per portion)	Model 1	1.12 (0.90; 1.39)	1.00 (ref)	0.69 (0.46; 1.03)	0.89 (0.63; 1.27)
	Model 2	1.18 (0.95; 1.46)	1.00 (ref)	0.68 (0.44; 1.06)	0.95 (0.64; 1.40)
Intake of red meat (per portion)	Model 1	1.42 (0.41; 4.86)	1.00 (ref)	0.54 (0.09; 3.44)	0.41 (0.05; 3.46)
	Model 2	1.82 (0.52; 6.30)	1.00 (ref)	0.36 (0.06; 2.24)	0.31 (0.03; 3.00)
Intake of coffee (per cup)	Model 1	1.04 (0.92; 1.18)	1.00 (ref)	0.91 (0.77; 1.08)	0.94 (0.77; 1.14)
	Model 2	1.03 (0.90; 1.17)	1.00 (ref)	0.91 (0.74; 1.11)	0.88 (0.71; 1.10)
Residential traffic intensity (heavy/extreme vs. rare/considerable)	Model 1	1.13 (0.71; 1.78)	1.00 (ref)	1.25 (0.49; 3.21)	1.60 (0.99; 2.58)
	Model 2	1.10 (0.70; 1.74)	1.00 (ref)	1.25 (0.51; 3.09)	1.30 (0.76; 2.23)
Mental distress (per 10 points)	Model 1	0.97 (0.85; 1.09)	1.00 (ref)	1.19 (0.93; 1.51)	0.86 (0.72; 1.02)
	Model 2	0.99 (0.87; 1.12)	1.00 (ref)	1.18 (0.92; 1.51)	0.86 (0.72; 1.03)
GDRS (per 10 points)	Unadjusted	**0.98 (0.97; 1.00)**	1.00 (ref)	**1.03 (1.01; 1.06)**	**1.07 (1.04; 1.10)**

Table 2: Continued.

Risk factor at baseline		Regression to normoglycemia	Remained prediabetic	Progression to Undiagnosed diabetes	Progression to Diagnosed diabetes
Metabolic markers					
HDL cholesterol (per 10 mg/dl)	Model 1	**1.16 (1.01; 1.33)**	1.00 (ref)	0.87 (0.69; 1.08)	**0.74 (0.62; 0.89)**
	Model 2	**1.17 (1.02; 1.35)**	1.00 (ref)	0.90 (0.71; 1.14)	0.85 (0.70; 1.04)
Triglycerides (per 10 mg/dl)	Model 1	0.98 (0.96; 1.01)	1.00 (ref)	**1.04 (1.01; 1.06)**	**1.03 (1.01; 1.05)**
	Model 2	0.99 (0.96; 1.01)	1.00 (ref)	**1.03 (1.01; 1.06)**	1.02 (1.00; 1.04)
GGT (per 1 U/l)	Model 1	1.00 (0.98; 1.02)	1.00 (ref)	**1.02 (1.01; 1.04)**	**1.03 (1.02; 1.05)**
	Model 2	1.00 (0.98; 1.02)	1.00 (ref)	**1.02 (1.00; 1.03)**	**1.03 (1.01; 1.04)**
ALT (per 1 U/l)	Model 1	1.00 (0.97; 1.03)	1.00 (ref)	**1.07 (1.03; 1.12)**	**1.08 (1.04; 1.12)**
	Model 2	1.02 (0.98; 1.05)	1.00 (ref)	**1.06 (1.01; 1.10)**	**1.07 (1.03; 1.10)**
hs-CRP (per 1 mg/l)	Model 1	1.02 (0.99; 1.06)	1.00 (ref)	0.95 (0.84; 1.08)	1.02 (0.98; 1.05)
	Model 2	1.02 (0.99; 1.06)	1.00 (ref)	0.91 (0.76; 1.08)	0.98 (0.95; 1.02)

Bold numbers indicate statistically significant ORs ($p < 0.05$). For all individual risk factors, *model 1* was adjusted for age and sex. For anthropometric markers, *model 2* was additionally adjusted for educational level, lifestyle factors, residential traffic intensity, and mental distress. For lifestyle factors, residential traffic intensity, mental distress, and metabolic markers, *model 2* was additionally adjusted for educational level, anthropometric markers, lifestyle factors, residential traffic intensity, and mental distress.

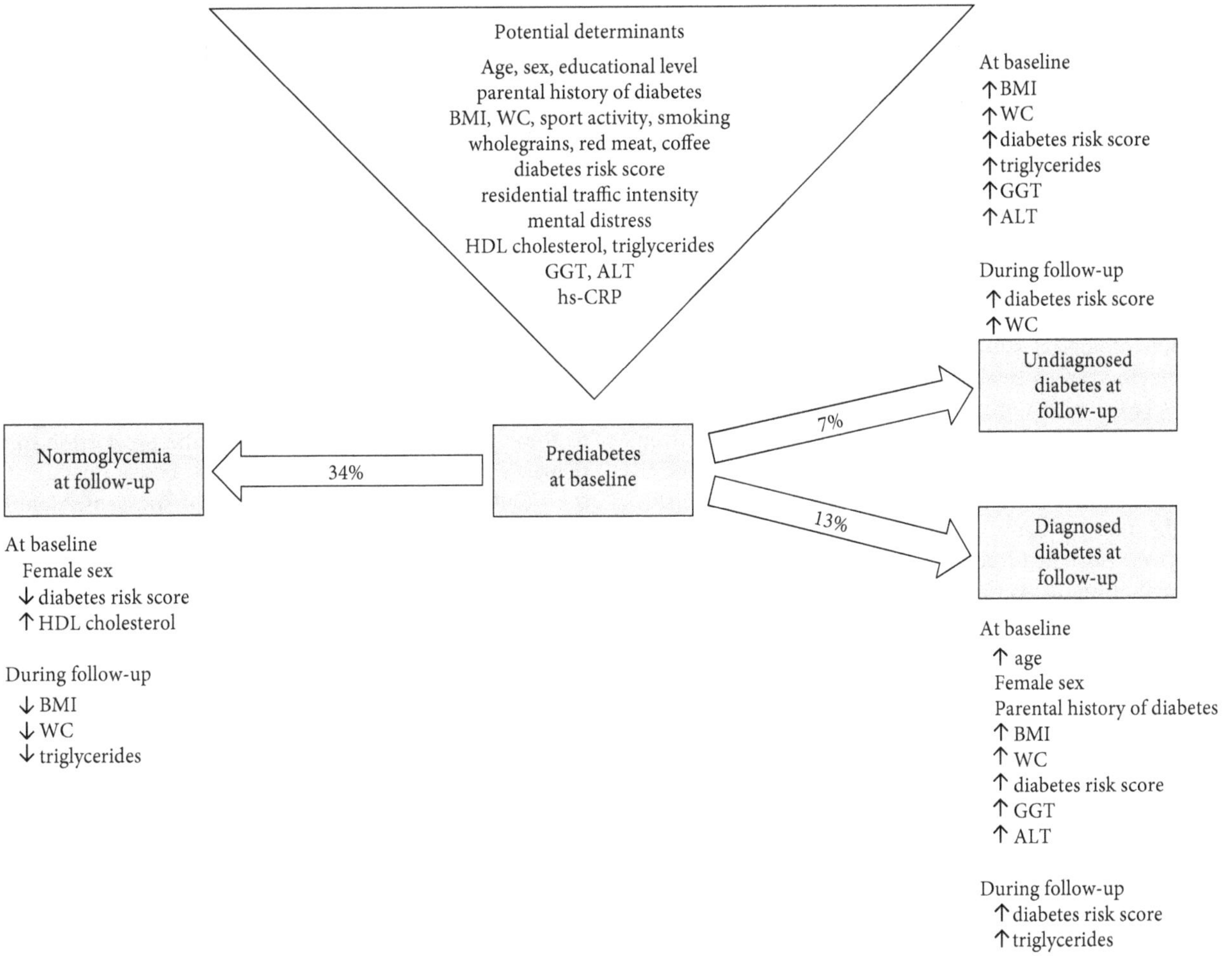

FIGURE 2: Overview on hypothesized determinants and study results. ↑ is equivalent to "higher at baseline/increase during follow-up"; ↓ is equivalent to "lower at baseline/decrease during follow-up"; BMI: body mass index; WC: waist circumference; HDL: high-density lipoprotein; GGT: gamma-glutamyl transferase; ALT: alanine aminotransferase; hs-CRP: high-sensitivity C-reactive protein.

diagnosed diabetes. Among potentially modifiable risk factors considered in the current study at baseline, favorable HDL cholesterol levels were related to a regression to normoglycemia. Less favorable levels of anthropometric markers and liver enzymes were associated with a progression to undiagnosed diabetes and diagnosed diabetes. In addition, less favorable triglyceride levels were related to a progression to undiagnosed diabetes. Higher values of the diabetes risk score as a summary measure of predominantly modifiable risk factors were associated with a progression to undiagnosed diabetes and diagnosed diabetes, whereas lower values were related to a regression to normoglycemia.

4.1. Discussion of Main Results. In this cohort, women had a higher chance of both a regression to normoglycemia and a progression to diagnosed diabetes. This finding might reflect a higher utilization of healthcare and greater health consciousness among women compared to men [32]. Higher age was associated with progression to diagnosed diabetes, confirming the well-known positive association between aging and the risk of type 2 diabetes. In addition, our findings related to a parental history of diabetes are consistent with findings from previous studies, indicating that individuals with a family history of diabetes are more likely to have their glucose level tested [33] and that a family history of diabetes probably affects an individual's knowledge of having diabetes [34].

Our findings regarding BMI and waist circumference mostly comport with findings from previous studies examining progression from IFG or IGT to diabetes [8, 11, 13, 14]. In contrast with our findings, previous studies from India and South Africa did not detect an association between waist circumference and a progression to diabetes [6, 35]. This disparity in results might be partly explained by the different ethnic groups included in the study populations. In our study, only decreases in BMI and waist circumference during follow-up but not their baseline values determined regression to normoglycemia. This finding is consistent with results of regional cohort studies of individuals with IFG or IGT in Germany [12] or the UK [4].

Interestingly, in multivariate analyses, none of the considered lifestyle factors was significantly associated with glycemic changes. This was also the case for fruit or vegetable intake and consumption of sugar-sweetened beverages or alcohol (data not shown). For physical activity, our null finding is consistent with the majority of previous studies that define glycemic status based on IFG, IGT [4, 6, 7, 9, 10, 15, 17], or HbA1c [17]. Only a few prior studies have investigated the association between dietary behaviors and changes in glycemic status in individuals with prediabetes, and the results have been inconsistent [7, 16]. The same is true for the association between smoking status and changes in glycemic status in individuals with prediabetes [6–10]. Differences in results might be explained by differences in the accuracy of the assessment methods used. In most epidemiological studies, including the present study, lifestyle factors are assessed through self-reporting, which is considered a rather imprecise method and is moreover prone to social desirability and recall bias [36, 37]. Given the high potential for misclassification, existing associations between lifestyle factors and change in glycemic status might not be detected [4]. In the case of physical activity, we also had to combine the assessed 5 categories into a dichotomous variable due to the relatively small sample sizes in certain categories, which might have been too broad to identify existing associations. Of particular relevance to dietary intake, a further explanation for our null finding might be that the influence of individual dietary components is fairly small and therefore difficult to detect. In the present study, values of the diabetes risk score had the expected associations with glycemic changes. These findings could not be fully explained by waist circumference or age (as two main score components) and thus highlight the value of a multifactorial diabetes risk assessment. In addition, a recent interventional study suggests that among individuals with prediabetes, there might be a high-risk phenotype that does not respond to lifestyle interventions such as dietary counseling and exercise [38–40].

Despite their discussed role in diabetes pathophysiology, traffic intensity and mental distress were also not related to glycemic changes among prediabetic adults in multivariate analyses. While we did not find a comparable study on traffic-related exposures, one study showed that mental loss as assessed by the mental component score of the SF-12 questionnaire was associated with a progression to diabetes in adults with IFG or IGT [41].

Similar to our findings, previous studies of individuals with IFG found higher baseline levels [7, 8, 10] or an increase in triglycerides [7] to be associated with a progression in glycemic status. However, the results that show a progression in glycemic status are less consistent for studies that analyze individuals with IFG and IGT together [6, 9, 35]. Only a few previous studies have explored measures of lipid metabolism with respect to a regression in glycemic status from IFG or IGT, and the findings have been inconsistent [9, 10]. The findings of the current study for liver enzymes, i.e., the association of higher GGT and ALT levels with progression in glycemic status, are in line with findings for GGT observed for individuals with IFG or IGT in a South African cohort [35]. With respect to hs-CRP, a study among Chinese adults with IGT found that higher levels of hs-CRP indicated a progression to diabetes [42], whereas no association with glycemic changes was observed in our study.

4.2. Limitations. This nationwide cohort study comprised participants from the general adult population in Germany covering a wide age range. However, the follow-up rate was rather moderate and the GNHIES98 participants who took part in the follow-up survey had some different characteristics from those who did not reparticipate or were deceased [24]. To account for differences arising from nonparticipation, a weighting factor was computed following the approach described above [27] and applied to all analyses in the present study.

Despite the application of a weighting factor, our study population might have been healthier compared to other studies. This was reflected by a higher proportion (34%) of individuals who reverted to normoglycemia compared to some other studies. For example, the proportion of participants with a regression was 4.4% based on data from the Whitehall II study, which applied the same definition for prediabetes but had a shorter follow-up time [17]. On the other hand, similar to that in our study, the proportion of individuals with a progression to diabetes was approximately one-fifth of participants in the Atherosclerosis Risk in Communities (ARIC) study, which used the same prediabetes definition and a similar follow-up length [43] as those of our study. One reason for the rather high proportion of individuals who reverted to normoglycemia in our study might be the relatively high proportion of individuals at the lower threshold of HbA1c-defined prediabetes. Thus, in a sensitivity analysis, we applied a stricter definition to identify only *relevant* changes in glycemic status. Nonetheless, the results remained largely unchanged.

Moreover, the proportion of participants with a migration background was rather low, and therefore, ethnicity could not be taken into account as a potential determining factor for glycemic changes [44]. We also had no information on whether participants only temporarily progressed to diabetes or regressed to normoglycemia between baseline and follow-up [45]. Further, we cannot rule out that the observed associations between changes in risk factors and changes in glycemic status in the additional analyses might be biased from reverse causation. Moreover, we did not adjust for multiple testing since analyses were exploratory.

Based on HbA1c measures and information about diabetes diagnosis, the present study permitted the identification of similarities and differences in the progression to diagnosed and undiagnosed diabetes. However, due to the lack of additional markers of glucose metabolism, we were unable to directly compare findings between individuals whose prediabetes was based on HbA1c and those whose prediabetes was defined by glucose criteria (e.g., IFG or IGT). The definition of prediabetes based on either of these measures might be too narrow, and a more refined identification of subgroups at high risk of developing diabetes remains a challenge with high relevance for the development of effective case finding and prevention strategies [38, 39, 46].

5. Conclusion

In this nationwide cohort of German adults who were followed for 12 years, approximately one-third of the individuals with HbA1c-based prediabetes reverted to normoglycemia and one-fifth progressed to self-reported diagnosed or HbA1c-based undiagnosed diabetes. Measures of anthropometry and lipid metabolism at baseline or as change during follow-up showed the most consistent associations with changes in glycemic status in both directions. In addition, elevated liver enzymes were related to the future development of undiagnosed or diagnosed diabetes; older age and a family history of diabetes were further associated with future diagnosed diabetes. In contrast with results from previous studies that primarily relied on glucose-based definitions of prediabetic states, the findings of the current study appear to be more variable for metabolic than for anthropometric markers. This difference is not surprising, given that the use of different diagnostic criteria to define glycemic status is likely to represent different pathophysiological states of glucose dysregulation. Our results further support the relevance of the HbA1c criterion in the definition of prediabetes and also demonstrate the need for more refined case finding strategies for diabetes prevention.

Abbreviations

ADA: American Diabetes Association
ALT: Alanine aminotransferase
DEGS1: German Health Interview and Examination Survey for Adults
GGT: Gamma-glutamyl transferase
GNHIES98: German National Health Interview and Examination Survey 1998
GDRS: German Diabetes Risk Score
hs-CRP: High-sensitivity C-reactive protein
IFG: Impaired fasting glucose
IGT: Impaired glucose tolerance.

Data Availability

The data set used in the study cannot be made publicly available because informed consent from study participants did not cover public access to the data. However, the minimal data set underlying the findings presented in this study is archived in the "Health Monitoring" Research Data Centre at the Robert Koch Institute (RKI) and may be accessed by all interested researchers. On-site access to the data set is possible at the Secure Data Center of the RKI's "Health Monitoring" Research Data Centre. Requests should be submitted to fdz@rki.de.

Conflicts of Interest

The authors declare that there is no conflict of interest regarding the publication of this paper.

Acknowledgments

The survey GNHIES98 and the primary part of DEGS1 were funded by the German Federal Ministry of Health. This study was supported by research grants from the German Federal Ministry of Health (FKZ: GE20130320).

References

[1] J. S. Skyler, G. L. Bakris, E. Bonifacio et al., "Differentiation of diabetes by pathophysiology, natural history, and prognosis," *Diabetes*, vol. 66, no. 2, pp. 241–255, 2017.

[2] A. G. Tabak, C. Herder, W. Rathmann, E. J. Brunner, and M. Kivimaki, "Prediabetes: a high-risk state for diabetes development," *Lancet*, vol. 379, no. 9833, pp. 2279–2290, 2012.

[3] J. W. Stevens, K. Khunti, R. Harvey et al., "Preventing the progression to type 2 diabetes mellitus in adults at high risk: a systematic review and network meta-analysis of lifestyle, pharmacological and surgical interventions," *Diabetes Research and Clinical Practice*, vol. 107, no. 3, pp. 320–331, 2015.

[4] D. H. Bodicoat, K. Khunti, B. T. Srinivasan et al., "Incident type 2 diabetes and the effect of early regression to normoglycaemia in a population with impaired glucose regulation," *Diabetic Medicine*, vol. 34, no. 3, pp. 396–404, 2017.

[5] American Diabetes Association, "2. Classification and diagnosis of diabetes: *standards of medical care in diabetes - 2018*," *Diabetes Care*, vol. 41, Supplement 1, pp. S13–S27, 2018.

[6] R. M. Anjana, C. S. Shanthi Rani, M. Deepa et al., "Incidence of diabetes and prediabetes and predictors of progression among Asian Indians: 10-year follow-up of the Chennai Urban Rural Epidemiology Study (CURES)," *Diabetes Care*, vol. 38, no. 8, pp. 1441–1448, 2015.

[7] S. S. Rasmussen, C. Glumer, A. Sandbaek, T. Lauritzen, and K. Borch-Johnsen, "Determinants of progression from impaired fasting glucose and impaired glucose tolerance to diabetes in a high-risk screened population: 3 year follow-up in the ADDITION study, Denmark," *Diabetologia*, vol. 51, no. 2, pp. 249–257, 2008.

[8] G. A. Nichols, T. A. Hillier, and J. B. Brown, "Progression from newly acquired impaired fasting glusose to type 2 diabetes," *Diabetes Care*, vol. 30, no. 2, pp. 228–233, 2007.

[9] X. Song, M. Qiu, X. Zhang et al., "Gender-related affecting factors of prediabetes on its 10-year outcome," *BMJ Open Diabetes Research & Care*, vol. 4, no. 1, article e000169, 2016.

[10] L. de Abreu, K. L. Holloway, M. A. Kotowicz, and J. A. Pasco, "Dysglycaemia and other predictors for progression or regression from impaired fasting glucose to diabetes or normoglycaemia," *Journal of Diabetes Research*, vol. 2015, Article ID 373762, 8 pages, 2015.

[11] S. L. Edelstein, W. C. Knowler, R. P. Bain et al., "Predictors of progression from impaired glucose tolerance to NIDDM: an analysis of six prospective studies," *Diabetes*, vol. 46, no. 4, pp. 701–710, 1997.

[12] B. Kowall, W. Rathmann, M. Heier et al., "Impact of weight and weight change on normalization of prediabetes and on persistence of normal glucose tolerance in an older population: the KORA S4/F4 study," *International Journal of Obesity*, vol. 36, no. 6, pp. 826–833, 2011.

[13] A. Gautier, R. Roussel, P. H. Ducluzeau et al., "Increases in waist circumference and weight as predictors of type 2 diabetes in individuals with impaired fasting glucose: influence of baseline BMI: data from the DESIR study," *Diabetes Care*, vol. 33, no. 8, pp. 1850–1852, 2010.

[14] A. F. Ishola, H. C. Gerstein, J. C. Engert et al., "Longitudinal relationships between glycemic status and body mass index

in a multiethnic study: evidence from observational and genetic epidemiology," *Scientific Reports*, vol. 6, no. 1, article 30744, 2016.

[15] S. Engberg, C. Glumer, D. R. Witte, T. Jorgensen, and K. Borch-Johnsen, "Differential relationship between physical activity and progression to diabetes by glucose tolerance status: the Inter99 study," *Diabetologia*, vol. 53, no. 1, pp. 70–78, 2010.

[16] P. Lecomte, S. Vol, E. Cacès et al., "Five-year predictive factors of type 2 diabetes in men with impaired fasting glucose," *Diabetes & Metabolism*, vol. 33, no. 2, pp. 140–147, 2007.

[17] K. Faerch, D. R. Witte, E. J. Brunner et al., "Physical activity and improvement of glycemia in prediabetes by different diagnostic criteria," *The Journal of Clinical Endocrinology and Metabolism*, vol. 102, no. 10, pp. 3712–3721, 2017.

[18] D. Vistisen, D. R. Witte, E. J. Brunner et al., "Risk of cardiovascular disease and death in individuals with prediabetes defined by different criteria: the Whitehall II study," *Diabetes Care*, vol. 41, no. 4, pp. 899–906, 2018.

[19] W. Thefeld, H. Stolzenberg, and B.-M. Bellach, "German National Health Interview and Examination Survey: Response, composition of participants, and analysis of non-respondents," *Gesundheitswesen*, vol. 61, pp. S57–S61, 1999.

[20] C. Scheidt-Nave, P. Kamtsiuris, A. Gosswald et al., "German Health Interview and Examination Survey for Adults (DEGS) - design, objectives and implementation of the first data collection wave," *BMC Public Health*, vol. 12, no. 1, p. 730, 2012.

[21] Diabetes Control and Complications Trial Research Group, D. M. Nathan, S. Genuth et al., "The effect of intensive treatment of diabetes on the development and progression of long-term complications in insulin-dependent diabetes mellitus," *The New England Journal of Medicine*, vol. 329, no. 14, pp. 977–986, 1993.

[22] C. Heidemann, Y. Du, R. Paprott, M. Haftenberger, W. Rathmann, and C. Scheidt-Nave, "Temporal changes in the prevalence of diagnosed diabetes, undiagnosed diabetes and prediabetes: findings from the German Health Interview and Examination Surveys in 1997-1999 and 2008-2011," *Diabetic Medicine*, vol. 33, no. 10, pp. 1406–1414, 2016.

[23] R. Paprott, K. Mühlenbruch, G. B. M. Mensink et al., "Validation of the German Diabetes Risk Score among the general adult population: findings from the German Health Interview and Examination Surveys," *BMJ Open Diabetes Research & Care*, vol. 4, no. 1, article e000280, 2016.

[24] C. Heidemann, H. Niemann, R. Paprott, Y. Du, W. Rathmann, and C. Scheidt-Nave, "Residential traffic and incidence of type 2 diabetes: the German Health Interview and Examination Surveys," *Diabetic Medicine*, vol. 31, no. 10, pp. 1269–1276, 2014.

[25] M. J. Kelly, F. D. Dunstan, K. Lloyd, and D. L. Fone, "Evaluating cutpoints for the MHI-5 and MCS using the GHQ-12: a comparison of five different methods," *BMC Psychiatry*, vol. 8, no. 1, p. 10, 2008.

[26] K. Mühlenbruch, T. Ludwig, C. Jeppesen et al., "Update of the German Diabetes Risk Score and external validation in the German MONICA/KORA study," *Diabetes Research and Clinical Practice*, vol. 104, no. 3, pp. 459–466, 2014.

[27] P. Kamtsiuris, M. Lange, R. Hoffmann et al., "The first wave of the German health interview and examination survey for adults (DEGS1): sample design, response, weighting and representativeness," *Bundesgesundheitsblatt Gesundheitsforschung Gesundheitsschutz*, vol. 56, no. 5-6, pp. 620–630, 2013.

[28] S. Greenland, J. Pearl, and J. M. Robins, "Causal diagrams for epidemiologic research," *Epidemiology*, vol. 10, no. 1, pp. 37–48, 1999.

[29] P. A. Berglund, "Multiple imputation using the fully conditional specification method: a comparison of SAS®, Stata, IVEware, and R. Paper 2081-2015," 2015, http://support.sas.com/resources/papers/proceedings15/2081-2015.pdf.

[30] T. E. Bodner, "What improves with increased missing data imputations?," *Structural Equation Modeling: A Multidisciplinary Journal*, vol. 15, no. 4, pp. 651–675, 2008.

[31] B. Ratitch, I. Lipkovic, and M. O'Kelly, *Combining Analysis Results from Multiply Imputed Categorical Data*, PharmaSUG 2013-Paper SP03, 2013.

[32] A. Oksuzyan, K. Juel, J. W. Vaupel, and K. Christensen, "Men: good health and high mortality. Sex differences in health and aging," *Aging Clinical and Experimental Research*, vol. 20, no. 2, pp. 91–102, 2008.

[33] H. J. Murff, R. L. Rothman, D. W. Byrne, and S. Syngal, "The impact of family history of diabetes on glucose testing and counseling behavior in primary care," *Diabetes Care*, vol. 27, no. 9, pp. 2247-2248, 2004.

[34] R. Valdez, P. W. Yoon, T. Liu, and M. J. Khoury, "Family history and prevalence of diabetes in the U.S. population: the 6-year results from the National Health and Nutrition Examination Survey (1999-2004)," *Diabetes Care*, vol. 30, no. 10, pp. 2517–2522, 2007.

[35] T. E. Matsha, D. J. Soita, M. S. Hassan et al., "Three-year's changes in glucose tolerance status in the Bellville South cohort: rates and phenotypes associated with progression," *Diabetes Research and Clinical Practice*, vol. 99, no. 2, pp. 223–230, 2013.

[36] J. R. Hebert, L. Clemow, L. Pbert, I. S. Ockene, and J. K. Ockene, "Social desirability bias in dietary self-report may compromise the validity of dietary intake measures," *International Journal of Epidemiology*, vol. 24, no. 2, pp. 389–398, 1995.

[37] L. S. Freedman, A. Schatzkin, D. Midthune, and V. Kipnis, "Dealing with dietary measurement error in nutritional cohort studies," *Journal of the National Cancer Institute*, vol. 103, no. 14, pp. 1086–1092, 2011.

[38] N. Stefan, H. Staiger, R. Wagner et al., "A high-risk phenotype associates with reduced improvement in glycaemia during a lifestyle intervention in prediabetes," *Diabetologia*, vol. 58, no. 12, pp. 2877–2884, 2015.

[39] N. Stefan, A. Fritsche, F. Schick, and H. U. Haring, "Phenotypes of prediabetes and stratification of cardiometabolic risk," *The Lancet Diabetes and Endocrinology*, vol. 4, no. 9, pp. 789–798, 2016.

[40] V. Schmid, R. Wagner, C. Sailer et al., "Non-alcoholic fatty liver disease and impaired proinsulin conversion as newly identified predictors of the long-term non-response to a lifestyle intervention for diabetes prevention: results from the TULIP study," *Diabetologia*, vol. 60, no. 12, pp. 2341–2351, 2017.

[41] M. Hunger, R. Holle, C. Meisinger, W. Rathmann, A. Peters, and M. Schunk, "Longitudinal changes in health-related qual-

ity of life in normal glucose tolerance, prediabetes and type 2 diabetes: results from the KORA S4/F4 cohort study," *Quality of Life Research*, vol. 23, no. 9, pp. 2515–2520, 2014.

[42] K. C. B. Tan, N. M. S. Wat, S. C. F. Tam, E. D. Janus, T. H. Lam, and K. S. L. Lam, "C-reactive protein predicts the deterioration of glycemia in Chinese subjects with impaired glucose tolerance," *Diabetes Care*, vol. 26, no. 8, pp. 2323–2328, 2003.

[43] E. Selvin, M. W. Steffes, E. Gregg, F. L. Brancati, and J. Coresh, "Performance of A1C for the classification and prediction of diabetes," *Diabetes Care*, vol. 34, no. 1, pp. 84–89, 2010.

[44] N. Abate and M. Chandalia, "The impact of ethnicity on type 2 diabetes," *Journal of Diabetes and its Complications*, vol. 17, no. 1, pp. 39–58, 2003.

[45] L. Perreault, Q. Pan, K. J. Mather et al., "Effect of regression from prediabetes to normal glucose regulation on long-term reduction in diabetes risk: results from the Diabetes Prevention Program Outcomes Study," *Lancet*, vol. 379, no. 9833, pp. 2243–2251, 2012.

[46] M. E. Bowen, "Rethinking diabetes screening and case finding strategies in clinical practice: who's really at risk?," 2016, https://cme.utsouthwestern.edu/sites/cme.utsouthwestern.edu/files/em1608e_082616_protocol_bowen.pdf.

10

Comparative Biochemical and Histopathological Studies on the Efficacy of Metformin and Virgin Olive Oil against Streptozotocin-Induced Diabetes in Sprague-Dawley Rats

Khadijah Saeed Balamash,[1] Huda Mohammed Alkreathy,[2] Elham Hamed Al Gahdali,[1] Sawsan Omer Khoja,[1] and Aftab Ahmad[3]

[1]*Department of Biochemistry, Faculty of Science, King Abdulaziz University, Jeddah, Saudi Arabia*
[2]*Department of Pharmacology, Faculty of Medicine, King Abdulaziz University, Jeddah, Saudi Arabia*
[3]*Health Information Technology Department, Jeddah Community College, King Abdulaziz University, P.O. Box 80283, Jeddah 21589, Saudi Arabia*

Correspondence should be addressed to Huda Mohammed Alkreathy; halkreathy@kau.edu.sa

Academic Editor: Raffaele Marfella

Treatment of diabetic patients with antioxidant, such as extra virgin olive oil (EVOO), may be beneficial in numerous debilitating complexities. This study was aimed at assessing the protective role of virgin olive oil in reducing hyperglycemia in streptozotocin- (STZ-) induced diabetic rats. Thirty-six healthy male Sprague-Dawley rats were divided into six groups (6 rats per group) including nondiabetic control (NC), diabetic control (DC), and animals treated with metformin, olive oil, and a combination of olive oil and metformin, respectively. The protective effect of olive oil was evaluated by determining the biochemical parameters (lipid profile, liver, and kidney) and by studying the histopathological alterations in pancreas, liver, and kidney tissues. The results showed a significant increase in alanine aminotransferase (ALT) and alkaline phosphatase (ALP) levels in diabetic rats. ALP levels remained significantly elevated in the diabetic rats that were treated with metformin and/or olive oil, and the highest level was noted in the group treated with olive oil (568.33 U/L). Contrarily, pretreatment with olive oil significantly decreased ALT (67.64 U/L) and ALP (226.17 U/L) levels. Histopathological data revealed that all the disorganized islets of Langerhans along with the clusters of inflammatory cells were absent in the group pretreated with the combination of virgin olive oil and metformin, which shows that prophylactic administration of this combination reduces the diabetic complications in a much better way. Therefore, pretreatment with olive oil with or without metformin is an encouraging approach for diabetes therapy with immense potential.

1. Introduction

The incidence of diabetes, a metabolic disorder, has soared globally in the last three decades mainly due to lifestyle modifications [1, 2]. It is estimated that by the year 2040, the number of diabetic adults worldwide would reach 642 million [3].

Diabetes mellitus (DM) is a global health issue with an ever increasing prevalence. The primary causes for the global ascendancy in DM are as follows: increase in aged population, stationary way of life, expanding patterns towards obesity, and unhealthy diet [1, 2]. The symptoms of DM consist of increased hunger, increased thirst, weight loss, polyuria, obscuring of vision, irregularities of lipoprotein metabolism, and hypertension. Severe complexities of diabetes mellitus like nonketotic hyperosmolar state or ketoacidosis might develop and may cause stupor, coma, and death [4]. The long-standing effects of diabetes mellitus involve a gradual advancement of the particular complexities of retinopathy with potential visual impairment, nephropathy that may prompt renal impairment, and/or neuropathy with danger of foot ulcers, Charcot joints, and features of autonomic dysfunction [5].

Since diabetes is known to induce an increase in free radical production that further leads to oxidative stress and damage of cell components, it is hypothesized that an antioxidant therapy could help to prevent diabetic complications [6]. Antioxidants might prevent the development of diabetes by repressing the peroxidation chain reaction [7, 8]. Numerous routine antioxidants like vitamin E and phenolic compounds are known to have hypoglycemic and/or hypolipidemic activities [9]. Though many antidiabetic medications are available, safer organic sources are preferred by diabetic patients.

Olive oil is one such natural agent that is a high source of phenols and is known to induce protective effects against many diseases [10]. The phenolic compounds of olive oil have anti-inflammatory and antioxidant properties and also have favorable impact on different physiological parameters, such as antimicrobial actions, bone validity, inflammatory markers, oxidative harm, plasma lipoproteins, and platelet and cell capacity [10–12]. Diet rich in olive oil is also known to mitigate diabetes [13, 14].

Therefore, this study is aimed at assessing the protective role of virgin olive oil in reducing hyperglycemia in STZ-induced diabetic rats by determining serum biochemical parameters and by studying the histopathological alterations of the pancreas, liver, and kidney.

2. Materials and Methods

2.1. Materials. Virgin olive oil (VOO) was obtained from Aladhara agricultural project, Al-Jouf, Kingdom of Saudi Arabia (KSA). Streptozotocin (STZ) was purchased from Sigma-Aldrich, USA. Metformin as glucophage (1000 mg tablet) was procured from a local pharmacy and was dissolved in distilled water containing 0.9% (wt/vol) sodium chloride for oral administration.

2.2. Animals. A total of 36 male Sprague-Dawley rats weighing 200-250 g were used for the study. The rats were housed in plastic cages at a controlled temperature of 22 ± 3°C with a 12-hour light/dark cycle for two weeks. Animals were fed with standard chow and supplied with drinking water ad libitum. The study lasted for a total of 6 weeks.

The protocol of this study was approved by the Unit of Biomedical Ethics, Faculty of Medicine, King Abdulaziz University, Jeddah, Saudi Arabia. All animal procedures and experiments were performed according to King Abdulaziz University's policy and international ethical guidelines on the care and use of laboratory animals (the National Research Council of the National Academy of Sciences, 2011).

2.3. Methods

2.3.1. Induction of Diabetes. Streptozotocin (STZ) was dissolved in 0.05 M citrate buffer (pH 4.5; 1 mL). Diabetes was induced by giving a single intraperitoneal (IP) injection of STZ (40 mg/kg bw). [15]. After STZ injection, rats were given 10% (wt/vol) ad libitum fructose solution for 3 days. Blood glucose level was measured after 3 days. Animals with blood glucose level above 250 mg/dL were considered diabetic and were used in the experiment. Rats were divided into six groups: group 1 comprised of nondiabetic control (NC) rats that were given normal saline, group 2 included diabetic control (DC) rats, group 3 had diabetic rats treated with metformin (DM) (the initial dose was 300 mg/kg bw/day given by oral gavage for 2 weeks which was then increased to 500 mg/kg bw/day for 4 weeks), group 4 included diabetic rats that were given olive oil (DO) (1 mL/100 g bw/day), group 5 had diabetic rats treated with olive oil and metformin (DOM) (diabetic rats were given olive oil (1 mL/100 g bw/day) orally for six weeks, and then the rats were treated daily with metformin (300 mg/kg bw/day) by oral gavage for two weeks followed by increasing the dose of metformin to 500 mg/kg bw/day for four weeks), and group 6 included diabetic rats that were given olive oil pretreatment (DOP) (1 mL/100 g bw/day) for 2 weeks before the induction of diabetes.

2.3.2. Oral Glucose Tolerance Test. Prior to overnight fasting and administration of D-glucose, blood was collected from the tail tip after 0, 30, 60, 90, and 120 minutes of administration.

2.4. Biochemical Analysis. Blood for biochemical analysis was collected via intraorbital sinus, and serum preparation was done by centrifugation (Sigma-Aldrich, USA) at 4000 rpm for 10 minutes. The serum was kept at −80°C for biochemical analysis.

2.4.1. Lipid Profile. Cholesterol, high-density lipoprotein (HDL), low-density lipoprotein (LDL), and triacylglycerol (TAG) were measured in serum using CHOL Flex® Reagent Cartridge, LDL Flex® Reagent Cartridge, and TRIG Flex® Reagent Cartridge (Siemens Healthcare Diagnostics Inc., Newark, USA), respectively, and measurements were taken according to the manufacturer's instructions.

2.4.2. Determination of Liver Function. Alkaline phosphatase (ALP), aspartate aminotransferase (AST), alanine aminotransferase (ALT), albumin (ALB), bilirubin (BIL), and total protein (TP) were measured using ALP Flex® Reagent Cartridge, AST Flex® Reagent Cartridge, ALTI Flex® Reagent Cartridge, ALB Flex® Reagent Cartridge, BIL Flex® Reagent Cartridge, and TP Flex® Reagent Cartridge (Siemens Healthcare Diagnostics Inc., Newark, USA), respectively, and experiments were performed according to the manufacturer's instructions.

2.4.3. Determination of Kidney Function. Creatinine (CREA), uric acid (URCA), and blood urea nitrogen (BUN) were measured using CREA Flex® Reagent Cartridge, URCA Flex® Reagent Cartridge, and BUN Flex® Reagent Cartridge (Siemens Healthcare Diagnostics Inc., Newark, USA), respectively. All experiments were performed according to the manufacturer's instructions.

2.5. Histopathological Examination. The liver, kidney, and pancreas from all the six groups of rats were fixed with 10%

TABLE 1: Lipid profiles of different groups of rats during the experiment and after the induction of diabetes by streptozotocin. Data was expressed as mean ± standard deviation (SD). Significances among different groups were determined by using the one-way analysis of variance (ANOVA) test. [1]***P***: significance versus control, [2]***P***: significance versus diabetic control.

Rat groups	Cholesterol (mmol/L)	High-density lipoprotein (mmol/L)	Low-density lipoprotein (mmol/L)	Triacylglycerol (mmol/L)
Group 1: nondiabetic control (NC)	1.37 ± 0.13	1.30 ± 0.10	0.23 ± 0.02	0.63 ± 0.13
Group 2: diabetic control (DC)	1.39 ± 0.10 $^1P = 0.899$	1.11 ± 0.21 $^1P = 0.127$	0.33 ± 0.03 $^1P = 0.097$	0.82 ± 0.17 $^1P = 0.540$
Group 3: diabetic and metformin (DM)	1.47 ± 0.23 $^1P = 0.486$, $^2P = 0.590$	1.31 ± 0.19 $^1P = 0.943$, $^2P = 0.111$	0.30 ± 0.06 $^1P = 0.196$, $^2P = 0.658$	1.98 ± 0.65 $^1\mathbf{P = 0.0001}$, $^2\mathbf{P = 0.0001}$
Group 4: diabetic and olive oil (DO)	1.42 ± 0.42 $^1P = 0.719$, $^2P = 0.828$	1.31 ± 0.22 $^1P = 0.954$, $^2P = 0.114$	0.36 ± 0.04 $^1\mathbf{P = 0.025}$, $^2P = 0.599$	1.15 ± 0.47 $^1P = 0.077$, $^2P = 0.273$
Group 5: diabetic, olive oil, and metformin (DOM)	1.36 ± 0.25 $^1P = 0.955$, $^2P = 0.857$	1.26 ± 0.09 $^1P = 0.722$, $^2P = 0.230$	0.31 ± 0.12 $^1P = 0.144$, $^2P = 0.782$	1.42 ± 0.44 $^1\mathbf{P = 0.009}$, $^2P = 0.052$
Group 6: diabetic and olive oil pretreatment (DOP)	1.34 ± 0.29 $^1P = 0.848$, $^2P = 0.757$	1.20 ± 0.19 $^1P = 0.387$, $^2P = 0.472$	0.42 ± 0.22 $^1\mathbf{P = 0.001}$, $^2P = 0.126$	1.04 ± 0.53 $^1P = 0.164$, $^2P = 0.466$

buffered formalin for 24 hours. Tissues were embedded in paraffin blocks and sectioned at approximately 3-5 μm thickness and were then stained with hematoxylin and eosin (H&E). Stained sections were examined for histological changes using light microscopy (Olympus BX51TF), and representative images were captured with an Olympus DP 72 camera.

2.6. Statistical Analysis. All the data were analyzed using SPSS (Statistical Package for the Social Sciences) version 20.0 software (SPSS Inc., Chicago, IL, USA). The data were presented as mean ± standard deviation (SD). Significance among different groups was determined by using the one-way analysis of variance (ANOVA) test. A P value of less than 0.05 was taken as having a statistically significant difference.

3. Results

3.1. Effect of Olive Oil on the Biochemical Parameters of STZ-Induced Diabetic Rats

3.1.1. Effect on the Lipid Profile. Nonsignificant changes were observed in the serum lipid profile of DC rats when compared to NC rats. The serum level of LDL in DO and DOP groups was significantly higher than that in the NC group ($P = 0.025$ and $P = 0.001$, respectively), but there was no significant difference in DM and DOM groups. The TAG serum level was significantly higher in the DM group than in NC and DC groups ($P = 0.0001$ and $P = 0.0001$, respectively), while it was higher in the DOM group than in the NC group ($P = 0.009$). TAG levels were not significantly different in DO and DOP groups when compared to NC and DC groups. No significant differences in the CHO and HDL serum level were observed among all the treated groups when compared to NC and DC groups (Table 1).

3.1.2. Effect on Liver Function. There was a nonsignificant difference in the serum AST, TP, BIL, and ALB of DC rats when compared to NC rats. The AST serum level in the DM group was significantly higher than that in NC and DC groups ($P = 0.001$ and $P = 0.029$, respectively). The AST level was also significantly higher in the DOM group than in the NC group ($P = 0.049$); however, there was no remarkable difference in DO and DOP groups when compared to NC and DC groups. On the other hand, the ALT serum level in DC, DM, DO, DOM, and DOP groups was noticeably more than that in the NC group ($P = 0.0001$, $P = 0.0001$, $P = 0.0001$, $P = 0.0001$, and $P = 0.022$, respectively) but was considerably lower in the DOP group than in the DC group ($P = 0.0001$). The ALP serum level in DC, DM, DO, DOM, and DOP groups was notably more than that in the NC group ($P = 0.0001$, $P = 0.0001$, $P = 0.0001$, $P = 0.0001$, and $P = 0.023$, respectively). It was also significantly higher in the DO group but lower in the DOP group than in the DC group ($P = 0.0001$ and $P = 0.015$, respectively). No meaningful differences in BIL serum level were observed among all the treated groups when compared to NC and DC groups. But the TP serum level was remarkably higher in the DO group than in NC and DC groups ($P = 0.017$ and $P = 0.004$, respectively) but was appreciably higher in the DOP group than in the DC group ($P = 0.020$); also, the changes were nonsignificant for the DOM group. The ALB serum level was significantly higher in DO and DOM groups than in the DC group ($P = 0.019$ and $P = 0.004$, respectively) but was not significantly different in DM and DOP groups when compared to NC and DC groups (Table 2).

3.1.3. Effect on Kidney Function. There was a nonsignificant difference in the serum BUN, CREA, and URCA of DC rats when compared to NC rats. BUN and URCA serum levels in the DM group were significantly higher ($P = 0.041$ and $P = 0.006$, respectively) but were not

TABLE 2: Liver functions of different groups of rats during the experiment and after the induction of diabetes by streptozotocin. Data was expressed as mean ± standard deviation (SD). Significances among different groups were determined by using the one-way analysis of variance (ANOVA) test. ^{1}**P**: significance versus control, ^{2}**P**: significance versus diabetic control.

Rat groups	Aspartate aminotransferase (U/L)	Alanine aminotransferase (U/L)	Alkaline phosphatase (U/L)	Bilirubin (μmol/L)	Total protein (g/L)	Albumin (g/L)
Group 1: nondiabetic control (NC)	114.01 ± 8.27	49.20 ± 11.84	134.20 ± 21.79	2.83 ± 0.41	70.00 ± 2.28	11.17 ± 1.72
Group 2: diabetic control (DC)	127.00 ± 18.83 $^{1}P = 0.274$	106.00 ± 14.25 ^{1}**P = 0.0001**	329.25 ± 24.19 ^{1}**P = 0.0001**	2.60 ± 0.89 $^{1}P = 0.663$	68.40 ± 2.79 $^{1}P = 0.505$	9.60 ± 1.95 $^{1}P = 0.070$
Group 3: diabetic and metformin (DM)	153.52 ± 27.24 ^{1}**P = 0.001**, ^{2}**P = 0.029**	92.60 ± 18.40 ^{1}**P = 0.0001**, $^{2}P = 0.105$	302.00 ± 73.70 ^{1}**P = 0.0001**, $^{2}P = 0.506$	3.50 ± 1.22 $^{1}P = 0.197$, $^{2}P = 0.099$	65.83 ± 3.87 $^{1}P = 0.074$, $^{2}P = 0.287$	10.50 ± 1.87 $^{1}P = 0.411$, $^{2}P = 0.291$
Group 4: diabetic and olive oil (DO)	134.00 ± 14.37 $^{1}P = 0.081$, $^{2}P = 0.554$	91.16 ± 13.05 ^{1}**P = 0.0001**, $^{2}P = 0.074$	568.33 ± 110.32 ^{1}**P = 0.0001**, ^{2}**P = 0.0001**	3.33 ± 1.21 $^{1}P = 0.331$, $^{2}P = 0.176$	75.67 ± 4.89 ^{1}**P = 0.017**, ^{2}**P = 0.004**	11.67 ± 1.37 $^{1}P = 0.537$, ^{2}**P = 0.019**
Group 5: diabetic, olive oil and metformin (DOM)	136.67 ± 34.05 ^{1}**P = 0.049**, $^{2}P = 0.414$	96.00 ± 11.47 ^{1}**P = 0.0001**, $^{2}P = 0.223$	348.68 ± 94.53 ^{1}**P = 0.0001**, $^{2}P = 0.635$	2.83 ± 0.41 $^{1}P = 1.000$, $^{2}P = 0.663$	72.50 ± 2.17 $^{1}P = 0.277$, $^{2}P = 0.092$	12.17 ± 0.98 $^{1}P = 0.220$, ^{2}**P = 0.004**
Group 6: diabetic and olive oil pretreatment (DOP)	114.60 ± 15.37 $^{1}P = 0.958$, $^{2}P = 0.296$	67.64 ± 12.10 ^{1}**P = 0.022**, ^{2}**P = 0.0001**	226.17 ± 53.05 ^{1}**P = 0.023**, ^{2}**P = 0.015**	3.00 ± 1.10 $^{1}P = 0.744$, $^{2}P = 0.457$	74.17 ± 3.76 $^{1}P = 0.074$, ^{2}**P = 0.020**	11.00 ± 0.63 $^{1}P = 0.836$, $^{2}P = 0.104$

TABLE 3: Kidney functions of different groups of rats during the experiment and after the induction of diabetes by streptozotocin. Data was expressed as mean ± standard deviation (SD). Significances among different groups were determined by using the one-way analysis of variance (ANOVA) test. ^{1}**P**: significance versus control, ^{2}**P**: significance versus diabetic control.

Rat groups	Blood urea nitrogen (mmol/L)	Creatinine (μmol/L)	Uric acid (μmol/L)
Group 1: nondiabetic control (NC)	7.23 ± 0.79	42.83 ± 5.38	55.17 ± 7.83
Group 2: diabetic control (DC)	7.84 ± 1.79 $^{1}P = 0.597$	49.80 ± 8.90 $^{1}P = 0.055$	48.80 ± 4.09 $^{1}P = 0.281$
Group 3: diabetic and metformin (DM)	10.25 ± 1.73 ^{1}**P = 0.008**, ^{2}**P = 0.041**	47.67 ± 5.54 $^{1}P = 0.159$, $^{2}P = 0.549$	65.83 ± 11.84 $^{1}P = 0.062$, ^{2}**P = 0.006**
Group 4: diabetic and olive oil (DO)	7.22 ± 2.14 $^{1}P = 0.988$, $^{2}P = 0.587$	48.67 ± 2.50 $^{1}P = 0.091$, $^{2}P = 0.750$	49.33 ± 15.32 $^{1}P = 0.300$, $^{2}P = 0.927$
Group 5: diabetic, olive oil, and metformin (DOM)	7.02 ± 1.48 $^{1}P = 0.843$, $^{2}P = 0.474$	48.17 ± 5.27 $^{1}P = 0.121$, $^{2}P = 0.646$	55.67 ± 7.79 $^{1}P = 0.929$, $^{2}P = 0.245$
Group 6: diabetic and olive oil pretreatment (DOP)	8.93 ± 3.43 $^{1}P = 0.125$, $^{2}P = 0.343$	45.83 ± 3.97 $^{1}P = 0.378$, $^{2}P = 0.268$	52.67 ± 7.39 $^{1}P = 0.655$, $^{2}P = 0.510$

significantly different in DO, DOM, and DOP groups in comparison to NC and DC groups. No significant differences in CREA serum level were observed among all the treated groups when compared to NC and DC groups (Table 3).

3.2. *Effect of Olive Oil on the Histopathology of the Pancreas, Liver, and Kidney of STZ-Induced Diabetic Rats*

3.2.1. Effect on the Histopathology of the Endocrine Pancreas (Islets of Langerhans). Histopathological examination of pancreatic tissue revealed that in untreated nondiabetic control (NC) rats, the islets of Langerhans as well as circumscribed masses surrounded by deeply stained pancreatic exocrine acini appeared normal (Figure 1(a)). β-cells could be identified partially with their location and their smaller dark nuclei, relative to those of α-cells. The cell clusters were separated by thin-wall blood sinusoids. In the pancreas of untreated diabetic control (DC) rats, islets of Langerhans appeared disorganized. β-cells showed an unstained vacuolated cytoplasm and dark-stained degenerated nuclei. Clusters of inflammatory cells could also be seen among the cells (Figure 1(b)). In contrast, the DM group showed that islets of Langerhans have a more or less normal cell population with the absence of degenerative changes as observed in the DC group. Blood

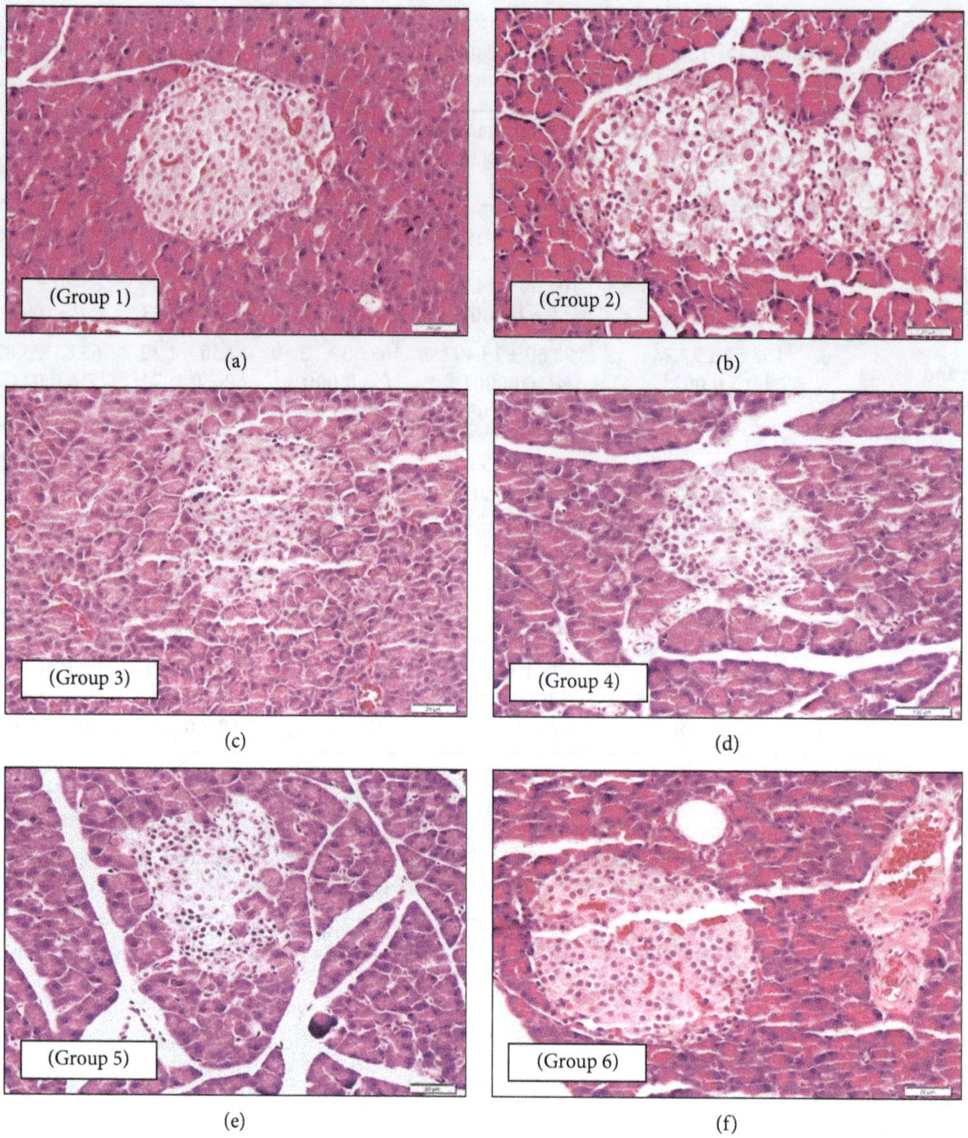

FIGURE 1: Photomicrographs of a section of the endocrine pancreatic tissue of rats: (a—group 1: NC) normal pancreatic structure and exocrine acini surrounding the islets of Langerhans (400x magnification); (b—group 2: DC) disorganized islets of Langerhans and clusters of inflammatory cells (β-cells show an unstained vacuolated cytoplasm and dark-stained degenerated nuclei) (400x magnification); (c—group 3: DM) normal islets of Langerhans and blood sinusoids (100x magnification); (d—group 4: DO) islets of Langerhans with a normal-looking population of β-cells (100x magnification); (e—group 5: DOM) normal islets of Langerhans with a normal population of β-cells and absence of any degenerative change (400x magnification); (f—group 6: DOP) normal islets of Langerhans with a normal β-cell population similar to that of group 1 (NC) indicating protection from the damaging effect of STZ (400x magnification). All sections were stained with H and E stain and viewed with a light microscope.

sinusoids also appeared to be normal (Figure 1(c)). Light microscopy examination of the pancreatic tissue of the DO group revealed that islets of Langerhans have a normal-looking population of β-cells (Figure 1(d)). The pancreatic tissue of the DOM group showed normal islets of Langerhans with a normal population of β-cells and absence of any degenerative changes observed in the DC group (Figure 1(e)). In the DOP group, islets of Langerhans appeared normal with a normal β-cell population, much like the NC group indicating protection from the damaging effect of STZ (Figure 1(f)).

3.2.2. Effect on the Histopathology of the Liver. Observation of the hepatic tissue of the untreated nondiabetic control (NC) rats showed histological features like radially arranged hepatocytes around the central vein. The cells have an acidophilic cytoplasm and rounded central vesicular euchromatic nuclei with well-defined nucleoli. The hepatocyte plates are separated by thin-walled blood sinusoids lined by flat endothelial cells. Occasionally, the prominent nuclei of von Kupffer cells were observed (Figure 2(a)). The section of the hepatic tissue of untreated diabetic control (DC) rats showed an increase in apoptotic hepatocytes (shrunken and dark-stained cells with

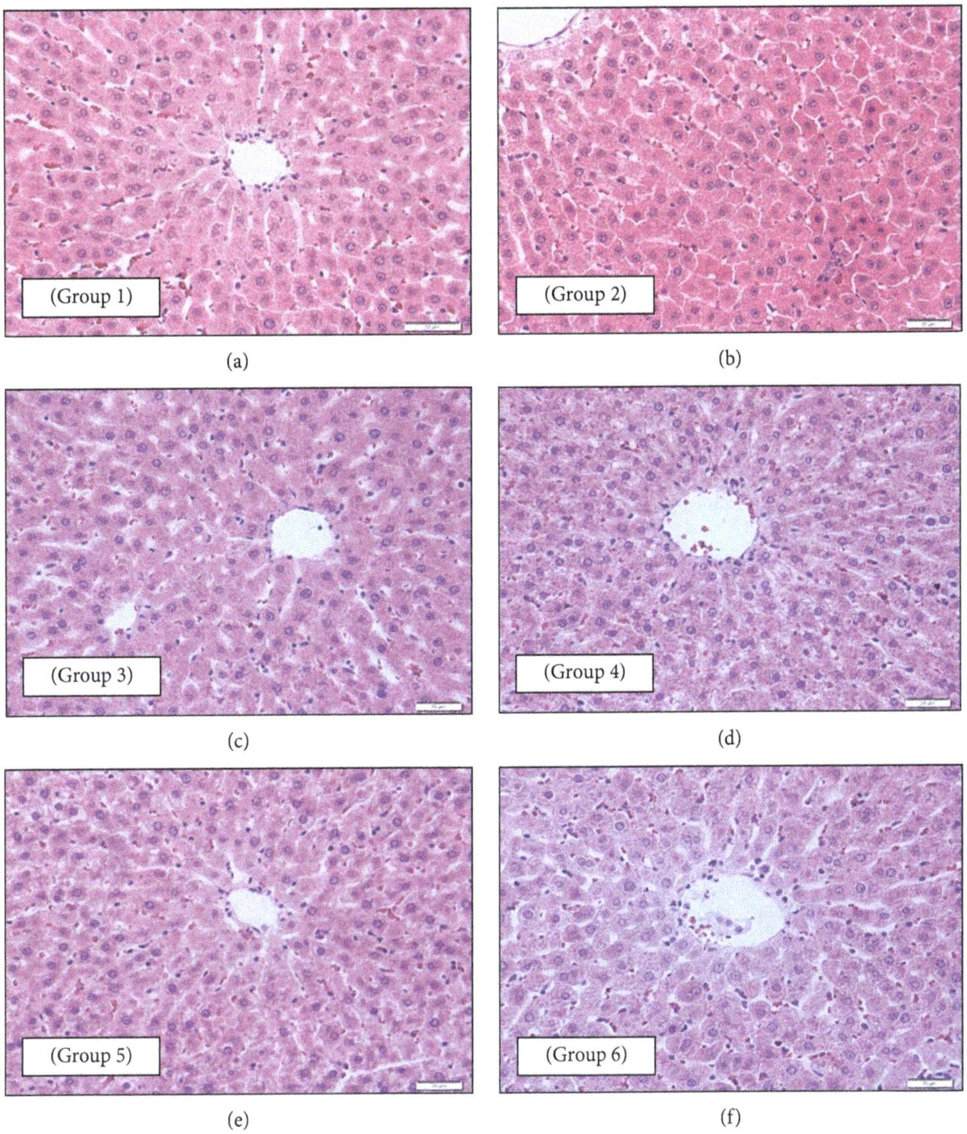

FIGURE 2: Photomicrographs of a section of the liver tissue of rats: (a—group 1: NC) almost normal hepatic structure (hepatocytes being radially arranged around the central vein and presence of von Kupffer cells lining the sinusoidal spaces) (200x magnification); (b—group 2: DC) numerous apoptotic dark-stained shrunken hepatocytes with small degenerated nuclei (400x magnification); (c—group 3: DM) nearly normal radially arranged hepatocytes around the central vein (it also shows that blood sinusoidal spaces and their von Kupffer cells are like those of the NC group) (400x magnification); (d—group 4: DO) almost normal hepatic structure with radially arranged hepatocytes around the central vein with the absence of any degenerated apoptotic cells (it also shows that hepatic sinusoidal spaces and von Kupffer cells are like those of the NC group) (400x magnification); (e—group 5: DOM) almost normal hepatic structure with radially arranged hepatocytes around the central vein (it also shows the presence of von Kupffer cells lining the sinusoidal spaces) (400x magnification); (f—group 6: DOP) almost normal hepatic structure with radially arranged hepatocytes around the central vein (it also shows active and healthy hepatocytes with active vesicular nuclei like that of the NC group) (400x magnification). All sections were stained with H and E stain and viewed with a light microscope.

small degenerated nuclei) (Figure 2(b)). The liver tissue sectioned from the DM rats showed nearly normal radially arranged hepatocytes around the central vein. Blood sinusoidal spaces and their von Kupffer cells are similar to those of the NC group (Figure 2(c)). The liver tissue taken from the DO rats exhibited almost normal hepatic structure with radially arranged hepatocytes around the central vein with the absence of any degenerated apoptotic cells. The hepatic sinusoidal spaces and von Kupffer cells are similar to those of the NC group (Figure 2(d)). Interestingly, the hepatic tissue of the DOM rat revealed relatively normal hepatic structure with radially arranged hepatocytes around the central vein. von Kupffer cells lining sinusoidal spaces were evident (Figure 2(e)). Meanwhile, the liver tissue of the DOP rat showed almost normal radially arranged hepatocytes around the central vein. Hepatocytes looked active and healthy with active vesicular nuclei similar to those observed in the NC group. The normal appearance of sinusoidal spaces and their lining by von Kupffer cells were exhibited (Figure 2(f)).

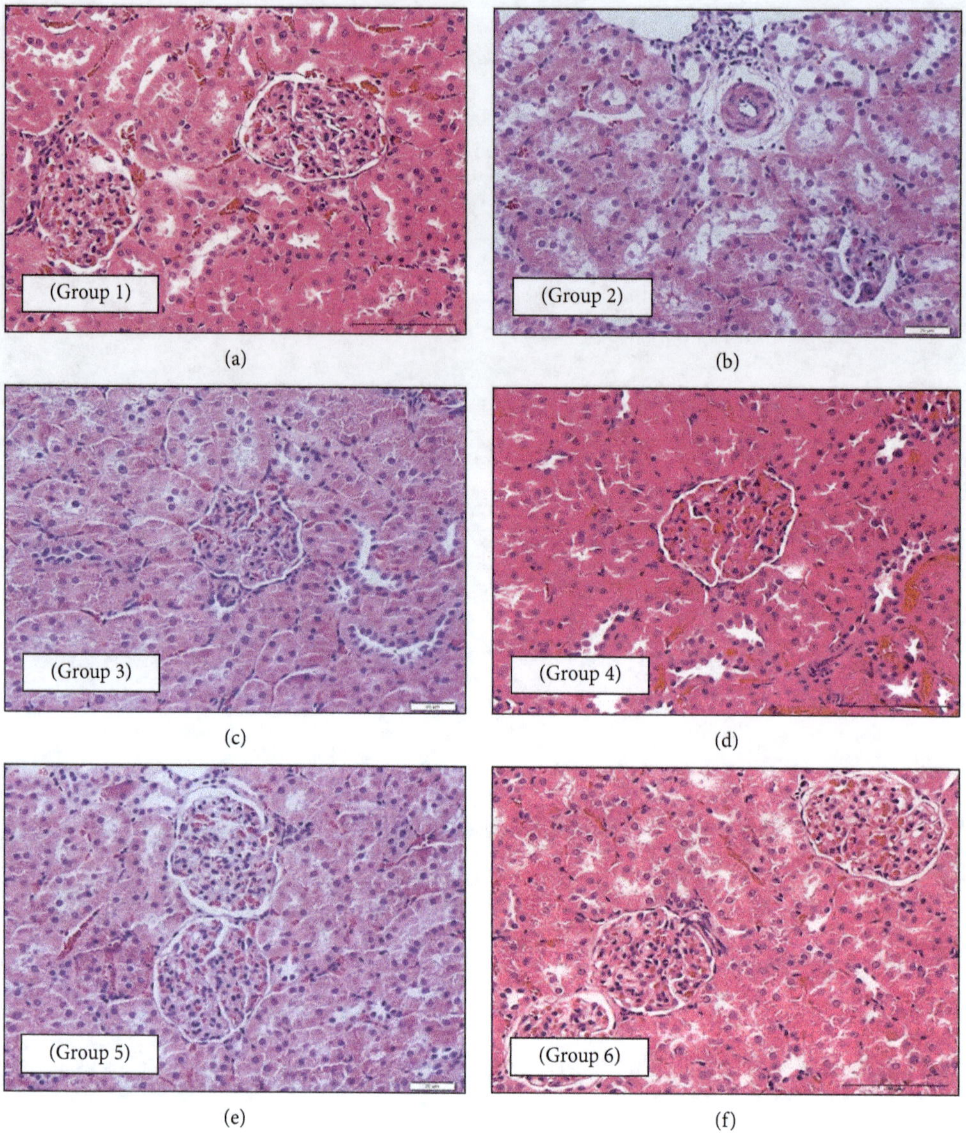

FIGURE 3: Photomicrographs of a section of the kidney tissue of rats: (a—group 1: NC) normal renal corpuscles with normal glomerular capillaries and renal tubules (40x magnification); (b—group 2: DC) deformity of renal corpuscle with atrophy of glomerular capillaries and unstained degenerated cytoplasmic regions in the renal tubular epithelium and arterioles showing diffused muscular media thickening with perivascular edema, fibrosis, and minimal interstitium lymphocytic infiltrate (400x magnification); (c—group 3: DM) normal renal corpuscles and glomeruli (it also shows normal renal tubules) (400x magnification); (d—group 4: DO) marked protection from diabetic changes with renal corpuscle, glomeruli, and tubules looking like those of the NC group (200x magnification); (e—group 5: DOM) marked protection against diabetic changes (it also shows normal and healthy renal corpuscles, glomeruli, and tubules) (400x magnification); (f—group 6: DOP) marked protection against diabetic changes (it also shows normal and healthy renal corpuscles, glomeruli, and tubules like those of the NC group) (200x magnification). All sections were stained with H and E stain and viewed with a light microscope.

3.2.3. Effect on the Histopathology of the Kidney. Renal histopathology showed that nondiabetic control (NC) rats have a normal cortex and medulla (Figure 3(a)). Renal corpuscles are the main histological feature of the cortex. The outer layer of Bowman's capsule lined by the simple squamous epithelium was clearly shown. The glomerulus looked as clusters of capillaries covered by the inner layer of Bowman's capsule. Renal tubules in the cortex include mainly the proximal and distal parts of the nephron. These are lined by the cuboidal epithelium. They differ from each other in the height of the cells and width of the lumen. Capillaries were seen between tubules. The section from the untreated diabetic control (DC) rat kidney tissue showed deformed renal corpuscles with atrophy of glomerular capillaries. Renal tubules showed that the lining cells exhibited unstained degenerated cytoplasmic regions. Arterioles showing diffused muscular media thickening with perivascular edema, fibrosis, and minimal interstitium lymphocytic infiltrate were shown (Figure 3(b)). The kidney tissue of the DM rats showed that normal renal corpuscles and glomeruli were dominating

(Figure 3(c)). Renal tubules also looked normal. Sections of the kidney from DO rats showed marked protection from diabetic changes (Figure 3(d)). Renal corpuscles, glomeruli, and tubules looked similar to those seen in the NC group. The renal tissue of the DOM group revealed marked protection against diabetic changes (Figure 3(e)). Renal corpuscles, glomeruli, and tubules looked normal and healthy like those of the NC group. The renal tissue of DOP rats showed marked protection against diabetic changes (Figure 3(f)).

4. Discussion

The protective effect of virgin olive oil was investigated in this study by observing the histopathological changes and biochemical parameters against STZ-induced diabetic rats. An abnormality in the lipid profile is one of the commonest complications associated with diabetes mellitus [16]. In the present study, it has been observed that there were nonsignificant differences in the serum lipid profile of DC rats when compared to NC rats. Also, no significant differences in CHO and HDL serum levels were observed among all the treated groups when compared to NC and DC groups. This could be attributed to the short experimental period. In this study, TAG in diabetic rats treated with metformin (DM) in combination with olive oil (DOM) was significantly increased after 6 weeks when compared with that in the NC group. Also, LDL in diabetic rats treated with olive oil (DO) and in diabetic rats pretreated with olive oil (DOP) was significantly increased after 6 weeks when compared with that in the NC group. Our findings are consistent with the study where the absence of lipid abnormalities in DC rats was found [17]. In accordance with our results, a significant increase was observed in TAG level in DM rats in another study when compared to the NC group [18]. However, other researchers have reported significant changes in lipid abnormalities [19].

The liver function test revealed no significant variation in the serum level of AST in the DC group compared to the NC group. In contrast, the serum level of ALT in DC and all the treated groups was significantly higher ($P = 0.0001$) than that in the NC group. The serum level of ALT decreased significantly ($P = 0.0001$) in the DOP group when compared to the DC group. The serum level of AST was significantly increased ($P = 0.001$ and $P = 0.029$, respectively) in the DM group when compared to NC and DC groups and in the DOM ($P = 0.049$) group when compared to the NC group.

Moreover, in the present study, some biochemical tests reflecting hepatocyte function, such as serum BIL, ALB, TP, and ALP, were performed. ALP is a potent anti-inflammatory mediator that can protect tissues from damage resulting from injury. Elevated activity of ALP ($P = 0.0001$) was observed in the DC group of rats when compared to the NC group. This observation of our study is supported by a previous study which reported increased ALP activity in experimentally diabetic rats [20]. The increased activity of this enzyme in serum may be a result of diabetes-induced damage to the tissues. In the present study, it has been shown that the serum level of ALP remained elevated in DM and DOM groups ($P = 0.0001$ and $P = 0.0001$, respectively) when compared to the NC group and in the DO group ($P = 0.0001$ and $P = 0.0001$, respectively) when compared to NC and DC groups. In contrast, the serum level of ALP in the DOP group was significantly decreased ($P = 0.015$) when compared to the DC group and significantly increased ($P = 0.023$) when compared to the NC group. Moreover, no significant variation has been observed in the serum BIL, TP, and ALB levels between the NC group and the DC group. The serum level of BIL among all groups was within normal range. Treatment of diabetic rats with olive oil (DO) caused a noticeable elevation in the serum TP level ($P = 0.017$ and $P = 0.004$, respectively) as compared to NC and DC groups. The serum level of ALB was found to be significantly increased in DO and DOM groups ($P = 0.019$ and $P = 0.004$, respectively) when compared to the DC group. These results agree with the study which reported that treatment of rats with STZ alone did not cause any significant changes in levels of TP, AST, and ALT [21].

The serum BUN, CREA, and URCA levels are the markers of nephrotoxicity implicated in the diagnosis of kidney damage [22]. In the present study, no significant variation in the serum BUN, CREA, and URCA levels between the NC and the DC rats as well as the treated rats was observed. This could be attributed to the species of rats being studied or the short experimental period. The results of this study showed that there is no significant increase in the level of serum CREA in all the treated groups when compared to the NC group. In contrast, the level of serum BUN in the DM group was significantly higher ($P = 0.008$ and $P = 0.041$, respectively) when compared to NC and DC groups. However, CREA is a more reliable indicator of renal function than BUN because BUN is not the most sensitive indicator of renal damage and is more likely to be affected by dietary and physiologic conditions that are not related to renal function [23].

Our findings are consistent with the study of Menon et al. where it was found that there was no significant increase in serum CREA and URCA levels in the DC group when compared to the NC group [23]. However, serum BUN levels in the DC group were found to be significantly increased when compared to those in the NC group. However, the observed significant increase in BUN in the DC and treated diabetic groups may be unrelated to renal function. However, contrary to our results, some researchers have observed that there was a significant increase in serum concentrations of BUN, UACA, and CREA in the DC group when compared to the NC group [24].

In this study, the histopathological examination of the sections of the pancreas, liver, and kidney from the DC group of rats showed massive pathological changes as compared to the normal structure observed in the NC group. The pancreatic tissue showed disorganization of the endocrine islets of Langerhans with β-cells showing an unstained vacuolated cytoplasm and dark-stained degenerated nuclei. Clusters of inflammatory cells could also be seen among the cells. The histopathological changes observed in the DC group were like those reported previously [25]. In contrast, the pancreatic tissue of the DM group showed a more or less normal population of islets of Langerhans, while the absence of degenerative changes was observed in the DC group. Further, this result agrees with the study where the same results were reported [26]. The pancreatic tissue of the DO group showed islets of Langerhans with a normal-looking population of β-cells. This finding is in agreement with the report of Al-Janabi et al. which reported a more healthy architecture of islets of Langerhans and acinar cells after the treatment with olive leaf extracts [26]. Treatment with metformin (DM) in combination with olive oil (DOM) showed an improvement in islets of Langerhans and normal population of β-cells, and the absence of any degenerative changes was observed in the DC group. These findings suggest that olive oil potentiates the effect of metformin to protect diabetic rat pancreas against oxidative stress and damage. Meanwhile, the pancreatic sections from the DOP group showed normal islets of Langerhans with a normal β-cell population that was much similar to that of the NC group indicating that olive oil exerted a protective effect against the destructive effect of STZ. Therefore, this protective effect may be attributed to the prophylactic intake of olive oil.

Vital organ examination, especially of the liver and kidney, showed that they are target organs for diabetic complication. Histopathological examination of the liver from the DC group showed pathological changes indicating degenerative change such as the presence of numerous dark-stained shrunken hepatocytes and small dark nuclei (apoptosis). Treatment with metformin (DM), olive oil (DO), and a combination of olive oil and metformin (DOM), respectively, restored the normal structural organization of the liver tissue in STZ diabetic rats, thereby exhibiting a protective role against hepatic damage. These histopathological changes observed in the DO group were similar to those reported previously [27]. Pretreatment with olive oil (DOP) was found to preserve the normal structure of the rat liver indicating a preventive or prophylactic role of olive oil.

In the present study, the kidney tissue of the DC group showed deformity of renal corpuscles with atrophy of glomerular capillaries. Additionally, renal tubules showed unstained degenerated cytoplasmic regions of the lining epithelium, while arterioles showed diffuse muscular media thickening with perivascular edema, fibrosis, and minimal interstitium lymphocytic infiltrate. These results are well supported by the study of Gopal et al. (2013) which showed severe destruction as well as glomerular sclerosis in the kidney of diabetic rats [28]. Furthermore, the DOP group in the present study showed protection against diabetic changes. Renal corpuscles, glomeruli, and tubules looked healthy like those in the NC group. These findings indicate the beneficial use of olive oil as a protective measure to decrease the risk of developing diabetes.

The histopathological data from this study strongly implies that the combination of olive oil with oral hypoglycemic agents may be a valuable adjuvant therapy to achieve and/or maintain glycemic control and possibly reduce or delay the onset of diabetic complications. We recommend further investigations on humans to study the complementary effect of the combination of olive oil and metformin on other body tissues.

4.1. Significance of the Study. This study shows the ameliorative effect of olive oil on diabetic rats that can be beneficial to maintain a glycemic control in diabetes and prevent the onset of diabetic complications. This study will further help in the research to uncover the critical area of how to achieve the management of diabetes and prevention of secondary diseases arising out of hyperglycemia. Thus, a new theory of pretreatment with olive oil as an adjuvant and a prophylactic supplement against diabetes and in antioxidant therapy in combination with hypoglycemic drugs in the management of diabetes mellitus may be arrived at.

Conflicts of Interest

The authors declare no conflict of interest associated with this work.

Acknowledgments

The authors acknowledge King Abdulaziz City for Science and Technology (KACST) for the technical and financial support (Grant no. P-S-35-37). We are also grateful to Professor Soad Ali Shaker, Department of Anatomy, Faculty of Medicine, KAU, for her help in carrying out the histopathological study of this work.

References

[1] C. T. Wu, Y. T. Tsai, J. G. Lin, S. L. Fu, and J. N. Lai, "Chinese herbal products and the reduction of risk of breast cancer among females with type 2 diabetes in Taiwan: a case-control study," *Medicine (Baltimore)*, vol. 97, no. 31, article e11600, 2018.

[2] NCD Risk Factor Collaboration (NCD-RisC), "Effects of diabetes definition on global surveillance of diabetes prevalence and diagnosis: a pooled analysis of 96 population-based studies with 331 288 participants," *The Lancet Diabetes & Endocrinology*, vol. 3, no. 8, pp. 624–637, 2015.

[3] L. H. Lau, J. Lew, K. Borschmann, V. Thijs, and E. I. Ekinci, "Prevalence of diabetes and its effects on stroke outcomes: a meta-analysis and literature review," *Journal of Diabetes Investigation*, 2018.

[4] American Diabetes Association, "Diagnosis and classification of diabetes mellitus," *Diabetes Care*, vol. 28, Supplement 1, pp. s37–s42, 2011.

[5] Emerging Risk Factors Collaboration, N. Sarwar, P. Gao et al., "Diabetes mellitus, fasting blood glucose concentration, and risk of vascular disease: a collaborative meta-analysis of 102 prospective studies," *The Lancet*, vol. 375, no. 9733, pp. 2215–2222, 2010.

[6] H. Y. Hung, K. Qian, S. L. Morris-Natschke, C. S. Hsu, and K. H. Lee, "Recent discovery of plant-derived anti-diabetic natural products," *Natural Product Reports*, vol. 29, no. 5, pp. 580–606, 2012.

[7] Y. Kajimoto and H. Kaneto, "Role of oxidative stress in pancreatic β-cell dysfunction," *Annals of the New York Academy of Sciences*, vol. 1011, no. 1, pp. 168–176, 2004.

[8] H. Kaneto, N. Katakami, D. Kawamori et al., "Involvement of oxidative stress in the pathogenesis of diabetes," *Antioxidants & Redox Signaling*, vol. 9, no. 3, pp. 355–366, 2007.

[9] A. Drissi, J. Girona, M. Cherki et al., "Evidence of hypolipemiant and antioxidant properties of argan oil derived from the argan tree (Argania spinosa)," *Clinical Nutrition*, vol. 23, no. 5, pp. 1159–1166, 2004.

[10] K. L. Tuck and P. J. Hayball, "Major phenolic compounds in olive oil: metabolism and health effects," *The Journal of Nutritional Biochemistry*, vol. 13, no. 11, pp. 636–644, 2002.

[11] J. López-Miranda, F. Pérez-Jiménez, E. Ros et al., "Olive oil and health: summary of the II international conference on olive oil and health consensus report, Jaen and Cordoba (Spain) 2008," *Nutrition, Metabolism and Cardiovascular Diseases*, vol. 20, no. 4, pp. 284–294, 2010.

[12] S. Cicerale, L. J. Lucas, and R. S. Keast, "Biologic0al activities of phenolic compounds present in virgin olive oil," *International Journal of Molecular Sciences*, vol. 11, no. 2, pp. 458–479, 2010.

[13] M.-I. Covas, K. Nyyssönen, H. E. Poulsen et al., "The effect of polyphenols in olive oil on heart disease risk factors: a randomized trial," *Annals of Internal Medicine*, vol. 145, no. 5, pp. 333–341, 2006.

[14] J. Salas-Salvado, M. Bullo, N. Babio et al., "Reduction in the incidence of type 2 diabetes with the Mediterranean diet: results of the PREDIMED-Reus nutrition intervention randomized trial," *Diabetes Care*, vol. 34, no. 1, pp. 14–19, 2011.

[15] S. Arora, S. K. Ojha, and D. Vohora, "Characterisation of streptozotocin induced diabetes mellitus in Swiss albino mice," *Global Journal of Pharmacology*, vol. 3, no. 2, pp. 81–84, 2009.

[16] N. Soltani, M. Keshavarz, and A. R. Dehpour, "Effect of oral magnesium sulfate administration on blood pressure and lipid profile in streptozocin diabetic rat," *European Journal of Pharmacology*, vol. 560, no. 2-3, pp. 201–205, 2007.

[17] B. Zhu, H. Shen, J. Zhou, F. Lin, and Y. Hu, "Effects of simvastatin on oxidative stress in streptozotocin-induced diabetic rats: a role for glomeruli protection," *Nephron. Experimental Nephrology*, vol. 101, no. 1, pp. e1–e8, 2005.

[18] H. B. H. Khan, K. S. Vinayagam, S. Palanivelu, and S. Panchanatham, "Anti-diabetic effect of Semecarpus anacardium Linn. nut milk extract in a high fat diet STZ-induced type 2 diabetic rat model," *Comparative Clinical Pathology*, vol. 21, no. 6, pp. 1395–1400, 2012.

[19] I. Fki, Z. Sahnoun, and S. Sayadi, "Hypocholesterolemic effects of phenolic extracts and purified hydroxytyrosol recovered from olive mill wastewater in rats fed a cholesterol-rich diet," *Journal of Agricultural and Food Chemistry*, vol. 55, no. 3, pp. 624–631, 2007.

[20] P. S. M. Prince, V. P. Menon, and L. Pari, "Effect of Syzigium cumini extracts on hepatic hexokinase and glucose-6-phosphatase in experimental diabetes," *Phytotherapy Research*, vol. 11, no. 7, pp. 529–531, 1997.

[21] S.-C. Hsi, Y.-P. Kao, P.-Y. Wang et al., "Grape seed procyanidins improve diabetic symptoms in mice with streptozotocin-induced diabetes," *The Open Physiology Journal*, vol. 2, no. 1, pp. 6–13, 2009.

[22] N. Khan and S. Sultana, "Abrogation of potassium bromate-induced renal oxidative stress and subsequent cell proliferation response by soy isoflavones in Wistar rats," *Toxicology*, vol. 201, no. 1-3, pp. 173–184, 2004.

[23] N. Menon, J. Sparks, and F. Omoruyi, "Hypoglycemic and hypocholesterolemic activities of the aqueous preparation of Kalanchoe pinnata leaves in streptozotocin-induced diabetic rats," *Asian Pacific Journal of Tropical Biomedicine*, vol. 5, no. 1, pp. 3–9, 2015.

[24] A. R. Amr and E. E.-K. Abeer, "Hypoglycemic effect of hazelnut and its effect on some sex hormones in alloxan induced diabetic in female rats," *Pakistan Journal of Nutrition*, vol. 12, no. 3, pp. 229–238, 2013.

[25] S. M. Ali Sangi, M. I. Sulaiman, M. F. Abd El-wahab, E. I. Ahmedani, and S. S. Ali, "Antihyperglycemic effect of thymoquinone and oleuropein, on streptozotocin-induced diabetes mellitus in experimental animals," *Pharmacognosy Magazine*, vol. 11, no. 44, pp. 251–257, 2015.

[26] O. S. I. Al-Janabi, M. S. Amer, and M. H. Khayri, "Effects of the extracts of olive and Morus alba leaves on experimentally STZ induced diabetes in male rats," *International Journal of Science and Research*, vol. 4, no. 3, pp. 1526–1532, 2013.

[27] H. Jemai, A. El Feki, and S. Sayadi, "Antidiabetic and antioxidant effects of hydroxytyrosol and oleuropein from olive leaves in alloxan-diabetic rats," *Journal of Agricultural and Food Chemistry*, vol. 57, no. 19, pp. 8798–8804, 2009.

[28] S. C. Mandal, V. Gopal, and V. Mandal, "Biochemical investigation of standardized Wattakaka volubilis leaf petroleum ether cold macerated extract against experimentally induced diabetes in the rat," *Pharmacologia*, vol. 4, no. 5, pp. 391–399, 2013.

11

Glycaemic Control after Metformin Discontinuation in Diabetic Patients with a Declining Renal Function

Theresa Leyco,[1] Davin Ryanputra,[2] Ray Peh,[2] Alexphil Ponce,[3] and Chin Meng Khoo[1]

[1]*Department of Medicine, National University Hospital, Singapore*
[2]*Yong Loo Lin School of Medicine, National University of Singapore, Singapore*
[3]*Higher Education Department, Centre for International Education, Cebu, Philippines*

Correspondence should be addressed to Chin Meng Khoo; chin_meng_khoo@nuhs.edu.sg

Academic Editor: Andrea Flex

Metformin is contraindicated in diabetic patients with declining renal function. This study examined the glycaemic control in diabetic patients with chronic kidney disease when metformin was discontinued. This was a retrospective study. We screened 2032 diabetic patients who attended the Diabetes Clinic at a tertiary hospital between 1 September 2014 and 30 September 2015. We analyzed the data on 69 patients whom metformin was discontinued due to declining renal function and had a complete 6-month follow-up. There was no significant difference in the HbA1c and body weight at 6-month follow-up compared to baseline after metformin discontinuation. The eGFR was significantly lower at 6-month follow-up compared to baseline. Upon metformin discontinuation, the majority of patients had their diabetes medication uptitrated (in particular insulin or sulphonylurea). Patients with an improved glycaemia at 6-month follow-up had further declined in eGFR compared to patients with worsened glycaemia. 17% of the study patients experienced hypoglycaemia. Upon metformin discontinuation, glycaemic control could be optimised with uptitration but should be balanced against the risk of hypoglycaemia. Further improvement in the glycaemic control might indicate further deterioration in the renal function.

1. Introduction

The rising prevalence of type 2 diabetes mellitus (T2DM) is considered one of the most challenging public health problems. More than 400 million people will be affected by T2DM by the year 2030, with the greatest increase expected in Asian populations [1, 2]. Metformin is the recommended first-line antidiabetic therapy for all patients in addition to lifestyle change. Metformin is a very effective antidiabetic agent, widely available and affordable. Its most common side effect is gastrointestinal irritation. T2DM is associated with dismal micro- and macrovascular complications. One of the most dreadful microvascular complications is diabetic nephropathy, which is often characterised by declining estimated glomerular filtration rate (eGFR) and proteinuria. Declining renal function prohibits many medications for fear of potential side effects from lower renal clearance. As such, it is recommended that metformin should be discontinued when the eGFR falls to 30 ml/minute/1.73 m^2 or below [3], in anticipation of a higher risk of lactic acidosis. Other antidiabetic agents including sulfonylureas, meglitinides, dipeptidyl peptidase-4 inhibitors, and insulin have been shown to be safe in patients with declining renal function [4].

This study aimed to examine the effect of metformin discontinuation on glycaemic control among diabetic patients with declining renal function. We hypothesised that the glycaemic control would worsen with metformin discontinuation. We also examined the various treatment strategies employed in a real-world practice to mitigate the worsening of glycaemic control upon metformin discontinuation.

2. Materials and Methods

2.1. Study Design and Subjects. This is a retrospective study conducted in the Diabetes Clinic, National University Hospital, Singapore. Data on all adult patients with T2DM (aged 21

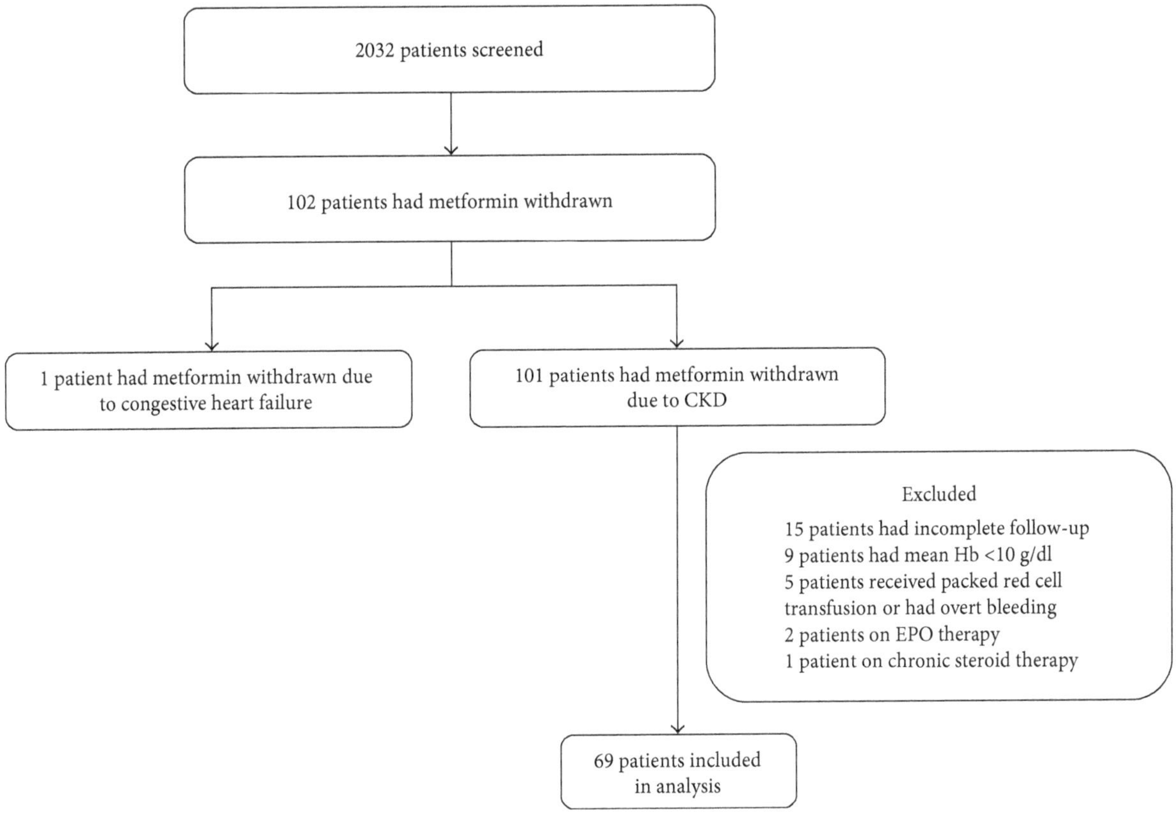

FIGURE 1: Recruitment of study population.

years and above) who had attended the diabetes clinic between 1 September 2014 and 30 September 2015 were screened for metformin withdrawal. We selected patients whom metformin was withdrawn due to worsening renal function and had a complete 6 months of follow-up after metformin discontinuation. Patients were excluded if they fulfilled any of the following criteria during the period when metformin was withdrawn: were on erythropoietin (EPO) therapy, received steroid therapy for at least 1 week, had an average haemoglobin level of less than 10 g/dL, had episode(s) of active bleeding or received packed red cell transfusion, or received renal replacement therapy.

2.2. Data Collection. This study was approved by Singapore's National Healthcare Group Domain Specific Review Board (DSRB Ref number C2016/00283). Data collected included age, sex, ethnicity, duration of diabetes, weight in kg, height in m, blood pressure (BP) in mmHg, average haemoglobin level, lipid profile, glycosylated haemoglobin (HbA1c) concentration, and serum creatinine. HbA1c concentration was measured using the Siemens/Bayer DCA 2000+ Analyser point-of-care management platform. The estimated glomerular filtration rate (eGFR) was calculated using the CKD-EPI equation. Data on hypertension, hyperlipidemia, ischemic heart disease (IHD), cerebrovascular disease (CVD), peripheral vascular disease (PVD), diabetic retinopathy, diabetic neuropathy, and medication history were also obtained. Hypoglycaemic episodes were recorded based on available self-monitoring blood glucose data or based on a physician's assessment during the clinic visit. All the data were collected at the clinical visit when metformin was withdrawn (baseline) and at 3 and 6 months after metformin withdrawal (follow-up). In contrast to the available recommendation to discontinue metformin, there were no guidelines on the management plan upon metformin discontinuation. Thus, diabetes management following metformin discontinuation was at the discretion of the physician-in-charge.

2.3. Statistical Analysis. Data analysis was performed using Minitab (version 16 for Windows; Minitab Inc., State College, PA) and SPSS (version 16 for Windows; SPSS, Inc., Chicago, IL). Values are expressed as means [standard deviation (SD)] unless stated otherwise. The paired t-test was used to examine the changes in HbA1c at 3 and 6 months from baseline. A repeated measure ANOVA was used to examine the change in HbA1c, body weight, and eGFR throughout the 6-month follow-up following metformin discontinuation. Wilcoxon signed-rank and Mann-Whitney U tests were used to examine the change in the diabetes treatment regime at baseline and at 3 months of follow-up. A p value <0.05 was considered statistically significant.

3. Results

A total of 2032 patients who attended the Diabetes Clinic, National University Hospital, Singapore between 1 September 2014 to 30 September 2015 were screened (Figure 1). There were 102 patients (5.02%) who had metformin discontinued. One patient had metformin discontinued due to congestive heart failure and was excluded from the analysis. The remaining 101 (4.97%) had metformin discontinued due to worsening renal function. Of these, 15 patients were excluded for incomplete follow-up data, nine patients for haemoglobin (Hb) concentration less than 10 g/dl, five patients for having received transfusion of packed red cells or had overt bleeding during the study period, two patients for having received EPO injection, and one patient for being on chronic steroid therapy.

Baseline patients' characteristics are shown in Table 1. Relevant to this study, the mean serum creatinine (SD) was 186.1 μmol/L (56.9 μmol/L) with the corresponding mean eGFR was 29.7 ml/min/1.73 m^2 (13.0 ml/min/1.73 m^2) at metformin discontinuation. Twenty-eight patients (40%) had metformin discontinued even when their baseline eGFR was between 30 and 60 ml/min/1.73 m^2. Body weight did not change significantly throughout the 6-month study period ($p = 0.148$). However, the mean eGFR declined significantly from 29.7 ml/min/1.73 m^2 (13.7 ml/min/1.73 m^2) to 26.4 ml/min/1.73 m^2 (11.2 ml/min/1.73 m^2) ($p = 0.049$). The mean HbA1c was 8.8% (2.3%) at baseline, 9.2% (2.2%) at three months, and 9.0% (2.2%) at 6-month follow-up ($p = 0.262$).

We identified two groups that had improved ($n = 25$, HbA1c decreased >0.5% at 6-month follow-up from baseline) and worsened glycaemic control ($n = 25$, HbA1c increased >0.5% at 6-month follow-up from baseline) (Table 2). There were 19 patients whose HbA1c change was less than 0.5% during the 6-month follow-up. Compared to the improved glycaemia group, worsened glycaemia group had a significantly longer duration of diabetes but lower mean HbA1c at baseline. Majority of the patients in both groups were on insulin therapy. There was no significant difference between groups in the use of oral antidiabetic agents at baseline. The eGFR remained stable in the group with worsened glycaemia but further declined significantly in the group with improved glycaemia.

Figures 2(a) and 2(b) show the changes in the diabetes treatment regime following metformin discontinuation. Upon discontinuation of metformin, the majority of the patients in the improved and worsened glycaemia group had their medication uptitrated or add-on another medication (in particular DPP-IV inhibitor). Compared to baseline, a large proportion of patients in the worsened glycaemia group had uptitration in medication dose (in particular insulin) ($p < 0.001$) at 3 months of follow-up after metformin discontinuation. In the improved glycaemia group, there were significant differences in the decrease in the proportion of patients with uptitration in medication ($p < 0.001$) and in the increase in the proportion of patients with downtitration of medication ($p = 0.046$) at 3 months of follow-up compared to baseline.

Twelve out of the 69 patients (17%; 5 from worsened glycaemia group, 5 from improved glycaemia group, and 2 with a HbA1c change of less than 0.5% in 6 months) reported hypoglycaemic episodes. All patients were on insulin therapy.

TABLE 1: Study patients characteristics.

	N	(%)	Mean	SD
Age, years			66.7	10.9
40–49	3	4		
50–59	19	28		
60–69	19	28		
70–79	20	29		
80–89	7	10		
90–99	1	2		
Male	37	54		
Ethnicity				
Chinese	37	54		
Malay	28	41		
Asian-Indian	4	6		
Diabetes duration, years			18.2	8.3
HbA1c, %			8.8	2.3
Weight, kg			71.8	12.9
Height, m			1.56	0.1
Body mass index, kg/m^2			28.0	5.8
Hypertension	65	94		
Hyperlipidemia	62	90		
Total cholesterol, mmol/L			4.9	19.6
Triglyceride, mmol/L			2.2	1.4
HDL, mmol/L			1.2	0.3
LDL, mmol/L			2.7	1.2
Ischemic heart disease	40	58		
Cardiovascular disease	12	17		
Peripheral vascular disease	12	17		
Diabetic retinopathy	22	32		
Diabetic neuropathy	7	10		
Serum creatinine, μmol/L			186.1	56.9
eGFR, ml/min/1.73 m^2			29.7	13.0
Hemoglobin, g/dl			11.8	1.4

4. Discussion

We reported the changes in the glycaemia level and glycaemia management among diabetic patients in whom metformin was discontinued due to declining renal function. It is recommended that metformin should be discontinued once eGFR falls below 30 ml/min/1.73 m^2 and to decrease the metformin dose in mild to moderate renal impairment (eGFR 30–60 ml/min/1.73 m^2). We noted that 40% of the study subjects had metformin prematurely withdrawn when eGFR was between 30 and 60 ml/min/1.73 m^2, and therefore they were potentially deprived of the overall reduction in morbidity and mortality, low hypoglycaemia risk, and cardiovascular benefits of metformin [5, 6].

While there is a clear recommendation on metformin discontinuation when renal function declines, there is no recommendation on how to manage the glycaemia upon metformin discontinuation. We found that there was no significant change in the glycaemic control at 6-month

Table 2: Characteristics of the patients with improved glycaemia (HbA1c decreased >0.5% at 6-month follow-up from baseline) and worsened glycaemia (HbA1c increased >0.5% at 6-month follow-up from baseline) following metformin discontinuation.

	Total cohort ($n = 69$)	Worsened glycaemia ($n = 25$)	Improved glycaemia ($n = 25$)	p value comparing worsened versus improved glycaemia
Age, years	66.7 (10.9)	68.1 (9.13)	65.0 (13.3)	0.339
Male, %	54	60	64	0.771
Diabetes duration, years	18.2 (8.3)	20.4 (7.48)	15.3 (7.4)	**0.020**
Medications at metformin discontinuation, %				
Insulin	51	52	56	0.776
Sulfonylurea	42	40	36	0.771
DPP-IV inhibitor	7	8	8	1.000
HbA1c, %				
At baseline	8.8 (2.3)	8.1 (2.0)	10.1 (2.5)	**0.002**
At 3 months	9.2 (2.2)	9.8 (2.6)[a]	9.1 (2.3)	
At 6 months	9.0 (2.2)	10.4 (2.6)[b]	8.3 (1.7)[b]	
Body weight, kg				
At baseline	71.8 (12.9)	75.3 (14.4)	68.7 (14.4)	0.107
At 3 months	72.4 (13.0)	75.5 (13.9)	71.4 (13.6)	
At 6 months	72.8 (12.2)	76.4 (13.1)	71.1 (14.0)	
eGFR, ml/minute/1.73 m^2				
eGFR at baseline	29.7 (13.0)	29.6 (8.5)	33.0 (12.3)	0.250
eGFR at 3 months	27.5 (10.8)	30.1 (14.7)	25.9 (10.5)[a]	
eGFR at 6 months	26.3 (11.2)	29.8 (17.2)	23.8 (9.1)[b]	

Values are in mean (SD) unless stated otherwise. $^a p < 0.05$ for comparison between baseline and at 3-month follow-up. $^b p < 0.05$ for comparison between baseline and at 6-month follow-up.

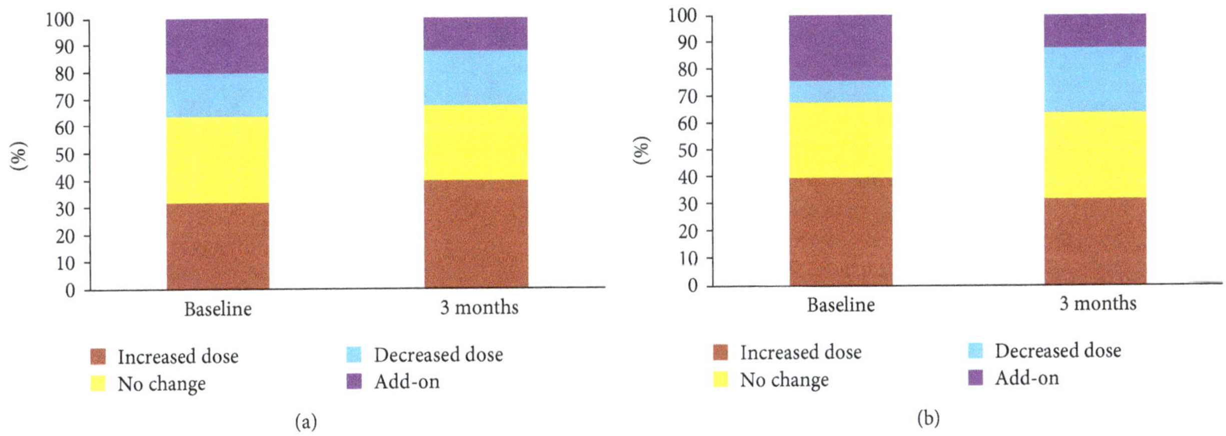

Figure 2: (a) Changes in diabetes treatment regime following metformin discontinuation in group with worsened glycaemia (HbA1c increased >0.5% at the 6-month follow-up from baseline). $p < 0.05$ comparing proportion of increased dose between 3 months and baseline. (b) Changes in diabetes treatment regime following metformin discontinuation in group with improved glycaemia (HbA1c decreased >0.5% at 6-month follow-up from baseline). $p < 0.05$ comparing proportion of increased dose or decreased dose between 3 months and baseline.

follow-up after metformin discontinuation. Majority of the patients had their medication uptitrated or had an additional antidiabetic agent when metformin was discontinued.

Although we did not find a significant change in the glycaemic control 6 months after metformin discontinuation, we observed that the glycaemic control deteriorated in the first 3 months after metformin discontinuation. Interestingly, we found that there were two groups of patients that experienced worsening or improvement in the glycaemic control at 6-month follow-up. The worsening of glycaemia was expected after metformin discontinuation, but optimisation of antidiabetic agents at metformin discontinuation and 3 months of follow-up did not stem off the worsening of glycaemia at 6-month follow-up in the group with worsened glycaemia. Similar treatment optimisation was observed in the group with improved glycaemia, and in fact, the treatment regimen was downtitrated at 3-month follow-up. A further decline in the renal function in the improved glycaemia group likely contributes to the improvement in glycaemia and explains the downtitration of treatment regimen at 3-month follow-up.

Glucose homoeostasis is complex in diabetic nephropathy. Insulin resistance plays a key role in the worsening of glycaemic control in patients with a decline renal function [7–9]. The increased insulin resistance is the effect of accumulated uremic toxins and increased oxidative stress [10]. Among the many antiglycaemic actions of metformin is an improvement in insulin sensitivity directly by increasing insulin tyrosine kinase receptor activity and indirectly by reducing lipotoxicity [11]. Thus, discontinuation of metformin in diabetic individuals will result in greater insulin resistance and worsening glycaemic control. Beside metformin and PPAR-gamma agonist, there is no other antidiabetic agent that would address the pathophysiologic insulin resistance. Thus, increasing the dose of insulin or sulphonylurea or the addition of a DPP-IV inhibitor might not be so effective in controlling glycaemia after metformin discontinuation. This was evident in the group with worsening glycaemia after metformin discontinuation in this study. However, consistent with the current opinion, improvement in the glycaemia in patients with diabetic kidney disease might suggest a further decline in renal function, and this is observed in our study. The decrease in the renal capacity of gluconeogenesis reduced clearance of antidiabetic agents, and poor nutrition might contribute to the improvement in glycaemic control or recurrent hypoglycaemia in patients with declining renal function [12–15].

Importantly, the optimisation of antidiabetic treatment must take into consideration the risk of hypoglycaemia. About 20% of our patients experienced hypoglycaemia within 6 months of optimisation of antidiabetic treatment. Aside from poor renal function, other risk factors for hypoglycaemia were seen in these patients such as old age, long duration of diabetes, high glycosylated haemoglobin, and the use of insulin. In the group with improved glycaemia, there was less treatment intensification at 3 months of follow-up, and this might have mitigated the hypoglycaemia risk in this group.

This study has several limitations. It is a retrospective study. We could not validate compliance to medications and dietary restriction. Our study has a small sample size, and this is due to our strict inclusion and exclusion criteria. We did not take into consideration patients whom metformin dose was reduced given the early decline in renal function (eGFR between 30 and 60 ml/minute/1.73 m^2). None of our patients were on PPAR-agonist or GLP-1 agonists. Thus, our interpretation of the data is limited to increasing the dose or addition of insulin, sulphonylurea, or DPP-IV inhibitor upon metformin discontinuation.

In conclusion, upitration of existing insulin or sulphonylurea or addition of DPP-IV inhibitor might help to mitigate deterioration in glycaemic control upon metformin discontinuation due to declining renal function. In patients with continuous improvement in glycaemic control, it is important to follow the renal function closely, as this may be a harbinger of a rapid decline in renal function toward end-stage kidney disease. Also, the optimisation of diabetes treatment should take into consideration the risk of hypoglycaemia in patients with a declining renal function.

Conflicts of Interest

The authors declare that they have no competing interests.

References

[1] C. S. Cockram, "The epidemiology of diabetes mellitus in the Asia-Pacific region," *Hong Kong Medical Journal*, vol. 6, no. 1, pp. 43–52, 2000.

[2] K. H. Yoon, J. H. Lee, J. W. Kim et al., "Epidemic obesity and type 2 diabetes in Asia," *The Lancet*, vol. 368, no. 9548, pp. 1681–1688, 2006.

[3] S. E. Inzucchi, K. J. Lipska, H. Mayo, C. J. Bailey, and D. K. McGuire, "Metformin in patients with type 2 diabetes and kidney disease: a systematic review," *JAMA*, vol. 312, no. 24, pp. 2668–2675, 2014.

[4] National Kidney Foundation, "KDOQI clinical practice guideline for diabetes and CKD: 2012 update," *American Journal of Kidney Diseases*, vol. 60, no. 5, pp. 850–886, 2012.

[5] Guideline development group, H. Bilo, L. C. C. Couchoud et al., "Clinical practice guideline on management of patients with diabetes and chronic kidney disease stage 3b or higher (eGFR < 45 mL/min)," *Nephrology Dialysis Transplantation*, vol. 30, no. 2, pp. ii1–ii142, 2015.

[6] W. G. Herrington and J. B. Levy, "Metformin: effective and safe in renal disease?," *International Urology and Nephrology*, vol. 40, no. 2, pp. 411–417, 2008.

[7] S. Kobayashi, K. Maesato, H. Moriya, T. Ohtake, and T. Ikeda, "Insulin resistance in patients with chronic kidney disease," *American Journal of Kidney Diseases*, vol. 45, no. 2, pp. 275–280, 2005.

[8] M.-T. Liao, C.-C. Sung, K.-C. Hung, C.-C. Wu, L. Lo, and K.-C. Lu, "Insulin resistance in patients with chronic kidney disease," *Journal of Biomedicine and Biotechnology*, vol. 2012, Article ID 691369, 12 pages, 2012.

[9] B. Spoto, A. Pisano, and C. Zoccali, "Insulin resistance in chronic kidney disease: a systematic review," *American Journal of Physiology - Renal Physiology*, vol. 311, no. 6, pp. F1087–F1108, 2016.

[10] R. Pecoits-Filho, H. Abensur, C. C. R. Betônico et al., "Interactions between kidney disease and diabetes: dangerous liaisons," *Diabetology & Metabolic Syndrome*, vol. 8, p. 50, 2016.

[11] R. Giannarelli, M. Aragona, A. Coppelli, and S. Del Prato, "Reducing insulin resistance with metformin: evidence today," *Diabetes & Metabolism*, vol. 29, no. 4, Part 2, pp. 6S28–6S35, 2003.

[12] M. Alsahli and J. Gerich, "Hypoglycemia in patients with diabetes and renal disease," *Journal of Clinical Medicine*, vol. 4, no. 5, pp. 948–964, 2015.

[13] C. Glorda, A. Ozzello, S. Gentile et al., "Incidence and correlates of hypoglycemia in type 2 diabetes. The Hypos-1 Study," *Journal of Diabetes and Metabolism*, vol. 5, no. 3, pp. 1–8, 2014.

[14] D. Tschope, P. Bramlage, C. Binz, M. Krekler, E. Deeg, and A. K. Gitt, "Incidence and predictors of hypoglycemia in type 2 diabetes – an analysis of the prospective DiaRegis registry," *BMC Endocrine Disorders*, vol. 12, p. 23, 2012.

[15] S. G. Bruderer, M. Bodmer, S. S. Jick, G. Bader, R. G. Schlienger, and C. R. Meier, "Incidence of and risk factors for severe hypoglycemia in treated type 2 diabetes mellitus in patients in the UK – a nested case-control analysis," *Diabetes, Obesity and Metabolism*, vol. 16, no. 9, pp. 801–811, 2014.

12

The Role of Serum Procalcitonin, Interleukin-6, and Fibrinogen Levels in Differential Diagnosis of Diabetic Foot Ulcer Infection

Pınar Korkmaz,[1] Havva Koçak,[2] Kevser Onbaşı,[3] Polat Biçici,[4] Ahmet Özmen,[5] Cemile Uyar,[5] and Duru Mıstanoğlu Özatağ[1]

[1]*Department of Clinical Microbiology and Infectious Diseases, Dumlupınar University Faculty of Medicine, 43020 Kutahya, Turkey*
[2]*Department of Biochemistry, Dumlupınar University Faculty of Medicine, Kutahya, Turkey*
[3]*Department of Endocrinology and Metabolism, Dumlupınar University Faculty of Medicine, Kutahya, Turkey*
[4]*Department of Plastic Surgery, Kütahya Dumlupınar Training and Research Hospital, Kutahya, Turkey*
[5]*Department of Clinical Microbiology and Infectious Diseases, Kütahya Dumlupınar Training and Research Hospital, Kutahya, Turkey*

Correspondence should be addressed to Pınar Korkmaz; drpinarkor@gmail.com

Academic Editor: Sergiu Catrina

Aims. We aimed to evaluate the roles of interleukin-6 (IL-6), PCT, and fibrinogen levels in the differential diagnosis of the patients with infected diabetic foot ulcer (IDFU) and noninfected diabetic foot ulcer (NIDFU) and to compare those with C-reactive protein (CRP), white blood cell (WBC), and erythrocyte sedimentation rate (ESR). *Methods.* Patients over 18 years with a diagnosis of type 2 diabetes mellitus and DFU who were followed up in our hospital between 1 January 2016 and 1 January 2017 were included in the study. In addition to this patient group, patients with diabetes but without DFU were determined as the control group. *Results.* Thirty-eight patients with IDFU, 38 patients with NIDFU, and 43 patients as the control group were included in the study. Fifty-six point three percent of the patients who participated in the study were males, and the mean age was 61.07 ± 11.04 years. WBC, ESR, CRP, IL-6, and fibrinogen levels of the cases with IDFU were determined to be significantly higher compared to the cases in NIDFU ($p < 0.01$). The area under the ROC curve (AUROC) value was highest for CRP (0.998; $p < 0.001$), and the best cut-off value for CRP was 28 m/L. The best cut-off values for fibrinogen, IL-6, ESR, and WBC were 480 mg/dL, 105.8 pg/mL, 31 mm/h, and 11.6 (10^3 μ/L), respectively. *Conclusion.* Serum PCT levels were not found to be effective in the discrimination of IDFU and NIDFU. Serum IL-6 and fibrinogen levels seem to be two promising inflammatory markers in the discrimination of IDFU.

1. Introduction

Foot infection in diabetic patients is a gradually increasing problem, and it can cause severe sequelae [1]. Infected diabetic foot ulcer (IDFU) usually develops based on the presence of skin ulceration after peripheral neuropathy or trauma. The wound is colonized by many microorganisms, and they may penetrate down to the deeper tissues and bone in consequence of the spread of infection. In cases of a progression of infection, the hospitalization of the patients, surgical resection, and amputation may be required [1]. Unfortunately, the life quality of patients undergoing lower extremity amputation is quite poor, and the five-year mortality is similar to that of some of the most mortal cancer types [2].

In a patient with a diabetic foot wound, first, the presence of infection should be assessed, and if present, the severity of the infection should be classified [3]. The classification systems of the Infectious Diseases Society of America (IDSA) and the International Working Group on the Diabetic Foot (IWGDF) are used to determine the severity of infection [1]. In the studies performed, the classification schemes used to detect the infection were found to be effective for prognosis and for the need for amputation in patients with diabetic foot ulcers [4–6].

An IDFU diagnosis should not be based on microbiological findings; clinical findings should also be used in the diagnosis [1, 7]. Since infection may rapidly deteriorate the patient's condition [2], it is necessary to diagnose IDFU rapidly [8]. However, always, it is not easy to diagnose IDFU [9]. Despite the presence of severe diabetic infection, an elevation in body temperature and leukocyte levels and in the erythrocyte sedimentation rate (ESR) may not be observed [1].

Procalcitonin (PCT) is the protein precursor of calcitonin, synthesized and released by C-cells in the thyroid gland. It is suggested that PCT production after inflammation is performed by the liver and peripheral blood mononuclear cells and is modulated by lipopolysaccharides and sepsis-related cytokines. It is also reported that PCT is a more accurate marker for a differential diagnosis of bacterial infections compared to C-reactive protein (CRP) [10]. Some studies have shown that serum PCT levels might play a role in the differential diagnosis of IDFU [11–13]. But, in another study, the role of serum PCT levels in the treatment and follow-up of infected ulcers was primarily evaluated, and then, it was reported that it had no role in the discrimination of diabetic ulcers with mild to moderate infection and severe infection [14].

Interleukin-6 (IL-6) is one of the proinflammatory cytokines that can be detected in serum in the early stages of infection. It plays a critical role, especially in the induction of CRP and fibrinogen synthesis in the liver during the course of bacterial infection. Therefore, it was suggested that this cytokine could increase earlier than CRP during bacterial infection and that it could enable an earlier diagnosis [15, 16]. There is a limited number of studies evaluating the role of serum IL-6 levels in diabetic ulcers [14, 17]. Fibrinogen and fibrin play important roles in blood clotting, fibrinolysis, cellular and matrix interactions, inflammation, wound healing, and neoplasia [18]. It was reported that serum fibrinogen levels were increased as an acute-phase protein in diabetic ulcers [17, 19].

Since there is a limited number of studies related to the use of serum IL-6, PCT, and fibrinogen levels in the diagnosis of IDFU and the results obtained are also contradictory, more advanced studies are needed on this subject. In this study, we also aimed to evaluate the roles of serum IL-6, PCT, and fibrinogen levels in the differential diagnosis both of patients with IDFU and of those with noninfected diabetic foot ulcers (NIDFU) and to compare those with other commonly used inflammatory markers like CRP, white blood cell (WBC), and ESR.

2. Materials and Methods

Patients over 18 years of age with a diagnosis of type 2 diabetes mellitus and diabetic foot ulcer and who were followed-up in infectious disease, internal medicine, and plastic reconstructive surgery polyclinics and clinics of our hospital between 1 January 2016 and 1 January 2017 were included in the study.

In addition to this patient group, patients with diabetes but without DFU were determined as the control group. The study was approved by the local ethics committee, and each patient was included in the study after obtaining written consent and then was informed about the study.

Patients were assessed regarding IDFU by a team including infectious disease specialists, internal medicine specialists, and plastic reconstructive surgeons. The presence of purulent discharge or two or more findings of inflammation (erythema, local warmth, local tenderness, pain, and induration) in diabetic ulcer were considered to be evidence of infection. Discrimination of IDFU and NIDFU was performed according to Infectious Diseases Society of America guidelines [19]. The patients followed up with the diagnosis of type 2 diabetes mellitus and who had no diabetic foot ulcer were determined to be the control group.

The following patients were not included in the study: the patients with other systemic or localized infectious diseases like sepsis, urinary system infection, pneumonia, and meningitis; the patients with a history of surgery within the last 6 weeks; the patients with hematological or solid malignancies; the patients with systemic inflammatory diseases like inflammatory bowel disease; the patients with rheumatoid arthritis or other rheumatic diseases; and the patients receiving ongoing immunosuppressive treatment and who received efficacious antibiotherapy earlier.

Demographic data, duration of diabetes, drugs used related to diabetes, concomitant diseases, depth of wound (superficial or deep), localization of wound (toe, metatarsal, or midfoot/heel), presence of purulent discharge, a positive probe-to-bone test, history of antibiotic use, and presence of fever were noted during admittance. Culture specimens for microbiological analysis were taken with deep tissue sampling. Osteomyelitis was assessed with the probe-to-bone test and plain-radiography [20]. Magnetic resonance imaging (MRI) was performed in patients requiring imaging examination. Blood samples were taken after 8–10 hours of overnight fasting, and complete blood count, ESR, HbA1c, fasting blood glucose, CRP, PCT, IL-6 and fibrinogen levels were studied. Complete blood count, ESR, HbA1c, fasting blood glucose, CRP, and fibrinogen levels were studied on the same day. Blood specimens for serum PCT and IL-6 levels were centrifuged at 4000 rpm for 10 minutes after storage for 30–60 minutes. Serum samples obtained were stored at −80°C until biochemical analyses were performed. Serum interleukin-6 measurements were performed by using a DiaSource Human IL-6 Elisa kit (DIAsource ImmunoAssays S.A., Belgium). Absorbance readings were performed by using a ChemWell 2910 Automated EIA and Chemistry Analyzer (Awareness Technology Inc., Martin Hwy., Palm City, USA). Results were reported as pg/mL. Serum PCT measurements were performed by using a Cobas e411 Immunoassay Analyzer (ROCHE), the electrochemiluminescence immunoassay (ECLIA) method, and Roche Diagnostics kit. The reference intervals of serum PCT levels were 0–0.05 ng/mL. Fibrinogen measurements in plasma were performed by using a coagulometer device (ACL TOP 700) and suitable kit (HemosIL Q.F.A. Thrombin). The reference intervals of serum fibrinogen levels were

TABLE 1: Demographic characteristics of the patients.

Characteristics		Total	Diabetic groups DFI ($n = 38$)	NDFI ($n = 38$)	Control ($n = 43$)	p
Age (year)	Min–max (median)	29–84 (61)	40–84 (62.5)	39–81 (63)	29–80 (59)	
	Mean ± SD	61.07 ± 11.04	62.97 ± 11.47	62.24 ± 10.93	58.35 ± 10.46	0.124
Gender, n (%)	Male	67 (56.3)	26 (68.4)	25 (65.8)	16 (37.2)	
	Female	52 (43.7)	12 (31.6)	13 (34.2)	27 (62.8)	**0.007**
Duration of diabetes (year)	Min–max (median)	1–35 (10)	2–35 (14)	1–32 (15)	1–21 (6)	
	Mean ± SD	11.60 ± 7.73	14.11 ± 7.65	13.47 ± 8.30	7.72 ± 5.61	**0.001**
Use of insulin, n (%)	Absent	52 (43.7)	9 (23.7)	10 (26.3)	33 (76.7)	
	Present	67 (56.3)	29 (76.3)	28 (73.7)	10 (23.3)	**0.001**
Use of oral antidiabetic, n (%)	Absent	64 (53.8)	29 (76.3)	25 (65.8)	10 (23.3)	
	Present	55 (46.2)	9 (23.7)	13 (34.2)	33 (76.7)	**0.001**
Not receiving antidiabetic treatment, n (%)	No	103 (86.6)	28 (73.7)	35 (92.1)	40 (93.0)	
	Yes	16 (13.4)	10 (26.3)	3 (7.9)	3 (7.0)	**0.019**
Hypertension, n (%)	Absent	58 (48.7)	14 (36.8)	24 (63.2)	20 (46.5)	
	Present	61 (51.3)	24 (63.2)	14 (36.8)	23 (53.5)	0.067
Cerebrovascular accident, n (%)	Absent	115 (96.6)	37 (97.4)	36 (94.7)	42 (97.7)	
	Present	4 (3.4)	1 (2.6)	2 (5.3)	1 (2.3)	0.836
Peripheral vascular disease, n (%)	Absent	105 (88.2)	27 (71.1)	35 (92.1)	43 (100.0)	
	Present	14 (11.8)	11 (28.9)	3 (7.9)	0 (0.0)	**0.001**
Chronic obstructive pulmonary disease, n (%)	Absent	114 (95.8)	35 (92.1)	36 (94.7)	43 (100.0)	
	Present	5 (4.2)	3 (7.9)	2 (5.3)	0 (0.0)	0.187
Chronic renal failure, n (%)	Absent	111 (93.3)	34 (89.5)	36 (94.7)	41 (95.3)	
	Present	8 (6.7)	4 (10.5)	2 (5.3)	2 (4.7)	0.656
Coronary artery disease, n (%)	Absent	86 (72.3)	23 (60.5)	31 (81.6)	32 (74.4)	
	Present	33 (27.7)	15 (39.5)	7 (18.4)	11 (25.6)	0.113
Fasting blood glucose	Min–max (median)	61–718 (190)	98–718 (230.5)	61–509 (195)	62–320 (141)	
	Mean ± SD	209.82 ± 111.76	253.32 ± 128.26	223.08 ± 115.23	159.65 ± 66.76	**0.001**
HbA1c	Min–max (median)	5.60–18 (9)	6.3–13.4 (9.2)	5.6–18 (9.35)	5.8–12.8 (7.2)	
	Mean ± SD	9.18 ± 2.30	9.55 ± 1.73	9.89 ± 2.68	8.23 ± 2.11	**0.002**

IDFU: infected diabetic foot ulcer; NIDFU: non-infected diabetic foot ulcer.

200–393 mg/dL. Serum complete blood count, ESR, HbA1c, fasting blood glucose, and CRP levels were studied in the biochemistry laboratory of our hospital. All tests were performed in a blinded manner.

NCSS (Number Cruncher Statistical System) 2007 (Kaysville, Utah, USA) program was used for the statistical analysis. During the evaluation of the study data, regarding the comparisons of descriptive statistical methods (mean, standard deviation, median, frequency, ratio, and minimum and maximum) as well as quantitative data, the Mann Whitney U test was used for the intergroup comparisons of parameters without normal distribution. One-way ANOVA test was used for the comparisons of the groups three or more with normal distribution, and the Bonferroni test was used to determine the group causing the difference if variances were homogenous but the Games-Howell test was used if variances were not homogenous; the Kruskal Wallis test was used for the comparisons of the groups three or more without normal distribution, and the Mann Whitney U test was used to determine the group causing the difference.

Pearson's chi-square test and the Fisher-Freeman-Halton test were used for the comparison of qualitative data. Diagnostic screening tests (sensitivity, specificity, positive predictive value, and negative predictive value) and ROC curve analysis were applied for the determination of cut-off points for parameters. Significance was evaluated at a level of $p < 0.05$.

3. Results

Thirty-eight patients with IDFU, 38 patients with NIDFU, and 43 patients as the control group were included in the study. Fifty-six point three percent of the patients ($n = 67$) who participated in the study were males, and the mean age was determined to be 61.07 ± 11.04 years. Demographic data of the patients who participated in the study are shown in Table 1. Wound characteristics in the groups with IDFU and NIDFU are shown in Table 2. A positive probe-to-bone test was observed in a total of 9 cases, and osteomyelitis was determined in 4 of these cases with MRI. We detected

Table 2: Evaluation of wound characteristics in the groups with diabetic ulcer.

Characteristics		Total ($n = 76$) n (%)	DFI ($n = 38$) n (%)	NDFI ($n = 38$) n (%)
Localization of ulcer	Toe	26 (34.2)	12 (31.6)	14 (36.8)
	Metatarsal	32 (42.1)	19 (50.0)	13 (34.2)
	Midfoot/heel	18 (23.7)	7 (18.4)	11 (28.9)
Depth of ulcer	Superficial	51 (67.1)	16 (42.1)	35 (92.1)
	Deep	25 (32.9)	22 (57.9)	3 (7.9)
Secretion	No	59 (77.6)	21 (55.3)	38 (100.0)
	Yes	17 (22.4)	17 (44.7)	0 (0.0)
Positive probe-to-bone test	No	67 (88.2)	29 (76.3)	38 (100.0)
	Yes	9 (11.8)	9 (23.7)	0 (0.0)
History of antibiotic use	No	58 (76.3)	20 (52.6)	38 (100.0)
	Yes	18 (23.7)	18 (47.4)	0 (0.0)
Fever	No	62 (81.6)	24 (63.2)	38 (100.0)
	Yes	14 (18.4)	14 (36.8)	0 (0.0)

IDFU: infected diabetic foot ulcer; NIDFU: noninfected diabetic foot ulcer.

Table 3: Inflammatory markers in infected diabetic foot ulcer (DFI), noninfected diabetic foot ulcer (NDFI), and control groups.

	Total	[1]DFI ($n = 38$)	[2]NDFI ($n = 38$)	[3]Control ($n = 43$)	p	$^{1\text{-}2}p$	$^{1\text{-}3}p$	$^{2\text{-}3}p$
WBC								
Min–max (median)	4–44.3 (9.6)	5–44.3 (13.7)	4–15.3 (9)	4.4–12.8 (8.4)				
Mean ± SD	10.7 ± 5.5	15.2 ± 7.5	9 ± 2.3	8.4 ± 2	**0.001**	**0.001**	**0.001**	0.237
ESR								
Min–max (median)	2–109 (24)	6–109 (56.5)	2–64 (26)	2–30 (11)				
Mean ± SD	31.66 ± 25.89	58.34 ± 24.68	27.21 ± 16.44	12.02 ± 7.23	**0.001**	**0.001**	**0.001**	**0.001**
CRP								
Min–max (median)	0.5–309 (8.7)	28–309 (195)	0.5–44 (9.1)	0.5–9 (2.7)				
Mean ± SD	62.43 ± 92.35	181.17 ± 76.36	10.52 ± 7.53	3.37 ± 2.6	**0.001**	**0.001**	**0.001**	**0.001**
IL-6								
Min–max (median)	4.4–1717.9 (40.8)	30.7–1717.9 (191.4)	6.6–576.7 (35.35)	4.4–152.2 (24.4)				
Mean ± SD	116.22 ± 221.98	275.12 ± 331.44	55.81 ± 90.21	29.18 ± 24.35	**0.001**	**0.001**	**0.001**	**0.004**
PCT								
Min–max (median)	0.02–10.30 (0.14)	0.02–10.3 (0.15)	0.02–0.41 (0.12)	0.04–0.64 (0.17)				
Mean ± SD	0.31 ± 0.98	0.6 ± 1.7	0.15 ± 0.09	0.19 ± 0.14	0.468	0.261	0.708	0.341
Fibrinogen								
Min–max (median)	105–1182 (357)	387–1182 (627)	105–840 (350.5)	200–568(293)				
Mean ± SD	436.54 ± 204.73	663.21 ± 185.24	360.34 ± 119.6	303.56 ± 71.28	**0.001**	**0.001**	**0.001**	**0.005**

IDFU: infected diabetic foot ulcer; NIDFU: noninfected diabetic foot ulcer; CRP: C-reactive protein; IL-6: interleukin-6; WBC: white blood cell; ESR: erythrocyte sedimentation rate; PCT: procalcitonin.

the characteristic findings of diabetic foot osteomyelitis on MRI, decreased signal intensity of the affected bone on T1-weighted images and increased intensity on T2-weighted and postcontrast images, in these patients. Deep tissue culture was taken from 17 cases with IDFU, and microbial growth was detected in 10 (58.8%) of them. The results of microbial growth were as follows: *S. aureus* in 4 cases, *P. aeruginosa* in 2 cases, *E. cloacae* and *E. coli* in 1 case, *Streptococcus* spp. in 1 case, and *P. vulgaris* in 1 case. The results related to inflammatory markers in the groups included in the study are shown in Table 3.

WBC levels of the cases with IDFU were determined to be significantly higher compared to the cases in NIDFU ($p < 0.01$) and diabetic control groups. ESR values of the cases with IDFU were determined to be significantly higher compared to the cases with NIDFU ($p < 0.01$) and diabetic control groups. ESR values of the cases with NIDFU were determined to be significantly higher compared to the cases

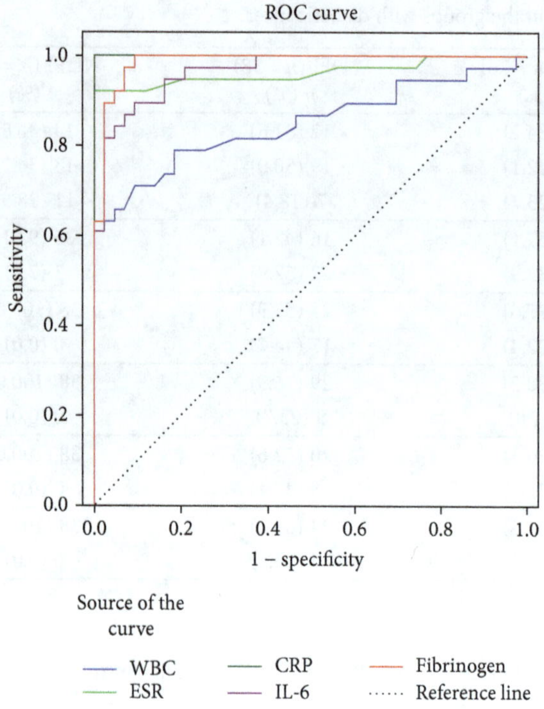

FIGURE 1: Receiver operating characteristic curves of inflammatory markers.

in the diabetic control group ($p < 0.01$). Serum CRP levels of the cases with IDFU were determined to be significantly higher compared to the cases with NIDFU ($p < 0.01$) and diabetic control groups ($p < 0.01$).

Serum CRP levels of the cases with NIDFU were determined to be significantly higher compared to the cases in the diabetic control group ($p < 0.01$).

Serum IL-6 levels of the cases with IDFU were determined to be significantly higher compared to the cases with NIDFU ($p < 0.01$) and diabetic control groups ($p < 0.01$). Serum IL-6 levels of the cases with NIDFU were determined to be significantly higher compared to the cases in the diabetic control group ($p < 0.01$). No statistically significant difference was determined between serum PCT measurements of the cases with IDFU compared to the cases with NIDFU ($p > 0.05$) and the cases in the diabetic control group ($p > 0.05$). Serum fibrinogen levels of the cases with IDFU were determined to be significantly higher compared to the cases with NIDFU ($p < 0.01$) and diabetic control groups ($p < 0.01$). Serum fibrinogen levels of the cases with NIDFU were determined to be significantly higher compared to the cases in the diabetic control group ($p < 0.01$).

The area under the ROC curve (AUROC) was measured to estimate the presence of bacterial infection in the cases with diabetic ulcer (Figure 1). AUROC value was highest for CRP (0.998; $p < 0.001$), followed by ESR (0.962; $p < 0.001$), fibrinogen (0.941; $p < 0.001$), IL-6 (0.904; $p < 0.001$) and WBC (0.849; $p < 0.001$), respectively. The best cut-off values for CRP, fibrinogen, IL-6, ESR, and WBC were 28 mg/L, 480 mg/dL, 105.8 pg/mL, 31 mm/h, and 11.6 ($10^3\,\mu$/L), respectively. Maximum sensitivity, specificity, and positive and negative predictive values are shown in Table 4.

4. Discussion

The role of various inflammatory markers like WBC, ESR, CRP, PCT, IL-6, and fibrinogen in the discrimination of IDFU was evaluated in this study. It was shown that all inflammatory markers evaluated in our study except PCT had a role in the discrimination of IDFU. Contrary to our study, in the study performed by Uzun et al. [12], the highest discriminatory power was defined for PCT in the diagnosis of IDFU (AUROC: 0.859). In another study performed by Jonaidi Jafari et al. [9] who evaluated the role of serum PCT levels in the discrimination of IDFU and NIDFU, sensitivity and specificity were determined to be 70% and 74%, respectively, for 0.21 ng/mL value of PCT. However, in the same study, the marker with the highest discriminatory power for IDFU and NIDFU was ESR and it was followed by CRP, PCT, and WBC. The authors state that serum PCT levels may have a role in the discrimination of IDFU in the case of the combination of markers like ESR and CRP [9]. Similarly, in another study performed by Massara et al. [13], the authors stated that the highest sensitivity and specificity in the discrimination of IDFU and NIDFU could be provided with a combination of at least two markers (CRP and PCT or ESR and PCT). Also in the study performed by Jeandrot et al. [11] evaluating the role of serum CRP and PCT levels in the discrimination of mildly infected and noninfected diabetic foot ulcer, the highest AUC value (AUROC: 0.947) was obtained with the combination of CRP and PCT.

In the majority of these studies evaluating the role of serum PCT levels, the patients not receiving antibiotic 6 months before admission were included in the study. When considering the natural history of IDFU in clinical practice, this is not a frequently encountered condition. In a review, the role of serum PCT levels in the discrimination of IDFU was evaluated and it was stated that the studies were heterogeneous and the patients receiving an antibiotic within the last 6 months were excluded in many of them. They also stated that serum PCT levels might have a potential role in the discrimination of IDFU but it could not discriminate severe infection from less severe infection [21]. Also in another review evaluating IDFU, it was stated that in the absence of systemic manifestations of localized infection, serum PCT levels could not discriminate acute infection from acute ischemia or noninfectious conditions or osteomyelitis from soft tissue infections [22]. Serum PCT levels have some limitations such as the following: they cannot be studied in the laboratory of many hospitals and they are expensive markers, able to show change according to age, pathogen, and type of infection [9]. Further studies are required for routine use of serum PCT levels in IDFU diagnosis.

As far as the literature can be reviewed so far, there are only two studies related to the use of serum IL-6 levels in IDFU diagnosis. The first one was a study including also type 1 diabetes patients; it was determined in this study that serum IL-6 levels were effective in ulcer classification according to

TABLE 4: Sensitivity, specificity, negative predictive value, and positive predictive value of inflammatory marker.

	Cut-off	Sensitivity	Specificity	Positive predictive value	Negative predictive value
CRP (mg/L)	≥28	100.00	97.37	97.40	100.00
Fibrinogen (mg/dL)	≥480	89.47	92.11	91.90	89.70
IL-6 (pg/mL)	≥105.8	76.32	94.74	93.50	80.00
ESR (mm/h)	≥42	73.68	84.21	82.40	76.20
WBC (10^3 μ/L)	≥11.6	71.05	90.70	87.10	78.00

CRP: C-reactive protein; IL-6: interleukin-6; WBC: white blood cell; ESR: erythrocyte sedimentation rate; PCT: procalcitonin.

Texas classification but it was not an independent variable for the determination of infection severity [17].

The second one was a study including only the patients with IDFU; it was determined in this study that serum IL-6 levels were increased in correlation with CRP and the other inflammatory markers and serum IL-6 levels were decreased in the patients recovered with antibiotic treatment. However, this study includes only the patients followed up with the diagnosis of IDFU, and since there is no control group, it is not possible to compare baseline serum IL-6 levels of the IDFU group and the NIDFU group [14]. As far as the literature could be evaluated, it was shown for the first time in our study that serum IL-6 levels were effective for the discrimination of infected and noninfected ulcer in a study including only type 2 diabetes patients. While this shows us that serum IL-6 levels might have a role in the diagnosis of IDFU, since the number of studies related to serum IL-6 levels is extremely limited, further studies are required.

In the study performed by Rattan et al. [23], it was reported that serum fibrinogen levels were elevated in the patients with diabetic ulcer compared to the patients without diabetic ulcer. As far as the literature related to the use of serum fibrinogen levels in IDFU could be evaluated, only two studies were found. The first one of these was the study performed by Weigelt et al. [17], and it was shown that there was no significant difference between the patients with and without diabetic ulcer regarding serum fibrinogen levels. The second one of these was the study performed by Li et al. [19], and serum fibrinogen levels were found to be associated with the severity of diabetic foot ulcer and undergoing amputation. In our study, serum fibrinogen levels were found to be effective for discriminating infected diabetic foot ulceration from uninfected diabetic foot ulceration.

CRP is an acute phase reactant whose levels elevate during inflammatory processes occurring in the body; elevated serum CRP levels can also be detected in the conditions not caused by bacterial infection [12]. In a study performed, elevated serum CRP levels were determined in diabetic patients compared to nondiabetic patients and again in the patients with DFU compared to the patients without DFU. However, in this study, serum CRP levels were not found to be statistically significant especially in the discrimination of IDFU and NIDFU [12]. On the contrary, in our study, serum CRP level is the inflammatory marker which has the highest discriminatory power in the discrimination of IDFU and NIDFU. In harmony with our study, serum CRP level was determined to be the inflammatory marker with the highest discriminatory power in the discrimination of mildly IDFU and NIDFU [11]. In another study indicating that serum CRP levels were more effective than the other inflammatory markers, 123 IDFUs were evaluated and the roles of serum PCT and CRP levels in IDFU were evaluated and only serum CRP levels were found to be effective in grading the severity of the infection [24].

There are some limitations in our study; since anaerobic culture was not accessible in our hospital, anaerobic pathogens were not studied in diabetic foot ulcers. Also, the diagnosis of osteomyelitis in our study was based on imaging reports rather than bone biopsy, which is a more definite diagnostic method.

As a result, serum CRP, ESR, IL-6, fibrinogen, and WBC levels were determined to be useful parameters in the diagnosis of IDFU in our study. Serum PCT levels were not found to be effective in the discrimination of IDFU and NIDFU. Serum IL-6 and fibrinogen levels seem to be two promising inflammatory markers in the discrimination of IDFU. The efficiency of serum IL-6 levels for the discrimination of infected and noninfected ulcer in infections of ulcers associated with type 2 diabetes was shown for the first time in our study. Since serum IL-6 levels have been used in a limited number of studies, further studies are required in order to understand its role in the diagnosis of IDFU. Since especially fibrinogen can be reached easily, test results can be obtained rapidly and it is cheap; it seems to be a useful inflammatory marker in the diagnosis of IDFU. As the studies related to the role of serum fibrinogen levels in IDFU increase, the cut-off point can be determined and it may play a role in the diagnosis of IDFU together with the other inflammatory markers.

Conflicts of Interest

The authors declare that they have no conflicts of interest.

Acknowledgments

This study was supported by a grant from the Scientific Research Project of Dumlupinar Üniversitesi (Project no. 2016-61).

References

[1] B. A. Lipsky, A. R. Berendt, P. B. Cornia et al., "2012 Infectious Diseases Society of America clinical practice guideline for the diagnosis and treatment of diabetic foot infections," *Clinical Infectious Diseases*, vol. 54, pp. 132–173, 2012.

[2] D. G. Armstrong, J. Wrobel, and J. M. Robbins, "Guest editorial: are diabetes-related wounds and amputations worse than cancer?," *International Wound Journal*, vol. 4, no. 4, pp. 286-287, 2007.

[3] N. C. Schaper, J. J. Van Netten, J. Apelqvist, B. A. Lipsky, K. Bakker, and International Working Group on the Diabetic Foot, "Prevention and management of foot problems in diabetes: a Summary Guidance for Daily Practice 2015, based on the IWGDF Guidance Documents," *Diabetes Metabolism Research and Reviews*, vol. 32, Supplement S1, pp. 7–15, 2016.

[4] L. A. Lavery, D. G. Armstrong, D. P. Murdoch, E. J. Peters, and B. A. Lipsky, "Validation of the Infectious Diseases Society of America's diabetic foot infection classification system," *Clinical Infectious Diseases*, vol. 44, no. 4, pp. 562–565, 2007.

[5] D. K. Wukich, K. B. Hobizal, and M. M. Brooks, "Severity of diabetic foot infection and rate of limb salvage," *Foot & Ankle International*, vol. 34, no. 3, pp. 351–358, 2013.

[6] A. H. Widatalla, S. E. Mahadi, M. A. Shawer, H. A. Elsayem, and M. E. Ahmed, "Implementation of diabetic foot ulcer classification system for research purposes to predict lower extremity amputation," *International Journal of Diabetes in Developing Countries*, vol. 29, no. 1, pp. 1–5, 2009.

[7] N. C. Schaper, "Diabetic foot ulcer classification system for research purposes: a progress report on criteria for including patients in research studies," *Diabetes/Metabolism Research and Reviews*, vol. 20, pp. S90–S95, 2004.

[8] J. Aragón-Sánchez, "Seminar review: a review of the basis of surgical treatment of diabetic foot infections," *The International Journal of Lower Extremity Wounds*, vol. 10, no. 1, pp. 33–65, 2011.

[9] N. Jonaidi Jafari, M. Safaee Firouzabadi, M. Izadi, M. S. Safaee Firouzabadi, and A. Saburi, "Can procalcitonin be an accurate diagnostic marker for the classification of diabetic foot ulcers?," *International Journal of Endocrinology and Metabolism*, vol. 12, article e13376, 2014.

[10] L. Simon, F. Gauvin, D. K. Amre, P. Saint-Louis, and J. Lacroix, "Serum procalcitonin and C-reactive protein levels as markers of bacterial infection: a systematic review and meta-analysis," *Clinical Infectious Diseases*, vol. 39, no. 2, pp. 206–217, 2004.

[11] A. Jeandrot, J. L. Richard, C. Combescure et al., "Serum procalcitonin and C-reactive protein concentrations to distinguish mildly infected from non-infected diabetic foot ulcers: a pilot study," *Diabetologia*, vol. 51, no. 2, pp. 347–352, 2008.

[12] G. Uzun, E. Solmazgul, H. Curuksulu et al., "Procalcitonin as a diagnostic aid in diabetic foot infections," *The Tohoku Journal of Experimental Medicine*, vol. 213, no. 4, pp. 305–312, 2007.

[13] M. Massara, G. De Caridi, R. Serra et al., "The role of procalcitonin as a marker of diabetic foot ulcer infection," *International Wound Journal*, vol. 14, no. 1, pp. 31–34, 2017.

[14] F. A. Altay, İ. Sencan, G. Ç. Şentürk et al., "Does treatment affect the levels of serum interleukin-6, interleukin-8 and procalcitonin in diabetic foot infection? A pilot study," *Journal of Diabetes and its Complications*, vol. 26, no. 3, pp. 214–218, 2012.

[15] C. Buck, J. Bundschu, H. Gallati, P. Bartmann, and F. Pohlandt, "Interleukin-6: a sensitive parameter for the early diagnosis of neonatal bacterial infection," *Pediatrics*, vol. 93, no. 1, pp. 54–58, 1994.

[16] R. C. Silveira and R. S. Procianoy, "Evaluation of interleukin-6, tumour necrosis factor-α and interleukin-1β for early diagnosis of neonatal sepsis," *Acta Paediatrica*, vol. 88, no. 6, pp. 647–650, 1999.

[17] C. Weigelt, B. Rose, U. Poschen et al., "Immune mediators in patients with acute diabetic foot syndrome," *Diabetes Care*, vol. 32, no. 8, pp. 1491–1496, 2009.

[18] M. W. Mosesson, K. R. Siebenlist, and D. A. Meh, "The structure and biological features of fibrinogen and fibrin," *Annals of the New York Academy of Sciences*, vol. 936, pp. 11–30, 2001.

[19] X. H. Li, L. Y. Guan, H. Y. Lin et al., "Fibrinogen: a marker in predicting diabetic foot ulcer severity," *Journal of Diabetes Research*, vol. 2016, Article ID 2358321, 5 pages, 2016.

[20] M. L. Grayson, G. W. Gibbons, K. Balogh, E. Levin, and A. W. Karchmer, "Probing to bone in infected pedal ulcers. A clinical sign of underlying osteomyelitis in diabetic patients," *Journal of the American Medical Association*, vol. 273, no. 9, pp. 721–723, 1995.

[21] K. Saeed, N. Ahmad, and M. Dryden, "The value of procalcitonin measurement in localized skin and skin structure infection, diabetic foot infections, septic arthritis and osteomyelitis," *Expert Review of Molecular Diagnostics*, vol. 14, no. 1, pp. 47–54, 2014.

[22] A. W. Glaudemans, I. Uçkay, and B. A. Lipsky, "Challenges in diagnosing infection in the diabetic foot," *Diabetic Medicine*, vol. 32, no. 6, pp. 748–759, 2015.

[23] R. Rattan and D. Nayak, "High levels of plasma malondialdehyde, protein carbonyl, and fibrinogen have prognostic potential to predict poor outcomes in patients with diabetic foot wounds: a preliminary communication," *The International Journal of Lower Extremity Wounds*, vol. 7, no. 4, pp. 198–203, 2008.

[24] J. H. Park, D. H. Suh, H. J. Kim, Y. I. Lee, I. H. Kwak, and G. W. Choi, "Role of procalcitonin in infected diabetic foot ulcer," *Diabetes Research and Clinical Practice*, vol. 128, pp. 51–57, 2017.

13

Differentially Expressed MicroRNAs in the Development of Early Diabetic Retinopathy

Qiaoyun Gong, Jia'nan Xie, Yang Liu, Ying Li, and Guanfang Su

Eye Center, The Second Hospital of Jilin University, No. 218 Ziqiang Street, Changchun, Jilin 130021, China

Correspondence should be addressed to Guanfang Su; sugf2012@163.com

Academic Editor: Patrizio Tatti

The pathological mechanisms of diabetic retinopathy (DR), a leading cause of blindness in adults with diabetes mellitus, remain incompletely understood. Because microRNAs (miRNAs) represent effective DR therapeutic targets, we identified aberrantly expressed miRNAs associated with cellular dysfunction in early DR and detected their potential targets. We exposed human retinal endothelial cells (HRECs) and a cell line of retinal pigment epithelial (RPE) cells to high glucose (25 mmol/L, 1–7 days) to mimic DR progression and used streptozotocin-injected rats (4–8 weeks) for an in vivo diabetes model. HREC/RPE viability decreased after 24 h incubation and diminished further over 6 days, and Hoechst staining revealed hyperglycemia-induced HREC/RPE apoptosis. Although miR-124/-125b expression decreased with DR progression in vitro and in vivo, miR-135b/-199a levels decreased in retinal cells under hyperglycemia exposure, but increased in diabetic retinas. Moreover, miR-145/-146a expression decreased gradually in high-glucose-treated HRECs, but increased in hyperglycemia-exposed RPE cells and in diabetic rats. Our findings suggested that aberrant miRNA expression could be involved in hyperglycemia-induced retinal-cell dysfunction, and the identified miRNAs might vary in different retinal layers, with expression changes associated with DR development. Therefore, miRNA modulation and the targeting of miRNA effects on transcription factors could represent novel and effective DR-treatment strategies.

1. Introduction

Diabetic retinopathy (DR) is currently the main cause of visual disability and blindness in working-age adults (20–65 years old) [1, 2]. DR results from abnormal retinal blood vessels that are either nonproliferative or proliferative. The blood-retinal barrier (BRB), which comprises the retinal vasculature and the retinal pigment epithelium, excludes the neural elements of the retina and the cytotoxic products from circulating inflammatory cells, thereby protecting and allowing the retina to regulate its extracellular chemical composition [3]. The inner BRB formed by retinal capillaries features endothelial cells harboring tight junctions that are almost impermeable to protein transport [4]. Endothelial cells are responsible for maintaining the BRB, and their impairment causes increased vascular permeability [5]. The outer BRB, which is formed by retinal pigment epithelial (RPE) cells, is located between retinal photoreceptors and the choroid. RPE cells play a crucial role in fluid balance within the retina [6] by forming the outer BRB and supporting the function of photoreceptors, with RPE cells capable of activation via milieu changes [7]. In the pathogenesis of diabetic complications, the primary causal factor is considered to be lasting exposure to hyperglycemia [8]. Exposure to high glucose (HG) and the resultant damage are pivotal to the BRB imbalance that leads to the leakage of fluids and lipids into the retina and contributes to DR progression. Therefore, to investigate the molecular changes induced by HG and assess the effects of glucose on the retina, we conducted in vitro studies using human retinal endothelial cells (HRECs) and RPE cells cultured under hyperglycemia conditions for different periods. Furthermore, for in vivo studies, we established a rat model of diabetes mellitus (DM) by intraperitoneally injecting the animals with streptozotocin (STZ).

DR pathogenesis is a multifactorial process, and numerous protein-encoding genes related to hyperglycemia-linked pathways have been investigated in DR progression [1, 9]. However, emerging data also suggest that an enormous number of noncoding RNAs, which exhibit little or no protein-coding potential, are expressed and play critical roles in DR pathogenesis [10–12], with microRNAs (miRNAs), in particular, receiving considerable research attention. miRNAs are a group of short (~21–23 nucleotides), highly conserved endogenous RNAs that do not encode proteins. miRNAs modulate gene expression through transcriptional or posttranscriptional regulation, inducing mRNA degradation or inhibiting protein translation by binding to the seed region in the 3′-untranslated region (3′-UTR) of target genes [13–15]. Notably, miRNAs are involved in the proliferation, migration, and apoptosis of retinal cells and in DR-related neovascularization, and miRNAs that exhibit increased or decreased expression during DR pathogenesis have been identified [10]. Modulation of miRNA levels exerts beneficial effects on slowing DR progression and could potentially be employed in DR-therapeutic strategies. However, few studies have focused on or elucidated the progressive changes in miRNA levels in DR. Wu et al. [11] reported that the expression of certain miRNAs either increases (e.g., miR-182) or decreases (e.g., miR-10b) in parallel with DR progression in the retinas of rats with STZ-induced DM; however, no study has been conducted thus far to investigate miRNA variations in human retinal cells under prolonged HG exposure. To effectively use miRNAs in clinical applications for DR, it is crucial to identify the continuous alterations of miRNAs related to DR development and pathogenesis. Here, based on the results of bioinformatics analysis, we examined the expression of hsa-miR-124-3p, -125b-5p, -135b-5p, -145-5p, -146a-5p, and -199a-5p in HRECs or RPE cells under hyperglycemic conditions or in vivo in diabetic rats.

In this study, we also focused on specificity protein 1 (SP1), which could represent a previously unknown target of miR-125b-5p. SP1 belongs to a family of transcription factors that harbors GC-rich promoters and is involved in basal promoter activity. SP1 positively regulates the expression of diverse genes encoding various angiogenesis-related factors, including vascular endothelial growth factor (VEGF) and fibrogenic cytokine, which are related to cell proliferation and migration, BRB damage and neovascularization, and, eventually, visual impairment. These factors can be detected in the vitreous fluid collected from patients with proliferative DR [16]. Therefore, combined miRNA and SP1 targeting to manipulate the pathways regulated by the transcription factor might represent a favorable strategy in the treatment of DR.

Our objectives were to discover the detailed alterations of additional miRNAs associated with the dysfunction and apoptosis of retinal cells in the early stage of DR. Furthermore, we analyzed the potential of therapeutic strategies based on targeting miRNA effects on transcription factors in the DR process. In addition to revealing the roles of miRNAs in DR, our study provides insights into miRNA expression in chronic diseases and potentially helps improve the development of therapeutic strategies used for these diseases.

2. Materials and Methods

2.1. Cell Culture. HRECs were purchased from ANGIO-PRO TEOMIE (Boston, MA, USA) and maintained in endothelial cell medium containing 5% fetal bovine serum (FBS) and 1% endothelial cell growth supplement (ScienCell, Carlsbad, CA, USA). The human RPE cell line ARPE-19 was purchased from American Type Culture Collection (ATCC, Manassas, VA, USA) and cultured according to the manufacturer's instructions. The cells were maintained in Dulbecco's modified Eagle medium/F-12 (Hyclone, Beijing, China) containing 10% FBS (Gibco; Thermo Fisher Scientific, Waltham, MA, USA). HREC and ARPE-19 cultures were maintained at 37°C in a humidified atmosphere containing 5% CO_2.

2.2. Hyperglycemia Treatment. HRECs and ARPE-19 cells were plated at 2500 cells/cm^2 in 6-well plates (Corning; Acton, MA, USA) and treated with normal glucose (NG; 5.5 mmol/L) as a control or with HG (25 mmol/L) or the osmotic control mannitol (MN; 19.5 mmol/L MN together with NG) under normoxic conditions for 1, 3, 5, and 7 days to mimic the chronic disease course in the early stage of DR. The cells were cultured in NG first and then in HG or in MN according to the number of HG days. The media were changed daily to eliminate metabolic byproducts and to provide the nutrients necessary for the cells.

2.3. Animal Model. Animal experiments were conducted according to the guidelines specified by the Animal Care and Use Committee of Jilin University. Male Sprague-Dawley rats (~200 g; 8 weeks old) were obtained from the Animal Center, College of Basic Medical Sciences, Jilin University, and housed in standard plastic rodent cages under a controlled environment (24°C; 12/12 h light/dark cycle). Diabetes was induced by injecting the animals once intraperitoneally with STZ [65 mg/kg, in citrate buffer (pH 4.5)]. Control rats received an identical volume of citrate buffer. Rats were regarded as diabetic when their blood glucose level exceeded 16.7 mmol/L at 72 h and 1 week post-STZ administration. Body weights of the rats were also monitored throughout the study. Control and diabetic rats were maintained for 4, 6, and 8 weeks ($n = 6$/group).

2.4. Cell Viability Assay. Cell viability was assessed using 3-(4,5-dimethylthiazol-2-yl)-5-(3-carboxy-methoxyphenyl)-2-(4-sulfophenyl)-2H–tetrazolium (MTS; Promega, Shanghai, China) according to the manufacturer's protocol. HRECs or ARPE-19 cells were seeded at a density of 2×10^3 cells/well in 96-well plates and treated with NG or HG for 1, 2, 3, 4, 5, and 6 days. Before detection, 100 μL of medium was replaced with fresh medium and 20 μL of MTS was added to cells. Following incubation for 1.5 h at 37°C, the absorbance at 490 nm was measured.

2.5. Assessment of Hyperglycemia-Induced Apoptosis. To distinguish the type of cell death under hyperglycemia conditions, nuclear morphology was examined by means of Hoechst 33258 staining and fluorescence microscopy. HRECs and ARPE-19 cells were treated with HG for 1, 3, 5, and 7 days, washed twice with 1× phosphate-buffered saline, incubated with 0.1 μg/mL Hoechst 33258 (Sigma-Aldrich, St. Louis, MO, USA) for 15 min in the dark, and examined under a microscope (Olympus, Tokyo, Japan). Cells harboring fragmented or condensed pyknotic nuclei were counted as apoptotic cells, and data are presented here as apoptotic cell percentages (apoptotic cells/total cells × 100).

2.6. miRNA Mimics and Transfection. The hsa-miR-125b-5p mimic and a scrambled negative-control miRNA were chemically synthesized by GenePharma (Shanghai, China). The sequences were, respectively, 5′-UCCCUGAGACCCUAACU UGUGA-3′ and 5′- UUCUCCGAACGUGUCACGUTT-3′. ARPE-19 cells in the logarithmic growth phase were seeded in 6-well plates and cultured under HG for 2 days before transfection. Upon reaching ~70% to 80% confluence, cells were transfected with miR-125b mimic or scramble-control miRNA (both at 50 nmol/L) using Lipofectamine RNAiMAX (Invitrogen, Carlsbad, CA, USA) transfection reagent. At 5 h after transfection, the medium was changed to fresh HG medium, and at 48 h and 72 h after transfection, the cells were harvested for mRNA and protein analysis, respectively.

2.7. Total RNA Isolation and Identification. Total RNA was extracted from HRECs and ARPE-19 cells cultured under different conditions or from rat retinal tissues. An Eastep Super total RNA extraction kit (Promega) was used according to manufacturer protocol, and RNA concentration and purity were measured using a NanoDrop 2000c spectrophotometer (Thermo Fisher Scientific). RNA samples featuring an A260/A280 value of ~2.0 were generally used for further analysis. The integrity of RNA samples was assessed through 1% agarose-gel electrophoresis.

2.8. Determination of miRNA- or mRNA-Expression Levels. To analyze miRNA-expression levels, 1.5 μg of total RNA was polyadenylated and reverse transcribed using an All-in-One miRNA first-strand cDNA synthesis kit (GeneCopoeia, Rockville, MD, USA). The obtained cDNA was diluted 1 : 5 for further quantitative real-time polymerase chain reaction (PCR). miRNA levels were measured using an All-in-One miRNA quantitative PCR (qPCR) detection kit with specific primers (GeneCopoeia). Measurements were performed in triplicate on a LightCycler 480 (Roche Diagnostics, Basel, Switzerland), and RNA U6 was used as a normalization control for miRNA expression.

For mRNA analysis, 500 ng of total RNA was reverse transcribed using a Perfect real-time RT reagent kit (Takara Bio, Beijing, China) in a 20 μL reaction volume, after which qPCR was performed using a reaction mixture that contained 1 μL of the cDNA, 10 μmol/L gene-specific primers (forward and reverse, mixed together), and 10 μL of 2× Fast SYBR Green master mix (Roche Diagnostics). Three replicates for each biological mixture were used, and reactions were performed on a LightCycler 480 (Roche Diagnostics). For each miRNA or mRNA run, we included two negative controls containing water instead of the template. The relative expression levels of miRNAs and mRNAs were calculated using the $2^{-\Delta\Delta Ct}$ method, in which the ratio of expression between an experimental group and the control group was determined.

2.9. Western Blot. Total protein was collected from ARPE-19 cells by lysing the cells for 30 min on ice in a cell-lysis buffer [radioimmunoprecipitation assay buffer containing phenylmethylsulfonyl fluoride (Dingguo Changsheng, Beijing, China)], treating the lysates with ultrasound and then centrifuging the lysates at 12,000 rpm for 10 min at 4°C. Protein concentrations were determined using a bicinchoninic acid protein assay kit (Beyotime, Jiangsu, China). Supernatant proteins were collected, denatured, concentrated in 5% sodium dodecyl sulfate-polyacrylamide gel electrophoresis (SDS-PAGE) stacking gels, separated in 10% SDS-PAGE gels, and transferred to polyvinylidene difluoride membranes. The membranes were blocked in 5% skim milk for 1 h, incubated with primary antibodies against SP1 (1 : 150; Santa Cruz Biotechnology, Dallas, TX, USA) and β-actin (1 : 1000; CMC-TAG, Milwaukee, WI, USA) at 4°C overnight, and then incubated with secondary antibodies (1 : 5000; Boster, Wuhan, China) for 40 min. An enhanced chemiluminescence plus kit (Millipore, Billerica, MA, USA) was used to visualize stained bands, and the densities of the grey bands were determined using ImageJ software (National Institutes of Health, Bethesda, MD, USA).

2.10. Statistical Analysis. Each experiment was repeated at least three times. Experimental data are presented as means ± standard deviation. Analyses for statistical significance were performed using Prism 6.0 software (GraphPad Software, San Diego, CA, USA). To assess statistical differences between groups in multiple comparisons, we used one-way analysis of variance, followed by the Student-Newman-Keuls post hoc test. The presented P values are two-sided, and results were considered statistically significant at a $P < 0.05$.

3. Results

3.1. Effect of Hyperglycemia on HREC and ARPE-19 Cell Viability and Apoptosis. Our aim was to identify miRNAs exhibiting altered expression during the progression of early DR. Therefore, we conducted experiments on HRECs and ARPE-19 cells exposed to hyperglycemia (25 mmol/L glucose).

MTS assay results showed that with an increase in the time of hyperglycemia treatment up to 6 days, the viability of HRECs and RPE cells decreased significantly (Figures 1(a) and 1(b)). We also examined how HG exposure altered the phenotype of these cells. Hoechst DNA-dye nuclear staining indicated that hyperglycemia induced nuclear condensation or fragmentation, particularly after incubation for 5 and 7 days. Representative apoptotic HRECs and RPE cells harboring condensed nuclei are indicated by arrowheads in Figures 1(c) and 1(d). The results of statistical analysis confirmed the observed increase in apoptosis of HRECs and RPE cells under HG exposure (Figures 1(e) and 1(f)).

3.2. Hyperglycemia-Induced Changes in miRNA Expression in HRECs and RPE Cells. To investigate the relevance of the miRNAs exhibiting expression changes with DR progression, we measured miRNA levels in HRECs cultured under HG exposure for different periods. Real-time qPCR analysis revealed that the levels of several miRNAs changed during the early stage of DR. Although the expression of miR-124-

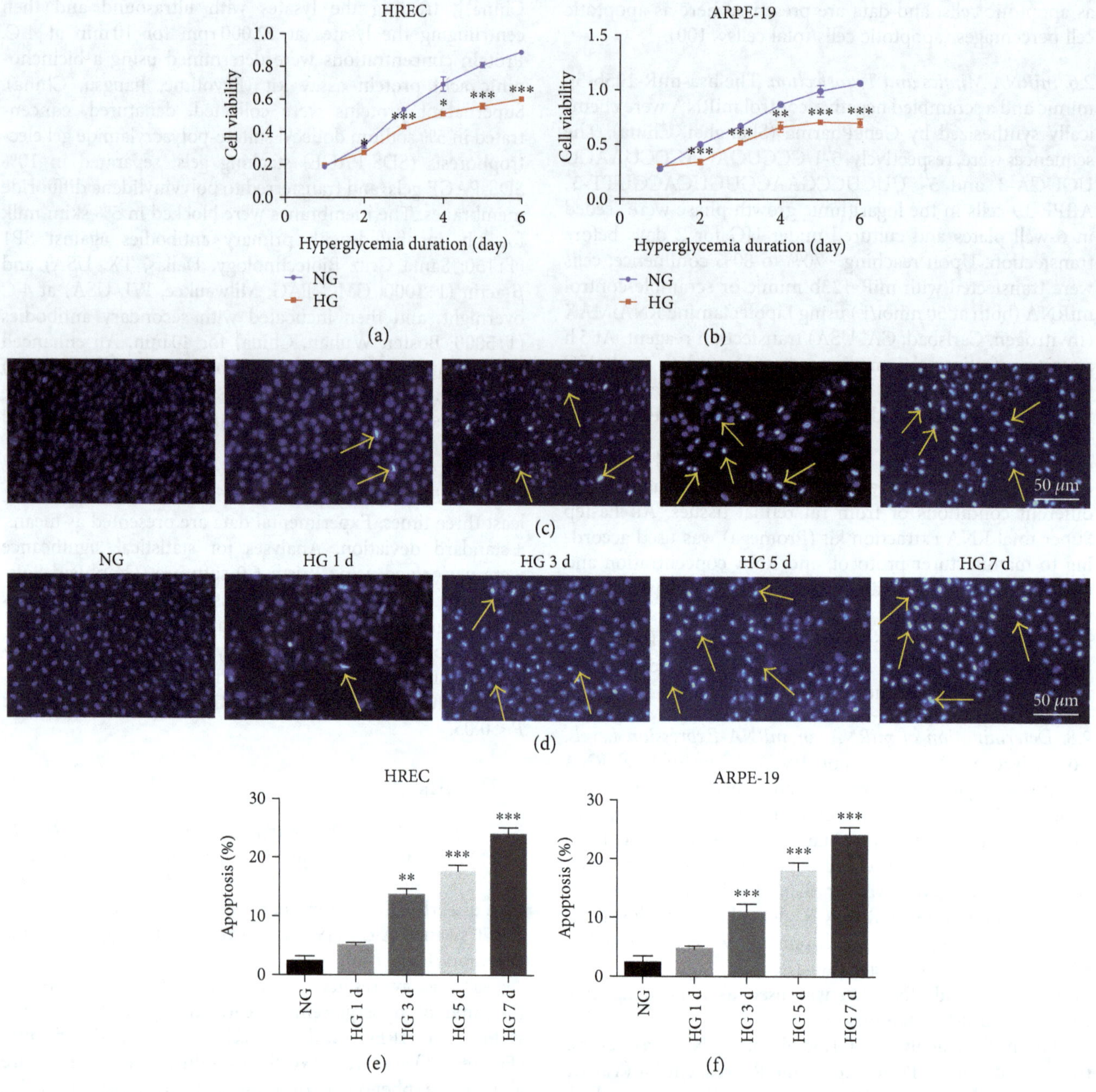

FIGURE 1: Effects of high glucose (HG) on the viability and apoptosis of HRECs and ARPE-19 cells. (a, b) Time-dependent increase in hyperglycemia-induced inhibition of HRECs and RPE proliferation. (c, d) Representative images of HRECs and RPE cells treated with normal glucose (NG) or HG. The number of apoptotic cells harboring condensed or fragmented nuclei (yellow, *arrowheads*) increased along with an increase in HG-treatment time. (e, f) Statistical analysis of apoptotic HRECs and RPE cells under different conditions. Quantification was performed using ImageJ software. $^{*}P < 0.05$; $^{**}P < 0.01$; $^{***}P < 0.001$.

3p and -125b-5p decreased gradually with an increase in HG-exposure time and concomitant with the early development of DR, miR-135b-5p, -145-5p, -146a-5p, and -199a-5p were upregulated on the first day and then downregulated on the following days (Figure 2(a)). These changes indicated that over the course of further DR development, the identified miRNAs might perform distinct (perhaps even opposite) functions. Our results suggested that miRNA levels likely vary during DR progression and that the roles played by miRNAs in retinal endothelial cells are complex and warrant further investigation.

We then exposed ARPE-19 cells to HG for different periods in an identical manner as HRECs to mimic the course of DR. The results of qPCR analysis showed that some of the miRNAs identified here were expressed in a manner distinct from that in HRECs. The expression of miR-124-3p, -125b-5p, -135b-5p, and -199a-5p decreased gradually along with an increase in HG-exposure time, whereas the

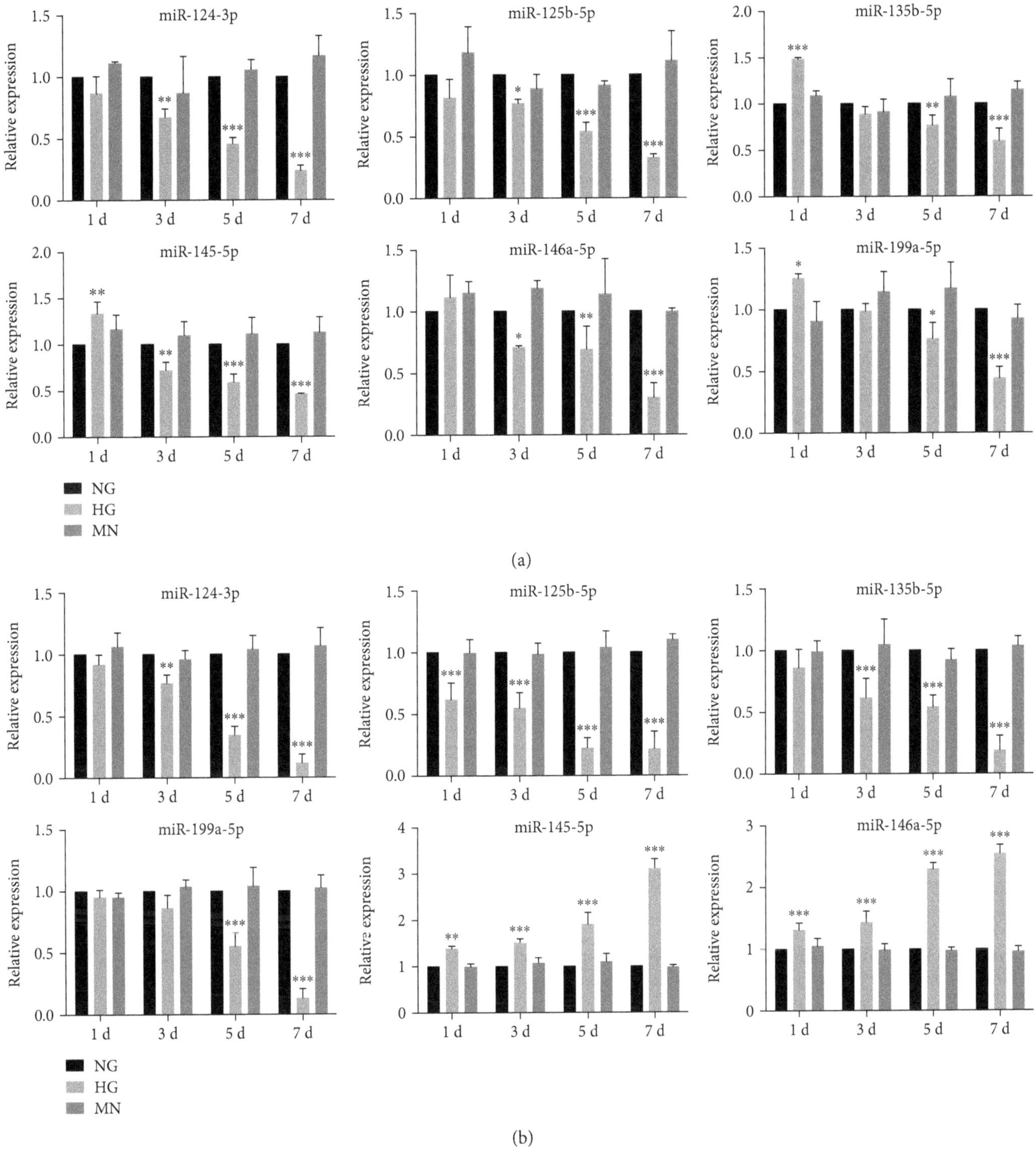

Figure 2: Aberrant levels of miRNAs in HRECs and ARPE-19 cells under hyperglycemia exposure for different periods. (a) In HRECs, miR-124-3p and -125b-5p were downregulated along with an increase in HG-exposure time, whereas miR-135b-5p, -145-5p, -146a-5p, and -199a-5p were first upregulated and then downregulated as compared to levels observed following NG treatment. (b) In RPE cells, HG treatment caused a gradual decline in the levels of miR-124-3p, -125b-5p, -135b-5p, and -199a-5p relative to levels observed after NG exposure. By contrast, miR-145-5p and -146a-5p levels were continually upregulated in RPE cells upon HG exposure. Treatment of HRECs and RPE cells with mannitol (MN) revealed that osmotic change exerted no effect on miRNA expression. $^{*}P < 0.05$; $^{**}P < 0.01$; $^{***}P < 0.001$.

expression of miR-145-5p and -146a-5p was elevated from day 1 to 7 (Figure 2(b)), with the levels of these two miRNAs on day 7 > 2.5-fold higher than those in the NG-exposed group. Moreover, in the MN osmotic-control group, no notable changes were detected in any of the miRNAs analyzed. Therefore, our results suggested that the levels of aberrantly

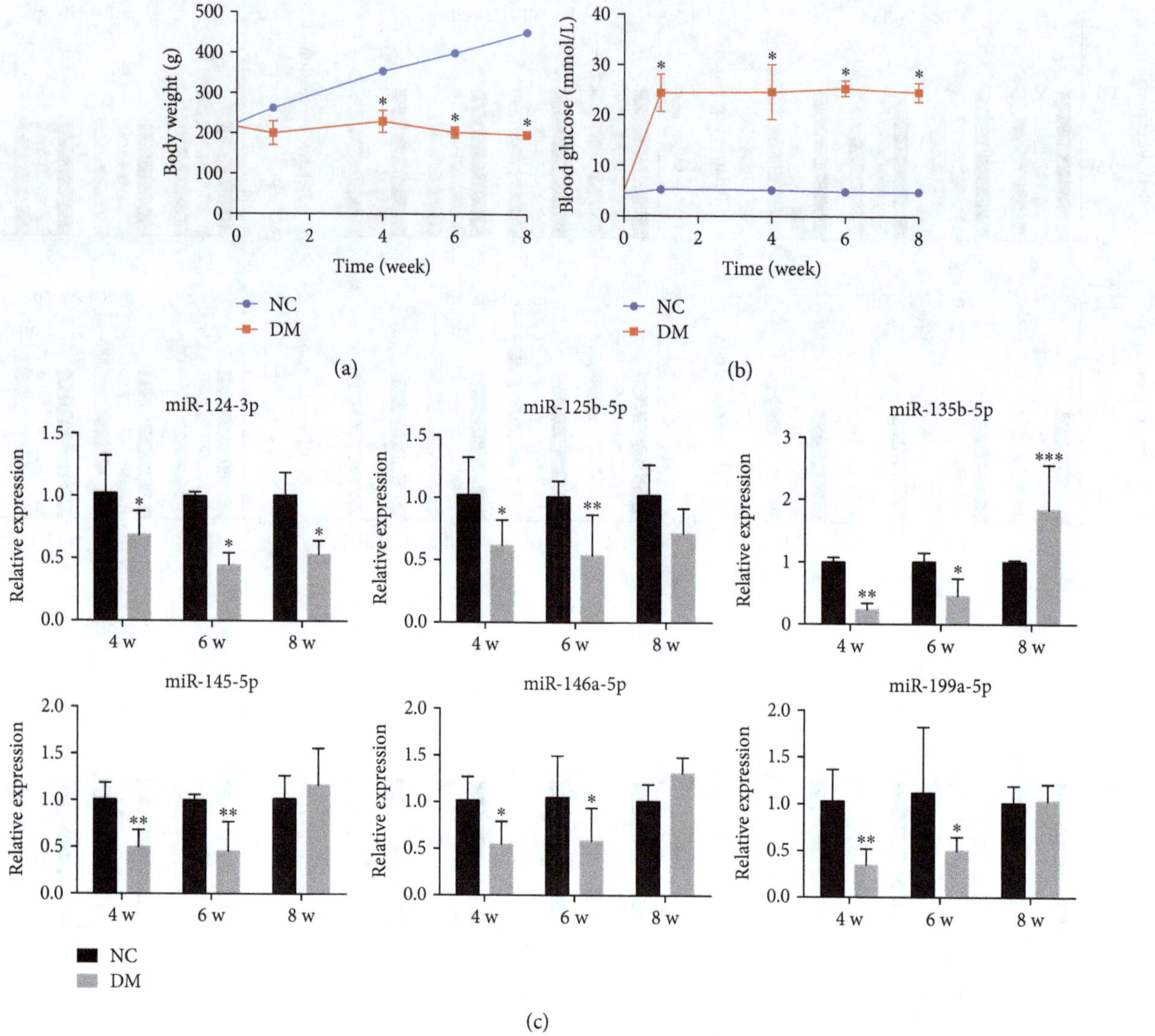

FIGURE 3: Abnormal expression of miRNAs in the retinas of rats with STZ-induced diabetes. (a) Body weight and (b) blood glucose levels of normal control (NC) and DM rats ($n = 6$/group). After intraperitoneal injection of STZ (65 mg/kg) in citrate buffer (pH 4.5), the body weight of DM rats was significantly lower and blood glucose levels increased 5-fold relative to the corresponding values measured for NC rats. (c) Expression of miR-124-3p and -125b-5p was downregulated in parallel with DR progression, whereas the levels of miR-135b-5p, -145-5p, -146a-5p, and -199a-5p decreased during the early stage of DR before increasing in the later stages of DR. $^{*}P < 0.05$; $^{**}P < 0.01$; $^{***}P < 0.001$, compared with NC.

expressed miRNAs varied in retinal cells concomitantly with DR development. These findings indicated that at different stages of DR, miRNA-based therapy should be based on the miRNAs that can be modulated functionally and markedly.

3.3. Aberrantly Expressed miRNAs in the Retinas of Diabetic Rats. To examine abnormal expression of miRNAs in the DM retina, we established an animal model of DM by injecting rats with STZ. These DM rats exhibited significant weight loss as compared with age-matched control rats (Figure 3(a)), with weight loss detected at 1 week post-STZ injection remaining low over the course of DR progression. Moreover, blood glucose levels were markedly elevated in STZ-treated rats during the first week after injection (Figure 3(b)), with levels >5-fold higher than those in normal control rats.

We then used retinal tissues from diabetic and control rats for miRNA validation through real-time PCR analysis. Unexpectedly, the expression of only miR-124-3p and -125b-5p was lower in the retina of DM rats in relation to DR development. By contrast, miR-135b-5p, -145-5p, -146a-5p, and -199a-5p levels were lower at 4 and 6 weeks post-STZ injection before increasing after 8 weeks to levels exceeding even those of the controls (Figure 3(c)). These results and those presented in the preceding subsection together showed that both in vitro and in vivo, the expression of miR-124 and -125b decreased in correspondence with DR progression, but that of miR-135b and -199a decreased in

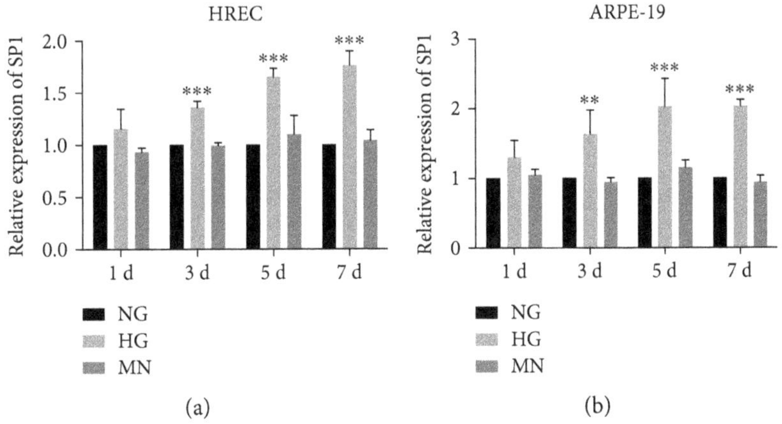

FIGURE 4: Quantitative reverse transcription PCR analysis showing SP1 mRNA upregulation in both HRECs and RPE cells exposed to hyperglycemia. SP1 expression in (a) HRECs and (b) RPE cells increased with HG-exposure time. SP1 mRNA levels were normalized relative to the mRNA levels of PUM1 and PPIA in HRECs and RPE cells, respectively. Culturing of HRECs and RPE cells with MN revealed that osmotic change did not affect SP1 expression. $^{**}P < 0.01$; $^{***}P < 0.001$, compared with NG.

retinal cells under hyperglycemia exposure and increased in the DM retina. Moreover, miR-145 and -146a were downregulated gradually in HG-treated HRECs, but were upregulated in RPE cells exposed to hyperglycemia and in DM rats.

3.4. The Role of SP1, a Previously Unknown Potential Target of miR-125b-5p, in DR Progression. Previous work revealed miR-125b-5p as one of the most abundant miRNAs in the retina, with this miRNA exhibiting an inherent ability to regulate cell differentiation, growth, and development [17, 18]. In this study, we confirmed that miR-125b was expressed at low levels in both HRECs and ARPE-19 cells under hyperglycemia exposure and in the DM retina. Therefore, modulation of miR-125b in early DR might exert beneficial effects with regard to slowing DR progression and DR-associated impairment. Furthermore, it is critical to study miR-125b-target genes related to the DR pathogenesis; however, only a few mRNAs have thus far been verified as miR-125b targets involved in DR pathogenesis [17]. According to the prediction obtained using TargertScan (http://www.targetscan.org/vert_71/), we identified SP1 as a target of miR-125b-5p; therefore, to examine potential regulatory interactions between miR-125b and SP1 during the course of DR, we used qPCR to measure SP1 mRNA levels in HG-treated HRECs and RPE cells. Subsequently, we transfected an miR-125b-5p mimic into ARPE-19 cells under hyperglycemia exposure, confirmed miR-125b upregulation, and determined the SP1-expression level at both the mRNA and protein levels.

Over increasing durations of hyperglycemia exposure, SP1 mRNA levels were evaluated in HRECs (Figure 4(a)) and ARPE-19 cells (Figure 4(b)) after normalization relative to the mRNA levels of Pumilio homolog 1 (PUM1) and peptidylprolyl isomerase A (PPIA), respectively. PUM1 in HRECs and PPIA in ARPE-19 cells were selected for normalization based on our previous analysis [19, 20]. In the MN osmotic-control groups, SP1 levels did not change significantly; however, when HRECs and ARPE-19 cells were exposed to HG, SP1 levels increased and remained high until days 5 and 7. This increase in SP1 expression along with DR progression was the opposite of that observed with miR-125b levels. As shown in Figure 5(a), putative interaction sites for miR-125b are present in the 3′-UTR of SP1 mRNA; therefore, we directly tested the effect of an miR-125b mimic on SP1 levels. Transfection of the miR-125b mimic led to a 25-fold increase in the level of miR-125b relative to a level in cells transfected with scramble-control miRNA (Figure 5(b)). Notably, after introduction of miR-125b into cells, SP1 expression was significantly inhibited at both the protein and mRNA levels (Figures 5(c) and 5(d)). These results strongly suggested that SP1 is a previously unidentified direct target of miR-125b associated with the progression of DR. Therefore, we propose that miR-125b could restrict SP1 levels in cells and that this modulation might affect its downstream targets and thereby ameliorate DR progression. These possibilities will be further and specifically tested in future studies.

4. Discussion

An uncontrolled high level of blood glucose is the leading cause of type 2 DM and related complications. DR is a chronic and serious eye complication associated with DM, and people with DR present an increased risk of other microvascular and macrovascular complications associated with diabetes [21]. Hyperglycemia is closely related to the pathologic changes related to DR, which are responsible for induction of neovascularization, inflammation, oxidative stress, apoptosis, and cell proliferation [22, 23]. In the early stages of DR, HRECs and RPE cells, which are components of the BRB, are affected and impaired by the adverse effects of HG, subsequently inducing BRB dysfunction and contributing to DR progression. Retinal-cell dysfunction is characterized by a decrease in cell viability and increase in apoptosis [24]. In this study, HRECs and RPE cells exposed to 25 mmol/L glucose for various periods exhibited diminished cell viability and increased apoptosis. These observed changes agreed with the findings reported in the previous studies.

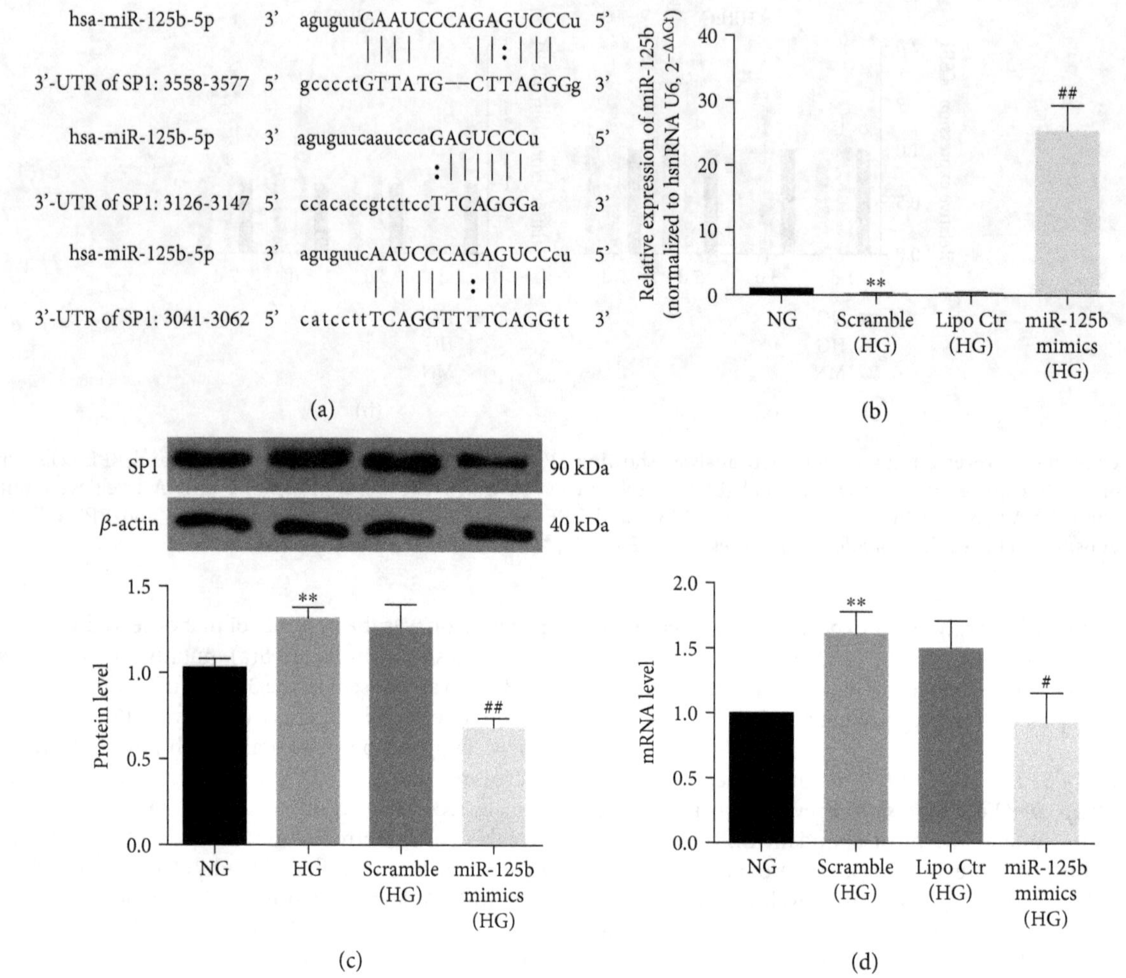

FIGURE 5: SP1 might represent a previously unknown target of miR-125b and suppression of high levels of SP1 expression by miR-125b in RPE cells under hyperglycemia. (a) Three representative predicted seed regions of miR-125b in the 3′ UTR of SP1 mRNA. (b) Expression of miR-125b was significantly increased after transfection with an miR-125b mimic (as compared to levels after transfection with a scramble-control miRNA) in RPE cells cultured under HG exposure. Lipofectamine did not affect miR-125b expression. (c, d) Hyperglycemia-induced increases in SP1 levels in RPE cells were alleviated by miR-125b upregulations, which was confirmed by (c) western blot and (d) quantitative reverse transcription PCR. Endogenous β-actin was used as a reference for protein expression, and SP1 mRNA level was normalized relative to PPIA mRNA level. $^{**}P < 0.01$, compared with NG; $^{\#}P < 0.05$; $^{\#\#}P < 0.01$, compared with scramble control.

Noncoding RNAs have been investigated in diverse diseases, including neuronal diseases, cardiovascular diseases, and cancer, with miRNAs, in particular, playing key roles in these diseases. Increasing numbers of miRNAs aberrantly expressed during DR progression have been identified, with some even applied to clinical therapies [10] or, in the case of circulating miRNAs, used as DR biomarkers [25]. To identify the potential role played by miRNAs in glucose-induced retinal-cell dysfunction/apoptosis, we analyzed miRNA expression related to DR by conducting in vitro studies on cells exposed to hyperglycemia and in vivo studies on a rat model of type 2 DM. Initial results obtained from the in vitro study (on HG-treated HRECs and ARPE-19 cells) showed that miRNAs were markedly dysregulated under hyperglycemic conditions. Among the identified miRNAs, miR-124-3p, -125b-5p, -135b-5p, and -199a-5p showed a gradual decrease in expression in either HRECs or RPE cells along with an increase in HG-treatment time, whereas miR-145-5p and -146a-5p exhibited opposite expression changes (downregulation in HRECs and upregulation in RPE cells) in response to HG exposure for increasing durations. Moreover, the same miRNA could be distinctly expressed in the different layers of the retina under the same conditions. Independent analysis of the miRNA data from the in vivo study on diabetic rats revealed changes in miRNA expression associated with DR progression. Although miR-124-3p and -125b-5p remained downregulated during the different periods of DR examined, miR-135b-5p, -145-5p, -146a-5p, and -199a-5p exhibited increases in expression along with DR development. These four miRNAs were expressed at lower levels than those observed in control rats at 4 and 6 weeks post-STZ induction, followed by an increase to levels exceeding those of controls at week 8. These findings implied that the same miRNAs might play opposite roles during DR development, a possibility also supported by previous studies. In a rat model of STZ-induced diabetes, miR-146a was downregulated in retinal endothelial cells at 1 month after diabetes onset [26], but was upregulated in the retina and in retinal endothelial cells at 3 months after diabetes onset [27], which agreed with our findings. The alteration of miRNAs in early stages of DR has been observed not only in human retinal cells, but also in the retinas of diabetic rats. The underlying reason for these findings could be that the pathologic changes associated with DR progression exert distinct effects on miRNA biogenesis, resulting in either upregulation or downregulation at different stages of DR. Therefore, the application of miRNAs in clinical therapy should be based on the modulation of miRNAs for which stable and confirmed changes in expression have been reported.

Among the miRNAs studied here, miR-124-3p and -125b-5p were found to be downregulated during DR progression both in vitro and in vivo. MiR-124, which was identified as a tumor suppressor, has been confirmed to be downregulated in cancers and investigated for its role in regulating cell proliferation and apoptosis by targeting different genes in distinct types of cancer [28–30]. Moreover, miR-135b was identified as a biomarker for colorectal cancer [31] and reported to modulate apoptosis by targeting large tumor-suppressor kinase 2 [32]. However, the role of these miRNAs in glucose-induced retinal-cell dysfunction during DR progression has not been studied previously. MiR-145 was shown to participate in the insulin-resistance pathway involving AKT/protein kinase B, which is strongly associated with type 2 DM [33]. The potential functions of miR-124, -135b, and -145 warrant further investigation regarding their roles in DR pathogenesis. Previous work showed that miR-146a was upregulated and functioned in negative-feedback regulation of the nuclear factor (NF)-κB-activation pathway in the retinal endothelial cells of diabetic rats at 3 months after diabetes onset [27]. The negative-feedback effect on NF-κB activation suggests that miR-146a could serve as an alternative target for DR treatment through NF-κB inhibition. Moreover, miR-199a-dependent cross-talk between VEGF and hypoxia-inducible factor 1α was validated in the diabetic retina [34], and miR-199a targeting could alleviate DR progression. Given that a single miRNA can regulate multiple genes, and one gene can potentially be regulated by multiple miRNAs, the aberrantly expressed miRNAs investigated in this study could be modulated in different pathways and, thus, might function in the development of DR.

We also found that miR-125b downregulation was correlated with the upregulation of a target gene, with our results suggesting SP1 as a previously unrecognized miR-125b-5p target. Accordingly, in ARPE-19 cells, miR-125b upregulation abolished the high levels of SP1 induced by hyperglycemia. SP1 is a key transcription factor; therefore, aberrant SP1 expression is involved in various types of diseases and plays vital roles in angiogenesis, inflammation, and cell proliferation, migration/invasion, and survival. Interactions between miRNAs and transcription factors are closely related during disease progression, and modulation of this network might exert beneficial effects [35, 36]. Investigation of SP1 at different stages of DR progression revealed that SP1 is tightly associated with angiogenesis-related factors, especially VEGF, and positively regulates their expression [16, 37, 38]. SP1 mRNA is also highly expressed in epiretinal membranes in proliferative DR, with SP1 protein mainly colocalized with VEGF [37]. Furthermore, SP1 binds to the VEGF-A promoter and upregulates VEGF-A expression during DR induced by hyperglycemia [38]. However, additional SP1-related downstream molecules need to be identified in association with DR pathogenesis. Given that modulation of SP1 expression could alleviate DR progression, the application of miR-125b or other miRNAs to target SP1 and other downstream targets might produce beneficial effects in DR treatment.

5. Conclusions

This study demonstrated that hyperglycemia induced a decrease in cell viability and an increase in apoptosis of HRECs and RPE cells. The miRNAs identified here showed changes in expression in HRECs and RPE cells along with increases in the duration of hyperglycemia exposure and in the retinas of DM rats along with the development of DR. Furthermore, these miRNAs could exhibit distinct alterations in different layers of the retina or during the different stages of DR. Moreover, SP1 was identified as a potential target of miR-125b-5p associated with DR progression. These results indicated the considerable potential of miRNAs for application in DR-specific therapeutic strategies.

Conflicts of Interest

The authors declare no conflict of interest.

Acknowledgments

This study was supported by all of the members of the Central Laboratory of the Second Hospital at Jilin University.

References

[1] D. A. Antonetti, R. Klein, and T. W. Gardner, "Diabetic retinopathy," *The New England Journal of Medicine*, vol. 366, pp. 1227–1239, 2012.

[2] B. A. Mysona, S. Matragoon, M. Stephens et al., "Imbalance of the nerve growth factor and its precursor as a potential biomarker for diabetic retinopathy," *BioMed Research International*, vol. 2015, Article ID 571456, 12 pages, 2015.

[3] T. W. Gardner, D. A. Antonetti, A. J. Barber, K. F. LaNoue, and S. W. Levison, "Diabetic retinopathy: more than meets the eye," *Survey of Ophthalmology*, vol. 47, Supplement 2, pp. S253–S262, 2002.

[4] J. G. Cunha-Vaz and A. Travassos, "Breakdown of the blood-retinal barriers and cystoid macular edema," *Survey of Ophthalmology*, vol. 28, no. Suppl, pp. 485–492, 1984.

[5] T. A. Ciulla, A. G. Amador, and B. Zinman, "Diabetic retinopathy and diabetic macular edema: pathophysiology, screening, and novel therapies," *Diabetes Care*, vol. 26, pp. 2653–2664, 2003.

[6] N. Miyamoto, Y. de Kozak, J. C. Jeanny et al., "Placental growth factor-1 and epithelial haemato-retinal barrier breakdown: potential implication in the pathogenesis of diabetic retinopathy," *Diabetologia*, vol. 50, pp. 461–470, 2007.

[7] O. Strauss, "The retinal pigment epithelium in visual function," *Physiological Reviews*, vol. 85, pp. 845–881, 2005.

[8] D. Aronson and E. J. Rayfield, "How hyperglycemia promotes atherosclerosis: molecular mechanisms," *Cardiovascular Diabetology*, vol. 1, p. 1, 2002.

[9] R. N. Frank, "Diabetic retinopathy," *The New England Journal of Medicine*, vol. 350, pp. 48–58, 2004.

[10] R. Mastropasqua, L. Toto, F. Cipollone, D. Santovito, P. Carpineto, and L. Mastropasqua, "Role of microRNAs in the modulation of diabetic retinopathy," *Progress in Retinal and eye Research*, vol. 43, pp. 92–107, 2014.

[11] J. H. Wu, Y. Gao, A. J. Ren et al., "Altered microRNA expression profiles in retinas with diabetic retinopathy," *Ophthalmic Research*, vol. 47, pp. 195–201, 2012.

[12] B. Yan, Z. F. Tao, X. M. Li, H. Zhang, J. Yao, and Q. Jiang, "Aberrant expression of long noncoding RNAs in early diabetic retinopathy," *Investigative Ophthalmology & Visual Science*, vol. 55, pp. 941–951, 2014.

[13] D. P. Bartel, "MicroRNAs: genomics, biogenesis, mechanism, and function," *Cell*, vol. 116, pp. 281–297, 2004.

[14] D. P. Bartel, "MicroRNAs: target recognition and regulatory functions," *Cell*, vol. 136, pp. 215–233, 2009.

[15] J. Krol, I. Loedige, and W. Filipowicz, "The widespread regulation of microRNA biogenesis, function and decay," *Nature Reviews. Genetics*, vol. 11, pp. 597–610, 2010.

[16] Y. Mitamura, C. Harada, and T. Harada, "Role of cytokines and trophic factors in the pathogenesis of diabetic retinopathy," *Current Diabetes Reviews*, vol. 1, pp. 73–81, 2005.

[17] A. Arora, J. Guduric-Fuchs, L. Harwood, M. Dellett, T. Cogliati, and D. A. Simpson, "Prediction of microRNAs affecting mRNA expression during retinal development," *BMC Developmental Biology*, vol. 10, p. 1, 2010.

[18] R. K. Kutty, W. Samuel, C. Jaworski et al., "MicroRNA expression in human retinal pigment epithelial (ARPE-19) cells: increased expression of microRNA-9 by N-(4-hydroxyphenyl)-retinamide," *Molecular Vision*, vol. 16, pp. 1475–1486, 2010.

[19] X. Liu, J. Xie, Z. Liu, Q. Gong, R. Tian, and G. Su, "Identification and validation of reference genes for quantitative RT-PCR analysis of retinal pigment epithelium cells under hypoxia and/or hyperglycemia," *Gene*, vol. 580, pp. 41–46, 2016.

[20] J. Xie, X. Liu, Y. Li, Y. Liu, and G. Su, "Validation of RT-qPCR reference genes and determination of Robo4 expression levels in human retinal endothelial cells under hypoxia and/or hyperglycemia," *Gene*, vol. 585, pp. 135–142, 2016.

[21] C. K. Kramer, T. C. Rodrigues, L. H. Canani, J. L. Gross, and M. J. Azevedo, "Diabetic retinopathy predicts all-cause mortality and cardiovascular events in both type 1 and 2 diabetes: meta-analysis of observational studies," *Diabetes Care*, vol. 34, pp. 1238–1244, 2011.

[22] S. Saker, E. A. Stewart, A. C. Browning, C. L. Allen, and W. M. Amoaku, "The effect of hyperglycaemia on permeability and the expression of junctional complex molecules in human retinal and choroidal endothelial cells," *Experimental eye Research*, vol. 121, pp. 161–167, 2014.

[23] L. Wang, J. Wang, J. Fang, H. Zhou, X. Liu, and S. B. Su, "High glucose induces and activates toll-like receptor 4 in endothelial cells of diabetic retinopathy," *Diabetology & Metabolic Syndrome*, vol. 7, p. 89, 2015.

[24] C. M. Sena, A. M. Pereira, and R. Seica, "Endothelial dysfunction - a major mediator of diabetic vascular disease," *Biochimica et Biophysica Acta*, vol. 1832, pp. 2216–2231, 2013.

[25] M. V. Joglekar, A. S. Januszewski, A. J. Jenkins, and A. A. Hardikar, "Circulating microRNA biomarkers of diabetic retinopathy," *Diabetes*, vol. 65, pp. 22–24, 2016.

[26] B. Feng, S. Chen, K. McArthur et al., "miR-146a-mediated extracellular matrix protein production in chronic diabetes complications," *Diabetes*, vol. 60, pp. 2975–2984, 2011.

[27] B. Kovacs, S. Lumayag, C. Cowan, and S. Xu, "MicroRNAs in early diabetic retinopathy in streptozotocin-induced diabetic rats," *Investigative Ophthalmology & Visual Science*, vol. 52, pp. 4402–4409, 2011.

[28] D. Deng, L. Wang, Y. Chen et al., "MicroRNA-124-3p regulates cell proliferation, invasion, apoptosis, and bioenergetics by targeting PIM1 in astrocytoma," *Cancer Science*, vol. 107, pp. 899–907, 2016.

[29] S. Liu, C. Hu, Y. Wang, G. Shi, Y. Li, and H. Wu, "miR-124 inhibits proliferation and invasion of human retinoblastoma cells by targeting STAT3," *Oncology Reports*, vol. 36, pp. 2398–2404, 2016.

[30] Q. Yuan, T. Sun, F. Ye, W. Kong, and H. Jin, "MicroRNA-124-3p affects proliferation, migration and apoptosis of bladder cancer cells through targeting AURKA," *Cancer Biomarkers*, vol. 19, pp. 93–101, 2017.

[31] K. Lee and L. R. Ferguson, "MicroRNA biomarkers predicting risk, initiation and progression of colorectal cancer," *World Journal of Gastroenterology*, vol. 22, pp. 7389–7401, 2016.

[32] Y. He, J. Wang, J. Wang et al., "MicroRNA-135b regulates apoptosis and chemoresistance in colorectal cancer by targeting large tumor suppressor kinase 2," *American Journal of Cancer Research*, vol. 5, pp. 1382–1395, 2015.

[33] C. Chakraborty, C. G. Doss, S. Bandyopadhyay, and G. Agoramoorthy, "Influence of miRNA in insulin signaling pathway and insulin resistance: micro-molecules with a major role in type-2 diabetes," *Wiley Interdisciplinary Reviews RNA*, vol. 5, pp. 697–712, 2014.

[34] S. Ling, Y. Birnbaum, M. K. Nanhwan, B. Thomas, M. Bajaj, and Y. Ye, "MicroRNA-dependent cross-talk between VEGF and HIF1alpha in the diabetic retina," *Cellular Signalling*, vol. 25, pp. 2840–2847, 2013.

[35] S. Safe, "MicroRNA-specificity protein (Sp) transcription factor interactions and significance in carcinogenesis," *Current Pharmacology Reports*, vol. 1, pp. 73–78, 2015.

[36] G. Zhang, H. Shi, L. Wang et al., "MicroRNA and transcription factor mediated regulatory network analysis reveals critical regulators and regulatory modules in myocardial infarction," *PloS One*, vol. 10, article e0135339, 2015.

[37] N. Yoshida-Hata, Y. Mitamura, T. Oshitari et al., "Transcription factor, SP1, in epiretinal membranes of patients with proliferative diabetic retinopathy," *Diabetes Research and Clinical Practice*, vol. 87, pp. e26–e28, 2010.

[38] K. Donovan, O. Alekseev, X. Qi, W. Cho, and J. Azizkhan-Clifford, "O-GlcNAc modification of transcription factor Sp1 mediates hyperglycemia-induced VEGF-A upregulation in retinal cells," *Investigative Ophthalmology & Visual Science*, vol. 55, pp. 7862–7873, 2014.

14

Health Literacy Status and Understanding of the Prescription Instructions in Diabetic Patients

Shivangini Singh,[1] Sahana Devadasa Acharya ,[1] Ashwin Kamath ,[1] Sheetal D. Ullal,[1] and Rathnakar P. Urval[2]

[1] *Department of Pharmacology, Kasturba Medical College, Mangalore, Manipal Academy of Higher Education, Karnataka 575001, India*
[2] *Department of Pharmacology, Kanachur Institute of Medical Sciences, Mangalore, Karnataka, India*

Correspondence should be addressed to Sahana Devadasa Acharya; sahana.acharya@manipal.edu

Academic Editor: Janet H. Southerland

This study aimed to assess the health literacy (HL) of patients having diabetes mellitus, their understanding of prescription instructions (PI), and the correlation between HL and understanding of PI. A cross-sectional survey was conducted in 263 adult diabetic patients who were assessed for their understanding of route of intake of the prescribed medication(s), frequency of intake, number of medication(s) to be consumed each time, indication for the medication(s), and the relation of drug intake with food. The HL of the patients was assessed by using Rapid Estimate of Adult Literacy in Medicine, a screening test comprising of 66 health-related words. The number of correctly pronounced words was used to assign a grade-equivalent reading level. There was a significant difference in the understanding of PI in patients with low and high HL levels. A significant difference was observed between the mean total score for interpreting PI in patients with 7 or fewer years of education compared with the other groups with a higher educational status ($P < 0.001$). To conclude, diabetic patients with low HL level will have difficulty in understanding PI. Hence, an alternative comprehensive strategy needs to be adopted in clinical practice in these patients to provide them the instructions to take medications properly.

1. Introduction

Health literacy (HL) is an individual proficiency that includes the skill to acquire, comprehend, and act on suitable health information [1]. In any health care system, patient involvement plays a key role in effective disease management, especially in cases of lifestyle-related diseases which require extensive ongoing self-care [2]. In diabetics, adequate glycemic control aimed at primary and secondary prevention of diabetic complications is necessary for which the patients need to follow strict dietary restrictions, lifestyle modification, and drug regimen. For adherence to these treatment requirements, patients have to understand the physician's instructions. When compared with patients with adequate HL, those who have limited HL find it harder to comprehend their medical condition and its management [3–6]. Understanding one's medication includes the knowledge of drug indication, required dosage, the frequency of drug intake, and for certain medications, some special instructions [7]. The correlation of HL status with the understanding of prescription instructions (PI) in diabetic patients has not been well studied. Determining the presence of any such potential correlation may help in formulating measures for better disease management. The objective of our study was to assess the HL status of diabetic patients, determine their ability to understand the PI, and study the correlation between the HL status and understanding of PI. We hypothesized that diabetic patients with high HL status would understand the PI better.

2. Materials and Methods

A cross-sectional study was conducted in adult patients (>18 years of age) with diabetes mellitus who attended the outpatient department of the tertiary care hospitals affiliated to a medical college in India. The study protocol was approved by the institutional ethics committee. All patients provided a written informed consent prior to participation, and the study was conducted in accordance with the Declaration of Helsinki. Patients with severely impaired vision, hearing problems, and those who had not completed even a single year of schooling were excluded from the study.

After the patients completed their consultation with the physician, their understanding of the PI was assessed. The patients were asked the following questions: what is the route of intake for the prescribed medication(s)? What is the frequency of intake of the medication(s)? What is the number of medication(s) units to be taken each time? Should the medication(s) be taken before, with, or after food? And, what is the indication for the prescribed medication(s)? A correct response received a score of 1, and an incorrect or incomplete response received 0 score.

HL was assessed using Rapid Estimate of Adult Literacy in Medicine (REALM), a screening test comprising of 66 health-related words [8]. It assesses an individual's ability to read health-related words. It helps to estimate the level of HL and, hence, can be used to instruct and educate the patients [9]. The number of correctly pronounced words was used to assign a grade-equivalent reading level. The HL scores were categorized into two groups: 0–60: lower literacy level and 61–66: higher literacy level, assuming that these patients would be capable of reading most of the patient education materials.

Three hundred nineteen diabetic patients were screened, and 263 eligible patients were recruited into the study; the recruitment was completed in 4 months. The sample size of 263 patients was calculated with reference to P (proportion of patients correctly inferring one or more label instructions among patients with adequate health literacy) 29% [10], 95% confidence interval (CI), and 80% power. The formula used was $n = Z^2_\alpha P(1 - P)/E^2$, where $Z_\alpha = 1.96$ at 95% CI; $P = 29\%$; $E = 0.2$ (error % of power).

2.1. Statistical Analysis. The analysis of study data was done using Statistical Package for Social Sciences, IBM Corporation, version 16.0. Descriptive statistics like proportion, mean ± standard deviation (SD), or median and interquartile range, wherever suitable, were calculated for the different demographic characteristics. The HL score categories were compared with respect to the various demographic characteristics. One-way ANOVA and independent *t*-test were used to analyze the continuous variables. Chi-square test was used to analyze the categorical variables. A P value of less than 0.05 was considered as statistically significant.

3. Results

Two hundred sixty-three patients with a prior diagnosis of diabetes mellitus were interviewed for determining their HL status and ability to understand PI. The mean age of the patients was 59.3 ± 11.67 years; 187 (71.1%) patients were males. Based on the REALM scores, patients were grouped into different grade ranges as given in Table 1 [11]. Nine percent of the patients had an HL score in the range of 61–66 (higher literacy level) with a grade equivalent to high school education, 28% had an HL score in the range of 45–60 (marginal literacy level) with a grade equivalent to 7th-8th grade, and 63% had a HL score in the range of 0–44 (low literacy level) with a grade below 6.

No significant difference was found between the patients in the higher and lower HL groups with respect to the demographic features, except for the educational status ($P < 0.001$) (Table 2). Forty-one percent of the patients with lower literacy level had 7 years of schooling or less, and 67% of the patients with higher literacy level were graduates.

The educational status and the grade-equivalent HL scores of the study population are shown in Table 3. Out of the 24 patients with HL scores in the range 61–66, 18 were graduates or postgraduates. Table 4 shows the proportion of patients with lower and higher HL who correctly answered the questions on PI. There was a significant difference ($P < 0.001$) in the understanding of PI between the patients with lower and higher HL levels, with the score for understanding PI increasing with HL level. Among the patients with lower HL, the mean total score for interpreting PI was better in patients with HL grade 7-8 (4.7 ± 0.8) compared with that of patients with HL grade 4–6 (3.83 ± 1.48, $P < 0.001$) and HL grade ≤ 3 (2.31 ± 2.18, $P < 0.001$) (Figure 1). The mean score for understanding PI in patients with 7 or less years of education was (2.21 ± 2.14), which was significantly less compared with the mean score of patients with 8–10 years of education (3.92 ± 1.68, $P < 0.001$), those with preuniversity (4.44 ± 1.26, $P < 0.001$), graduation (4.94 ± 0.23, $P < 0.001$), and master's degree (5 ± 0.00, $P < 0.046$) (Figure 2).

Percentage of patients receiving one medication per prescription was 84.8%, two medications per prescription was 14.4%, and three medications per prescription was 0.76%. The mean total score for interpreting PI was 3.36 ± 2.07, 4.26 ± 1.31, and 5 in patients receiving one, two, and three medications per prescription, respectively. There was a significant difference in mean score for understanding PI between patients receiving one and two medications per prescription ($P < 0.027$). There were only two patients who received three medications per prescription. Patients receiving insulin therapy had a significantly lesser score for interpreting PI when compared with those receiving only oral antidiabetics (3.07 ± 2.16 versus 3.76 ± 1.89; $P = 0.02$). Male patients had a higher score for interpreting PI compared with female patients (3.69 ± 1.87 versus 3.05 ± 2.22; $P = 0.001$). The duration of the disease did not have an effect on the PI interpretation scores.

4. Discussion

In this study, we investigated the HL status of diabetic patients and its relationship with the ability to understand PI. Overall, the proportion of patients having low literacy was higher in this study when compared with other studies [7, 9]. Most patients with a higher literacy level were graduates, which suggests that patients with higher educational status have a better HL score than patients with lesser years of

Table 1: Scores and grade equivalents for the REALM questionnaire.

Health literacy score	Grade range
0–18	Third grade and below; they will not be able to read most low literacy materials; they will need repeated oral instructions
19–44	Fourth to sixth grade; they will need low literacy materials; they may not be able to read prescription labels
45–60	Seventh to eighth grade; they will struggle with most patient education materials; they will not be offended by low literacy materials
61–66	High school; they will be able to read most patient education materials

Table 2: Demographic characteristics of diabetic patients based on their health literacy levels.

Characteristics	Health literacy level Low ($n = 239$) Scores 0–60	High ($n = 24$) Scores 61–66	P value
Age (mean ± SD)	59.04 ± 11.81	61.92 ± 9.93	0.251
Male (%)	170 (71.9)	17 (70.8)	0.976
Female (%)	69 (28.9)	7 (29.2)	
Education (%) 7 years or less	97 (40.6)	1 (4.2)	<0.001*
8–10 years	91 (38.1)	1 (4.2)	
11-12 years	30 (12.6)	4 (16.7)	
Graduation	20 (8.4)	16 (66.7)	
Masters	1 (0.4)	2 (8.3)	
Number of patients on insulin (%)	104 (43.5)	6 (25)	0.08
Number of patients on OHA (%)	147 (61.5)	19 (79.2)	0.087
Number of patients both insulin and OHA (%)	13 (5.4)	1 (4.2)	0.791
Total number of medication per day (mean ± SD)	1.15 ± 0.37	1.21 ± 0.51	0.52
Duration of disease (median (IQR))	8 (4, 13)	10 (5.25, 12)	0.519

SD: standard deviation; IQR: interquartile range; OHA: oral hypoglycemic agents; *significant association between educational status and literacy level when applied Chi-square test.

Table 3: Grade-equivalent health literacy scores and education levels of diabetic patients.

Educational level	HL score (grade equivalent) 0–18 (3rd grade) (%)	19–44 (4th–6th grade) (%)	45–60 (7th–8th grade) (%)	61–66 (High school) (%)
Masters	0	0	1 (33.3)	2 (66.7)
Graduation	0	2 (5.6)	18 (50)	16 (44.4)
Preuniversity college	6 (17.6)	5 (14.7)	19 (55.9)	4 (11.8)
8–10 years of schooling	35 (38)	28 (30.4)	28 (30.4)	1 (1.1)
7 or fewer years of schooling	77 (78.6)	13 (13.3)	7 (7.1)	1 (1)

Table 4: Correct interpretation of prescription medication instruction by diabetic patients based on their health literacy levels.

Questions	Health literacy level Low ($n = 239$) Scores 0–60	High ($n = 24$) Scores 61–66	P value
For route of administration (%)	183 (76.6)	24 (100)	0.008
Frequency of intake in a day (%)	161 (67.4)	24 (100)	0.001
Number of tablets per dose (%)	148 (61.9)	24 (100)	<0.001
Relation of intake of drug with food (%)	151 (63.2)	24 (100)	<0.001
Drug is for diabetes or other condition (%)	161 (67.4)	24 (100)	0.001

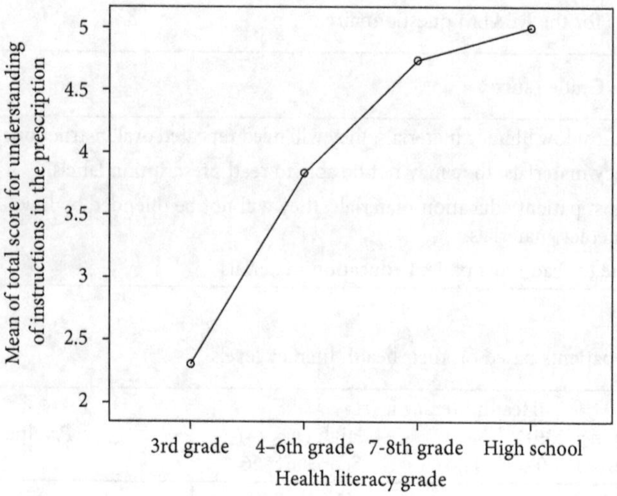

FIGURE 1: Relationship between understanding of the prescription instructions and health literacy grade among diabetic patients.

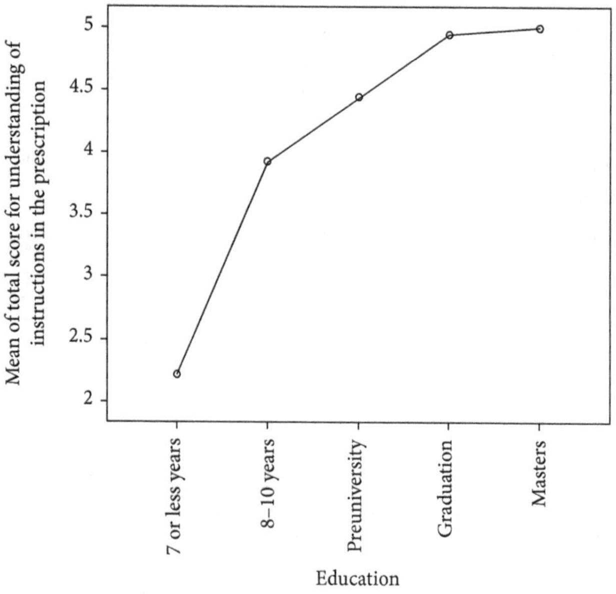

FIGURE 2: Relationship between understanding of the prescription instructions and education level of diabetic patients.

schooling as seen in an earlier study [10]. Fifty percent of the graduates also had a lower literacy level, which may be influenced by the medium of education [9]. There was no difference in the literacy levels between males and females in this study. A similar finding was noted in other studies, but it is difficult to draw any conclusion as the proportion of female patients (28.1%) was less in this study [12].

In this study, patients with lower HL had difficulty in understanding all the five questions regarding PI. All the patients in the higher literacy group answered these questions correctly. Seventy-seven percent of the patients in the lower literacy group knew the route of intake of the drug, but the proportion of patients who knew the number of tablets to be taken per dose was the least (62%), which means that the functional HL regarding the prescription medication was poor in diabetic patients who had lower HL scores. These findings might be important in the management of diabetic patients, especially those with lower HL. The findings emphasize the need for adopting specific strategies to improve the understanding of PI. Among the 239 patients with lower literacy level, 117 (49%) answered all the five prescription-related questions correctly which means that HL alone may not influence the understanding of PI. Age and duration of the disease did not influence the understanding of the PI in this study. The lack of age-related difference in the scores for understanding PI could, at least partly, be due to the lesser percentage of patients in the age group of 20–45 years in this study. Unlike in the study by Davis et al., the understanding of PI was better in patients with more number of prescription medications [13].

Our study has limitations. We could not study the impact of HL on the outcome of diabetes treatment because of the cross-sectional study design. The percentage of female patients and those with educational qualification more than preuniversity level was less in this study which could have influenced the findings.

5. Conclusion

Diabetic patients with lower HL level will have difficulty in understanding the PI. Hence, an alternative, comprehensive strategy needs to be adopted in clinical practice to provide instructions regarding proper medication use in these patients.

Conflicts of Interest

The authors declare that there is no conflict of interest regarding the publication of this article.

Acknowledgments

The authors thank the support provided by the Short Term Studentship (STS) program of Indian Council of Medical Research (ICMR) in carrying out this study.

References

[1] R. Parker and S. C. Ratzan, "Health literacy: a second decade of distinction for Americans," *Journal of Health Communication*, vol. 15, Supplement 2, pp. 20–33, 2010.

[2] H. Ishikawa, E. Yano, S. Fujimori et al., "Patient health literacy and patient–physician information exchange during a visit," *Family Practice*, vol. 26, no. 6, pp. 517–523, 2009.

[3] T. C. Davis and M. S. Wolf, "Health literacy: implications for family medicine," *Family Medicine*, vol. 36, no. 8, pp. 595–598, 2004.

[4] R. Y. Torres and R. Marks, "Relationships among health literacy, knowledge about hormone therapy, self-efficacy, and

decision-making among postmenopausal health," *Journal of Health Communication*, vol. 14, no. 1, pp. 43–55, 2009.

[5] M. S. Wolf, T. C. Davis, J. T. Cross, E. Marin, K. Green, and C. L. Bennett, "Health literacy and patient knowledge in a Southern US HIV clinic," *International Journal of STD & AIDS*, vol. 15, no. 11, pp. 747–752, 2004.

[6] J. A. Gazmararian, M. V. Williams, J. Peel, and D. W. Baker, "Health literacy and knowledge of chronic disease," *Patient Education and Counseling*, vol. 51, no. 3, pp. 267–275, 2003.

[7] S. Kripalani, L. E. Henderson, E. Y. Chiu, R. Robertson, P. Kolm, and T. A. Jacobson, "Predictors of medication self-management skill in a low-literacy population," *Journal of General Internal Medicine*, vol. 21, no. 8, pp. 852–856, 2006.

[8] T. C. Davis, S. W. Long, R. H. Jackson et al., "Rapid estimate of adult literacy in medicine: a shortened screening instrument," *Family Medicine*, vol. 25, no. 6, pp. 391–395, 1993.

[9] U. P. Rathnakar, M. Belman, A. Kamath, B. Unnikrishnan, K. Ashok Shenoy, and A. L. Udupa, "Evaluation of health literacy status among patients in a tertiary care hospital in coastal Karnataka, India," *Journal of Clinical and Diagnostic Research*, vol. 7, no. 11, pp. 2551–2554, 2013.

[10] T. C. Davis, A. D. Federman, P. F. Bass III et al., "Improving patient understanding of prescription drug label instructions," *Journal of General Internal Medicine*, vol. 24, no. 1, pp. 57–62, 2009.

[11] R. S. Safeer and J. Keenan, "Health literacy: the gap between physicians and patients," *American Family Physician*, vol. 72, no. 3, pp. 463–468, 2005.

[12] P. N. Peterson, S. M. Shetterly, C. L. Clarke et al., "Health literacy and outcomes among patients with heart failure," *Journal of the American Medical Association*, vol. 305, no. 16, pp. 1695–1701, 2011.

[13] T. C. Davis, M. S. Wolf, P. F. Bass III et al., "Literacy and misunderstanding prescription drug labels," *Annals of Internal Medicine*, vol. 145, no. 12, pp. 887–894, 2006.

15

Therapeutic Potential of Fulvic Acid in Chronic Inflammatory Diseases and Diabetes

John Winkler and Sanjoy Ghosh

Department of Biology, IKBSAS, University of British Columbia-Okanagan, Canada

Correspondence should be addressed to Sanjoy Ghosh; sanjoy.ghosh@ubc.ca

Academic Editor: Craig S. Nunemaker

Chronic inflammatory diseases like diabetes are on a rise in the Western world. Based on the tsunami of new cases every year, new therapeutic measures must be considered. A promising avenue might involve the attenuation of underlying inflammation through natural health products (NHPs). This is because most NHPs have a rich history in traditional medicine and might be considered safer under appropriate doses and conditions. However, the biggest impediment in NHP research is that rarely do these products come with verified health benefits or dosing schedules established through modern scientific research. Fulvic acid (FvA), one such NHP, comes from humic substances produced by microorganisms in soil. Traditional medicine and modern research claim FvA can modulate the immune system, influence the oxidative state of cells, and improve gastrointestinal function; all of which are hallmarks of diabetes. This minireview outlines the available peer-reviewed research on FvA and examines its anecdotal health claims. We show that although available research has been minimal, there is substantial evidence to pursue FvA research in preventing chronic inflammatory diseases, including diabetes.

1. Introduction

Diseases associated with chronic inflammation such as diabetes, cardiovascular disease, and colitis have been increasing. For example, the number of people living with diabetes in Canada in 2015 was 3.4 million and is predicted to reach 5 million by 2025 [1]. Millions of dollars have been poured into the development of drugs to treat these diseases with little success [2]. Thus, it is time to explore new avenues in treating and preventing chronic inflammatory diseases. Natural health products (NHPs) may provide a promising route in this quest for alternatives. First, they require little to no development, and second, they are often accompanied by a history rich in traditional medicine [3]. Fulvic acid (FvA) is a publically available NHP that combines those two facts and may provide promising outcomes for chronic inflammatory diseases.

FvA is a subclass of diverse compounds known as humic substances, which are by-products of organic degradation from microorganisms [4]. What separates FvA from other humic substances (HS) is a set of physical and chemical properties shown in Figure 1(a), indicated by Stevenson [5] and followed by the International Humic Substance Society (IHSS; St. Paul, Minnesota, USA) [4, 6]. By definition, FvAs consist in small molecular weight, hydrophilic, carboxylic-containing molecules. The other HS have higher molecular weight and different solubility and oxygen content. The structure of FvA has been proposed by many authors to be a mixture of covalently linked phenolic, quinoid, and benzene carboxylic acid compounds [6]. It is important to note that FvA can change with geographic location. The parent material from which FvA originates influences oxygen, nitrogen, aromatic ring, and carbon content [7]. For example, in Israel, FvA isolated from clay contains ~2.0% (m/m) nitrogen, and FvA isolated from sand contains ~4.4% (m/m) nitrogen [7]. In addition, FvA isolated from Israel has ~49% (m/m) carbon whereas FvA from Italy has ~39% carbon content [7]. Health Canada indicates that FvA is consistent with the structure shown in Figure 1(b) [8].

FvA has been indirectly utilized in traditional Indian medicine ("Ayurveda") for roughly 3000 years [3]. The substance called Shilajit, a tar-like exudate from the Himalayas,

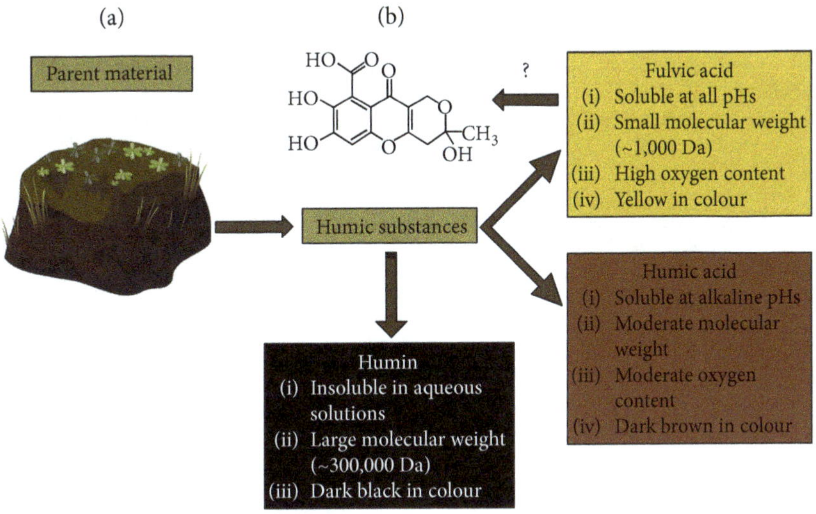

Figure 1: The characterization and classification of humic substances. Adapted from [5]. (a) Humic substances are isolated from various parent material like peat, coal, water, and soil through a series of precipitation/dissolution steps; their general characteristics are highlighted in each box [9, 10]. (b) Proposed composition of fulvic acid by Health Canada.

contains about 15–20% FvA and is used for medicinal purposes. As per ancient texts, Shilajit can have immune-modulation, antioxidant, diuretic, antihypertensive, and hypoglycaemic effects [3]. In addition, when applied externally, it is claimed to be an antiseptic and analgesic [11]. Reviews on Shilajit indicate that the intake is safe; however, the pharmacological dosing of such molecules remain unknown [3]. Despite such lack of information, Shilajit/FvA is currently available as a nutraceutical to the public [12]. The purpose of this review is to investigate and highlight the current knowledge base regarding FvA and its effects on animals and animal cells.

2. Immunomodulation by FvA

The most adequately researched claim of FvA is its ability to modulate the immune system. However, the outcomes of such studies remain controversial. FvA can be both proinflammatory and anti-inflammatory in animal systems. The available literature regarding the effects of FvA on the immune system is summarized in Figure 2.

2.1. Anti-inflammatory Effects of FvA. Asthma, allergies, and eczema, along with many other disorders, can be associated with overactive immune cells [13]. In these cases, anti-inflammatory drugs are critical for reducing symptoms. Several studies indicate that FvA can act as an anti-inflammatory by reducing the release of proinflammatory mediators from cells. First, Junek et al. show that FvA at 200 μg/mL can reduce tumour necrosis factor alpha (TNF-α) expression after exposure to the endotoxin Lipopolysaccharide (LPS) in differentiated human monocytes (U937) [14]. FvA also is shown to reduce cyclooxygenase 2 (COX2) and prostaglandin E2 (PGE2) secretion after homocysteine stimulation in primary human monocytes [15]. FvA from solubilized sludge (SS-FA) is shown to reduce B-hexosaminidase and histamine release in immunoglobulin-E-sensitized mast cells and basophil cells [16]. This information suggests that FvA can have anti-inflammatory and antiallergy effects. Yamada et al. also show SS-FA decreases TNF-α, interleukin-4 (IL-4), and IL-13 from mast cells.

Unfortunately, *in vivo* studies into the effects of FvA have been too few and sporadic. A pilot clinical study shows coal-derived FvA (oxifulvic acid) at 4.5% (w/w) reduces wheal and flare size after allergen challenge in humans [17]. The reduction by FvA shows similar results to 1% hydrocortisone. The anti-inflammatory properties of oxifulvic acid are also shown in mice [18]. In the study, mice sensitized with dinitrofluorobenzene on the ear and then again challenged 6 days later see a reduction in swelling with FvA treatment comparable to steroid medication. A patented isolation procedure yielding carbohydrate-derived fulvic acid (CHD-FvA) mimics the above information almost entirely. In a randomized clinical trial, topical administration of CHD-FvA is shown to significantly reduce eczema rash in humans [19]. However, a burning sensation was also reported in this study. In addition, oral ingestion of CHD-FvA isolated from South Africa at 100 mg/kg can reduce paw edema in rats at levels similar to nonsteroidal anti-inflammatory drugs [20]. Overall, the above studies promise the potential of FvA to treat overactive immune disorders, specifically eczema.

2.2. Proinflammatory Effects of FvA. The immune system is an integral part of human health and has evolved to be a complex organization in which we rely. It provides protection against pathogens and stops tumour growth by initiating the inflammatory response [21, 22]. Interestingly, FvA has been shown to enhance inflammation in animals too. In the same study by Sabi et al. [20], topically applied CHD-FvA can reduce the size of wounds infected with *Staphylococcus aureus*, thus stopping the progression of the infection. CHD-FvA is also suggested to reduce the size of wounds infected with antibiotic-resistant pathogens [23]. This suggests a bimodal effect of FvA that not only suppresses

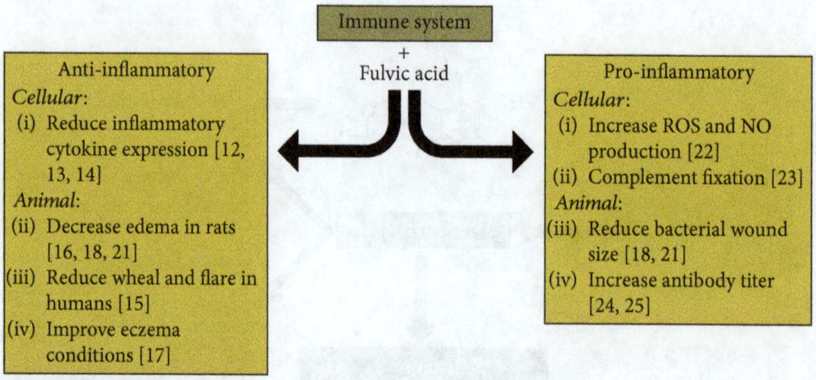

FIGURE 2: Known literature for the effects of fulvic acid on the immune system. Fulvic acid is shown to induce as well as reduce inflammation.

immune function but also stimulates it. Essentially, it provides evidence that FvA ensures proper immune function. Schepetkin et al. show that FvA can activate isolated murine macrophages from the peritoneal cavity. Nitric oxide (NO) and reactive oxygen species (ROS) important for killing bacteria and intracellular signalling increase in FvA-treated peritoneal macrophages [24]. They do however indicate cell viability is reduced with 100 μg/mL of FvA, questioning studies by Junek et al. [14]. In addition, Schepetkin et al. also show that IHSS FvA standards and low molecular-weight extracts from Nepal Shilajit can fix the complement system [25]. This gives rise to the thought that FvA can activate the immune system when needed to protect against infection and foreign pathogens.

2.3. Detrimental Immune Effects of FvA. Several studies indicate that FvA may be harmful too. FvA derived from Hungarian lignite can activate humoral immunity and reduce thyroid function in rats [26]. In this study, FvA increases antibody titre against ovalbumin 14 days and 26 days after challenge. They also indicate that lymphocyte diameter increases in rats, a sign of cellular activation [26]. These results are not isolated; Kunavue and Lien show increases in IgG antibodies in weanling pigs after FvA treatment [27]. No significant increase is found in lymphocyte, monocyte, or granulocyte numbers in the blood however. Unfortunately, Kunavue and Lien do not mention the location and isolation procedure of the FvA used.

Such discordant effects seem to result from variances in therapeutic dosages and/or the origin of FvA in the study. Thereby, it is an absolute must to establish safe dosing for FvA depending on its source in order to treat/prevent immune-modulatory disorders.

3. Oxidative Stress

Oxidative stress is closely linked to chronic inflammatory diseases [28]. Oxidative stress is described as an imbalance of highly reactive oxygen species (ROS) compared to antioxidants [29]. When the cellular equilibrium shifts towards higher ROS, endogenous antioxidants like glutathione (GSH) and superoxide dismutase (SOD) are outmatched. This leads to cellular dysfunction, lipid peroxidation, and possible cell death [30]. The effects of FvA on the oxidative state in cells and animals are summarized in Figure 3.

3.1. Antioxidant Capabilities of FvA. FvA has been shown to sequester superoxide radicals and other ROS outside of the cell [31]. Inside the cell though, FvA can uncouple the electron transport chain in liver mitochondria, which is associated with lowering ROS production [32]. In addition, the most promising *in vivo* study regarding the antioxidant ability of FvA is the reduction of oxidative stress markers after isoproterenol (ISO) induced myocardial damage in rats. Shikalgar and Naikwade show that FvA at 300 mg/kg/day for 4 weeks decreases lipid peroxidation and myocardial damage markers after ISO and significantly increases GSH, SOD, and catalase (CAT) levels [33]. Another study confirms this information in fish. After feeding FvA for 60 days, a decrease in lipid peroxidation and an increase in the expression of SOD, CAT, and glutathione peroxidase (GPx) are seen [34].

3.2. Oxidant Capabilities of FvA. Just like in inflammation, FvA can also cause oxidative damage instead of preventing it. FvA increases oxidative stress when exposed to isolated cartilage cells from 12-day-old embryonic chicks [35]. This study contrasts ones showing a decrease in lipid peroxidation and further suggests FvA as a causative factor in Kashin-Beck disease. An underlying factor for elevated oxidative stress is that FvA can increase cellular respiration rates at extended exposure in rat mitochondria, which may lead to the production of more oxygen radicals [30]. FvA has been shown to increase oxidative markers like hydrogen peroxide and nitric oxide and induce apoptosis in hepatic cancer cell lines [36]. Similarly, FvA can increase smooth muscle contractions, which can be linked to oxidative damage [37].

4. Gut Health

The gut forms the interphase of the outside world, the microbiome, and the host. Sufficient evidence shows that poor gut health can lead to inflammation and disease [38]. In agriculture, FvA has been shown to influence the soil microbe composition and be able to conjugate itself to various minerals,

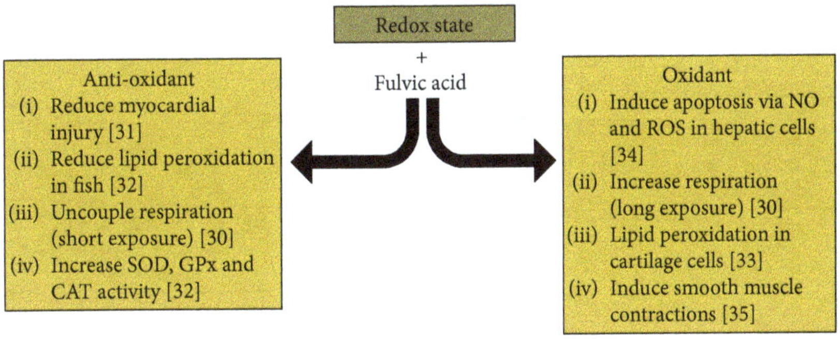

FIGURE 3: Known literature for the effects of fulvic acid on the redox state of cells. Fulvic acid is shown to have various effects which include increasing oxidative stress but also reducing it.

aiding in the uptake in plants [39, 40]. As a result, FvA is suggested to improve the gut flora, nutrient absorption, and heal adverse disorders related to the gut. Below is the available content regarding FvA effects on gut health and summarized in Figure 4.

4.1. Shifting the Microbiota. In regard to the microbiota, very little information is available in animals. A study by Gao et al. show that FvA at 1.5% (w/w) can modulate the gut microflora in loach (*Paramisgurnus dabryanus*) fish [34]. After 60 days of feeding, the abundance of Proteobacteria phyla decreases and Firmicute levels increase in the intestine. In addition, 10 bacteria genera were influenced by FvA treatment. Bacteria of note include an increase in *Variovorax*, *Lactococcus*, and *Lactobacillus* and a decrease in *Serratia* and *Acinetobacter*. This is the only study investigating the effect of FvA on the microbiome.

4.2. Enhancing Nutrient Absorption. Gao et al. [34] also show FvA increases the activity of digestive enzymes like lysozyme, proteases, and acid/alkaline phosphatases in fish. This is strengthened in part by an intensive study investigating nutrient digestibility in pigs [27]. FvA supplemented at 200 ppm in fed improved phosphorus and ash digestion but interestingly had no effect on fat and protein digestibility, contrasting data found in loach.

FvA is shown to influence the bioavailability of heavy metals in animal models as well. FvA can increase the absorption of copper in porcine oviductal epithelial cells and simultaneously reduces its toxicity [41]. In addition to nutrients, FvA has been shown to mediate drug delivery in rats too [42]. Carbamazepine (CBZ) a common anticonvulsant has a low bioavailability, but when conjugated to FvA, absorption across an everted rat intestinal sac increases along with concentrations of CBZ in the blood plasma. FvA has been shown to increase absorption of nutrients and drugs; thus, a concern is the absorption of pollutants and toxins into the blood. However, in a study by Qiang et al., FvA does not increase the absorption of perfluorooctanesulfonate (PFOS) in carp, a conclusion based on the amount of PFOS in the feces of fish compared to controls [43].

4.3. Improve Gut Disorders. A preliminary clinical study exists which investigates the efficacy of probiotics in combination with FvA in gastrointestinal (GI) disorders [44]. Unfortunately though, all groups including ones with FvA see no improvement in Gastrointestinal Quality of Life Index (GIQLI) and Visual Analogue Scale (VAS) scores for GI symptoms. This study does showcase the safety of FvA intake over a 12-week period. Even though FvA is not shown to have an effect in the previous study, FvA isolated from Shilajit shows promise to be antiulcerogenic during several battery tests in albino rats [45].

5. Potential of FvA in Diabetes

Type 2 Diabetes Mellitus (T2DM) is characterized by improper insulin signalling and attenuated glucose uptake into cells [46]. This can lead to prolonged hyperglycaemia after feeding and adverse symptoms [46]. The cause of diabetes remains a mystery, but research associates inflammation, oxidative stress, and changes in the gut microbiome among the many causative factors [47]. Shilajit, which contains FvA, has been shown to reduce hyperglycaemia in diabetic rats and increase SOD activity in pancreatic beta cells [48, 49]. Unfortunately though, there is no direct evidence in the English language showing only FvA in preventing T2DM symptoms. However, the accumulative effects highlighted in this review and the last two studies suggest its therapeutic potential.

Those with T2DM show signs of chronic inflammation and elevated proinflammatory cytokines in serum like TNF-α, IL-1, and IL-6 [47]. FvA is shown to reduce these types of cytokines and proinflammatory markers in animal models [14, 16]. In addition, a proposed treatment regime for T2DM involves nonsteroidal anti-inflammatory drugs (NSAIDs) to alleviate symptoms [50]. FvA might fit as an adjunct treatment to reduce markers of oxidative stress and inflammation as FvA can act in a similar manner to NSAIDs [20]. FvA might also reduce oxidative damage and increase antioxidant enzymes like SOD, CAT, and GPx [33]. Beta cells, which are responsible for insulin production, undergo oxidative damage during T2DM [51]. Protecting the redox state of beta cells may prove beneficial in preventing T2DM. Lastly, patients with T2DM are found with a change in gut microbial composition, and FvA may influence the bacterial community [34].

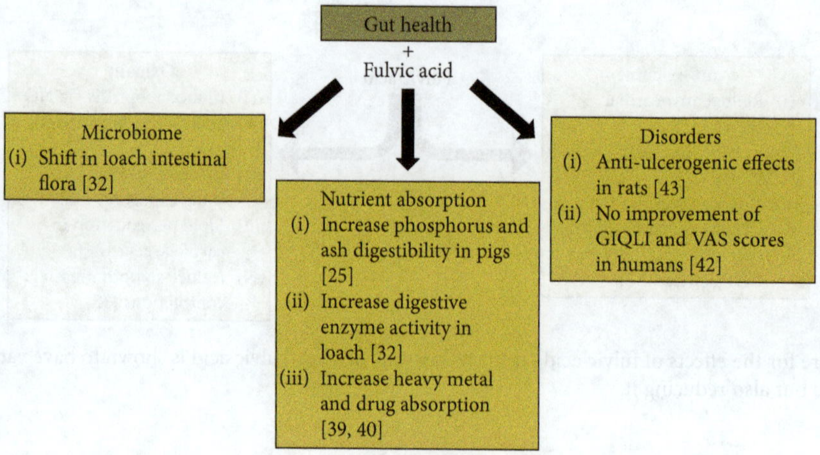

Figure 4: Known literature for the effects of fulvic acid on gut health. Fulvic acid has been shown to influence the microbiome, nutrient absorption, and gut disorders.

6. Conclusions

The information gathered in this review indicate that FvA can act as an immune modulator, influence the redox state, and potentially affect gut health. FvA is shown to decrease proinflammatory markers but also activate the immune system to kill bacteria. It is shown to reduce oxidative stress and even induce apoptosis in hepatic cancer lines. FvA is shown to also influence the microbiome and possibly improve gut function. FvA appears to have a yin-yang effect when it comes to these physiological states. This trend can be seen with most drugs and NHPs; however, toxicity may manifest itself at high intake and poor administration [52, 53].

Although the supporting literature is minimal, if considered in combination, the potential for FvA to be a candidate in preventing inflammatory diseases like diabetes arises. This is promising as our current approach to these kinds of diseases is lacking. It is important to note that FvA research in some cases is conflicting, which is thought to be a result of variance in dosage, parent material, and isolation procedure. In addition, there is no consensus on the structure of FvA, a standard isolation, or parent material. Thus, it is of paramount concern to reconcile these factors and establish dosing for age groups and differing FvA. This will help make conclusive statements regarding FvA function and its influence on immune-related diseases.

Conflicts of Interest

The authors declare that there is no conflict of interest regarding the publication of this article.

Acknowledgments

The authors would like to acknowledge the members of the Ghosh lab and Gibson lab from the University of British Columbia for their advice and continued support.

References

[1] Canadian Diabetes Association, "Diabetes statistics in Canada," June 2018, http://www.diabetes.ca/how-you-can-help/advocate/why-federal-leadership-is-essential/diabetes-statistics-in-canada.

[2] I. Tabas and C. K. Glass, "Anti-inflammatory therapy in chronic disease: challenges and opportunities," *Science*, vol. 339, no. 6116, pp. 166–172, 2013.

[3] E. Wilson, G. V. Rajamanickam, G. P. Dubey et al., "Review on shilajit used in traditional Indian medicine," *Journal of Ethnopharmacology*, vol. 136, no. 1, pp. 1–9, 2011.

[4] N. Senesi and E. Loffredo, "The chemistry of soil organic matter," in *Soil Physical Chemistry*, pp. 239–370, CRC Press, Boca Raton, FL, USA, 2nd edition, 1999.

[5] F. J. Stevenson, *Humus Chemistry: Genesis, Composition, Reactions*, John Wiley & Sons, 1994.

[6] R. L. Wershaw, D. J. Pinckney, and S. E. Booker, "Chemical structure of humic acids–part 1, a generalized structural model," *Journal of Research of the US Geological Survey*, vol. 5, no. 5, pp. 565–569, 1977.

[7] Y. Chen, N. Senesi, and M. Schnitzer, "Chemical and physical characteristics of humic and fulvic acids extracted from soils of the Mediterranean region," *Geoderma*, vol. 20, no. 2, pp. 87–104, 1978.

[8] Health Canada - Government of Canada, "Chemical substance-fulvic acid," July 2004, June 2018, http://webprod.hc-sc.gc.ca/nhpid-bdipsn/ingredReq.do?id=3223&lang=eng.

[9] N. Senesi, T. M. Miano, M. R. Provenzano, and G. Brunetti, "Characterization, differentiation, and classification of humic substances by fluorescence spectroscopy," *Soil Science*, vol. 152, no. 4, pp. 259–271, 1991.

[10] J. R. Ertel and J. I. Hedges, "The lignin component of humic substances: distribution among soil and sedimentary humic, fulvic, and base-insoluble fractions," *Geochimica et Cosmochimica Acta*, vol. 48, no. 10, pp. 2065–2074, 1984.

[11] H. Meena, H. K. Pandey, M. C. Arya, and Z. Ahmed, "*Shilajit:* a panacea for high-altitude problems," *International Journal of Ayurveda Research*, vol. 1, no. 1, pp. 37–40, 2010.

[12] E. M. Peña-Méndez, J. Havel, and J. Patočka, "Humic substances – compounds of still unknown structure: applications

in agriculture, industry, environment, and biomedicine," *Journal of Applied Biomedicine*, vol. 3, pp. 13–24, 2005.

[13] L. P. Ngoc, D. R. Gold, A. O. Tzianabos, S. T. Weiss, and J. C. Celedón, "Cytokines, allergy, and asthma," *Current Opinion in Allergy and Clinical Immunology*, vol. 5, no. 2, pp. 161–166, 2005.

[14] R. Junek, R. Morrow, J. I. Schoenherr et al., "Bimodal effect of humic acids on the LPS-induced TNF-α release from differentiated U937 cells," *Phytomedicine*, vol. 16, no. 5, pp. 470–476, 2009.

[15] S.-J. Chien, T.-C. Chen, H.-C. Kuo, C.-N. Chen, and S.-F. Chang, "Fulvic acid attenuates homocysteine-induced cyclooxygenase-2 expression in human monocytes," *BMC Complementary and Alternative Medicine*, vol. 15, no. 1, p. 61, 2015.

[16] P. Yamada, H. Isoda, J. K. Han, T. P. N. Talorete, T. Yamaguchi, and Y. Abe, "Inhibitory effect of fulvic acid extracted from Canadian sphagnum peat on chemical mediator release by RBL-2H3 and KU812 cells," *Bioscience, Biotechnology, and Biochemistry*, vol. 71, no. 5, pp. 1294–1305, 2007.

[17] J. R. Snyman, J. Dekker, S. C. K. Malfeld, and C. E. J. van Rensburg, "Pilot study to evaluate the safety and therapeutic efficacy of topical oxifulvic acid in atopic volunteers," *Drug Development Research*, vol. 57, no. 1, pp. 40–43, 2002.

[18] C. E. J. Van Rensburg, S. C. K. Malfeld, and J. Dekker, "Topical application of oxifulvic acid suppresses the cutaneous immune response in mice," *Drug Development Research*, vol. 53, no. 1, pp. 29–32, 2001.

[19] J. J. Gandy, J. R. Snyman, and C. E. J. van Rensburg, "Randomized, parallel-group, double-blind, controlled study to evaluate the efficacy and safety of carbohydrate-derived fulvic acid in topical treatment of eczema," *Clinical, Cosmetic and Investigational Dermatology*, vol. 4, pp. 145–148, 2011.

[20] R. Sabi, P. Vrey, and C. E. J. van Rensburg, "Carbohydrate-derived fulvic acid (CHD-FA) inhibits carrageenan-induced inflammation and enhances wound healing: efficacy and toxicity study in rats," *Drug Development Research*, vol. 73, no. 1, pp. 18–23, 2012.

[21] K. E. de Visser, A. Eichten, and L. M. Coussens, "Paradoxical roles of the immune system during cancer development," *Nature Reviews Cancer*, vol. 6, no. 1, pp. 24–37, 2006.

[22] A. Iwasaki and R. Medzhitov, "Regulation of adaptive immunity by the innate immune system," *Science*, vol. 327, no. 5963, pp. 291–295, 2010.

[23] Y. Zhao, P. Paderu, G. Delmas et al., "Carbohydrate-derived fulvic acid is a highly promising topical agent to enhance healing of wounds infected with drug-resistant pathogens," *Journal of Trauma and Acute Care Surgery*, vol. 79, no. 4, pp. S121–S129, 2015.

[24] I. A. Schepetkin, A. I. Khlebnikov, S. Y. Ah et al., "Characterization and biological activities of humic substances from mumie," *Journal of Agricultural and Food Chemistry*, vol. 51, no. 18, pp. 5245–5254, 2003.

[25] I. A. Schepetkin, G. Xie, M. A. Jutila, and M. T. Quinn, "Complement-fixing activity of fulvic acid from shilajit and other natural sources," *Phytotherapy Research*, vol. 23, no. 3, pp. 373–384, 2009.

[26] A. V. Vucskits, I. Hullár, A. Bersényi, E. Andrásofszky, M. Kulcsár, and J. Szabó, "Effect of fulvic and humic acids on performance, immune response and thyroid function in rats," *Journal of Animal Physiology and Animal Nutrition*, vol. 94, no. 6, pp. 721–728, 2010.

[27] N. Kunavue and T. F. Lien, "Effects of fulvic acid and probiotic on growth performance, nutrient digestibility, blood parameters and immunity of pigs," *Journal of Animal Science Advances*, vol. 2, no. 8, pp. 711–721, 2012.

[28] J. W. Baynes, "Role of oxidative stress in development of complications in diabetes," *Diabetes*, vol. 40, no. 4, pp. 405–412, 1991.

[29] H. Sies, "Oxidative stress: oxidants and antioxidants," *Experimental Physiology*, vol. 82, no. 2, pp. 291–295, 1997.

[30] Y. Dotan, D. Lichtenberg, and I. Pinchuk, "Lipid peroxidation cannot be used as a universal criterion of oxidative stress," *Progress in Lipid Research*, vol. 43, no. 3, pp. 200–227, 2004.

[31] N. C. Rodríguez, E. C. Urrutia, B. H. Gertrudis, J. P. Chaverri, and G. B. Mejía, "Antioxidant activity of fulvic acid: a living matter-derived bioactive compound," *Journal of Food, Agriculture & Environment*, vol. 9, pp. 123–127, 2011.

[32] S. A. Visser, "Effect of humic substances on mitochondrial respiration and oxidative phosphorylation," *Science of the Total Environment*, vol. 62, pp. 347–354, 1987.

[33] T. S. Shikalgar and N. S. Naikwade, "Evaluation of cardioprotective activity of fulvic acid against isoproterenol induced oxidative damage in rat myocardium," *International Research Journal of Pharmacy*, vol. 9, no. 1, pp. 71–80, 2018.

[34] Y. Gao, J. He, Z. He et al., "Effects of fulvic acid on growth performance and intestinal health of juvenile loach *Paramisgurnus dabryanus* (Sauvage)," *Fish & Shellfish Immunology*, vol. 62, pp. 47–56, 2017.

[35] A. Peng, W. H. Wang, C. X. Wang et al., "The role of humic substances in drinking water in Kashin-Beck disease in China," *Environmental Health Perspectives*, vol. 107, no. 4, pp. 293–296, 1999.

[36] K. Pant, A. Gupta, P. Gupta, A. Ashraf, A. Yadav, and S. Venugopal, "Anti-proliferative and anticancer properties of fulvic acid on hepatic cancer cells," *Journal of Clinical and Experimental Hepatology*, vol. 5, article S2, 2015.

[37] A. M. Beer, J. Lukanov, and P. Sagorchev, "The influence of fulvic and ulmic acids from peat, on the spontaneous contractile activity of smooth muscles," *Phytomedicine*, vol. 7, no. 5, pp. 407–415, 2000.

[38] J. L. Round and S. K. Mazmanian, "The gut microbiota shapes intestinal immune responses during health and disease," *Nature Reviews Immunology*, vol. 9, no. 5, pp. 313–323, 2009.

[39] M. Petrovic and M. Kastelan-Macan, "The uptake of inorganic phosphorus by insoluble metal-humic complexes," *Water Science & Technology*, vol. 34, no. 7-8, pp. 253–258, 1996.

[40] B. N. V. Priya, K. Mahavishnan, D. S. Gurumurthy, H. Bindumadhava, A. P. Upadhyay, and N. K. Sharma, "Fulvic acid (FA) for enhanced nutrient uptake and growth: insights from biochemical and genomic studies," *Journal of Crop Improvement*, vol. 28, no. 6, pp. 740–757, 2014.

[41] N. Sanmanee and M. Areekijseree, "The effects of fulvic acid on copper bioavailability to porcine oviductal epithelial cells," *Biological Trace Element Research*, vol. 135, no. 1-3, pp. 162–173, 2010.

[42] M. A. Mirza, N. Ahmad, S. P. Agarwal, D. Mahmood, M. Khalid Anwer, and Z. Iqbal, "Comparative evaluation of humic substances in oral drug delivery," *Results in Pharma Sciences*, vol. 1, no. 1, pp. 16–26, 2011.

[43] L. Qiang, M. Chen, L. Zhu, W. Wu, and Q. Wang, "Facilitated bioaccumulation of perfluorooctanesulfonate in common carp (*Cyprinus carpio*) by graphene oxide and remission mechanism

of fulvic acid," *Environmental Science & Technology*, vol. 50, no. 21, pp. 11627–11636, 2016.

[44] L. S. Kim, L. Hilli, J. Orlowski, J. L. Kupperman, M. Baral, and R. F. Waters, "Efficacy of probiotics and nutrients in functional gastrointestinal disorders: a preliminary clinical trial," *Digestive Diseases and Sciences*, vol. 51, no. 12, pp. 2134–2144, 2006.

[45] S. Ghosal, S. K. Singh, Y. Kumar et al., "Anti-ulcerogenic activity of fulvic acids and 4′-methoxy-6-carbomethoxybiphenyl isolated from shilajit," *Phytotherapy Research*, vol. 2, no. 4, pp. 187–191, 1988.

[46] B. C. Martin, J. H. Warram, A. S. Krolewski et al., "Role of glucose and insulin resistance in development of type 2 diabetes mellitus: results of a 25-year follow-up study," *The Lancet*, vol. 340, no. 8825, pp. 925–929, 1992.

[47] M. Y. Donath and S. E. Shoelson, "Type 2 diabetes as an inflammatory disease," *Nature Reviews Immunology*, vol. 11, no. 2, pp. 98–107, 2011.

[48] S. K. Bhattacharya, "Shilajit attenuates streptozotocin induced diabetes mellitus and decrease in pancreatic islet superoxide dismutase activity in rats," *Phytotherapy Research*, vol. 9, no. 1, pp. 41–44, 1995.

[49] N. A. Trivedi, B. Mazumdar, J. D. Bhatt, and K. G. Hemavathi, "Effect of shilajit on blood glucose and lipid profile in alloxan-induced diabetic rats," *Indian Journal of Pharmacology*, vol. 36, no. 6, p. 373, 2004.

[50] P. N. Bellucci, M. F. González Bagnes, G. Di Girolamo, and C. D. González, "Potential effects of nonsteroidal anti-inflammatory drugs in the prevention and treatment of type 2 diabetes mellitus," *Journal of Pharmacy Practice*, vol. 30, no. 5, pp. 549–556, 2017.

[51] R. P. Robertson, J. Harmon, P. O. T. Tran, and V. Poitout, "β-cell glucose toxicity, lipotoxicity, and chronic oxidative stress in type 2 diabetes," *Diabetes*, vol. 53, Supplement 1, pp. S119–S124, 2004.

[52] M. M. Wolfe, D. R. Lichtenstein, and G. Singh, "Gastrointestinal toxicity of nonsteroidal antiinflammatory drugs," *New England Journal of Medicine*, vol. 340, no. 24, pp. 1888–1899, 1999.

[53] C. S. Scott, G. Z. Retsch-Bogart, and M. M. Henry, "Renal failure and vestibular toxicity in an adolescent with cystic fibrosis receiving gentamicin and standard-dose ibuprofen," *Pediatric Pulmonology*, vol. 31, no. 4, pp. 314–316, 2001.

16

Fibrin Clot Strength in Patients with Diabetes Mellitus Measured by Thrombelastography

Benjamin T. Maatman, Glen Schmeisser, and Rolf P. Kreutz

Krannert Institute of Cardiology, Indiana University School of Medicine, Indianapolis, IN, USA

Correspondence should be addressed to Rolf P. Kreutz; rkreutz@iu.edu

Academic Editor: Giovanni de Gaetano

Background. Patients with diabetes mellitus (DM) exhibit increased risk of recurrent myocardial infarction. Maximal clot strength measured by thrombelastography (TEG) is a risk factor for recurrent ischemic events. We hypothesized that diabetic subjects exhibit increased fibrin clot strength in platelet-poor plasma and that glycemic control correlates with maximal fibrin clot strength. *Methods.* We collected plasma samples from subjects with known or suspected coronary artery disease undergoing cardiac catheterization ($n = 354$). We measured kaolin-activated TEG in platelet-poor citrate plasma. Time to fibrin formation (R), clot formation time (K), and maximal fibrin clot strength (MA) were recorded. *Results.* Plasma fibrin MA was increased among subjects with DM ($n = 152$) as compared to non-DM ($n = 202$) (37.0 ± 8 versus 34.1 ± 8 mm; $p < 0.001$). Hemoglobin A1c (HbA1c) ($\rho = 0.22$; $p = 0.001$) and fibrinogen ($\rho = 0.29$; $p < 0.001$) correlated with fibrin MA. In multivariable regression analysis, DM remained significantly associated with plasma MA after adjustment for fibrinogen level ($p = 0.003$). *Conclusions.* Subjects with diabetes mellitus exhibit increased maximal fibrin clot strength measured by TEG in platelet-poor plasma.

1. Introduction

Diabetes mellitus (DM) leads to increased risk of coronary artery disease (CAD) and is considered a CAD risk equivalent [1–5]. Hyperglycemia during acute coronary syndrome (ACS) has been associated with worse outcomes even in the absence of overt diabetes [6]. DM is associated with elevated fibrinogen, increased thromboxane A2, reduced platelet nitric oxide synthesis, as well as increased plasminogen activator inhibitor-1 (PAI-1) release from platelets leading to inhibition of thrombolysis [7–11].

Thrombelastography (TEG) is an established clinical laboratory method for analysis of coagulation and fibrinolysis and allows for quantitative measurement of the dynamic processes of clot formation and clot strength [12, 13]. We have previously demonstrated the feasibility of measurement of plasma fibrin clot strength by TEG in platelet-poor plasma and correlation with whole blood fibrin TEG measurements [14]. Elevated whole blood as well as platelet-poor plasma maximal clot strength by TEG (TEG-MA) has been associated with an increased risk of ischemic events after coronary stenting [15–17]. Subjects with high plasma clot strength showed a 3.8-fold increased risk for cardiovascular death or myocardial infarction after percutaneous coronary intervention [17].

We hypothesized that subjects with DM exhibit increased fibrin clot strength (TEG-MA) in platelet-poor plasma as compared with controls and that extent of glycemic control correlates with maximal fibrin clot strength.

2. Materials and Methods

2.1. Patients. The study protocol was approved by the Indiana University Institutional Review Board for Research. All enrolled individuals gave written informed consent. Subjects with known or suspected coronary artery disease who were referred for cardiac catheterization were included in this study. Blood samples were obtained prior to cardiac catheterization or hospital discharge. Plasma samples were stored as part of a biobank registry in patients with

Table 1: Baseline variables.

Patient characteristics	Total study population ($n = 354$)	No diabetes mellitus ($n = 202$)	Diabetes mellitus ($n = 152$)	p value
Age (years)	57.1 ± 9.9	55.8 ± 9.8	58.8 ± 9.7	0.005
BMI (kg/m^2)	32 ± 7.3	31.2 ± 7.6	33 ± 6.9	0.018
Male (%)	209/354 (59.3%)	124/202 (61.4%)	85/152 (55.9%)	0.3
African Americans (%)	95/354 (26.8%)	54/202 (26.7%)	41/109 (27%)	0.71
Hypertension (%)	320/354 (90.4%)	172/202 (85.1%)	148/152 (97.4%)	<0.001
Hyperlipidemia (%)	303/354 (85.6%)	160/202 (79.2%)	143/152 (94.1%)	<0.001
Coronary artery disease (%)	310/354 (87.6%)	171/202 (84.6%)	139/152 (91.4%)	0.06
History of myocardial infarction (%)	203/354 (57.3%)	118/202 (58.4%)	85/152 (55.9%)	0.64
History of percutaneous coronary intervention (%)	257/354 (72.6%)	147/202 (72.7%)	110/152 (72.4%)	0.93
History of coronary artery bypass grafting (%)	58/354 (16.4%)	27/202 (13.4%)	31/152 (20.4%)	0.08
Congestive heart failure (%)	63/354 (17.8%)	32/202 (15.8%)	31/152 (20.4%)	0.27
Smoking (%)	162/354 (45.8%)	106/202 (52.5%)	56/152 (36.8%)	0.003
Hemoglobin A1c (%)	n/a	5.82 ± 0.5	7.92 ± 1.8	<0.001
Insulin dependent (%)	n/a	n/a	50/152 (30%)	n/a
Daily insulin dose (units)	n/a	n/a	93 ± 74	n/a
Fibrinogen (mg/ml)	3.7 ± 3.1	3.2 ± 2	4.3 ± 4	0.027
Plasminogen activator inhibitor-1 (ng/ml)	120.8 ± 96	112 ± 89	134.8 ± 106	0.34
Factor XIIIa (%)	91.1 ± 30	92.1 ± 31	89.7 ± 29	0.48

cardiovascular disease (Genetics and Cardiac Catheterization (GENCATH) study).

2.2. Blood Samples. Whole blood was collected by peripheral venipuncture in 3.2% citrate after discarding of initial blood draw. We obtained platelet-poor plasma (PPP) by centrifugation at 2000 ×g for 15 min. Plasma was stored at −80°C and thawed immediately before analysis.

2.3. Subjects with Diabetes Mellitus. Hemoglobin A1c (HbA1c) was recorded if there was a value present during chart review within three months of the blood sample collection. Within the insulin-dependent subpopulation of the diabetic group, the total daily administered insulin dose was recorded and this was defined as the sum of short-acting plus long-acting insulin as obtained from the patient's medication list.

2.4. Thrombelastography (TEG). Kaolin-activated TEG (Haemonetics, USA) was performed in all subjects ($n = 354$) using platelet-poor citrate plasma samples according to the manufacturer's instructions. Citrate plasma was mixed with kaolin and then loaded in a heparinase-coated cup containing 20 ml of CaCl2 [18]. Thrombelastography was stopped after time to fibrin formation (R), clot formation time (K), and maximal clot strength (MA) were recorded. In a subset of subjects ($n = 74$), kaolin-activated TEG was also performed in the same fashion using whole blood citrate samples.

2.5. Enzyme-Linked Immuno Assays (ELISA). Fibrinogen (Fibrinogen (human) ELISA kit; Alpco Diagnostics, Salem, New Hampshire, USA), Plasminogen Activator Inhibitor-1 (PAI-1 (human) ELISA kit; Raybiotech, Norcross, Georgia, USA) and factor XIIIa (Zymutest Factor XIII-A, Aniara, West Chester, Ohio, USA) were measured by ELISA in citrate platelet-poor plasma according to the manufacturer's instructions.

2.6. Statistical Analysis. We conducted statistical analysis with SPSS 24 (IBM, USA). We defined statistical significance as a p value less than 0.05, with all tests being conducted two sided. All the values are mean ± SD. We used unpaired, two-sided Student's t-test to compare normally distributed continuous data between two groups after assessing normal distribution of continuous data by the Kolmogorov-Smirnov test. We used the χ^2 test to compare categorical variables. To calculate correlation between thrombelastography parameters (MA, R, and K) and other continuous variables, Spearman's rho was used. Multivariable linear regression analysis was performed with TEG-MA as the dependent variable and diabetes mellitus as the covariate with forward stepwise adjustment for remaining clinical variables and fibrinogen level.

3. Results

We enrolled 152 diabetic and 202 nondiabetic subjects (total $n = 354$). Baseline characteristics of the study subjects are displayed in Table 1. Diabetic subjects had higher body mass index (BMI) and higher prevalence of hypertension and hyperlipidemia but lower prevalence of smoking (Table 1). HbA1C was higher in the diabetic group as compared to nondiabetic subjects (7.92 ± 0.5% versus 5.82 ± 1.8%; $p < 0.001$) (Table 1). Among the insulin-dependent diabetic subjects, the average total daily dose of insulin was 93 units (Table 1).

TABLE 2: Thrombelastography measures.

	No diabetes mellitus ($n = 202$)	Diabetes mellitus ($n = 152$)	p value
Plasma TEG-R (min)	6.9 ± 3.8	6.6 ± 3.0	0.36
Plasma TEG-K (min)	1.47 ± 1.2	1.38 ± 1.3	0.49
Plasma TEG-MA (mm)	34.1 ± 7.5	37.0 ± 8.1	<0.001
Whole blood TEG-R (min)	5.1 ± 2.2	5.6 ± 1.6	0.26
Whole blood TEG-K (min)	1.5 ± 0.5	1.58 ± 0.5	0.45
Whole blood TEG-MA (mm)	66 ± 5.8	66.6 ± 5.6	0.61

TEG-R = time to fibrin formation; TEG-K = clot formation time; TEG-MA = maximal clot strength. Plasma TEG: $n = 354$. Whole blood TEG: $n = 74$.

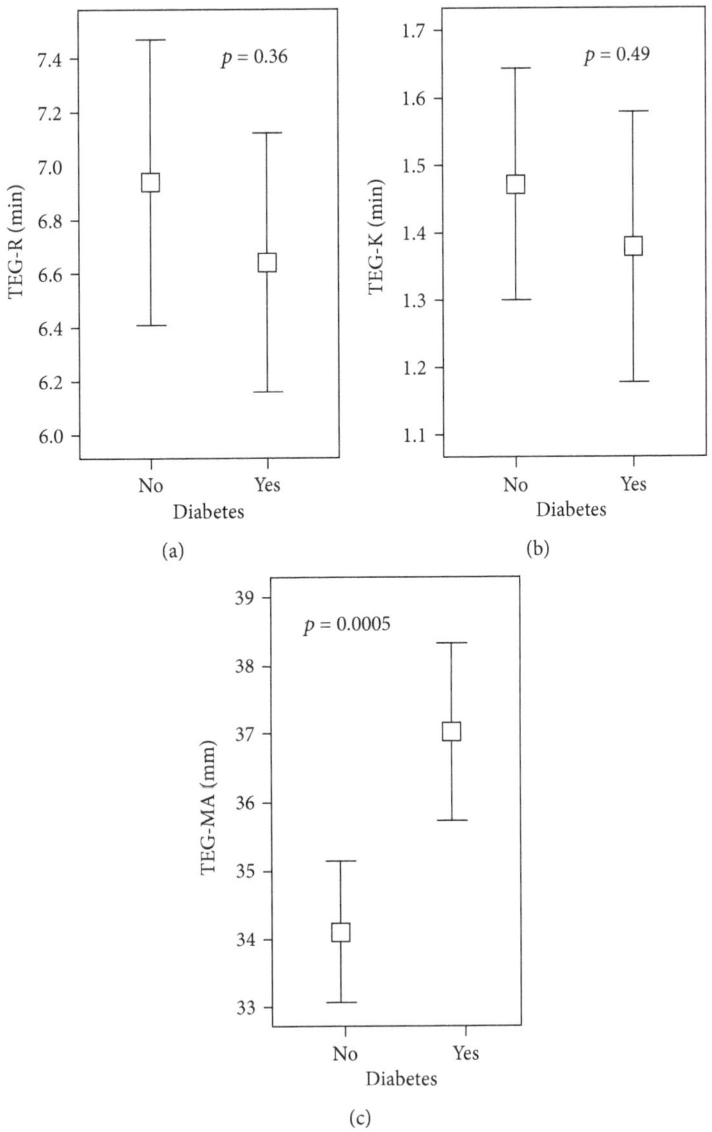

FIGURE 1: Thrombelastography measures between subjects with diabetes mellitus and without diabetes mellitus in platelet-poor plasma. (a) TEG-R: time to fibrin formation. (b) TEG-K: clot formation time. (c) TEG-MA: maximal fibrin clot strength. Mean ± 95% confidence interval.

Maximal fibrin clot strength in platelet-poor plasma (plasma TEG-MA) was higher among subjects with diabetes as compared to nondiabetics (37.0 ± 8 versus 34.1 ± 8 mm; $p < 0.001$) (Table 2, Figure 1). There was no significant difference in time to initial fibrin formation (plasma TEG-R) in the diabetic population (6.6 ± 3 versus 6.9 ± 3.8 min; $p = 0.36$) or clot formation time (plasma TEG-K) (1.38 ± 1.3 versus 1.47 ± 1.2 min; $p = 0.49$) (Figure 1, Table 2). Among

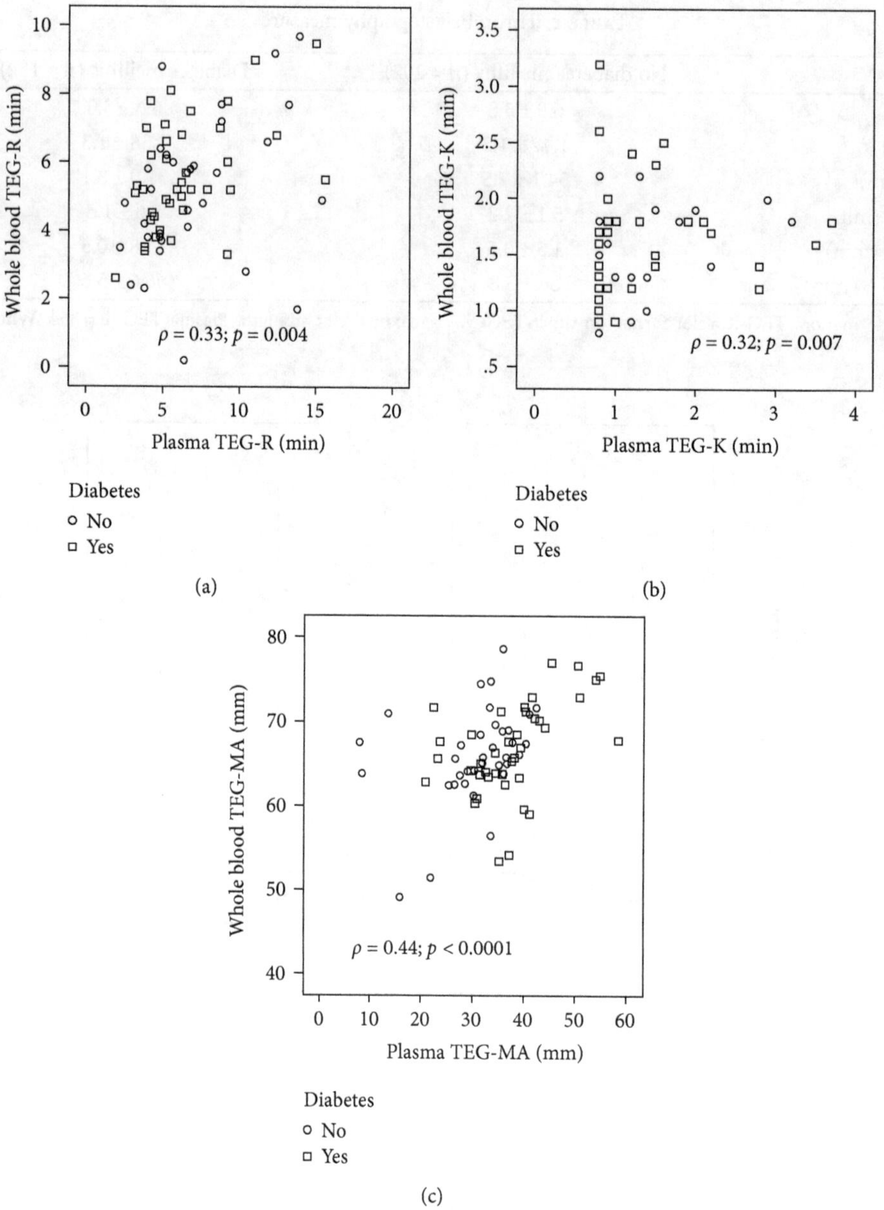

FIGURE 2: Correlation between whole blood and platelet-poor plasma TEG measurements in a subgroup of the overall study population ($n = 74$) divided between subjects with and without diabetes mellitus. (a) TEG-R: time to fibrin formation. (b) TEG-K: clot formation time. (c) TEG-MA: maximal clot strength.

the subgroup of individuals ($n = 74$) who had both plasma and whole blood TEG assays completed, there was no significant difference in whole blood TEG measurements between the DM and non-DM groups (Table 2). Whole blood and platelet-poor plasma TEG measurements correlated for all measures but most strongly for TEG-MA ($\rho = 0.44$; $p < 0.0001$) (Figure 2).

There was a nonsignificant trend towards shorter clot formation time (plasma TEG-K: 1.12 ± 0.6 versus 1.5 ± 1.4 min; $p = 0.08$) in insulin-dependent diabetics compared to non-insulin-dependent diabetics. There was no significant difference in plasma TEG-MA (38.1 ± 9 versus 36.5 ± 8 mm; $p = 0.27$) and time to fibrin formation between insulin-dependent and non-insulin-dependent diabetics (plasma TEG-R: 6.3 ± 2.3 versus 6.8 ± 3.3 min; $p = 0.37$) (Table 3). The differences in plasma TEG-MA remained unchanged between DM and non-DM subjects after exclusion of subjects with HbA1C in the prediabetic range (5.7–6.4% as defined by American Diabetes Association [19]) (plasma TEG-MA: 37.3 ± 8 versus 34.3 ± 7 mm; $p < 0.001$).

HbA1c correlated with plasma TEG-MA ($\rho = 0.22$, $p = 0.001$), with higher TEG-MA in subjects with elevated HbA1C and, hence, poorer control of their DM (Figure 3). There was no significant correlation between daily insulin dose and TEG-MA among patients with insulin-dependent DM ($\rho = -0.07$; $p = 0.64$) (Figure 3).

Fibrinogen was elevated in subjects with diabetes mellitus (4.3 ± 4 versus 3.2 ± 2 mg/ml, $p = 0.027$) (Table 1).

TABLE 3: Thrombelastography: insulin-dependent versus non-insulin-dependent diabetes mellitus.

	Insulin-dependent DM ($n = 50$)	Non-insulin-dependent DM ($n = 102$)	p value
Plasma TEG-R (min)	6.3 ± 2.3	6.8 ± 3.3	0.37
Plasma TEG-K (min)	1.12 ± 0.6	1.5 ± 1.4	0.08
Plasma TEG-MA (mm)	38.1 ± 9	36.5 ± 8	0.27

TEG-R = time to fibrin formation; TEG-K = clot formation time; TEG-MA = maximal fibrin clot strength.

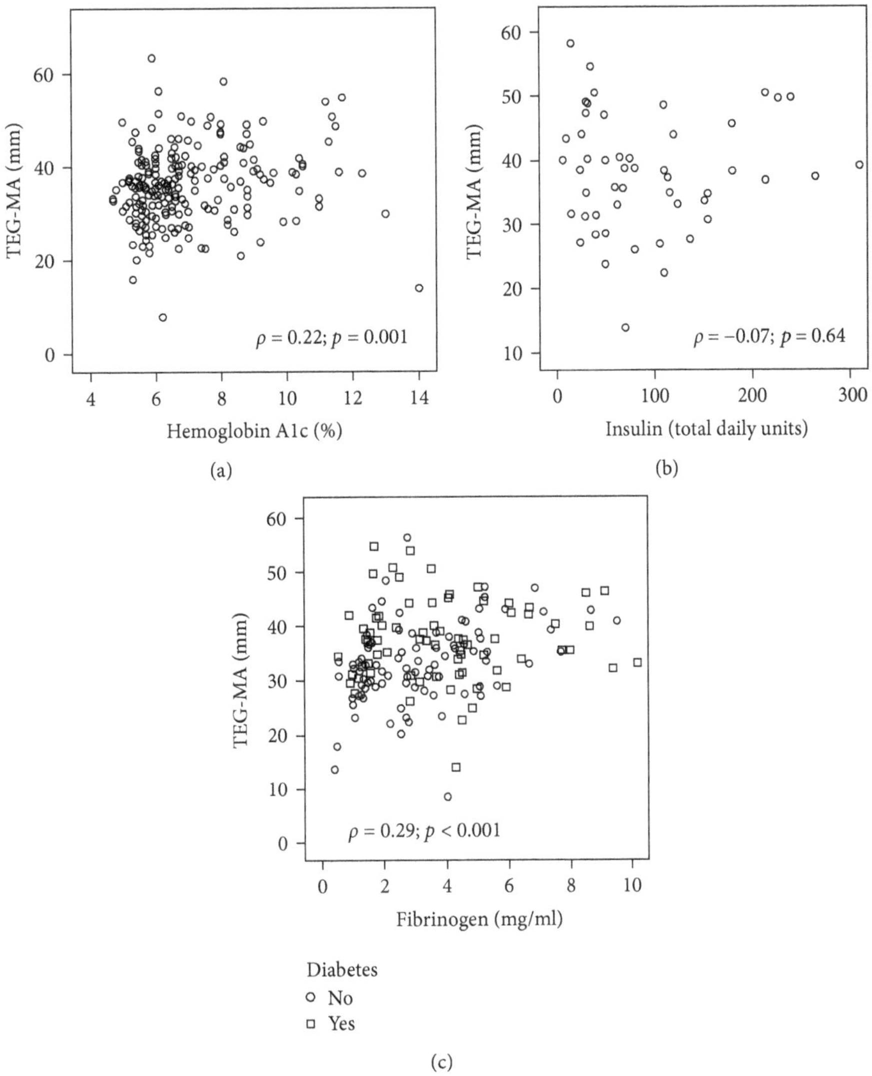

FIGURE 3: Scatterplot demonstrating maximal plasma fibrin clot strength (TEG-MA), hemoglobin A1c (a), insulin total daily dose (units) (b), and fibrinogen (c).

Fibrinogen correlated with plasma fibrin TEG-MA ($\rho = 0.29$; $p < 0.001$; Figure 3) but not whole blood TEG-MA ($\rho = 0.14$; $p = 0.45$). PAI-1 and factor XIIIa were not significantly different between subjects with and without DM (Table 1). PAI-1 did not correlate with plasma TEG-MA ($\rho = -0.034$; $p = 0.79$).

In multivariable linear regression analysis, DM ($p = 0.003$) and fibrinogen ($p = 0.019$) remained significantly associated with plasma TEG-MA after forward stepwise adjustment for clinical variables (Table 4).

4. Discussion

The results of our study demonstrate that subjects with diabetes mellitus have increased fibrin clot strength (MA) as measured by TEG in platelet-poor plasma compared to

Table 4: Multivariable linear regression analysis.

Variable	B	95% confidence interval for B	p value
Diabetes mellitus	3.5 ± 1.2	1.2–5.8	0.003
Fibrinogen	0.44 ± 0.2	0.07–0.8	0.019

Dependent variable: plasma TEG-MA.

nondiabetics. The association of diabetes mellitus with plasma fibrin clot strength persisted after adjustment for fibrinogen, which influences strength of clot formation measured by TEG. We have recently demonstrated that elevated fibrin clot strength measured by TEG in platelet-poor plasma is associated with increased risk of recurrent myocardial infarction and death after PCI, similar to the findings observed in studies using whole blood TEG assays [17].

In whole blood, maximal clot strength (MA) measured by TEG is the sum of the additive forces generated by aggregating and contracting platelets incorporated into the growing, initially soluble fibrin network, which is cross-linked and stabilized by FXIIIa [13, 20]. In a large cohort study of subjects with coronary artery disease by Lev et al., DM was also independently associated with whole blood (platelet-fibrin) clot strength measured by TEG [21].

In the subgroup of patients in our study who had both whole blood and plasma TEG studies performed, there was a moderate correlation between both measurements for TEG-MA and to a lesser degree for TEG-R and TEG-K. While plasma MA was significantly higher in diabetic subjects, we did not find a significant difference in whole blood MA in our study. This may be due to the smaller number of subjects with whole blood TEG assays completed, as well as possible differences in platelet contribution to clot strength in whole blood TEG between subjects with and without diabetes.

Fibrinogen is an important determinant of fibrin structure and of cross-linked fibrin network strength, and both fibrinogen and factor XIIIa activity influence maximal fibrin clot strength measured by TEG [22]. Fibrinogen has been previously shown to be elevated in subjects with diabetes mellitus [11, 23]. In our study, fibrinogen levels were also higher in subjects with DM, and fibrinogen remained a significant covariate in multivariable linear regression analysis. In contrast, PAI-1 and factor XIIIa were not significantly different between diabetics and nondiabetics.

We did not find any significant correlation between daily insulin dose and plasma TEG-MA among the insulin-dependent subpopulation, while elevated plasma MA was associated with worse glycemic control. Possible mechanisms linking hyperglycemia to a prothrombotic state include effects on gene transcription of coagulation factors, loss of the endothelial layer through glycosylation with a deficiency of nitric oxide, direct glycosylation of coagulation factors altering their activity [24, 25], as well as increased platelet activation [4, 26–29]. Combined hyperinsulinemia and hyperglycemia has been demonstrated to acutely increase circulating tissue factor procoagulant activity (TF-PCA) ninefold in previously healthy subjects [30].

Current recommendations in primary prevention of cardiovascular disease among patients with DM do not yet incorporate use of therapies targeted towards reduction of thrombin formation and fibrin stabilization. However, recent results from the COMPASS study demonstrate a significant reduction in cardiovascular death/myocardial infarction or stroke in patients with stable cardiovascular disease who were treated with rivaroxaban 2.5 mg twice daily in addition to aspirin as compared to patients who were treated with aspirin alone (HR 0.76; 95% CI: 0.66–0.86) [31]. The reduction in risk with rivaroxaban was more pronounced in the diabetic subgroup (HR 0.74; 95% CI: 0.61–0.9) [31]. Future studies will need to assess whether TEG parameters in diabetic patients could be used to risk stratify and develop treatment strategies in diabetic patients with known or suspected cardiovascular disease.

Limitations to our study include that HbA1C values were collected retrospectively and were not standardized to a collection at the time of TEG blood sample collection; as values were only recorded if collected within a three-month window, glycemic control at time of analysis was assumed to be equivalent. We were not able to assess thrombolysis characteristics of patients with DM, as spontaneous thrombolysis generally does not occur with TEG after activation with kaolin and CaCl2.

In conclusion, our data show that diabetes mellitus is associated with increased fibrin clot strength (TEG-MA) as measured in platelet-poor plasma, a marker of thrombotic risk in patients with coronary artery disease. Worse glycemic control as defined by an elevated HbA1C is moderately correlated with higher plasma TEG-MA, whereas there was no statistically significant correlation with use or dosage of insulin. Further studies are warranted to examine the mechanisms associated with increased plasma TEG-MA and to examine the utility of plasma TEG-MA in personalized approaches to guide antithrombotic therapies in patients with diabetes mellitus.

Disclosure

The contents of this manuscript have in part been presented as a poster at the Arteriosclerosis, Thrombosis, and Vascular Biology (ATVB) scientific meeting in 2015, and the corresponding abstract has been published in Arteriosclerosis, Thrombosis, and Vascular Biology, May 2015, Volume 35, Issue Suppl 1: A597.

Conflicts of Interest

Rolf P. Kreutz has served as scientific consultant for Roche Diagnostics, Coramed, and Haemonetics Corporation.

Acknowledgments

The study was supported in part by the Indiana University School of Medicine-IU Health Strategic Research Initiative, the IU Health Values Grant, and the CTSI Specimen Storage Facility (SSF), subsidized by the Indiana Clinical and Translational Sciences Institute which is supported, in part, by a NCRR Clinical and Translational Sciences Award (U54-RR025761; Anantha Shekhar, PI) and Indiana Clinical and Translational Sciences Institute SSF facility construction funded in part through a NCRR construction grant (C06-RR020128-01; R.S. Fife, PI, K. Cornetta, Co-I). Dr. Benjamin T. Maatman was supported by a travel grant from the Charles Fisch Cardiovascular Research Award endowed by Dr. Suzanne B. Knoebel of the Krannert Institute of Cardiology.

References

[1] W. B. Kannel and D. L. McGee, "Diabetes and glucose tolerance as risk factors for cardiovascular disease: the Framingham Study," *Diabetes Care*, vol. 2, no. 2, pp. 120–126, 1979.

[2] K. Pyörälä, M. Laakso, and M. Uusitupa, "Diabetes and atherosclerosis: an epidemiologic view," *Diabetes/Metabolism Research and Reviews*, vol. 3, no. 2, pp. 463–524, 1987.

[3] J. Stamler, O. Vaccaro, J. D. Neaton, D. Wentworth, and The Multiple Risk Factor Intervention Trial Research Group, "Diabetes, other risk factors, and 12-yr cardiovascular mortality for men screened in the multiple risk factor intervention trial," *Diabetes Care*, vol. 16, no. 2, pp. 434–444, 1993.

[4] S. M. Haffner, S. Lehto, T. Rönnemaa, K. Pyörälä, and M. Laakso, "Mortality from coronary heart disease in subjects with type 2 diabetes and in nondiabetic subjects with and without prior myocardial infarction," *The New England Journal of Medicine*, vol. 339, no. 4, pp. 229–243, 2015.

[5] E. Barrett-Connor, "Diabetes and heart disease," *Diabetes Care*, vol. 26, no. 10, pp. 2947–2958, 2003.

[6] P. Petursson, J. Herlitz, K. Caidahl et al., "Admission glycaemia and outcome after acute coronary syndrome," *International Journal of Cardiology*, vol. 116, no. 3, pp. 315–320, 2007.

[7] R. A. Rabini, R. Staffolani, P. Fumelli, B. Mutus, G. Curatola, and L. Mazzanti, "Decreased nitric oxide synthase activity in platelets from IDDM and NIDDM patients," *Diabetologia*, vol. 41, no. 1, pp. 101–104, 1998.

[8] G. Davì, I. Catalano, M. Averna et al., "Thromboxane biosynthesis and platelet function in type II diabetes mellitus," *The New England Journal of Medicine*, vol. 322, no. 25, pp. 1769–1774, 1990.

[9] Y. Zhu, P. Carmeliet, and W. P. Fay, "Plasminogen activator inhibitor-1 is a major determinant of arterial thrombolysis resistance," *Circulation*, vol. 99, no. 23, pp. 3050–3055, 1999.

[10] R. P. Kreutz, P. Nystrom, Y. Kreutz et al., "Inhibition of platelet aggregation by prostaglandin E1 (PGE1) in diabetic patients during therapy with clopidogrel and aspirin," *Platelets*, vol. 24, no. 2, pp. 145–150, 2013.

[11] W. B. Kannel, R. B. D'Agostino, P. W. F. Wilson, A. J. Belanger, and D. R. Gagnon, "Diabetes, fibrinogen, and risk of cardiovascular disease: the Framingham experience," *American Heart Journal*, vol. 120, no. 3, pp. 672–676, 1990.

[12] M. T. Ganter and C. K. Hofer, "Coagulation monitoring: current techniques and clinical use of viscoelastic point-of-care coagulation devices," *Anesthesia & Analgesia*, vol. 106, no. 5, pp. 1366–1375, 2008.

[13] A. Bitar and R. P. Kreutz, "Role of thrombelastography (TEG) in risk assessment and guidance of antithrombotic therapy in patients with coronary artery disease," *Drug Development Research*, vol. 74, no. 8, pp. 533–540, 2013.

[14] D. Lu, J. Owens, and R. P. Kreutz, "Plasma and whole blood clot strength measured by thrombelastography in patients treated with clopidogrel during acute coronary syndromes," *Thrombosis Research*, vol. 132, no. 2, pp. e94–e98, 2013.

[15] R. P. Kreutz, J. Owens, J. A. Breall et al., "C-reactive protein and fibrin clot strength measured by thrombelastography after coronary stenting," *Blood Coagulation & Fibrinolysis*, vol. 24, no. 3, pp. 321–326, 2013.

[16] P. A. Gurbel, K. P. Bliden, K. Guyer et al., "Platelet reactivity in patients and recurrent events post-stenting: results of the PREPARE POST-STENTING Study," *Journal of the American College of Cardiology*, vol. 46, no. 10, pp. 1820–1826, 2005.

[17] R. P. Kreutz, G. Schmeisser, B. Maatman et al., "Fibrin clot strength measured by thrombelastography and outcomes after percutaneous coronary intervention," *Thrombosis and Haemostasis*, vol. 117, no. 2, pp. 426–428, 2017.

[18] R. P. Kreutz, A. Bitar, J. Owens et al., "Factor XIII $Val_{34}Leu$ polymorphism and recurrent myocardial infarction in patients with coronary artery disease," *Journal of Thrombosis and Thrombolysis*, vol. 38, no. 3, pp. 380–387, 2014.

[19] American Diabetes Association, "Diagnosis and classification of diabetes mellitus," *Diabetes Care*, vol. 33, no. 4, article e57, 2010.

[20] O. N. Okafor and D. A. Gorog, "Endogenous fibrinolysis: an important mediator of thrombus formation and cardiovascular risk," *Journal of the American College of Cardiology*, vol. 65, no. 16, pp. 1683–1699, 2015.

[21] E. I. Lev, K. P. Bliden, Y. H. Jeong et al., "Influence of race and sex on thrombogenicity in a large cohort of coronary artery disease patients," *Journal of the American Heart Association*, vol. 3, no. 5, article e001167, 2014.

[22] V. G. Nielsen, W. Q. Gurley Jr, and T. M. Burch, "The impact of factor XIII on coagulation kinetics and clot strength determined by thrombelastography," *Anesthesia & Analgesia*, vol. 99, no. 1, pp. 120–123, 2004.

[23] G. Di Giovine, M. Verdoia, L. Barbieri et al., "Impact of diabetes on fibrinogen levels and its relationship with platelet reactivity and coronary artery disease: a single-centre study," *Diabetes Research and Clinical Practice*, vol. 109, no. 3, pp. 541–550, 2015.

[24] B. A. Lemkes, J. Hermanides, J. H. Devries, F. Holleman, J. C. Meijers, and J. B. Hoekstra, "Hyperglycemia: a prothrombotic factor?," *Journal of Thrombosis and Haemostasis*, vol. 8, no. 8, pp. 1663–1669, 2010.

[25] P. J. Grant, "Diabetes mellitus as a prothrombotic condition," *Journal of Internal Medicine*, vol. 262, no. 2, pp. 157–172, 2007.

[26] M. J. Price, D. J. Angiolillo, P. S. Teirstein et al., "Platelet reactivity and cardiovascular outcomes after percutaneous coronary intervention: a time-dependent analysis of the Gauging Responsiveness with a VerifyNow P2Y12 assay: Impact on Thrombosis and Safety (GRAVITAS) trial," *Circulation*, vol. 124, no. 10, pp. 1132–1137, 2011.

[27] M. E. Carr, "Diabetes mellitus: a hypercoagulable state," *Journal of Diabetes and its Complications*, vol. 15, no. 1, pp. 44–54, 2001.

[28] J. H. Jung, U. S. Tantry, P. A. Gurbel, and Y. H. Jeong, "Current antiplatelet treatment strategy in patients with diabetes mellitus," *Diabetes & Metabolism Journal*, vol. 39, no. 2, pp. 95–113, 2015.

17

The Effects of *Momordica balsamina* Methanolic Extract on Kidney Function in STZ-Induced Diabetic Rats: Effects on Selected Metabolic Markers

Anelisiwe Siboto, Ntethelelo Sibiya, Andile Khathi, and Phikelelani Ngubane

School of Laboratory Medicine and Medical Sciences, University of KwaZulu-Natal, Durban, South Africa

Correspondence should be addressed to Phikelelani Ngubane; ngubanep1@ukzn.ac.za

Academic Editor: Patrizio Tatti

Background. Studies suggest that *Momordica balsamina* (*intshungu*) possesses hypoglycaemic effects. The effects of *Momordica balsamina* on diabetic complications such as DN, however, have not been established. Accordingly, this study seeks to investigate the effects of *M. balsamina* on kidney function in STZ-induced diabetic rats. *Methods.* Methanolic extracts (ME) of *M. balsamina*'s leaves were used in this study. Short-term effects of *M. balsamina* methanolic extract on kidney function and MAP were studied in STZ-induced diabetic rats treated twice daily with *M. balsamina* methanolic extract (250 mg/kg), insulin (175 μg/kg, s.c.), and metformin (500 mg/kg) for 5 weeks. *Results. M. balsamina* methanolic extract significantly increased Na^+ excretion outputs in STZ-induced diabetic rats by comparison to STZ-diabetic control rats. *M. balsamina* methanolic extract significantly increased GFR in STZ-diabetic rats with a concomitant decrease in creatinine concentration and also reduced kidney-to-body ratio, albumin excretion rate (AER), and albumin creatinine ratio (ACR). *M. balsamina* methanolic extract significantly reduced MAP in STZ-diabetic animals by comparison with STZ-diabetic control animals. These results suggest that *M. balsamina* methanolic extract not only lowers blood glucose but also has beneficial effects on kidney function and blood pressure. *Conclusion.* These findings suggest that *M. balsamina* may have beneficial effects on some processes that are associated with renal derangement in STZ-induced diabetic rats.

1. Introduction

Diabetic nephropathy (DN), as a result of sustained hyperglycaemia, affects approximately 20–40% of individuals with diabetes mellitus [1]. Diabetic nephropathy is a leading common cause of chronic kidney disease (CKD) and kidney failure which are the major causes of morbidity and mortality associated with type 1 diabetes mellitus [2, 3]. The sustained hyperglycaemia is associated with the structural kidney abnormalities such as the thickening of the glomerular basement membrane, mesangial expansion, tubular hypertrophy, and extracellular matrix deposition [4, 5]. These structural abnormalities mediate the functional kidney abnormalities such as declining glomerular filtration rate, electrolyte imbalance, increased blood pressure, and increased protein excretion [6, 7].

Several mechanisms have been reported to contribute to the development and progression of diabetic nephropathy. These mechanisms include oxidative stress; the advanced glycation end product (AGE) receptor of the AGE pathway and the renin-angiotensin aldosterone system have been implicated to play a role in the development of diabetic nephropathy [8]. These metabolic flux or pathways are mainly activated by sustained hyperglycaemia. Taken together, the activation of these pathways cause the intrarenal haemodynamic's changes through the glycosylation of intrarenal proteins that induce hyperfiltration and glomerular dysfunction [1, 9].

Various agents such as oral antihyperglycaemic drugs, insulin, and antirenin-angiotensin system (RAS) are currently available for the prevention and management of DN; however, the efficacy of these agents is inadequate [10].

Insulin has been shown to normalise glomerular filtration rate (GFR) and oxidative status which helps delay the onset and progression of CKD [11]. However, the bolus administration of insulin in high doses is associated with sodium retention which often leads to the development of hyperinsulinaemic oedema and elevated blood pressure [12]. Other antidiabetic agents such as metformin and insulin secretagogues are at times unable to achieve glycaemic targets and may thus be unable to prevent the progression to DN. Therefore, there is a need to further explore other avenues as means of alternative treatment, thus achieving a holistic therapy for DN.

Medicinal plants have been used for treatment of DM and associated complications [13]. Studies in our laboratory have demonstrated that medicinal plants such as *Syzygium aromaticum* and *Syzygium cordutum* confer renoprotection in streptozotocin- (STZ-) induced diabetic rats [14, 15]. *Mormodica balsamina* (MB), our plant of interest, is fairly common and widespread in southern Africa and is closely related to *M. charantia* [16]. *M. charantia* has been shown to improve renal function by normalising oxidative status [17]. *M. balsamina* has been shown to have hypoglycaemic activity [18]. However, the renoprotective effects of *M. balsamina* have not yet been established. We envisage that evaluation of parameters such as GFR and electrolyte handling will shed some light on the therapeutic effects of *M. balsamina* regarding kidney function. The aim of the study therefore is to investigate the effects of *M. balsamina* on kidney function in STZ-induced diabetic rats.

2. Materials and Methods

2.1. Drugs and Chemicals. Drugs were sourced from standard pharmaceutical suppliers. All chemicals were of analytical grade and were purchased from standard commercial suppliers.

2.2. Plant Extraction

2.2.1. Plant Material. Momordica balsamina was identified by a botanist in the Department of Botany at the University of KwaZulu-Natal, Westville. The plant was harvested at the University of KwaZulu-Natal in Durban, South Africa. The leaves were washed three times with water to remove any residual dirt. The leaves were then grinded to a pulp using an electric grinder. Thereafter, the pulp was subjected to either methanolic or aqueous extraction as previously described [18].

2.2.2. Methanolic Extraction (ME). The pulp (1.15 kg) was extracted by cold percolation with methanol (95%, 6.9 L) for 24 h. The methanolic extract was recovered from the mixture and methanol was further added to the plant material for further extraction. This process was repeated three times to maximise the yield (609 g). The three extracts were pooled together and the combined extract was concentrated at reduced pressure (22–26 mmHg) at 45–60°C.

2.3. Animals. Male Sprague-Dawley rats weighing 250–300 g were used to carry out the study. The animals were bred and kept in the Biomedical Research Unit of the University of KwaZulu-Natal under normal laboratory conditions (temperature and humidity) in a 12 h day: 12 h night cycle. The animals were allowed access to water ad libitum and 40 g standard rat chow daily (Meadow Feeds, Pietermaritzburg, South Africa). All animal experiments were reviewed and accepted by the Animal Research Ethics Committee of the University of KwaZulu-Natal (AREC/049/016DM). Before the study commenced, the animals were allowed to acclimatise for 5 days in the metabolic cages.

2.3.1. Diabetes Induction. Type 1 diabetes mellitus was induced in male Sprague-Dawley rats by a single intraperitoneal injection of 60 mg/kg STZ in freshly prepared 0.1 M citrate buffer (pH 6.3). The control group received the vehicle, citrate buffer, through the same route. Seven days after the induction of diabetes, rats with a blood glucose concentration greater than 20 $mmol \cdot L^{-1}$ were considered diabetic.

2.4. Experimental Protocol. The short-term effects of *M. balsamina* were studied in separate groups of nondiabetic and STZ-induced diabetic male rats ($n = 6$) housed individually in Makrolon polycarbonate metabolic cages (Techniplast, Labotec, South Africa) for 5 weeks. ME (250 mg/kg, p.o.) was administered twice daily at 0900 h and 1500 h by means of a bulbed steel tube. Animals which received DMSO/saline (3 mL/kg, p.o.) served as controls, while those given metformin (500 mg/kg, p.o.) and insulin (200 μg/kg, s.c.) served as positive controls. Blood glucose measurements were made once every third day over the period of 5 weeks using the tail prick method. Glucose was determined using the Elite® glucometer (Elite (Pty) Ltd., Health Care Division, South Africa). Urine volume and urinary glucose concentrations, albumin, creatinine, urea, Na^+, K^+, Cl^-, body weight, 24-hour water intake, food consumption, and mean arterial pressure (MAP) were determined once every third day. MAP was monitored using a noninvasive tail cuff method with photoelectric sensors (IITC Model 31 Computerised Blood Pressure Monitor, Life Sciences, Woodland Hills, California, USA) as previously described [19]. The unit works with IITC hardware system to measure blood pressure and heart rate in conscious rats. The animals were warmed at ±30°C in an enclosed chamber (IITC Model 31 Computerised Blood Pressure Monitor, Life Sciences, Wood land Hills, California, USA) for 30 minutes before taking blood pressure readings. All measurements were conducted at 0900 h. Creatinine and albumin concentration were measured in plasma and urine samples at the Global Clinical and Viral Laboratory, Amanzimtoti, South Africa. GFR was calculated using a standard formula from measurements of the plasma and urinary concentrations of creatinine and urine flow rate in the fifth week.

2.5. Plasma and Tissue Collection. At the end of the 5-week experimental period, all animals were anaesthetised via a gas anaesthetic chamber (100 mg/kg) for 3 minutes using halothane. Blood samples were collected by cardiac puncture into single precooled heparinized containers for biochemical analysis. The blood was centrifuged at 10 ×g in a Hermle Laborechnic GmBH centrifuge (Wehingen, Germany) for plasma collection. The kidneys were removed, weighed, and then snap frozen in liquid nitrogen. Afterwards, the kidneys and plasma were stored in an Ultra Bio Freezer (Snijers Scientific, Tilburg, Netherlands) at −80°C.

2.6. Malondialdehyde (MDA) Measurements. MDA measurements were carried out as per a well-established protocol in our laboratory [15]. Briefly, tissues (50 mg) were homogenized in 500 μL of 0.2% phosphoric acid. The homogenate was centrifuged at 400 ×g for 10 min. Subsequently, 400 μL of the homogenate was supplemented with 400 mL 2% phosphoric acid and then separated into two glass tubes, each receiving equal volumes of the solution. Afterwards, 200 μL of 7% phosphoric acid was added into both glass tubes followed by 400 μL of thiobarbituric acid (TBA)/butylated hydroxytoluene (BHT) into one sample test glass tube and 400 μL of 3 mM hydrochloric acid (HCl) into the second glass tube which stood as a blank. Thereafter, 200 μL of 1 M HCl was then added to sample and blank test tubes to establish an acidic pH of 1.5. Both solutions were heated at 100°C for 15 min and allowed to cool to room temperature. 1.5 ML of butanol was then added to the cooled solution; the sample was vortexed for 1 min for rigorous mixing and allowed to settle until two phases could be differentiated. The top butanol layer was transferred to Eppendorf tubes and centrifuged at 13,200 ×g for 6 min. The samples were aliquoted into a 96-well microtiter plate in triplicates, and the absorbance was read at 532 nm using a BioTek mQuant spectrophotometer (Biotek, Johannesburg, South Africa). The absorbance from these wavelengths was used to calculate the concentration of MDA using Beer's law.

$$\text{Concentration} = \frac{\text{absorbance}_{\text{Final}}}{\text{absorption coefficient}\ \left(156\ \text{mmol}^{-1}\right)}. \tag{1}$$

2.7. Glutathione Peroxidase (GPx) and Superoxide Dismutase (SOD) Activity. Kidney GPx and SOD activity was measured using assay kits following the manufacturer's instructions (Elabscience and Biotechnology, WuHan).

2.8. Aldosterone. Plasma aldosterone was measured using an ELISA kit following the manufacturer's instructions (Elabscience and Biotechnology, WuHan).

2.9. Statistical Analysis. Data is expressed as means ± standard error of means (SEM). Statistical analysis was conducted using GraphPad Prism and InStat software (version 5.00, GraphPad Software, San Diego, California, USA). Energy balance parameters, MAP, and urine output were analysed using analysis of variance (ANOVA) for repeated measures, which was followed by the Bonferroni post hoc test. Terminal parameters were analysed using ANOVA followed by the Bonferroni post hoc test, which was used to analyse differences between the controls and the experimental groups. Values of $p < 0.05$ indicate statistical significance.

3. Results

3.1. Energy Balance. Nondiabetic controls, diabetic controls, and diabetic rats treated with MB, metformin, and insulin were assessed for body weight change and 24-hour water consumption weekly for 5 weeks (Table 1). Diabetic control rats exhibited severe weight loss despite the significantly higher weekly intake of food and water when compared to the normal nondiabetic control rats (DC versus ND, $p < 0.05$). In contrast, nondiabetic control rats progressively gained weight from the 2nd week of treatment until the end of the experimental period. MB-treated (250 mg/kg) STZ-diabetic rats, however, stabilised body weights by comparison to untreated STZ-diabetic controls from the 3rd week to the 5th week of the experimental period while significantly decreasing food intake ($p < 0.05$). The effects of metformin (500 mg/kg) were similar to those of MB. Administration of insulin (175 μg/kg) improved body weight and decreased food and water intake from the 3rd to the 5th week of the experimental period by comparison to untreated STZ-diabetic rats.

3.2. Mean Arterial Pressure (MAP). Figure 1 shows the mean arterial pressure (MAP) of nondiabetic controls; diabetic controls; and diabetic rats treated with MB, metformin, and insulin measured weekly over the 5-week experimental period. Diabetic control rats showed increased MAP over the period of 5 weeks by comparison to nondiabetic rats. However, the administration of MB stabilised MAP to normalcy from the 3rd week to 5th week by comparison to STZ-diabetic controls. The administration of insulin (175 μg/kg) also increased MAP by comparison to nondiabetic rats. The effects of metformin were similar to MB.

3.3. Urine Output. Figure 2 shows the 24 h urine output of nondiabetic controls, diabetic controls, and diabetic rats treated with MB, metformin, and insulin measured over the 5-week period. Diabetic controls showed increased urine output throughout the study by comparison to nondiabetic rats. The administration of MB (250 mg/kg) decreased urine output from the 4th week to the 5th week of the experimental period by comparison to STZ-diabetic rats. The effects of insulin and metformin were similar to those of MB.

3.4. Electrolyte Handling. Table 2 shows urinary and plasma biochemical parameters of nondiabetic controls, diabetic controls, and diabetic rats treated with *M. balsamina*, metformin, and insulin. On the 5th week of the experimental period, plasma creatinine concentrations were significantly ($p < 0.05$) elevated in STZ-diabetic rats in comparison with nondiabetic rats. On the other hand, urinary creatinine concentrations were significantly reduced at the same time point. Administration of *M. balsamina*, however, significantly reduced plasma creatinine concentrations while significantly increasing urinary creatinine concentrations by comparison with STZ-diabetic rats ($p < 0.05$). The effects of metformin and insulin on plasma creatinine and urinary urea were similar to *M. balsamina*. Plasma urea concentrations were significantly ($p < 0.05$) increased in STZ-diabetic rats, while plasma albumin was notably reduced by comparison with

Table 1: Comparison of food, water intake, and body weight (b.wt) change of nondiabetic controls, diabetic controls, and diabetic rats treated with MB, metformin, and insulin during a 5-week study ($n = 6$ in each group). Values are expressed as mean ± SEM.

Parameter	Treatment	Time (weeks) 1	2	3	4	5
Food intake (g/100 g)	NC	11.9 ± 3.4	12.2 ± 1.6	12.3 ± 1.7	13.0 ± 0.4	12.9 ± 0.9
	DC	27.6 ± 1.2	25.4 ± 1.4	16.7 ± 0.4	28.0 ± 1.1	24.8 ± 0.3
	MB	10.0 ± 2.1*	10.2 ± 2.6*	16.4 ± 1.1	26.47 ± 2.4*	18.9 ± 0.6
	INS	19.2 ± 2.2*	18.8 ± 1.9*	11.2 ± 0.8	15.5 ± 3.0*	14.2 ± 0.9*
	MTF	28.2 ± 0.6*	22.7 ± 0.5	21.8 ± 0.5	19.8 ± 0.7	26.8 ± 1.7
Water intake (mL/100 g)	NC	30 ± 8.2	35 ± 1.4	32.5 ± 8.5	45 ± 9.6	51.2 ± 7.2
	DC	60 ± 9.6	61.3 ± 12.9	95.0 ± 3.7	91.3 ± 3.4	96 ± 1.0
	MB	72.5 ± 2.5	67.0 ± 4.1	73.8 ± 8.3	78.7 ± 9.6	76 ± 1.0
	INS	73.0 ± 4.4	76.3 ± 9.4	76.3 ± 0.1	76.4 ± 4.8	74.2 ± 2.3
	MTF	68.8 ± 3.1	41.3 ± 7.5	45.6 ± 2.5	45.2 ± 2.3	43.8 ± 1.1
% b.wt change/week	NC	44.7 ± 9.4	69.7 ± 5.9	76 ± 8.6	90.7 ± 11.1	92.5 ± 9.9
	DC	−72 ± 8.6	−87.2 ± 20	−77.5 ± 9.8	−77.5 ± 12	−80 ± 7.4
	MB	−13.8 ± 8*	−11.1 ± 5*	−19.5 ± 6.2*	−15.3 ± 6.1*	−40.5 ± 11
	INS	18.5 ± 13.9*	3.2 ± 15.7*	30.0 ± 16.2*	38.3 ± 18.1*	28.3 ± 3.2*
	MTF	−23 ± 7.3	−6 ± 6.8	−32 ± 2.9	−11 ± 17.3	−37 ± 3.2
Glucose (mmol/L)	NC	5.1 ± 0.3	5.1 ± 0.4	4.9 ± 0.3	5.8 ± 0.5	5.3 ± 0.1
	DC	33.1 ± 1.5#	33.1 ± 0#	33.4 ± 0.2#	33.0 ± 0.8#	33.2 ± 0.2#
	MB	27.2 ± 0.3	29.1 ± 0.3	24.2 ± 1.9*	25.6 ± 0.6*	26.4 ± 1.0*
	INS	30.7 ± 0.8	23.2 ± 2.6	21.1 ± 2.3*	21.9 ± 1.6*	17.1 ± 0.9*
	MTF	28.0 ± 2.1	26.0 ± 1.4	25.7 ± 0.5*	24.6 ± 0.9*	24.8 ± 0.6*

#$p < 0.05$ by comparison with nondiabetic control and *$p < 0.05$ by comparison with diabetic control.

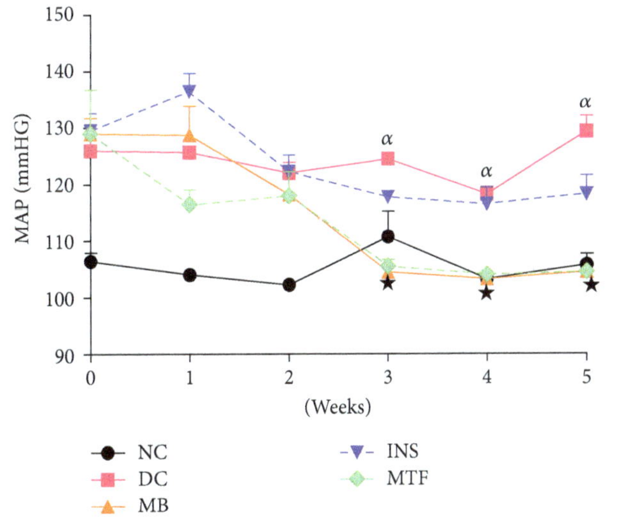

Figure 1: Mean arterial blood pressure of nondiabetic controls, diabetic controls, and diabetic rats treated with *M. balsamina*, metformin, and insulin over a period of 5 weeks. Values are expressed as mean ± SEM. $^{\alpha}p < 0.05$ by comparison to nondiabetic control; ★$p < 0.05$ by comparison with diabetic control.

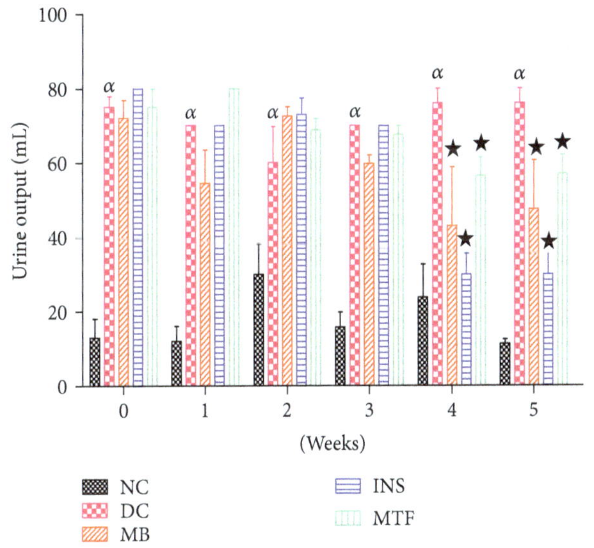

Figure 2: Urine output of nondiabetic controls, diabetic controls, and diabetic rats treated with *M. balsamina*, metformin, and insulin over a period of 5 weeks. Values are expressed as mean ± S EM. $^{\alpha}p < 0.05$ by comparison to nondiabetic control; ★$p < 0.05$ by comparison with diabetic control.

nondiabetic control rats. However, treatment with *M. balsamina* significantly ($p < 0.05$) decreased plasma urea concentration while significantly ($p < 0.05$) increasing plasma albumin in comparison with STZ-diabetic control rats. The effects of metformin and insulin on plasma urea and plasma albumin were similar to *M. balsamina*. STZ-diabetic control

Table 2: Comparison of plasma biochemical parameters and urinary electrolytes of nondiabetic controls, diabetic controls, and diabetic rats treated with MB, metformin, and insulin during a 5-week study ($n = 6$ in each group). Values are expressed as mean ± SEM.

Parameters	Groups				
	NC	DC	MB	INS	MTF
Urinary Na^+ (mmol/L)	66.8 ± 1.2	42.3 ± 3.5#	53.7 ± 1.3*	38.2 ± 1.2	66.0 ± 2.9*
Plasma Na^+ (mmol/L)	120.3 ± 3.3	134.0 ± 2.0#	121.5 ± 4.2*	133.2 ± 1.3	121.7 ± 1.4*
Urinary K^+ (mmol/L)	45.5 ± 1.7	25.5 ± 2.1#	53.7 ± 1.3*	38.2 ± 3.3*	55.5 ± 4.1*
Plasma K^+ (mmol/L)	9.9 ± 1.3	7.6 ± 0.6#	7.9 ± 0.3	9.5 ± 0.7*	8.4 ± 0.4*
Urinary urea (mmol/L)	654.3 ± 6.8	117.8 ± 4.8#	315.3 ± 5.8*	356 ± 9.9*	351 ± 8.0*
Plasma urea (mmol/L)	4.9 ± 0.3	17.5 ± 1.3#	7.0 ± 0.6*	7.6 ± 0.8*	6.4 ± 0.9*
Urinary albumin (g/L)	1.7 ± 0.2	3.5 ± 0.4#	3.2 ± 0.7	4.2 ± 0.7*	4.7 ± 1.1*
Plasma albumin (g/L)	16.5 ± 1.0	12.3 ± 0.6#	13.2 ± 0,6	14.3 ± 0.7*	14.3 ± 1.3*
Urinary creatinine (μmol/L)	9.9 ± 0.7	14.9 ± 0.3#	10.4 ± 0.2*	8.1 ± 0.4*	10.8 ± 0.2*
Creatinine (μmol/L)	32.5 ± 1.3	45.8 ± 1.1#	29.8 ± 1.0*	34.8 ± 1.9*	28.2 ± 0.8*
Aldosterone (pg/mL)	0.2 ± 0.02	0.4 ± 0.1#	0.3 ± 0.4*	0.4 ± 0.2	0.2 ± 0.1*

# $p < 0.05$ by comparison with nondiabetic control; * $p < 0.05$ by comparison with diabetic control.

Table 3: Effects of *M. balsamina* on the kidney-to-body weight ratio after a 5-week study ($n = 6$ in each group). Values are expressed as mean ± SEM.

Experimental groups	Final body weight (g)	Kidney weight (g)	Kidney : body weight ratio (%)
NC	342.5 ± 9.92	1.11 ± 0.081	0.32 ± 0.02
DC	170 ± 7.39#	1.37 ± 0.09#	0.80 ± 0.02#
MB	209 ± 11.33*	1.01 ± 0.031*	0.53 ± 0.03*
INS	278.5 ± 7.5*	1.14 ± 0.14*	0.41 ± 0.06*
MTF	212.5 ± 0.04*	0.97 ± 0.40*	0.46 ± 0.023*

# $p < 0.05$ by comparison with nondiabetic control; * $p < 0.05$ by comparison with diabetic control.

showed significantly increased plasma Na^+ concentration, aldosterone and decreased urinary Na^+ concentrations at week 5 by comparison with nondiabetic rats ($p < 0.05$). Administration of *M. balsamina*, however, significantly ($p < 0.05$) reduced plasma Na^+ and aldosterone concentrations, while urinary Na^+ concentrations significantly ($p < 0.05$) increased at week 5 by comparison to STZ-induced diabetic rats. The effects of metformin were similar to *M. balsamina*. Insulin administration increased plasma Na^+ and aldosterone concentrations while urinary Na^+ was decreased. Urinary K^+ concentrations were significantly ($p < 0.05$) decreased, while plasma K^+ concentrations were significantly ($p < 0.05$) elevated in STZ-diabetic rats by comparison to nondiabetic rats. Administration of *M. balsamina* significantly ($p < 0.05$) increased urinary K^+ output and decreased plasma K^+ concentrations on the 5th week of experimental period. The effects of *M. balsamina* on urinary K^+ output and plasma K^+ were comparable with those of metformin and insulin.

3.5. Kidney Weights. Table 3 shows kidney-to-body weight ratio of nondiabetic controls, diabetic controls, and diabetic rats treated with *M. balsamina*, metformin, and insulin measured after 5 weeks of treatment. The kidney-to-body weight ratio was significantly increased in STZ-diabetic rats by comparison to nondiabetic controls ($p < 0.05$). The administration of MB, insulin, or metformin did not affect the kidney-tobody weight ratio by comparison to STZ-diabetic controls.

3.6. Kidney Function. Table 4 shows factors of kidney function of nondiabetic controls, diabetic controls, and diabetic rats treated with *M. balsamina*, metformin, and insulin assessed after the 5-week experimental period. STZ-diabetic control animals showed significantly increased AER, ACR, and GFR in comparison with nondiabetic animals ($p < 0.05$). The administration of *M. balsamina*, however, significantly decreased AER, ACR, and GFR on the 5th week of experimental period ($p < 0.05$). The effects of insulin were similar to those of MB.

3.7. Oxidative Stress Markers. Table 5 shows kidney malondiadehyde (MDA) concentration and activities of SOD and GPx in nondiabetic controls; diabetic controls; diabetic rats treated with MB, metformin, and insulin measured after 5 weeks of experimental period. Diabetic control rats had significantly increased kidney MDA concentration and had a decrease activity of SOD and GPx in comparison with nondiabetic control ($p < 0.05$). STZ-diabetic rats treated with MB, insulin (175 μg/kg) or metformin (500 mg/kg) showed significantly decreased MDA levels and increased activity of SOD and GPx in kidneys by comparison with STZ-induced diabetic control rats ($p < 0.05$).

4. Discussion

The current study investigated the effects of *M. balsamina* on renal function in STZ-induced diabetic rats. The results herein indicate that *M. balsamina* is effective in ameliorating renal fluid and electrolyte handling in STZ-induced diabetic

Table 4: Comparison albumin excretion rate (AER), albumin creatinine ratio (ACR), and glomerular filtration rate (GFR) of nondiabetic controls, diabetic controls, and diabetic rats treated with MB, metformin, and insulin rats after a 5-week study ($n = 6$ in each group). Values are expressed as mean ± SEM.

Parameters	Groups				
	NC	DC	MB	INS	MTF
AER (mg/day)	0.024 ± 0.01	0.29 ± 0.03#	0.17 ± 0.01*	0.15 ± 0.01*	0.19 ± 0.03*
ACR	8.10 ± 013	27.03 ± 1.13#	15.72 ± 1.50*	13.48 ± 0.84*	19.23 ± 0.28*
GFR (mL/min/100 g)	33.5 ± 0.5	24.8 ± 1.3#	33.7 ± 1.5*	37.9 ± 1.3*	30.9 ± 2.1*

#$p < 0.05$ by comparison with nondiabetic control; *$p < 0.05$ by comparison with diabetic control.

Table 5: Effects of MB on MDA concentrations and activities of SOD and GPx in kidney tissues of non-diabetic controls, diabetic controls, and diabetic rats treated with MB, metformin, and insulin. Values are expressed as mean ± SEM.

Parameter measured	Treatment	Kidney
MDA (nmol·g^{-1} protein)	NC	0.994 ± 0.020
	DC	4.21 ± 0.12#
	INS	1.1 ± 0.01*
	MTF	1.19 ± 0.01*
	MB	1.14 ± 0.01*
SOD activity (pg/mL)	NC	13.43 ± 0.76
	DC	6.01 ± 0.09#
	INS	9.89 ± 0.10*
	MTF	10.11 ± 0.02*
	MB	10.08 ± 0.05*
GPx activity (ng/mL)	NC	2137.31 ± 0.03
	DC	1703.491 ± 0.03#
	INS	2062.21 ± 0.02*
	MTF	2125.75 ± 0.01*
	MB	21370.37 ± 0.03*

#$p < 0.05$ by comparison with nondiabetic control; *$p < 0.05$ by comparison with diabetic control.

rats. In addition, *M. balsamina* reduces oxidative stress and MAP in STZ-induced diabetic rats.

Diabetes is a metabolic disorder characterised by hyperglycaemia. Previous studies, however, have reported that medicinal plants have hypoglycaemic effects [14, 20]. In agreement with previous reports, the use of *M. balsamina* crude extract in STZ-induced diabetic rats significantly attenuated blood glucose concentration in this study. Diabetes mellitus is also associated with polyphagia, polydipsia, and reduction in body weight [21]. Treatment with *M. balsamina*, however, lowered food intake while improving body weight.

Sustained hyperglycaemia has been shown to activate the intrarenal renin aldosterone system which is thought to increase Na^+ retention at various sites of the kidney such as distal tubule and collecting duct of the nephron [22]. Na^+ retention, as assisted by increased aldosterone levels, has been shown to increase MAP in STZ-diabetic rats as also seen in this study [23]. *M. balsamina*, however, decreased MAP of STZ-induced diabetic rats possibly via the inhibition of intrarenal renin aldosterone system as *M. balsamina* administration resulted in decreased concentrations of plasma aldosterone in comparison to untreated STZ-diabetic rats [22, 23]. The results are of importance because diabetes is well known to lead to high blood pressure that eventually results in cardiovascular complications [24].

STZ-induced diabetes is associated with increased kidney weights, albumin excretion rate (AER), and albumin creatinine ratio (ACR) due to the accumulation of extracellular proteins and kidney damage [25]. Treatment with *M. balsamina*, however, attenuated kidney hypertrophy as evidenced by the reduced kidney to body ratio, AER, and ACR. The extracellular protein-induced kidney hypertrophy has been shown to cause structural changes such as the thickening of the glomerular basement membrane, thereby impairing kidney function which includes fluid and electrolyte imbalance in acute renal failure [25]. Furthermore, the impairment of kidney function as a result of the thickening of the glomerular basement membrane is also associated with elevated creatinine concentration with a reduction in GFR as seen in the STZ-diabetic rats in this study at the end of the experimental period. These changes, however, were attenuated in the *M. balsamina*-treated animals as *M. balsamina* increased urinary Na^+ outputs of STZ-diabetic rats and elevated GFR as assessed by creatinine clearance, suggesting an upregulation of renal function. GFR is an important marker of kidney function, and treatment-related increases in creatinine clearance indicate improvement of kidney function in experimental animals [11]. In addition, increases in AER and ACR are markers of the thickening basement membrane [25].

The significant increase in the excretion of Na^+ by *M. balsamina* may perhaps occur via the inhibition of increased proximal reabsorption of Na^+ which is often seen in DM [26]. Kidneys maintain the optimum chemical composition of body fluids by removing Na^+, K^+, urea, albumin, and creatinine [27, 28]. The concentration of these electrolytes, however, was increased in the plasma of STZ-diabetic animals possibly due to sustained hyperglycaemia [28]. Treatment with *M. balsamina*, however, was shown to increase excretion of urea and albumin in STZ-diabetic rats possibly via the amelioration of hyperglycaemia. Studies have shown that improved glycaemic control is beneficial in improving kidney function [28].

Hyperglycaemia-induced oxidative stress in diabetes is a major cause for the development and progression of diabetic microvascular complications such as diabetic nephropathy [29]. In diabetes mellitus, hyperglycaemia can simply inactivate antioxidant enzymes such as SOD and GPx by glycating these proteins and inducing oxidative stress which in turn causes lipid peroxidation [30]. Decreased antioxidant enzyme levels and enhanced lipid peroxidation have been well documented in STZ-induced diabetes [31]. In the enzymatic antioxidant defence system, SOD is one of the important enzymes which scavenge the superoxide radicals by converting them to H_2O_2 and molecular oxygen [8, 30]. The observed decrease in SOD activity in diabetic control rats could result from inactivation by H_2O_2 or by glycosylation of the enzyme, which has been reported to occur in diabetes [30]. GPx is also involved in the elimination of H_2O_2 [32, 33]. The decreased activity of SOD and GPx in the diabetic state may be due to inactivation caused by reactive oxygen species. The results herein showed that elevated concentrations of MDA, a marker of lipid peroxidation, were restored after 5 weeks of treatment with *M. balsamina*. The reduction of MDA levels could be due to improvement in glycaemic control and also increased antioxidant status since *M. balsamina* significantly stimulated the increased activity of SOD and GPx. Medicinal plant extracts have been shown to have antioxidant properties due to their phytochemicals such as alkaloids, polyphenols, saponins, vitamins (C and E), carotenoids, and flavonoids [13–15]. All these have protective roles against oxidative damage, thus preventing lipid peroxidation and protecting the kidneys from severe increases of reactive oxygen species and depletion of superoxide dismutase and reduced glutathione [15, 34, 35]. Studies in our laboratory have indeed shown that reduction of blood glucose may prevent oxidative stress and therefore delay the onset of diabetic complications [14, 15]. Taken together, these results suggest that *M. balsamina* protects the kidneys from damage that occurs in the STZ-induced diabetic animal model.

5. Conclusion

The results described in this study demonstrated that *M. balsamina* ameliorates kidney dysfunction associated with diabetes as shown by increased urinary Na^+ outputs and reduction of plasma creatinine with concomitant increase in GFR. These observations warrant further investigations on *M. balsamina* as a potential alternative remedy for diabetes-associated kidney dysfunction.

Conflicts of Interest

The authors declare no conflict of interest, and the work has not been published elsewhere.

Acknowledgments

The authors are grateful to the Biomedical Research Unit, University of KwaZulu-Natal for the supply of animals. This study was partly funded by NRF South Africa and the University of KwaZulu-Natal, Research Division.

References

[1] R. Rabkin, "Diabetic nephropathy," *Clinical Cornerstone*, vol. 5, no. 2, pp. 1–11, 2003.

[2] P. Stenvinkel, "Chronic kidney disease: a public health priority and harbinger of premature cardiovascular disease," *Journal of Internal Medicine*, vol. 268, no. 5, pp. 456–467, 2010.

[3] J. F. Navarro and C. Mora, "Diabetes, inflammation, proinflammatory cytokines, and diabetic nephropathy," *TheScientificWorldJOURNAL*, vol. 6, pp. 908–917, 2006.

[4] G. Wolf and F. N. Ziyadeh, "Cellular and molecular mechanisms of proteinuria in diabetic nephropathy," *Nephron Physiology*, vol. 106, no. 2, pp. p26–p31, 2007.

[5] H. Fujita, H. Fujishima, S. Chida et al., "Reduction of renal superoxide dismutase in progressive diabetic nephropathy," *Journal of the American Society of Nephrology*, vol. 20, no. 6, pp. 1303–1313, 2009.

[6] J. Coresh, B. C. Astor, T. Greene, G. Eknoyan, and A. S. Levey, "Prevalence of chronic kidney disease and decreased kidney function in the adult US population: third National Health and nutrition examination survey," *American Journal of Kidney Diseases*, vol. 41, no. 1, pp. 1–12, 2003.

[7] C. K. Kramer, C. B. Leitão, L. C. Pinto et al., "Risk factors for micro and macrovascular disease in black and white patients with type 2 diabetes mellitus," *Revista da Associação Médica Brasileira*, vol. 55, no. 3, pp. 308–314, 2009.

[8] A. Ceriello, "New insights on oxidative stress and diabetic complications may lead to a "causal" antioxidant therapy," *Diabetes Care*, vol. 26, no. 5, pp. 1589–1596, 2003.

[9] M. Brownlee, "Biochemistry and molecular cell biology of diabetic complications," *Nature*, vol. 414, no. 6865, pp. 813–820, 2001.

[10] M. J. Fowler, "Diabetes treatment, Part 1: diet and exercise," *Clinical Diabetes*, vol. 25, no. 3, pp. 105–109, 2007.

[11] P. Ruggenenti, A. Schieppati, and G. Remuzzi, "Progression, remission, regression of chronic renal diseases," *The Lancet*, vol. 357, no. 9268, pp. 1601–1608, 2001.

[12] V. N. Bas, S. Cetinkaya, S. Yilmaz Agladioglu et al., "Insulin oedema in newly diagnosed type 1 diabetes mellitus," *Journal of Clinical Research in Pediatric Endocrinology*, vol. 2, no. 1, pp. 46–48, 2010.

[13] G. Arumugam, P. Manjula, and N. Paari, "A review: anti diabetic medicinal plants used for diabetes mellitus," *Journal of Acute Disease*, vol. 2, no. 3, pp. 196–200, 2013.

[14] P. S. Ngubane, S. I. Hadebe, M. R. Serumula, and C. T. Musabayane, "The effects of transdermal insulin treatment of streptozotocin-induced diabetic rats on kidney function and renal expression of glucose transporters," *Renal Failure*, vol. 37, no. 1, pp. 151–159, 2014.

[15] B. N. Mkhwanazi, M. R. Serumula, R. B. Myburg, F. R. van Heerden, and C. T. Musabayane, "Antioxidant effects of maslinic acid in livers, hearts and kidneys of streptozotocin-induced diabetic rats: effects on kidney function," *Renal Failure*, vol. 36, no. 3, pp. 419–431, 2014.

[16] G. Thakur, M. Bag, B. Sanodiya et al., "*Momordica balsamina*: a medicinal and neutraceutical plant for health care management," *Current Pharmaceutical Biotechnology*, vol. 10, no. 7, pp. 667–682, 2009.

[17] M. Abdollahi, A. B. Z. Zuki, A. Rezaeizadeh, Y. M. Goh, and M. M. Noordin, "Effects of *Momordica charantia* aqueous extract on renal histopathological changes associated with

streptozotocin-induced diabetes mellitus type II in neonatal rats," *Journal of Medicinal Plants Research*, vol. 5, no. 9, pp. 1779–1787, 2011.

[18] N. Bhardwaj, V. Gauttam, and A. Kalia, "Evaluation of antidiabetic activity of *Momordica balsamina* Linn seeds in experimentally-induced diabetes," *Journal of Chemical and Pharmaceutical Research*, vol. 2, no. 5, pp. 701–707, 2010.

[19] H. P. Madlala, F. R. Van Heerden, K. Mubagwa, and C. T. Musabayane, "Changes in renal function and oxidative status associated with the hypotensive effects of oleanolic acid and related synthetic derivatives in experimental animals," *PLoS One*, vol. 10, no. 6, article e0128192, 2015.

[20] C. T. Musabayane, N. Mahlalela, F. O. Shode, and J. A. O. Ojewole, "Effects of *Syzygium cordatum* (Hochst.) [Myrtaceae] leaf extract on plasma glucose and hepatic glycogen in streptozotocin-induced diabetic rats," *Journal of Ethnopharmacology*, vol. 97, no. 3, pp. 485–490, 2005.

[21] T. L. van Belle, K. T. Coppieters, and M. G. von Herrath, "Type 1 diabetes: etiology, immunology and therapeutic strategies," *Physiological Reviews*, vol. 91, no. 1, pp. 79–118, 2011.

[22] W. A. Hsueh and K. Wyne, "Renin-angiotensin-aldosterone system in diabetes and hypertension," *The Journal of Clinical Hypertension*, vol. 13, no. 4, pp. 224–237, 2011.

[23] Y. Yang and H. Ma, "Aldosterone," *Research*, vol. 1, no. 5, pp. 89–93, 2009.

[24] S. I. McFarlane and J. R. Sowers, "Aldosterone function in diabetes mellitus: effects on cardiovascular and renal disease," *The Journal of Clinical Endocrinology & Metabolism*, vol. 88, no. 2, pp. 516–523, 2003.

[25] B. F. Palmer and D. J. Clegg, "Electrolyte and acid–base disturbances in patients with diabetes mellitus," *The New England Journal of Medicine*, vol. 373, no. 6, pp. 548–559, 2015.

[26] B. Feldt-Rasmussen, E. R. Mathiesen, T. Deckert et al., "Central role for sodium in the pathogenesis of blood pressure changes independent of angiotensin, aldosterone and catecholamines in type 1 (insulin-dependent) diabetes mellitus," *Diabetologia*, vol. 30, no. 8, pp. 610–617, 1987.

[27] C. G. Musso, J. Alvarez Gregori, J. R. Jauregui, and J. F. Macías Núñez, "Creatinine, urea, uric acid, water and electrolytes renal handling in the healthy oldest old," *World Journal of Nephrology*, vol. 1, no. 5, pp. 123–126, 2012.

[28] N. Hasona and A. Elasbali, "Evaluation of electrolytes imbalance and dyslipidemia in diabetic patients," *Medical Sciences*, vol. 4, no. 2, pp. 1–4, 2016.

[29] N. Kashihara, Y. Haruna, V. K. Kondeti, and Y. S. Kanwar, "Oxidative stress in diabetic nephropathy," *Current Medicinal Chemistry*, vol. 17, no. 34, pp. 4256–4269, 2010.

[30] S. Penckofer, D. Schwertz, and K. Florczak, "Oxidative stress and cardiovascular disease in type 2 diabetes: the role of antioxidants and pro-oxidants," *The Journal of Cardiovascular Nursing*, vol. 16, no. 2, pp. 68–85, 2002.

[31] X. Wang, X.-l. Ye, R. Liu et al., "Antioxidant activities of oleanolic acid in vitro: possible role of Nrf2 and MAP kinases," *Chemico-Biological Interactions*, vol. 184, no. 3, pp. 328–337, 2010.

[32] M. L. Onozato, A. Tojo, A. Goto, T. Fujita, and C. S. Wilcox, "Oxidative stress and nitric oxide synthase in rat diabetic nephropathy: effects of ACEI and ARB," *Kidney International*, vol. 61, no. 1, pp. 186–194, 2002.

[33] J. W. Baynes, "Role of oxidative stress in development of complications in diabetes," *Diabetes*, vol. 40, no. 4, pp. 405–412, 1991.

[34] A. P. Rolo and C. M. Palmeira, "Diabetes and mitochondrial function: role of hyperglycemia and oxidative stress," *Toxicology and Applied Pharmacology*, vol. 212, no. 2, pp. 167–178, 2006.

[35] M. Sani, S. Kouhsari, and L. Moradabadi, "Effects of three medicinal plants extracts in experimental diabetes: antioxidant enzymes activities and plasma lipids profiles in comparison with metformin," *Iranian Journal of Pharmaceutical Research*, vol. 11, no. 3, pp. 897–903, 2012.

18

Readiness of Sub-Saharan Africa Healthcare Systems for the New Pandemic, Diabetes

Bernardo Nuche-Berenguer[1] **and Linda E. Kupfer**[2]

[1]*National Institute of Diabetes and Digestive and Kidney Diseases, National Institutes of Health, Bethesda, MD 20892-1804, USA*
[2]*Fogarty International Center, National Institutes of Health, Bethesda, MD 20814, USA*

Correspondence should be addressed to Linda E. Kupfer; kupferl@mail.nih.gov

Academic Editor: Joseph P. O'hare

Background. Effective health systems are needed to care for the coming surge of diabetics in sub-Saharan Africa (SSA). *Objective.* We conducted a systematic review of literature to determine the capacity of SSA health systems to manage diabetes. *Methodology.* We used three different databases (Embase, Scopus, and PubMed) to search for studies, published from 2004 to 2017, on diabetes care in SSA. *Results.* Fifty-five articles met the inclusion criteria, covering the different aspects related to diabetes care such as availability of drugs and diagnostic tools, the capacity of healthcare workers, and the integration of diabetes care into HIV and TB platforms. *Conclusion.* Although chronic care health systems in SSA have developed significantly in the last decade, the capacity for managing diabetes remains in its infancy. We identified pilot projects to enhance these capacities. The scale-up of these pilot interventions and the integration of diabetes care into existing robust chronic disease platforms may be a feasible approach to begin to tackle the upcoming pandemic in diabetes. Nonetheless, much more work needs to be done to address the health system-wide deficiencies in diabetes care. More research is also needed to determine how to integrate diabetes care into the healthcare system in SSA.

1. Introduction

While the international community is certainly aware of sub-Saharan Africa (SSA) problems caused by malnutrition and HIV and other infectious diseases, awareness of the increasing burden of chronic noncommunicable diseases (NCDs) such as diabetes is still low [1–3]. However, diabetes is not rare in SSA. It is estimated that, in 2014, 20 million people in SSA had diabetes and 523,000 died because of this disease or conditions related to it, with 76% of them under the age of 60 [4]. Moreover, the demographic changes coming with increased age and urbanization of the population favor a continued upward trend of diabetes in the region [5]. The prediction is that for the year 2035, 41.5 million people in SSA will have diabetes [4]. This increase is much higher than in any other region in the world [4]. In terms of prevalence, the limited data available shows that the prevalence varies from 3 to 15% [5, 6] with an overall diabetes prevalence for SSA in 2013 of 4.8% predicted to rise to 5.3% in 2035 [4]. In SSA, it is estimated that 62% of diabetic patients remain undiagnosed [4], which, if correct, represents the highest number of undiagnosed cases in the world. It is suspected that the very low prevalence of type I diabetes might also be an underestimate [7], due in part to the short life expectancy for children diagnosed with this disease, which varies between 7 months and 7 years depending on the country [6]. In general, the lack of proper surveillance systems for NCDs in LMICs makes the real magnitude of diabetes unknown and the lack of data makes it difficult to get policy makers' attention so that they can develop policies to prevent and address the increasing burden of diabetes on the population.

Due to the lack of attention to diabetes by both policymakers and healthcare professionals, patients usually present late in the diabetes cascade with complications of the disease [3]. Even when symptoms lead patients to seek care, they are often misdiagnosed [8]. From 2007 to 2010, it was estimated that due to untreated diabetes in SSA, millions of persons developed eye complications [9], blindness [6, 10], kidney damage [10], cardiovascular disease [10], or had lost a foot because of amputation due to diabetes [10]. It is therefore easy to infer that diabetes has a high social and economic impact in the region [11, 12] and affects employers and national economies due to the loss of productivity [13, 14].

Although the diabetes pandemic keeps growing, the estimated yearly expenditure on healthcare for diabetes in SSA in 2009 is the lowest of any other region in the world [4]. Moreover, the international organizations and NGOs that have successfully addressed other pandemics, such as HIV, have not yet begun to systematically address NCDs in the region. There is no doubt that to address diabetes, sub-Saharan Africa will require robust healthcare systems able to diagnose, treat, and provide chronic care for the diabetic patients. These systems should include the provision of diagnostic and treatment capacity, a trained workforce, and the existence of proper surveillance systems and treatment guidelines. In this review, we analyze the capacity of healthcare systems in the region to confront this new pandemic. We also identify examples and opportunities to integrate diabetes care into other successful, chronic care health platforms, specifically those devoted to care for people living with HIV (PLHIV) in a cost-effective way.

2. Methods

The data methodology used for this study was a systematic review that followed the Cochrane Systematic Review protocol [15]. The review took place between August and September 2014, and it was updated in August 2017. We searched for studies on the management of diabetes in countries of SSA. This included reports on diagnostic and treatment capacity for diabetes. We also sought for studies reporting interventions aimed to increase this capacity. Finally, we included in our search studies covering the topic of integration of diabetes care into existing HIV platforms.

2.1. Eligibility Criteria. We included articles published in English between 2004 and 2017 in peer-reviewed journals. We considered relevance to the review studies covering diabetes care in SSA countries, following the criteria of the International Diabetes Federation [4]. The rationale of the search was to obtain studies providing an overview of the current capacity to manage diabetes in SSA and the current attempts to increase capacity.

2.2. Information Sources. Databases searched for this review were selected based on their level of comprehensiveness and coverage of the topic; they included PubMed, Scopus, and Embase. Several gray literature sources were also considered. Expert opinion and snowball sampling techniques were then employed to identify other relevant documents that may have been omitted from the initial search.

2.3. Search Strategy. For the initial, broad selection, we combined the medical subject headings (MeSH) "diabetes," "insulin," "hyperglycemia," and "type 1 or type 2 diabetes" and the region "sub-Saharan Africa" with terms such as, "health system," "healthcare workforce," "management," "early diagnosis," "treatment," "non-communicable diseases," "self-management," "provider management," "access to care," and "RAPIA"(Rapid Assessment Protocol for Insulin Access). To cover the topic of integration of diabetes care into an existing platform, the HIV platform, we also combined all these terms with "HIV" and "PEPFAR" and "AMPATH," two platforms supporting HIV care, prevention, and treatment in SSA.

2.4. Study Selection. A strategy was employed initially to identify English language studies that fulfilled a suitable combination of the following inclusion criteria: community-based; cross-sectional, randomized, cohort, case-control; reporting healthcare worker readiness for the management of diabetes; reported empowerment of patients for self-management of diabetes; and reporting efforts to integrate diabetes care in existing health infrastructures. In the first stage of the review, the initial selection of reports was screened and narrowed (see Table 1) to eliminate duplicates and those studies irrelevant to the main topic [16]. Then, the rest of the articles were screened based on the inclusion criteria. When multiple reports of the same study were retrieved, the most complete report was selected. Laboratory-based studies, anonymous reports, letters, commentaries, case studies, and reviews were excluded.

2.5. Data Collection Process and Data Items. After reading each article that appeared relevant and met the inclusion criteria, we made notes of the year of study and publication, objectives, study design, methodology, primary and secondary outcomes, location and year of study, population of interest, plan for future work, existence of national policies and/or guidelines for diabetes management, diagnostic and treatment capacity and availability for diabetics (availability of medicines, healthcare worker capacity), managing of diabetes care information (medical records), existence of linkage of diabetes care with care for other diseases, lessons learned from other disease platforms (e.g., PEPFAR) that could be applied to diabetes care, and recommendations issued by the authors. All the extracted data were reviewed by two independent researchers.

2.6. Risk of Bias in Individual Studies. To assess the risk of bias in each individual study, we collected the information on the limitations of each study as reported by the authors.

2.7. Summary Areas of Interest and Synthesis of Results. The principal areas of interest extracted from the studies were (1) diabetes diagnostic capacity; (2) access to medicines for diabetic patients; (3) capacity of healthcare workers; (4) pilot projects to enhance healthcare workers' capacity and (5) increase patients' adherence to treatment; (6) existence of electronic medical records; (7) provision of national guidelines for diabetes care; and (8) pilot projects to study integration of diabetes care into HIV and TB platforms. The results were synthesized and analyzed below following these areas.

Table 1: Examples of interventions to improve patient adherence to diabetes treatment in SSA.

Country	Summary of intervention	Outcomes
Mozambique [42] Rwanda [50]	Improvement of care through establishment of partnerships and systematic care	Increased information about diabetes and access to care for patients
Cameroon [27, 66] Kenya [33]	Integration of diabetes care into primary care facilities	Reduced transportation barriers and improved patient retention rates
Kenya [52] DRC [68]	Cell phone-based home glucose monitoring programs	The clinical outcomes have not been evaluated yet
Kenya [34] Nigeria [69]	Establishment of home-based screening for diabetes	No improvement in clinical outcomes
Kenya [35] Cameroon [70]	Introduction of self-monitoring blood glucose programs	No improvement in clinical outcomes
South Africa [67]	Establishing of mobile testing units	Improvement in linkage to care
Ghana [71]	Setting off electronic reminders on risk management for diabetic patients	Increased adherence to treatment and reducing of FBG
Cameroon [72, 73] Kenya [36, 44]	Different approaches to establish peer support for diabetes patients	Increased adherence to treatment and improvement in clinical outcomes

3. Results

A total of 3186 English language records were initially identified, plus an additional 3 were included via snowball sampling and expert opinion. A title or title and abstract screening of the initial 3186 articles narrowed these down to 318 articles for full text review; finally, 55 articles remained that met the eligibility criteria by including evaluation of different aspects on health system performance, interventions devoted to the improvement of diabetes care, and some mention of the integration of diabetes care in other disease care platforms. These articles were included in the final qualitative analysis (Figure 1).

The degree of integration of diabetes within health systems varied from little to no mention of integration to examples in which significant integration of diabetes was explicitly discussed. Based on the study questions, nine areas related to diabetes and healthcare systems emerged from the analysis: (1) capacity to diagnose diabetes; (2) access to medicines for diabetic patients; (3) capacity of healthcare workers; (4) pilot experiences designed to optimize the effectiveness of healthcare workers' capacity; (5) pilot experiences for increasing patients' adherence to treatment (Table 1); (6) existence of electronic medical records; (7) provision of national guidelines for diabetes care; and (8) integration of diabetes care into HIV and TB platforms (Table 2).

3.1. The Capacity to Diagnose Diabetes. Diagnostic capacity is crucial for an effective healthcare system. Most of the literature analyzed in our review describes the poor diagnostic capacity of the healthcare centers studied in the region. Health centers studied in Mozambique [17, 18], Zambia [17], Rwanda [19], South Africa [20–24], Ethiopia [25, 26], Cameroon [27–30], Malawi [31, 32], Swaziland [25], Kenya [29, 33–36], Nigeria [29], Senegal [29], Uganda [37, 38], Ghana [39], and Tanzania [29, 40, 41] reported, especially in primary care facilities, a scarcity of glucose meters, testing strips, and laboratory capacity to measure glycosylated hemoglobin (HbA1C), which is the most reliable tool to diagnose diabetes. The lack of access to HBA1C testing can result in poor glucose control as reported in a cross-sectional study in Cameroon and Guinea [30]. Some initiatives, such as the "twinning program between the Mozambique and the UK government" [41], consisted in a series of activities supporting the Ministry of Health in developing a training program for specialists in diabetes care, developing patients education materials, establishing guidelines, and increasing the health system capacity. This program resulted in an increase in the availability of glucose measuring tools in Mozambique health centers [42]. In South Africa, the 1994 implementation by the Government of the diabetes management program improved diagnostic capabilities and currently some of the health centers, especially those in urban areas [22, 43], have diabetes diagnostic tools. Other countries like Cameroon [27, 37] have also improved their diabetes diagnostic capacity, but the general perception is that there is a lot of work to be done in SSA, especially in rural areas.

3.2. Access to Medicines for Diabetic Patients. Although there have been significant improvements, access to medicines in SSA is still limited. There are three main problems referred to in the literature: lack of availability in the health centers, large expense for the patients, and/or inadequate storage conditions. The best example of accessibility and affordability of diabetes medication is South Africa [20–23] where health systems went through a great transition after Apartheid, and the main diabetes medicines (it refers to those included in the WHO Essentials Medicines List: http://www.who.int/medicines/publications/essentialmedicines/20th_EML2017.pdf?ua=1) are now available and provided for free. However, it is common in SSA that government initiatives do not reach the rural areas [23, 44] resulting in poor access to medicines is these settings [23, 39, 44]. Cameroon has diabetes drugs on their list of essential medicines [28, 45], which should make them available and free to patients. In other countries like

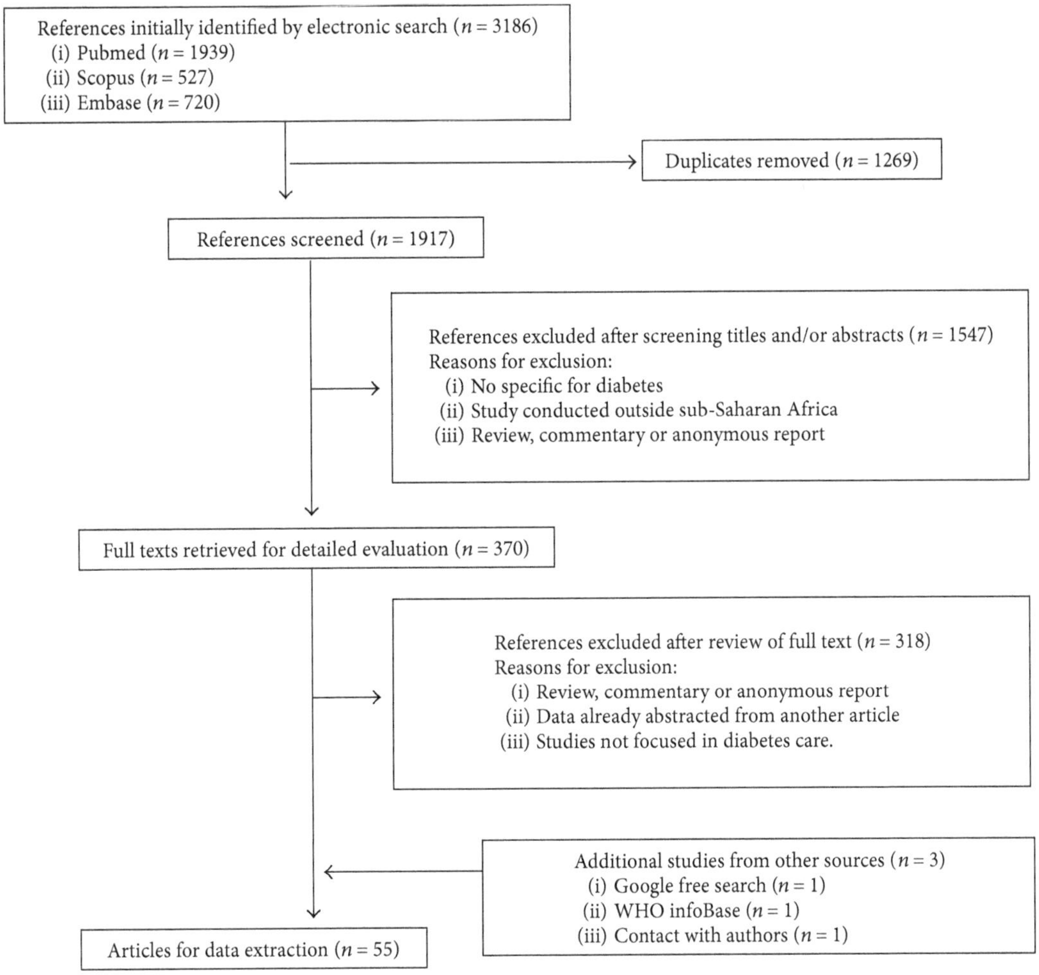

FIGURE 1: Flow diagram of the study selection procedure.

TABLE 2: Examples of integration of diabetes care into other health platforms in SSA.

Country	Platform	Actions taken
Malawi [31]	TB-integrate HIV, TB, and diabetes	(i) Improved patients' knowledge (ii) Facilitated access to treatment (iii) Created EMR
Kenya [34, 52]	PEPFAR platform (AMPATH)	(i) Trained healthcare workers in diabetes care (ii) Improved diagnostic capacity (iii) Created a database of diabetics (iv) Created home-based diabetes screening programs
Uganda [76]	Community-based HIV programs	(i) Screening of diabetes and other NCDs (ii) Achieved a 63% linkage to care for diabetes
South Africa [67]	Community-based HIV programs	(i) Screening of diabetes and other NCDs (ii) Use of mobile testing units to reduce transportation barriers
Kenya [33]	MSF HIV platform	(i) Integrated management of diabetes and HIV (ii) Educated patients in healthy lifestyles
Ethiopia [25]	International Center for Diabetes Care and Treatment programs (ICAP)	(i) Applied lessons learned from HIV care to diabetes (ii) Established EMRs for diabetes

Zambia and Mozambique, insulin is sold free of taxes and available at a subsidized price [17]. However, procurement of insulin is poorly coordinated and often not adapted to the needs of the region resulting in improper storage during transportation and poor distribution to rural areas [17]. A study conducted in Uganda showed that only hospitals had an acceptable storage of diabetes drugs, while the local and subregional hospitals lacked first-line therapy for diabetes, and stock-outs were commonly reported [37]. In Mozambique, a partnership program with the UK government resulted in a more optimized system improving the procurement systems for insulin and therefore its availability [42]. In Tanzania, diabetes drugs are generally available but some reports show that about 36% of patients have problems affording the medicines [46]. Another study in Tanzania reports occasional unavailability of medicine in the public sector that forces the patients to buy their medication in the private sector at a higher price [40]. In Ghana, insulin is paid for by National Health Insurance; however, 45% of people are not registered and have to pay out of pocket for insulin [47]. Moreover, two surveys in Nigeria [48, 49] have shown that the economic burden of diabetes is high for some patients due to the impact of out of pocket payments. In countries like Rwanda [19, 50, 51], Ethiopia [25, 26], Swaziland [25], Kenya [52], Nigeria [53] Burundi, Senegal [54], and the Democratic Republic of Congo [51] diabetes drugs are still unavailable or are too expensive to be accessible. This is identified by patients as one of the biggest reasons for nonadherence to treatment [54].

3.3. Capacity of Healthcare Workers. The capacity of healthcare workers to manage diabetes is uneven in different countries. Medical doctors are often better capacitated than other healthcare workers such as nurses, nurse practitioners, medical officers, and nonmedical doctors [37, 40, 55, 56] to diagnose and treat diabetes. In countries like Mozambique and Zambia, low capacity of healthcare workers to diagnose diabetes have often led to misdiagnosis [17]. Another study in Cameroon demonstrated that healthcare workers had some problems in diagnosing diabetes, especially when using an HBA1C test, and did not have adequate knowledge about treatment, drug prescriptions, and management of the complications and comorbidities of the disease [57]. A survey in Uganda estimated that half of the healthcare workers had only fair knowledge of diabetes and that they generally had little experience in managing diabetic patients [37]. Another study in Uganda showed that healthcare workers had little knowledge of the use of HBA1C testing compared to fasting blood glucose (FBG) [58]. Similar results were obtained in a survey in Malawi [32]. In some of the selected studies, the healthcare workers with diabetes training do not fully understand the disease and may have misconceptions regarding treatment. For example, in a South African study, doctors did not know how to properly use/prescribe insulin and had fears related to the induction of hypoglycemia [20]. Another study in Nigeria showed how physicians were prescribing medicines that were not appropriate for their patients [56]. Although South Africa has a good health system overall, reports show that the primary care system is still poor and there is a need to empower the primary care centers in order to reach the rural areas [43]. Documentation exists that in Rwanda [19, 51], Nigeria [55], Mozambique [18], Ghana [39, 47], Uganda [38] Tanzania [40, 41], Burundi, and the Democratic Republic of Congo [51], there is little preparation or training of the healthcare workforce when it comes to dealing with diabetes and effective training programs are needed. This is probably true in many countries across the continent.

3.4. Pilot Experiences Designed to Optimize Healthcare Workers' Capacity. Several pilot interventions have been recently conducted to improve diabetes diagnosis and control capacity of healthcare workers in SSA. The training is given by doctors or by other qualified personnel. Most of these interventions are based on the idea of enhancing the training of the existing healthcare workforce and then transferring some of the functions ("task shifting" [59]) done by medical doctors to other healthcare workers. Task shifting has several benefits. First, it can alleviate some of the effects of the paucity of doctors available [60]; second, because community health workers (CHW) and nurses work in the community, it brings care closer to the patients, reducing the distance they must travel for treatment and so on; finally, it frees up doctors for more complex tasks that other healthcare workers cannot perform. In the context of diabetes, task shifting is focused on improving the healthcare workers' capacity for diagnosis, prescription of medicines, and education of patients about healthy lifestyles. The hope is that task shifting will result in higher rates of diagnosis and treatment adherence of diabetic patients. Pilot studies conducted in Ethiopia [26], South Africa [21, 23, 61], and Cameroon [27, 28, 62] have demonstrated this approach to be effective in increasing the use of testing equipment and patient retention. In Mozambique, after the implementation of a partnership program with the UK government, there was a significant improvement in the capacity of the healthcare workers for managing diabetes [42] and some studies have documented improvements in glucose control with patients living in areas where task shifting have been implemented [23]. A training program in Tanzania [63] successfully resulted in the elaboration of diabetes educational materials for patients, and a task shifting program with nurses in Kenya [64] showed nurses were capable of adhering to protocols and guidelines for diabetes care. An intervention in South Africa capacitating primary healthcare workers in identifying signs of diabetes and providing appropriate referral not only had an impact in this healthcare workers' knowledge but also improved early detection and referral for high risk, poorly controlled patients [43]. Approaches aimed at training pharmacists about diabetes management have also been successful [65]. In another pilot experience in South Africa [22], doctors received a capitation fee in advance for caring for diabetic patients and participant centers were responsible for any additional costs due to poor management. This achieved major reductions in hospital admission rates for acute metabolic emergencies and a sustainable reduction in patient's HbA1C [22]. Independent of the approach used, in general, the authors of these articles stress the importance of providing continuous education to the healthcare workforce. This is especially important to counteract the high turnover of personnel, especially in rural areas.

3.5. Pilot Experiences for Increasing Patients' Adherence to Treatment. Improving patient adherence to treatment is another key component for achieving optimal diabetes control in SSA. Lack of adherence could be due to several factors such as the high cost of medicines (see Section 3.1), poor care by healthcare workers (see Section 3.2), behavioral and environmental difficulties involved with following a healthy lifestyle, and/or the difficulty of getting to a health center [42, 66, 67]. Some studies suggest that access to care is more important than quality of care for the improvement of glycemic control [29]. Our literature review found some examples of pilot interventions that sought to increase adherence of patients to treatment by lowering some of the barriers to care—see Table 1. The aforementioned UK-Mozambique twinning program [42] was successful in improving adherence to treatment by increasing the information that patients got about diabetes and by increasing the access to diabetes drugs and diagnostic tools. The integration of diabetes care in primary care facilities, which reduces, in many cases, the problems of transportation, is also an effective strategy to improve patient retention rates. This has been demonstrated in several studies conducted in Cameroon [27, 66] and Kenya [33]. Another way to reduce the barriers associated with transportation was tried in Kenya and the Democratic Republic of Congo [52, 68] with the introduction of a cell phone-based home glucose-monitoring program although the clinical outcomes of these interventions have not yet been evaluated. However, in other studies, the introduction of home-based screening for diabetes did not improve the retention rates when compared to community-based screenings [34] and self-monitoring blood glucose (SBMG) did not result in better outcomes for patients in Nigeria [69], Kenya [35], and Cameroon [70]. Infrequent SMBG testing, lack of glucose meters, and limited patient involvement are all associated with the suboptimal glycemic control achieved by SBMG in these studies [70]. Other studies have proposed to lower the transportation barrier by integrating the linkage to care using mobile testing units [67].

A randomized control (RCT) study in Ghana [71] evaluating the effect of electronic reminders on risk management among diabetic patients proved this intervention successful in increasing adherence to medical appointments and reducing FBG in the intervention group. The establishment of peer-support groups has also proven effective in increasing diabetic patients' adherence to treatment and in improving clinical outcomes, as demonstrated by a RCT in Cameroon [72], by a retrospective study in Kenya [44], and in the setting of a diabetes camp for children in Cameroon [73]. Recently, an intervention in Kenya [36] extended the peer-support approach by including peer/microfinance groups and an integration of community education which resulted in significant improvements in linkage to care and clinical outcomes. In summary, linkage to and retention in care is very important for chronic diseases, and although it is especially difficult to achieve in rural settings, there are several interventions, such as peer support, mobile testing, and electronic reminders, that have been shown to be successful in addressing these areas.

3.6. Existence of Electronic Medical Records. Electronic medical records (EMR) are the foundation for complete population-based epidemiological information. EMRs, many of which track medicines used, also enables the prediction of the need for medicines avoiding the medicine shortages or "stock-outs" that are common in SSA. There are examples of the existence of EMRs in the region. One of the clearest examples is South Africa where all centers belonging to the Centers of Diseases and Endocrinology (CDE) network have access to a customized Internet clinical management program that they are obliged to use for entering the medical history of the patients [22]. In recent years, efforts to implement EMRs with diabetes modules have been conducted through pilot studies in several countries [25, 31, 51, 52]. EMRs have allowed the collection of epidemiological and financial data related to diabetes. Most of the studies identified by our review reported paper-based medical records. However, these records are easily lost and make sharing and aggregating information, as well as patient tracking, much more complicated.

3.7. National Guidelines for Diabetes Care. The standardization of protocols in the diagnosis and treatment of diabetes is another important aspect in achieving successful management of diabetic patients. The literature shows little prevalence of diabetes guidelines in SSA. Guidelines for diabetes care are found in South Africa [21, 22, 43, 74], Mozambique [42], and Cameroon [66]. However, sometimes, even when the guidelines are established, they are not disseminated to primary care centers like in Ghana and Tanzania [40, 47] or they simply do not take into account budgetary constraints making them difficult to implement [24]. In Uganda, the availability of guidelines for diabetes care seems to be unevenly distributed among the healthcare facilities at different levels as was demonstrated in a recent study where guidelines were found to be common in hospitals but not in lower level facilities [37]. Per another study in Uganda, it is also essential to establish specific cut-off points for HBA1C that consider ethnic differences [58].

The development and dissemination of treatment guidelines, appropriate to low resource settings, need to be addressed in SSA. Several of the pilots reviewed suggest that the development of guidelines is key to achieving successful diabetes care. As a basis for their guidelines, countries can use the WHO guidelines for prevention and control of NCDs: *Guidelines for primary health care in low resource settings (2012).*

3.8. Integration of Diabetes Care into Existing HIV and TB Platforms. In SSA, there is a new opportunity to deliver chronic care for patients with diabetes through investments made in addressing other chronic diseases such as HIV and TB. A multicountry survey conducted in PEPFAR treatment centers showed how PEPFAR has laid the foundation for improving health system performance in health areas other than HIV, such as diabetes care [75]. In our literature search, we found reports of attempts to integrate diabetes care into the infrastructure built for care of other diseases and these findings are summarized in Table 2. For instance, in Malawi, efforts were conducted to use the infrastructure and also the lessons learned from a TB prevention and control program to also manage and monitor patients with diabetes [31]. In this program, diabetic patients, previously diagnosed, were also tested for HIV and TB, and the three diseases were managed in an integrated way. The program improved patients' knowledge about their condition, gave them access to treatment, and created a system of EMRs to track them over time. In Kenya, the innovative tools, structure, and interventions developed for the care of persons with HIV by the USAID-AMPATH program have facilitated the provision of basic diabetes care in the region: trained personnel, insulin, HbA1C, and point of care glucose testing devices have been added to HIV clinics [52]. This has revealed the poor quality of diabetes care, especially in insulin-dependent patients, and has helped to build a database of diabetics in the area. In Uganda [76, 77] and South Africa [67], community-based HIV testing campaigns also included screening and diagnosis for diabetes and other NCDs, which also, parenthetically, helped to reduce the stigma associated with persons who had HIV. This intervention identified new diabetic patients and the intervention in Uganda [76] achieved a 63% linkage of care to newly diagnosed diabetic patients.

The training of HIV health counselors to perform home-based diabetes and hypertension screening was also applied in Kenya [34] achieving success in the identification of new cases but a low yield (23%) in linking them to care. As a result of the success of this experience, the Kenyan Ministry of Health partnered with AMPATH and began the broad implementation of a diabetes- and hypertension-screening program [34]. Also in Kenya, hospitals ran by the NGO *Medecins Sans Frontieres* have been providing HIV-related services for several years, integrating hypertension and diabetes into their services to allow more holistic management of these diseases in a single patient [33].

However, the existence of a good HIV infrastructure by itself does not guarantee good provision of care for diabetic patients, as was demonstrated in two hospitals in Ethiopia and Swaziland [25]. In these two hospitals, despite a well-developed HIV infrastructure, only 26% of diabetic patients had optimal control of their disease. However, this same study demonstrated that after an intervention in the Ethiopian hospital, aimed to leverage HIV and diabetes services, important advances were made in increasing documented service delivery to diabetic patients and improving standards of care with no added staff [25]. Moreover, an EMR was generated based on the lessons learned from the existing HIV platform. This resulted in a general improvement in diabetic patients' attention and follow-up. However, as clinical outcomes were not measured for this intervention its comparison with similar initiatives is difficult.

4. Discussion

While the international community is certainly aware of SSA problems caused by malnutrition, HIV, and other infectious diseases, awareness of the increasing burden of noncommunicable diseases such as diabetes is still low [3–5]. It is "estimated" that, in 2014, 20 million people in sub-Saharan Africa had diabetes and 523,000 died because of this disease or conditions related to it with 76% of them under the age of 60 [4]. The prediction is that for the year 2035, 41.5 million people will have diabetes in SSA [4]. Thus, the number of diabetics in SSA will double in the next 20 years, an increase that is much higher than we see in any other region in the world [4]. It is important to highlight that the data on diabetes prevalence is based on estimations, since in 2009 only 15% of people with diabetes had been properly diagnosed [6] and although these numbers have improved significantly in 2013 [4], 62% of diabetic patients remain undiagnosed, which represents the highest number of undiagnosed cases in the world. Clearly, there is an urgent need to increase the capacity of health systems in SSA to manage diabetes.

Our review identified important flaws, but also successful interventions, in health systems in SSA that can affect care of diabetic patients. Diagnosis, access to diabetes medication, and trained healthcare workers are often unavailable, and EMRs and national guidelines for diabetes care are extremely limited. The combination of these factors explains the absence of necessary epidemiologic data, complicates tracking of patients, and hinders the ability to forecast future pharmaceutical and human resource needs [31]. Moreover, linkage and retention to care of diagnosed patients is hard because of the difficulties in the access to health centers, and the high prices or stock-outs of essential diabetes medicines [48, 49, 53, 66, 67]. Based on the findings in our review, we have modified the WHO health system building blocks (Figure 2) to represent the needs for effective management of diabetes in SSA.

In this review, we have found interventions that have been shown to be effective in SSA to address many of these issues. These include task shifting of healthcare personnel, reducing costs for and increasing access to care, ensuring the steady supply of drugs [17, 26, 40, 47, 55, 56], increasing diagnostic capacity [17, 34, 40], formulation, introduction, and adaptation of realistic clinical guidelines [24, 55, 58], implementation of diabetic modules for EMRs [31, 51], and education for both patients and healthcare personnel [17, 20, 33]. Especially in underserved areas [21], it is also recommended to train pharmacists or even traditional healers to tackle the lack of adequate healthcare workers to care for diabetics [18, 20, 23, 27, 28, 55, 65]. This training must be continuous to counteract the high turnover of personnel especially in rural areas [26, 56]. This can be achieved by increasing communication between doctors and other healthcare workers [43]. Some papers [78] recommend the creation of specific centers for the treatment of diabetes. However, it seems unrealistic to think that countries dealing with an unfinished agenda of infectious diseases should create vertical systems for the care of NCDs, especially because of the overlap in the continuum and chronicity of care of some of these diseases. Others recommend the establishment of partnerships with external organizations [19] or the integration of diabetes care in other disease platforms [25, 34, 40, 45, 52, 67, 76, 79]. One of the first efforts to achieve this integration was the application of the Directly Observed Therapy Short Course (DOTS) for tuberculosis which has been integrated to include diabetes care [79]. DOTS included political commitment, diagnosis, and standardized treatment by capable health workers, standardized monitoring and

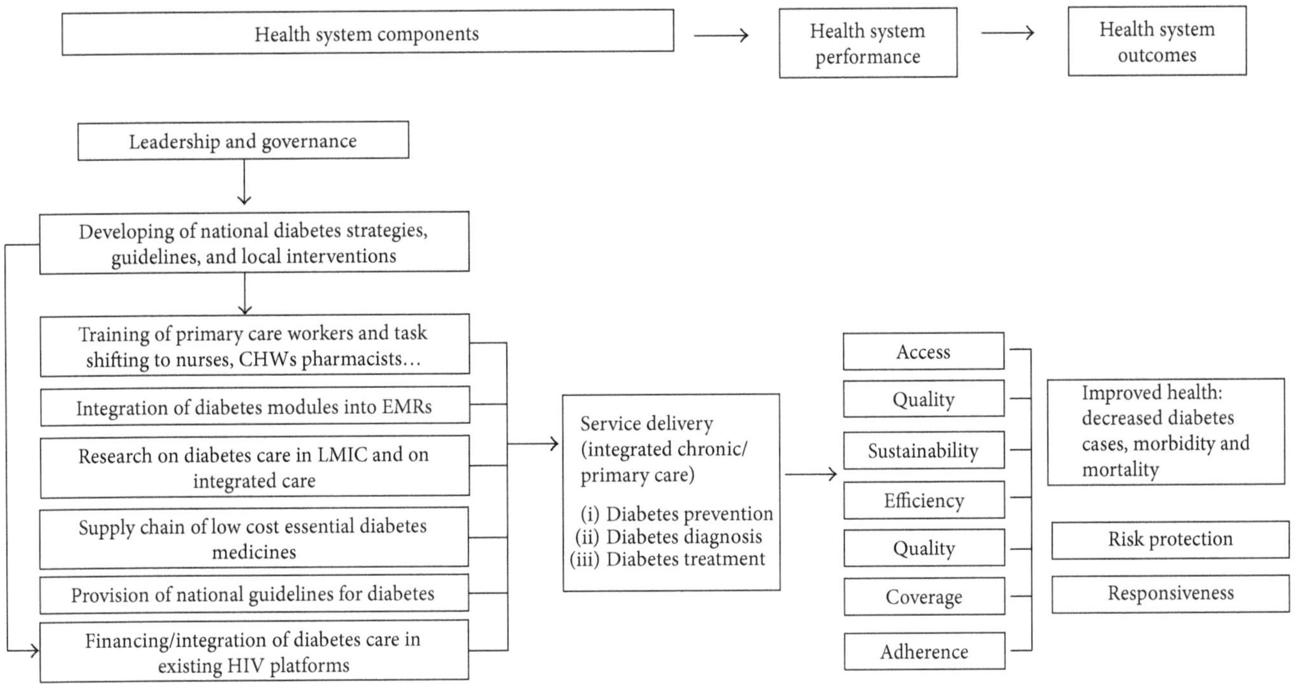

FIGURE 2: WHO health system building blocks based on the authors' recommendations.

evaluation system, and uninterrupted drug supplies. The adaptation of this for diabetes in Malawi allowed the implementation of an electronic record system for diabetic patients [31]. This integrated model facilitates and improves care for patients while avoiding competition between communicable and noncommunicable diseases for limited resources. In fact, healthcare platforms should probably be designed by the chronicity of care given, chronic versus acute, rather than by the disease itself. An analysis conducted in centers funded through PEPFAR showed how the infrastructure originally built for HIV care can help to improve the health systems performance to care for other diseases [75] suggesting that this platform could be used for provision of more general chronic care. The integration of diabetes care in HIV platforms has been attempted [33, 34, 67, 76], has a very low cost (less than 3$ per patient) [76], and seems like a good option for sub-Saharan African countries.

A number of countries have developed national strategies to address diabetes. These strategies have included some of the interventions mentioned above, population-based screening [18, 23, 33, 34, 42, 52, 65], task shifting by training primary healthcare workers [21, 23, 26–28, 61, 62, 64, 65], provision of free medicines [20, 21, 28] or at a subsidized price [17, 46], and empowerment of patients [27, 33, 34, 66]. Partnerships have also helped. For instance, *Novo Nordisk* offers insulin at a lower price to LMIC countries [17] and several NGOs like *Medecines sans Frontieres* are including diabetes care in their facilities [33]. The Mozambique-UK partnership program has also achieved important advances in diabetes care for that country [42].

The studies included in this systematic review had some limitations, as mentioned by their authors. These limitations include low number of participants [28, 43, 63, 65–67, 73], participants and centers not representative sample of the studied country [25, 29, 40, 45, 53, 54]. Other studies reported high loss to follow-up [27, 50]. In general, the interpretation of the studies included in this review was difficult because of incomplete information, missing baseline data, and bias. Studies analyzing intervention data should be interpreted with caution due to the "regression to the mean" phenomenon [28, 66]. In interventions in poorly controlled patients, high baseline blood glucose values could explain the big reduction in blood glucose overestimating the effectiveness of the intervention [23]. Poor access to diagnostic devices and their lack of standardization might have underestimated the prevalence of diabetes [18, 29, 34]. In some of the cohort studies, the follow-up time was short [21, 44] and in general as some papers recognize [28] the pilot experiences need to be validated with randomized trials.

Further, while articles discussing both, health systems and diabetes in some respect were included in this review; it may have not always been the articles' explicit intent to consider this relationship. In addition, only articles written in English were included in the final pool of articles; this could have excluded some important information. As the relationship between diabetes and health systems in SSA has not been previously explored, the groupings that emerged during analysis were intended to guide discussion, but they themselves are somewhat arbitrary and further analysis may be useful. Finally, while the search criteria was as inclusive as possible and was supplemented by both a snowball sampling technique and expert input, some areas may have been unintentionally skipped.

About the methodology used to perform this systematic review, we followed the recommendations provided by the Cochrane handbook for systematic reviews [15]. This protocol is the most commonly used in the fields of medicine and health system interventions [16]. In this review, we did not perform statistical techniques (meta-analysis) to combine results of the eligible interventions. This was due to the lack of data about diabetes in SSA and also because the interventions included in our review, aimed either to optimize effectiveness of healthcare workers' capacity or to increase patients' adherence to treatment, were often using different approaches and were difficult to include in the same meta-analysis. That is probably the reason for the scarcity of meta-analysis measuring the impact of interventions aimed to improve NCD management in SSA [80]. For instance, a recent systematic review on the role of CHWs treating diabetes in the United States [81] suggests that CHW interventions have significant impact in physical health outcomes. However, similar analysis of the interventions that are currently being developed in SSA would be an important contribution to inform policy makers about effective interventions for the improvement of diabetes care in the region.

5. Conclusions

In summary, although improvements have been achieved in SSA in the last years for the provision of chronic diabetes care, many challenges remain. Improving the control and treatment of diabetes is a goal that SSA healthcare systems must achieve in the years to come, as the impact of the disease will grow steeply in the region. This objective must be accomplished in settings that still have an unfinished agenda for infectious diseases. That is why optimizing the existing resources by integrating diabetes care with other disease platforms, like those currently providing care for chronic diseases such as HIV and TB, is a great opportunity to improve diabetes diagnostic systems, provision of medicines, training of health personnel, empowerment of patients, and tracking of the disease burden. Finally, research into the most cost-effective way to implement chronic diabetes care in SSA is needed to successfully confront the upcoming pandemic.

Conflicts of Interest

The authors declare that they have no conflicts of interest.

References

[1] D. G. McLarty, C. Pollitt, and A. B. Swai, "Diabetes in Africa," *Diabetic Medicine*, vol. 7, no. 8, pp. 670–684, 1990.

[2] A. A. Motala, M. A. K. Omar, and F. J. Pirie, "Epidemiology of diabetes in Africa," in *The epidemiology of diabetes mellitus*, J. Ekoe, M. Rewers, R. Williams and P. Zimmet, Eds., pp. 133–146, Wiley, Chichester, England, 2008.

[3] N. S. Levitt, "Diabetes in Africa: epidemiology, management and healthcare challenges," *Heart*, vol. 94, no. 11, pp. 1376–1382, 2008.

[4] *The Diabetes Atlas*, International Diabetes Federation, Brussels, Belgium, Sixth edition, 2013.

[5] J. C. Mbanya, A. A. Motala, E. Sobngwi, F. K. Assah, and S. T. Enoru, "Diabetes in sub-Saharan Africa," *The Lancet*, vol. 375, no. 9733, pp. 2254–2266, 2010.

[6] *The Diabetes Atlas*, International Diabetes Federation, Brussels, Belgium, Fourth edition, 2009.

[7] "End poverty 2015," in *Fact Sheet on MDG4: Reduce Child Mortality*, United Nations, New York, NY, USA, 2008.

[8] D. Beran and J. S. Yudkin, "Diabetes care in sub-Saharan Africa," *Lancet*, vol. 368, no. 9548, pp. 1689–1695, 2006.

[9] *The Diabetes Atlas*, International Diabetes Federation, Brussels, Belgium, Third edition, 2006.

[10] DiabCare-middle Africa 2008, *A Survey Study on Diabetes Management, Complications and Psychosocial Aspects of Diabetic Patients in Middle African Countries*, Bagsvaerd, Denmark, 2008.

[11] R. J. Barro, "Economic growth in a cross section of countries," *Quarterly Journal of Economics*, vol. 106, no. 2, pp. 407–443, 1991.

[12] J. M. Kirigia, H. B. Sambo, L. G. Sambo, and S. P. Barry, "Economic burden of diabetes mellitus in the WHO African region," *BMC International Health and Human Rights*, vol. 9, no. 1, p. 6, 2009.

[13] D. Bloom, D. Canning, and J. Sevilla, "The effect of health on economic growth: a production function approach," *World Development*, vol. 32, pp. 1–13, 2004.

[14] D. E. Bloom and J. D. Sachs, "Geography, demography, and economic growth in Africa," *Brookings Papers on Economic Activity*, vol. 2, pp. 207–295, 1998.

[15] The Cochrane Collaboration, *Cochrane handbook for systematic reviews of interventions*, London, UK, 2011.

[16] R. Atun, T. de Jongh, F. Secci, K. Ohiri, and O. Adeyi, "A systematic review of the evidence on integration of targeted health interventions into health systems," *Health Policy and Planning*, vol. 25, no. 1, pp. 1–14, 2010.

[17] D. Beran, J. S. Yudkin, and M. de Courten, "Access to care for patients with insulin-requiring diabetes in developing countries: case studies of Mozambique and Zambia," *Diabetes Care*, vol. 28, no. 9, pp. 2136–2140, 2005.

[18] C. Silva-Matos, A. Gomes, A. Azevedo, A. Damasceno, A. Prista, and N. Lunet, "Diabetes in Mozambique: prevalence, management and healthcare challenges," *Diabetes & Metabolism*, vol. 37, no. 3, pp. 237–244, 2011.

[19] F. Gishoma, "Restoring diabetes care in Rwanda: the need for effective partnerships," *World Hospitals and Health Services*, vol. 41, no. 4, pp. 36-37, 2005.

[20] M. Haque, S. H. Emerson, C. R. Dennison, M. Navsa, and N. S. Levitt, "Barriers to initiating insulin therapy in patients with type 2 diabetes mellitus in public-sector primary health care centres in cape town," *South African Medical Journal*, vol. 95, no. 10, pp. 798–802, 2005.

[21] G. V. Gill, C. Price, D. Shandu, M. Dedicoat, and D. Wilkinson, "An effective system of nurse-led diabetes care in rural Africa," *Diabetic Medicine*, vol. 25, no. 5, pp. 606–611, 2008.

[22] L. A. Distiller, M. A. Brown, B. I. Joffe, and B. D. Kramer, "Striving for the impossible dream: a community-based multi-practice collaborative model of diabetes management," *Diabetic Medicine*, vol. 27, no. 2, pp. 197–202, 2010.

[23] C. Price, D. Shandu, M. Dedicoat, D. Wilkinson, and G. V. Gill, "Long-term glycaemic outcome of structured nurse-led diabetes care in rural Africa," *QJM*, vol. 104, no. 7, pp. 571–574, 2011.

[24] K. Steyn, C. Lombard, N. Gwebushe et al., "Implementation of national guidelines, incorporated within structured diabetes and hypertension records at primary level care in Cape Town,

South Africa: a randomised controlled trial," *Global Health Action*, vol. 6, no. 1, article 20796, 2013.

[25] M. Rabkin, Z. Melaku, K. Bruce et al., "Strengthening health systems for chronic care: leveraging HIV programs to support diabetes services in Ethiopia and Swaziland," *Journal of Tropical Medicine*, vol. 2012, Article ID 137460, 6 pages, 2012.

[26] Y. Mamo, E. Seid, S. Adams, A. Gardiner, and E. Parry, "A primary healthcare approach to the management of chronic disease in Ethiopia: an example for other countries," *Clinical Medicine*, vol. 7, no. 3, pp. 228–231, 2007.

[27] N. D. Labhardt, J. R. Balo, M. Ndam, J. J. Grimm, and E. Manga, "Task shifting to non-physician clinicians for integrated management of hypertension and diabetes in rural Cameroon: a programme assessment at two years," *BMC Health Services Research*, vol. 10, no. 1, p. 339, 2010.

[28] A. P. Kengne, L. Fezeu, E. Sobngwi et al., "Type 2 diabetes management in nurse-led primary healthcare settings in urban and rural Cameroon," *Primary Care Diabetes*, vol. 3, no. 3, pp. 181–188, 2009.

[29] E. Sobngwi, M. Ndour-Mbaye, K. A. Boateng et al., "Type 2 diabetes control and complications in specialised diabetes care centres of six sub-Saharan African countries: the Diabcare Africa study," *Diabetes Research and Clinical Practice*, vol. 95, no. 1, pp. 30–36, 2012.

[30] A. Camara, N. M. Baldé, J. Sobngwi-Tambekou et al., "Poor glycemic control in type 2 diabetes in the south of the Sahara: the issue of limited access to an HbA1c test," *Diabetes Research and Clinical Practice*, vol. 108, no. 1, pp. 187–192, 2015.

[31] T. J. Allain, J. J. van Oosterhout, G. P. Douglas et al., "Applying lessons learnt from the 'DOTS' tuberculosis model to monitoring and evaluating persons with diabetes mellitus in Blantyre, Malawi," *Tropical Medicine & International Health*, vol. 16, no. 9, pp. 1077–1084, 2011.

[32] R. Wood, V. Viljoen, L. Van Der Merwe, and R. Mash, "Quality of care for patients with non-communicable diseases in the Dedza District, Malawi," *African Journal of Primary Health Care & Family Medicine*, vol. 7, no. 1, p. 8, 2015.

[33] A. Sobry, W. Kizito, R. Van den Bergh et al., "Caseload, management and treatment outcomes of patients with hypertension and/or diabetes mellitus in a primary health care programme in an informal setting," *Tropical Medicine & International Health*, vol. 19, no. 1, pp. 47–57, 2014.

[34] S. D. Pastakia, S. M. Ali, J. H. Kamano et al., "Screening for diabetes and hypertension in a rural low income setting in western Kenya utilizing home-based and community-based strategies," *Globalization and Health*, vol. 9, no. 1, p. 21, 2013.

[35] K. Wambui Charity, A. M. V. Kumar, S. G. Hinderaker, P. Chinnakali, S. D. Pastakia, and J. Kamano, "Do diabetes mellitus patients adhere to self-monitoring of blood glucose (SMBG) and is this associated with glycemic control? Experiences from a SMBG program in western Kenya," *Diabetes Research and Clinical Practice*, vol. 112, pp. 37–43, 2016.

[36] S. D. Pastakia, S. M. Manyara, R. Vedanthan et al., "Impact of bridging income generation with group integrated care (BIGPIC) on hypertension and diabetes in rural western Kenya," *Journal of General Internal Medicine*, vol. 32, no. 5, pp. 540–548, 2017.

[37] D. Katende, G. Mutungi, K. Baisley et al., "Readiness of Ugandan health services for the management of outpatients with chronic diseases," *Tropical Medicine & International Health*, vol. 20, no. 10, pp. 1385–1395, 2015.

[38] S. R. Whyte, S. J. Park, G. Odong, M. Ojara, and A. Lamwaka, "The visibility of non-communicable diseases in Northern Uganda," *African Health Sciences*, vol. 15, no. 1, pp. 82–89, 2015.

[39] K. Nyarko, D. K. Ameme, D. Ocansey, E. Commeh, M. T. Markwei, and S. A. Ohene, "Capacity assessment of selected health care facilities for the pilot implementation of package for essential non-communicable diseases (PEN) intervention in Ghana," *Pan African Medical Journal*, vol. 25, Supplement 1, p. 16, 2016.

[40] R. Peck, J. Mghamba, F. Vanobberghen et al., "Preparedness of Tanzanian health facilities for outpatient primary care of hypertension and diabetes: a cross-sectional survey," *The Lancet Global Health*, vol. 2, no. 5, pp. e285–e292, 2014.

[41] C. Leung, E. Aris, A. Mhalu et al., "Preparedness of HIV care and treatment clinics for the management of concomitant non-communicable diseases: a cross-sectional survey," *BMC Public Health*, vol. 16, no. 1, p. 1002, 2016.

[42] D. Beran, C. Silva Matos, and J. S. Yudkin, "The Diabetes UK Mozambique twinning programme. Results of improvements in diabetes care in Mozambique: a reassessment 6 years later using the rapid assessment protocol for insulin access," *Diabetic Medicine*, vol. 27, no. 8, pp. 855–861, 2010.

[43] I. Katz, H. Schneider, Z. Shezi et al., "Managing type 2 diabetes in Soweto-the South African chronic disease outreach program experience," *Primary Care Diabetes*, vol. 3, no. 3, pp. 157–164, 2009.

[44] K. B. Khabala, J. K. Edwards, B. Baruani et al., "Medication adherence clubs: a potential solution to managing large numbers of stable patients with multiple chronic diseases in informal settlements," *Tropical Medicine & International Health*, vol. 20, no. 10, pp. 1265–1270, 2015.

[45] J. O. Mekong, A. P. Kengne, M. Y. Dehayem, E. Sobngwi, and J. C. Mbanya, "Cardiovascular preventative therapies and outcomes of care among urban sub-Saharan Africans with type 2 diabetes: a cross-sectional study in Cameroon," *Journal of Clinical Outcomes Management*, vol. 19, no. 10, pp. 446–452, 2012.

[46] M. Justin-Temu, R. S. Nondo, K. Wiedenmayer, K. L. Ramaiya, and A. Teuscher, "Anti-diabetic drugs in the private and public sector in Dar es Salaam, Tanzania," *East African Medical Journal*, vol. 86, no. 3, pp. 110–114, 2009.

[47] J. Kratzer, "Structural barriers to coping with type 1 diabetes mellitus in Ghana: experiences of diabetic youth and their families," *Ghana Medical Journal*, vol. 46, no. 2, Supplement, pp. 39–45, 2012.

[48] I. L. Okoronkwo, J. N. Ekpemiro, E. U. Okwor, P. U. Okpala, and F. O. Adeyemo, "Economic burden and catastrophic cost among people living with type2 diabetes mellitus attending a tertiary health institution in south-east zone, Nigeria," *BMC Research Notes*, vol. 8, no. 1, p. 527, 2015.

[49] I. L. Okoronkwo, J. N. Ekpemiro, O. E. Onwujekwe, A. C. Nwaneri, and P. N. Iheanacho, "Socioeconomic inequities and payment coping mechanisms used in the treatment of type 2 diabetes mellitus in Nigeria," *Nigerian Journal of Clinical Practice*, vol. 19, no. 1, pp. 104–109, 2016.

[50] S. L. Marshall, D. V. Edidin, V. C. Arena et al., "Glucose control in Rwandan youth with type 1 diabetes following establishment of systematic, HbA1c based, care and education," *Diabetes Research and Clinical Practice*, vol. 107, no. 1, pp. 113–122, 2015.

[51] F. Verbeke, T. Hategekimana, G. Karara et al., "Information systems for monitoring the burden of chronic diseases in public reference health facilities in Rwanda, Burundi and eastern DRC," *Rwanda Medical Journal*, vol. 70, no. 1, pp. 26–30, 2013.

[52] S. D. Pastakia, R. Karwa, C. B. Kahn, and J. S. Nyabundi, "The evolution of diabetes care in the rural, resource-constrained setting of western Kenya," *The Annals of Pharmacotherapy*, vol. 45, no. 6, pp. 721–6, 2011.

[53] J. Fadare, M. Olamoyegun, and B. A. Gbadegesin, "Medication adherence and direct treatment cost among diabetes patients attending a tertiary healthcare facility in Ogbomosho, Nigeria," *Malawi Medical Journal*, vol. 27, no. 2, pp. 65–70, 2015.

[54] R. BeLue, K. Ndiaye, F. NDao, F. N. N. Ba, and M. Diaw, "Glycemic control in a clinic-based sample of diabetics in M'Bour Senegal," *Health Education & Behavior*, vol. 43, no. 1, Supplement, pp. 112S–116S, 2016.

[55] O. Alebiosu et al., "Original research: knowledge of diabetes and hypertension care among health care workers in southwest Nigeria," *Postgraduate Medicine*, vol. 121, no. 1, pp. 173–177, 2009.

[56] P. O. Erah and H. I. Eroje, "Prescribing of antidiabetic medicines to older diabetes type 2 patients in Lagos, Nigeria," *Nigerian Quarterly Journal of Hospital Medicine*, vol. 23, no. 1, pp. 12–16, 2013.

[57] A. M. Jingi, J. R. Nansseu, and J. J. Noubiap, "Primary care physicians' practice regarding diabetes mellitus diagnosis, evaluation and management in the West region of Cameroon," *BMC Endocrine Disorders*, vol. 15, no. 1, p. 18, 2015.

[58] R. W. Mayega, D. Guwatudde, F. E. Makumbi et al., "Comparison of fasting plasma glucose and haemoglobin A1c point-of-care tests in screening for diabetes and abnormal glucose regulation in a rural low income setting," *Diabetes Research and Clinical Practice*, vol. 104, no. 1, pp. 112–120, 2014.

[59] R. Joshi, M. Alim, A. P. Kengne et al., "Task shifting for non-communicable disease management in low and middle income countries – a systematic review," *PLoS One*, vol. 9, no. 8, article e103754, 2014.

[60] R. M. Scheffler, J. X. Liu, Y. Kinfu, and M. R. Dal Poz, "Forecasting the global shortage of physicians: an economic- and needs-based approach," *Bulletin of the World Health Organization*, vol. 86, no. 7, pp. 516–523, 2008.

[61] L. R. Fairall, N. Folb, V. Timmerman et al., "Educational outreach with an integrated clinical tool for nurse-led non-communicable chronic disease management in primary care in South Africa: a pragmatic cluster randomised controlled trial," *PLoS Medicine*, vol. 13, no. 11, article e1002178, 2016.

[62] A. Leke, C. Portwood, and M. Maboh, "Diabetes management: student nurses contribute using point-of-care testing," *Medical Education*, vol. 47, no. 11, p. 1122, 2013.

[63] E. P. Davila, Z. Suleiman, J. Mghamba et al., "Non-communicable disease training for public health workers in low- and middle-income countries: lessons learned from a pilot training in Tanzania," *International Health*, vol. 7, no. 5, pp. 339–347, 2015.

[64] D. Some, J. K. Edwards, T. Reid et al., "Task shifting the management of non-communicable diseases to nurses in Kibera, Kenya: does it work?," *PLoS One*, vol. 11, no. 1, article e0145634, 2016.

[65] S. I. Bello, K. A. Ganiyu, Y. O. Dakop, and P. O. Erah, "Pharmacist's intervention in the control of blood sugar levels in randomised diabetes patients at a primary health care setting in Benin City," *Nigerian Quarterly Journal of Hospital Medicine*, vol. 22, no. 4, pp. 245–248, 2012.

[66] N. D. Labhardt, J. R. Balo, M. Ndam, E. Manga, and B. Stoll, "Improved retention rates with low-cost interventions in hypertension and diabetes management in a rural African environment of nurse-led care: a cluster-randomised trial," *Tropical Medicine & International Health*, vol. 16, no. 10, pp. 1276–1284, 2011.

[67] D. Govindasamy, K. Kranzer, N. van Schaik et al., "Linkage to HIV, TB and non-communicable disease care from a mobile testing unit in Cape Town, South Africa," *PLoS One*, vol. 8, no. 11, article e80017, 2013.

[68] J. Van Olmen, M. Van Pelt, B. Malombo et al., "Process evaluation of a mobile health intervention for people with diabetes in low income countries – the implementation of the TEXT4DSM study," *Journal of Telemedicine and Telecare*, vol. 23, no. 1, pp. 96–105, 2017.

[69] S. O. Iwuala, M. A. Olamoyegun, A. A. Sabir, and O. A. Fasanmade, "The relationship between self-monitoring of blood glucose and glycaemic control among patients attending an urban diabetes clinic in Nigeria," *Annals of African Medicine*, vol. 14, no. 4, pp. 182–187, 2015.

[70] J. Claude Mbanya, P. Aschner, J. C. N. Chan, J. Jose Gagliardino, and J. Saji, "Self-monitoring of blood glucose (SMBG) and glycaemic control in Cameroon: results of the international diabetes management practices study (IDMPS)," *Diabetes Research and Clinical Practice*, vol. 126, pp. 198–201, 2017.

[71] D. N. Adjei, C. Agyemang, J. B. Dasah, P. Kuranchie, and A. G. B. Amoah, "The effect of electronic reminders on risk management among diabetic patients in low resourced settings," *Journal of Diabetes and its Complications*, vol. 29, no. 6, pp. 818–821, 2015.

[72] F. K. Assah, E. N. Atanga, S. Enoru, E. Sobngwi, and J. C. Mbanya, "Community-based peer support significantly improves metabolic control in people with type 2 diabetes in Yaoundé, Cameroon," *Diabetic Medicine*, vol. 32, no. 7, pp. 886–889, 2015.

[73] M. Y. Dehayem, R. Takogue, S. P. Choukem et al., "Impact of a pioneer diabetes camp experience on glycemic control among children and adolescents living with type 1 diabetes in sub-Saharan Africa," *BMC Endocrine Disorders*, vol. 16, no. 1, p. 5, 2016.

[74] A. Klisiewicz and F. Raal, "Sub-optimal management of type 2 diabetes mellitus—a local audit," *Metabolism and Diabetes of South Africa*, vol. 14, no. 1, pp. 13–16, 2009.

[75] M. E. Kruk, A. Jakubowski, M. Rabkin, B. Elul, M. Friedman, and W. El-Sadr, "PEPFAR programs linked to more deliveries in health facilities by African women who are not infected with HIV," *Health Affairs*, vol. 31, no. 7, pp. 1478–1488, 2012.

[76] G. Chamie, D. Kwarisiima, T. D. Clark et al., "Leveraging rapid community-based HIV testing campaigns for non-communicable diseases in rural Uganda," *PLoS One*, vol. 7, no. 8, article e43400, 2012.

[77] Search Collaboration, "Evaluating the feasibility and uptake of a community-led HIV testing and multi-disease health campaign in rural Uganda," *Journal of the International AIDS Society*, vol. 20, no. 1, article 21514, 2017.

[78] J. O. Adeleye, N. O. Agada, W. O. Balogun, O. R. Adetunji, and H. O. Onyegbutulem, "Diabetes care in Nigeria: time for a paradigm shift," *African Journal of Medicine and Medical Sciences*, vol. 35, no. 2, pp. 155–159, 2006.

[79] A. D. Harries, A. Jahn, R. Zachariah, and D. Enarson, "Adapting the DOTS framework for tuberculosis control to the management of non-communicable diseases in sub-Saharan Africa," *PLoS Medicine*, vol. 5, no. 6, article e124, 2008.

[80] K. G. Shojania, S. R. Ranji, K. M. McDonald et al., "Effects of quality improvement strategies for type 2 diabetes on glycemic control: a meta-regression analysis," *JAMA*, vol. 296, no. 4, pp. 427–440, 2006.

[81] L. J. Trump and T. J. Mendenhall, "Community health workers in diabetes care: A systematic review of randomized controlled trials," *Families, Systems & Heatlh*, vol. 35, no. 3, pp. 320–340, 2017.

19

Gene Expression Profiling Identifies Downregulation of the Neurotrophin-MAPK Signaling Pathway in Female Diabetic Peripheral Neuropathy Patients

Lin Luo,[1] Wen-Hua Zhou,[2] Jiang-Jia Cai,[1] Mei Feng,[3] Mi Zhou,[3] Su-Pei Hu,[4] Jin Xu,[1,3] and Lin-Dan Ji[1,5]

[1]*Zhejiang Key Laboratory of Pathophysiology, Medical School of Ningbo University, Ningbo 315211, China*
[2]*Laboratory of Behavioral Neuroscience, Ningbo Addiction Research and Treatment Center, Medical School of Ningbo University, Ningbo 315211, China*
[3]*Department of Preventive Medicine, Medical School of Ningbo University, Ningbo 315211, China*
[4]*Department of Research and Teaching, Ningbo No. 2 Hospital, Ningbo 315010, China*
[5]*Department of Biochemistry, Medical School of Ningbo University, Ningbo 315211, China*

Correspondence should be addressed to Jin Xu; xujin1@nbu.edu.cn and Lin-Dan Ji; jilindan@nbu.edu.cn

Academic Editor: Joseph F. Ndisang

Diabetic peripheral neuropathy (DPN) is a common complication of diabetes mellitus (DM). It is not diagnosed or managed properly in the majority of patients because its pathogenesis remains controversial. In this study, human whole genome microarrays identified 2898 and 4493 differentially expressed genes (DEGs) in DM and DPN patients, respectively. A further KEGG pathway analysis indicated that DPN and DM share four pathways, including apoptosis, B cell receptor signaling pathway, endocytosis, and Toll-like receptor signaling pathway. The DEGs identified through comparison of DPN and DM were significantly enriched in MAPK signaling pathway, NOD-like receptor signaling pathway, and neurotrophin signaling pathway, while the "neurotrophin-MAPK signaling pathway" was notably downregulated. Seven DEGs from the neurotrophin-MAPK signaling pathway were validated in additional 78 samples, and the results confirmed the initial microarray findings. These findings demonstrated that downregulation of the neurotrophin-MAPK signaling pathway may be the major mechanism of DPN pathogenesis, thus providing a potential approach for DPN treatment.

1. Introduction

Diabetes mellitus (DM) has become one of the largest global public health problems of this century. According to the World Health Organization global report on diabetes, over 8.5% of the global population, approximately 422 million adults, have diabetes [1]. Diabetes of all types can lead to complications in many parts of the body and can increase the overall risk of premature death. Potential complications include cardiomyopathy, vasculopathy, neuropathy, retinopathy, nephropathy, dermatopathy, and encephalopathy [2, 3]. Diabetic peripheral neuropathy (DPN) is characterized as a chronic symmetrical, progressive disorder with early symptoms of pain, allodynia, and paresthesia, and it affects approximately 50% of people with considerable morbidity, mortality, and diminished quality of life [4]. Despite the development of diagnostic methods and therapeutic modalities, DPN is still not diagnosed or managed properly in most patients [5].

Over the past decade, there have been many achievements in understanding the pathogenesis of DPN. However, controversy remains because of a multifactorial etiology involving both metabolic and vascular factors [6]. Chronic hyperglycemia used to be regarded as the major factor in the initiation of various metabolic events underlying DPN. Results from the Diabetes Control and Complication Trial

(DCCT) support the hypothesis that DPN develops as a result of increased blood glucose and have suggested that treating hyperglycemia in type 1 DM can markedly decrease the incidence of DPN, by up to 60 to 70% [7]. However, more recent studies have reported that intensive glucose control in patients with type 2 DM has no significant effect on the development of DPN [8]. Over 40% of type 2 DM patients develop DPN despite good glucose control, thus suggesting that hyperglycemia is only one of the many key events that cause nerve and microvascular injury [9]. Nevertheless, hyperglycemia has effects on several major, well-characterized biochemical pathways that include activation of the polyol pathway [10], formation of advanced glycation end products (AGEs) and their receptors [11], activation of protein kinase C (PKC) [12] and inducible nitric oxide synthase [13], increased poly(ADP-ribose) polymerase (PARP) activity [14], and elevated inflammation [15]. Furthermore, oxidative stress and mitochondrial dysfunction [16], hypoxia and ischemia [17], elevated cytokines [18], and deficiencies in neurotrophic factors [19] also play significant etiologic roles in DPN. Despite advances in delineating the etiology of DPN, few effective therapies exist to manage, delay, or prevent the development of painful DPN. Therefore, identifying precise mechanisms and related therapeutic drugs remains paramount.

Systems biology approaches, such as whole genome expression profiling, may provide new insights into the molecular mechanisms of DPN without preset bias. However, previous studies have identified global transcriptomic changes only in animal models [20]. In the present study, we used high-throughput genome-wide expression microarrays to identify alterations in the transcriptome, both common and distinct, between type 2 DM and DPN. The results may provide relevant information for the future development of new mechanism-based diagnostics and therapies.

2. Material and Methods

2.1. Study Design. A workflow was designed to identify candidate genes whose expression levels may differentiate among healthy controls (CN), DM patients, and DPN patients (Figure 1). After obtaining three individual differentially expressed gene (DEG) datasets (DM versus CN, DPN versus CN, and DPN versus DM), we used a Venn diagram to identify the shared and distinct gene expression changes between DPN and DM. Subsequently, several gene annotation databases were used to identify the potential biological functions and signaling pathways involved in DPN. Finally, DEGs of interest were further validated in an independent sample set.

2.2. Participants. The participants were recruited from hospitals affiliated with Ningbo University from April 2015 to June 2016. The healthy controls had no family history of diabetes or neurologic disorders, exhibited normal glucose tolerance, and were free of any major chronic diseases. Type 2 DM cases were defined as meeting at least one of the following criteria: fasting plasma glucose ≥ 7 mmol/L, 2 h plasma glucose after oral glucose tolerance test (OGTT) ≥ 11.1 mmol/L, and use of glucose-lowering drugs or physician-diagnosed diabetes. Diabetic peripheral neuropathy was diagnosed by a positive assessment through neurologic examinations and nerve conduction studies, as previously described [20]. In brief, the criteria for DPN were as follows: (1) confirmed type 2 DM patients; (2) decreased sensation and positive neuropathic sensory symptoms (including pricking, burning, stabbing, or aching pain) in the toes, feet, or legs; (3) decreased distal sensation and unequivocally decreased or absent ankle reflexes; (4) and abnormal motor and sensory nerve conduction. Patients with type 1 DM, cardiovascular diseases, previous history of neurologic disorders, peripheral vascular occlusive disease, autoimmune disease, or any other possible causes of peripheral neuropathy were excluded from all groups. Patients with any clinically observable diabetic complications were excluded from the DM group. The DPN patients involved in the present study were all new cases without any antineuropathy medication. Patients with any other major acute or chronic complication associated with diabetes or vitamin B12/folic acid deficiencies were excluded from the DPN group. The protocol of this study was approved by the medical ethics committee of Ningbo University. The health records and blood samples (2 mL) of the participants were collected after informed written consents were provided by the subjects. A total of 6 healthy controls, 6 DM patients, and 6 DPN patients were recruited for the microarray analysis. In the validation stage, another 26 healthy controls, 26 DM patients, and 26 DPN patients were included. An overview of the clinical and demographic characteristics of the participants can be found in Table 1.

2.3. RNA Preparation. Total RNA was isolated from peripheral blood mononuclear cells (PBMCs) by using a TaKaRa MiniBEST Universal RNA Extraction Kit according to the manufacturer's instructions. The RNA quality was determined on the basis of an optical density (OD) 260/280 ratio ≥ 1.8 and OD260/230 ratio ≥ 2.0 using a NanoDrop ND-1000 spectrophotometer. RNA integrity was determined using an Agilent 2100 Bioanalyzer. The intensity of the 18S and 28S rRNA bands was examined on a 1% formaldehyde-agarose gel. RNA samples with an RNA integrity number (RIN) of ≥ 6.0 and 28S/18S > 1.5 were subjected to microarray analysis.

2.4. Microarray Analysis. The microarray analysis was performed by BGI Inc., including RNA amplification, probe labeling, hybridization, and data extraction. Briefly, aliquots (100 ng) of total RNA were amplified and transcribed into fluorescent Cy5-labeled antisense RNAs (aRNAs) by using a OneArray Amino Allyl aRNA Amplification Kit (Phalanx Biotech, San Diego, CA) according to the manufacturer's instructions. The Cy5-labeled aRNAs were fragmented and then hybridized to the Human Whole Genome OneArray Version 6.0 (Phalanx Biotech, San Diego, CA). Nonspecific binding targets were washed out three times. The arrays were scanned by an Agilent G2505C Microarray Scanner (Agilent Technologies, Wilmington, DE). The fluorescence intensities of each spot were analyzed with Feature Extraction software

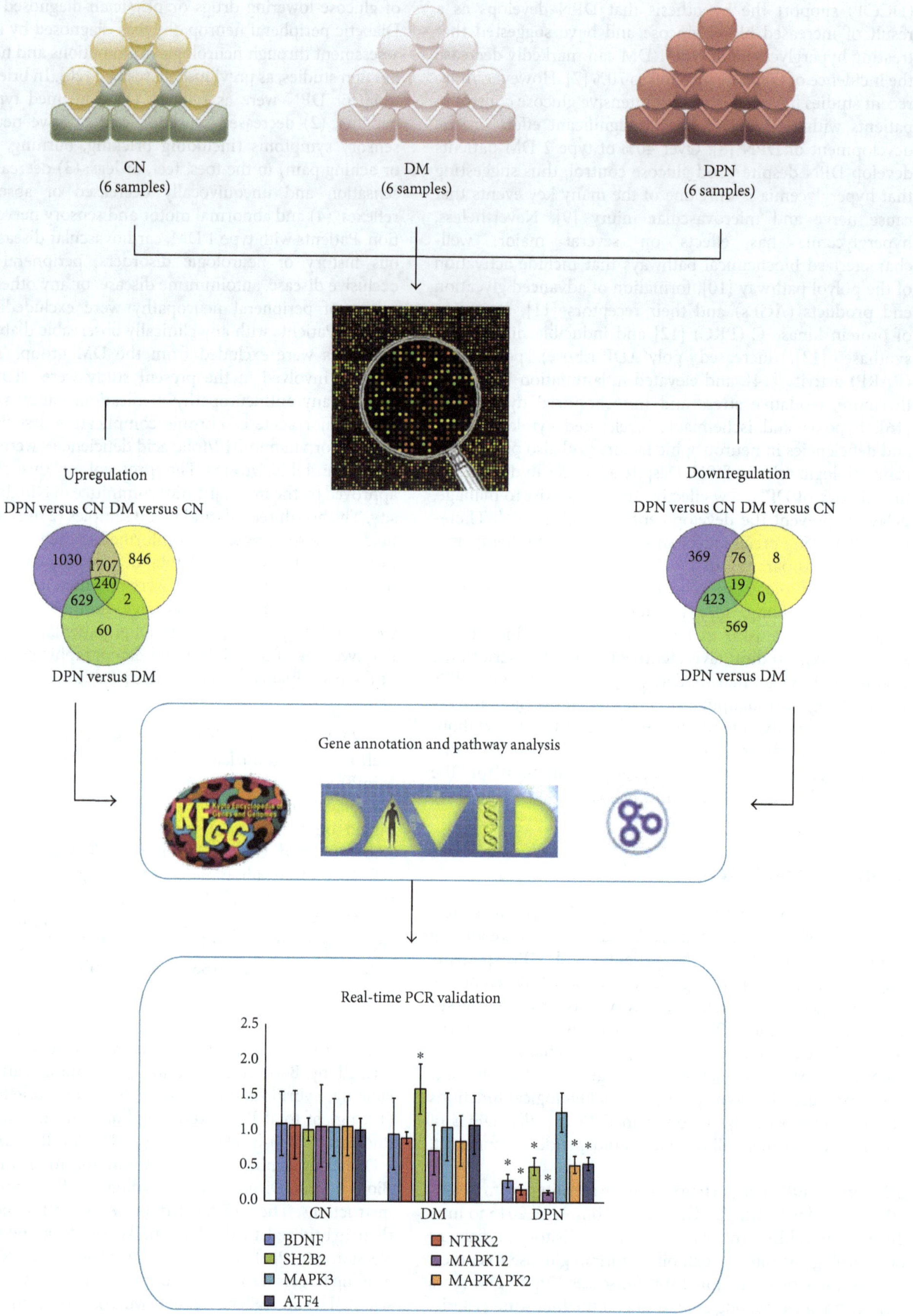

Figure 1: The workflow of the study. The asterisks represent statistical significance ($P < 0.05$) compared with the control group.

Table 1: Clinical and demographic characteristics of the participants.

	Control	T2DM	DPN
Discovery panel			
Number	6	6	6
Gender	Female	Female	Female
Age (y)	51.17 ± 6.08	53.83 ± 10.80	57.33 ± 7.92
Fasting glucose (mmol/L)	5.10 ± 0.21	9.23 ± 2.02*	9.95 ± 2.11*
Validation panel			
Number	26	26	26
Gender	Female	Female	Female
Age (y)	50.91 ± 5.60	51.25 ± 8.13	53.21 ± 11.15
Fasting glucose (mmol/L)	5.27 ± 0.59	8.96 ± 1.58*	9.72 ± 1.81*

The asterisks represent statistical significance ($P < 0.05$) compared with the control group.

(Agilent Technologies, Wilmington, DE). Overall, 18 microarray chips were analyzed in this study.

2.5. Statistical Analysis of the Microarray Data. The microarray data were normalized using the R/Bioconductor Limma package [21]. An empirical Bayes model was used to compare DEGs between groups, and the criteria for DEGs were FDR < 0.05 and $|\log_2 \text{(ratio)}| \geq 1$. Hierarchical clustering was performed to visualize distinguishable gene expression profiles among the samples. The gene annotation and biological interpretation of the identified DEGs were performed using the Database for Annotation, Visualization, and Integrated Discovery (DAVID) v6.8 [22]. Biological functions, represented by Gene Ontology terms (http://geneontology.org/) and Kyoto Encyclopedia of Genes and Genomes pathways (http://genome.jp/kegg/), were deemed significant at a Benjamini-Hochberg-corrected $P < 0.05$. The R/Bioconductor Pathview package was used for pathway-based gene data integration and visualization [23].

2.6. Quantitative Real-Time PCR (qRT-PCR). Seven representative genes selected from DEGs involved in the neurotrophin-MAPK signaling pathway were validated by qRT-PCR in another 26 independent samples from each group (CN, DM, and DPN). Total RNA was extracted as described above, and double-stranded cDNA was synthesized using a PrimeScript RT Reagent Kit (TaKaRa Biotechnology, Dalian, China) according to the manufacturer's instructions. Real-time PCR was performed using LightCycler 480 SYBR Green I Master mix (Roche, Mannheim, Germany). The $2^{-\Delta\Delta CT}$ method was used to quantify the relative expression of each gene, using GAPDH expression to normalize each sample. All experiments were run in triplicate and repeated three times. Differences in expression among groups were evaluated with a one-way analysis of variance (ANOVA) using SPSS 16.0 software. A significant difference was considered to be indicated by $P < 0.05$.

Table 2: Number of differentially expressed genes in different groups.

	DM versus CN	DPN versus CN	DPN versus DM
Upregulated	2795	3606	931
Downregulated	103	887	1011

3. Results

3.1. Identification of DEGs among DM Patients, DPN Patients, and Healthy Controls. The gene expression data from this study are available in the Gene Expression Omnibus (GEO, accession number GSE95849). Compared with healthy individuals, patients with DM and DPN exhibited 2795 and 3606 upregulated genes, respectively, whereas 103 genes and 887 genes were expressed at a lower level in DM and DPN patients compared with the healthy controls (Table 2). Among these DEGs, DM and DPN patients shared 1947 upregulated and 95 downregulated genes. In DPN patients, compared with DM patients, 1942 genes were differentially expressed, including 931 upregulated and 1011 downregulated genes (Table 2).

3.2. Functional Annotation and Enrichment Analysis of the DEGs. According to the GO analysis, the DEGs of DM and DPN patients were enriched in many similar GO terms as well as distinct GO terms (Figure 2). Compared with the profile of healthy controls, the DM-associated gene expression profile primarily included DEGs related to intracellular transport, immune response, cell activation, protein localization, and inflammatory response (Figure 2(a)). The DPN patients exhibited differential expression of genes involved in protein transport, protein localization, leukocyte activation, immune response, protein kinase cascades, and cell death (Figure 2(b)). Between the DPN and DM group, the differentially expressed genes were enriched in cell activation, cellular response to stress, and cell death as well as in the regulation of transcription and translation (Figure 2(c)).

KEGG pathway analysis revealed that, in comparison with healthy controls, DPN and DM shared four pathways (Table 2), including apoptosis (hsa04210), B cell receptor signaling pathway (hsa04662), endocytosis (hsa04144), and Toll-like receptor signaling pathway (hsa04620). Moreover, Fc gamma R-mediated phagocytosis (hsa04666), chemokine signaling pathway (hsa04062), and insulin signaling pathway (hsa04910) were enriched in the DM group, and NOD-like receptor signaling pathway (hsa04621), lysosome (hsa04142), valine, leucine and isoleucine degradation (hsa00280), and amino sugar and nucleotide sugar metabolism (hsa00520) were enriched in the DPN group. In contrast, for DEGs between DPN and DM patients, the most enriched pathway was MAPK signaling pathway (hsa04010), followed by NOD-like receptor signaling pathway (hsa04621) and neurotrophin signaling pathway (hsa04722). For the gene set lists of these three pathways, see electronic Supplementary Table 1 available online at https://doi.org/10.1155/2017/8103904. When the DEGs identified between DPN and DM patients were further

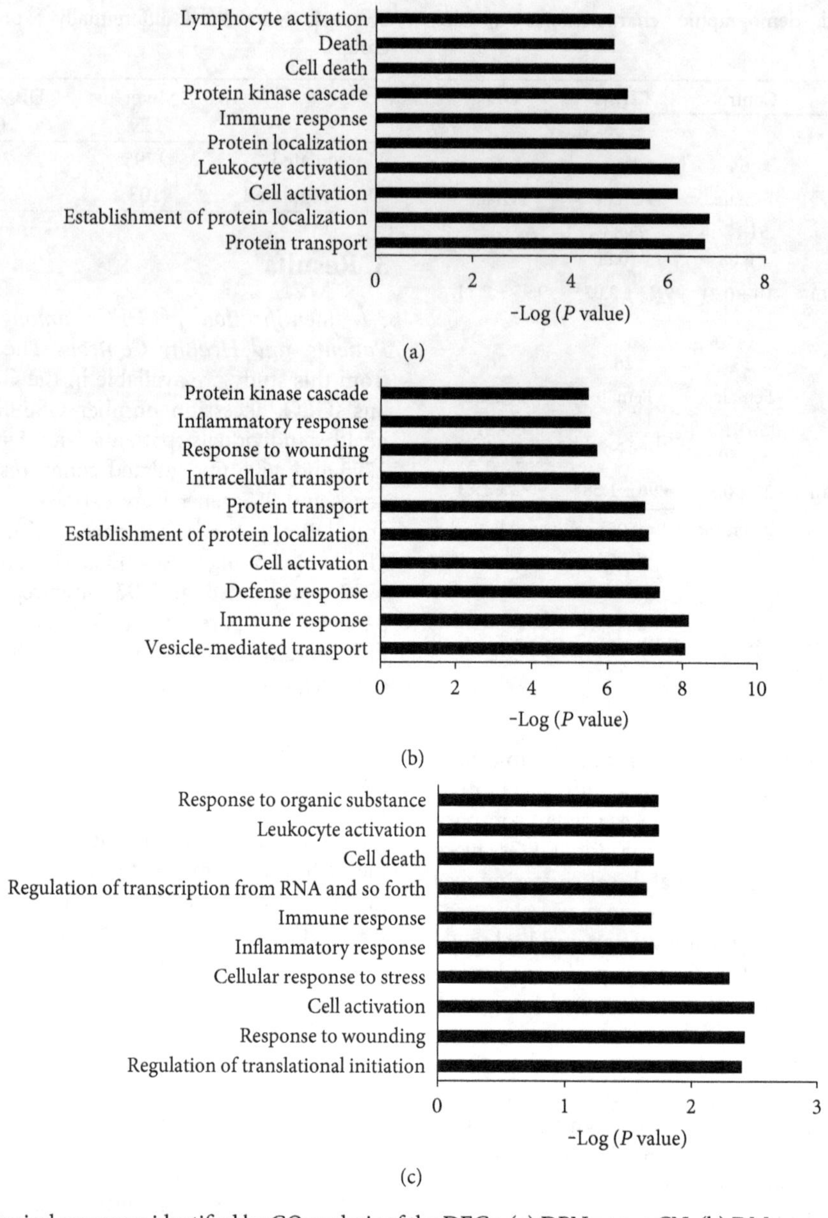

FIGURE 2: The top 10 biological processes identified by GO analysis of the DEGs: (a) DPN versus CN, (b) DM versus CN, and (c) DPN versus DM. Bars represent −log (*P* value).

analyzed with regard to upregulation and downregulation, the upregulated genes were enriched in the infectious disease category, whereas the downregulated genes were enriched in the "neurotrophin signaling pathway" and "MAPK signaling pathway" (Table 3). A KEGG Pathview analysis also showed that downregulation of the neurotrophin-MAPK signaling pathway was the major pathogenesic pathway in diabetic peripheral neuropathy patients (Figure 3).

3.3. Validation of DEGs in the Neurotrophin-MAPK Signaling Pathway. Seven DEGs selected from the "neurotrophin-MAPK signaling pathway" were further validated in an additional 78 participants by qRT-PCR. These genes are *BDNF* (brain-derived neurotrophic factor), *NTRK2* (neurotrophic tyrosine kinase type 2 receptor, also known as TrkB), *SH2B2* (SH2B adaptor protein 2, also known as rAPS), *MAPK3* (mitogen-activated protein kinase 3, also known as Erk), *MAPK12* (mitogen-activated protein kinase 12, also known as p38), *MAPKAPK2* (mitogen-activated protein kinase-activated protein kinase 2), and *ATF4* (activating transcription factor 4, also known as CREB). The results confirmed the initial microarray findings for all of the genes except *MAPK3*, whose expression was not changed in DM patients or in DPN patients (Figure 4).

4. Discussion

DPN is the most common complication of diabetes, affecting up to 50% of patients, and it contributes significantly to pain, loss of sensation, numbness, injury, and lower extremity amputation [4]. Because complex pathways are implicated in the pathophysiology of DPN, there are still no specific

Table 3: The significant KEGG pathways for the DEGs of DPN versus DM.

	KEGG pathway	Count	Benjamini q value
Upregulated	hsa05164: influenza A	25	0.001
	hsa05162: measles	21	0.001
	hsa00020: citrate cycle (TCA cycle)	9	0.008
	hsa05168: herpes simplex infection	23	0.009
Downregulated	hsa04722: neurotrophin signaling pathway	21	0.001
	hsa04010: MAPK signaling pathway	31	0.003
	hsa04668: TNF signaling pathway	18	0.003
	hsa04380: osteoclast differentiation	20	0.003
	hsa05169: Epstein-Barr virus infection	25	0.003
	hsa05166: HTLV-I infection	30	0.003
	hsa04660: T cell receptor signaling pathway	16	0.010
	hsa05215: prostate cancer	14	0.020
	hsa05142: Chagas disease (American trypanosomiasis)	15	0.029
	hsa05145: toxoplasmosis	16	0.031
	hsa04068: FoxO signaling pathway	17	0.039
	hsa04064: NF-kappa B signaling pathway	13	0.039
	hsa04621: NOD-like receptor signaling pathway	10	0.040

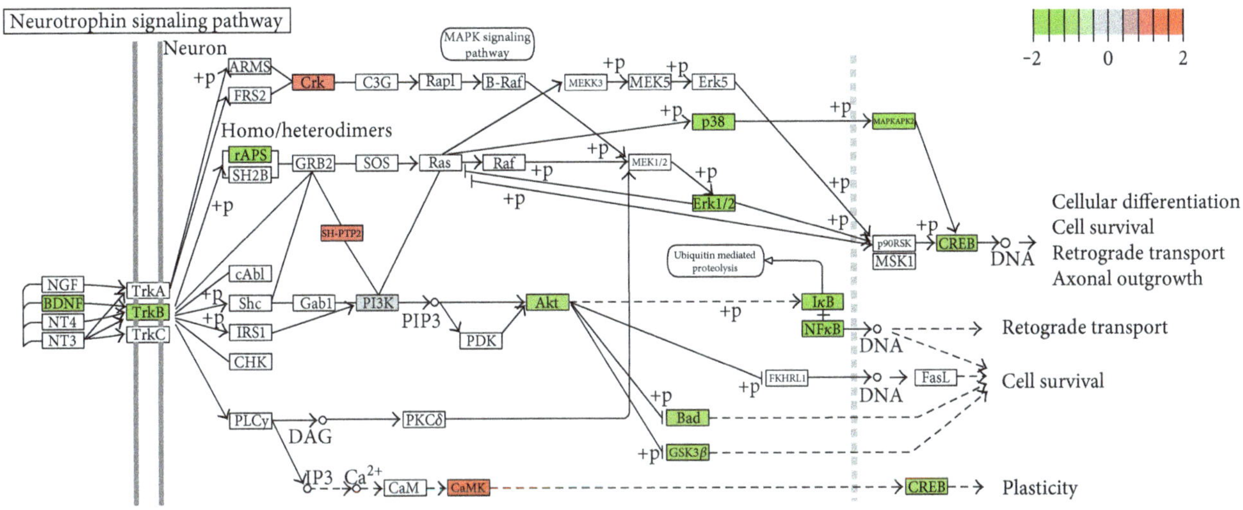

Figure 3: Downregulation of the neurotrophin-MAPK signaling pathway in DPN.

treatments and no means of predicting or preventing DPN onset or progression. Gene expression microarrays have been widely used in diabetic studies, because alterations in transcriptional profiles provide a robust and sensitive way to better understand the mechanisms of the disease and its complications. Microarray analyses have previously been used to investigate the mechanisms underlying diabetic cardiomyopathy [24], diabetic nephropathy [25], diabetic bone disease [26], and diabetic periodontitis [27] in diabetic patients or animal models. However, only one study has been conducted in patients with diabetic neuropathy to identify the DEGs and the related biological pathways responsible for the progression of diabetic neuropathy [28]. That study comprised a microarray experiment performed on human sural nerves collected from 50 patients with diabetic neuropathy during a 52-week clinical trial. Hyperglycemia may cause damage to the majority of the peripheral nerve system, not just the sural nerve. Moreover, as mentioned in that article, it is highly unlikely that future studies of diabetic neuropathy in patients will include the collection of sural nerve biopsies [28]. Therefore, performing new transcriptional microarray analyses with commonly used human sample material, such as PBMCs, to identify the gene expression signatures of DPN is necessary. Actually, transcriptome studies in PBMCs have been widely used in diabetic studies. Gene expression profiles in PBMCs can clinically stratify patients with recent-onset type 1 DM [29] and reflect the pathophysiology of type 2 DM [30]. In PBMCs from children with diabetes, the gene expression microarrays identified that type 1 and type 2 DM likely shared a common pathway for β-cell

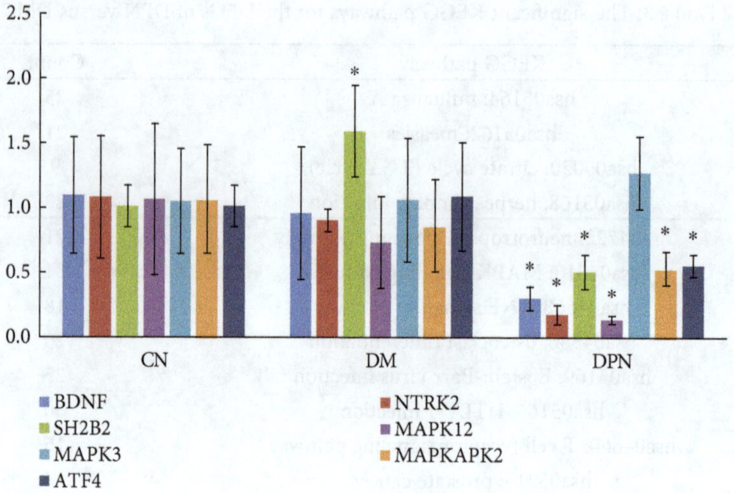

FIGURE 4: Microarray data were validated by qRT-PCR. The results are expressed as the mean ± SD. The asterisks represent statistical significance ($P < 0.05$) compared with the control group.

dysfunction that includes secretion of IL-1β and prostaglandins by immune effector cells [31]. Furthermore, a microarray study of gene expression in PBMCs identified that *THBS1* and *COX1* genes were upregulated, while *MMP9* and *COX2* genes were downregulated in patients with diabetic nephropathy [32].

The abovementioned microarray study on DPN identified DEGs that are functionally enriched in inflammatory responses and defense response pathways and may potentially be responsible for the progression of diabetic neuropathy [28]. In the current study, we found that DPN and DM shared four pathways, at least two of which were directly associated with immune-related functions, the "B cell receptor signaling pathway" and "Toll-like receptor signaling pathway." It is widely accepted that inflammation and immunity are crucially involved in diabetes and a majority of diabetic complications [33, 34]; therefore, changes in the immune response may not be a distinct mechanism of DPN. We further compared the expression profiles of DPN and DM patients and identified that DPN-specific DEGs were significantly enriched in "MAPK signaling pathway", "NOD-like receptor signaling pathway", and "neurotrophin signaling pathway". A stratification analysis further indicated that "neurotrophin signaling pathway" and "MAPK signaling pathway" were the top two pathways with downregulated DEGs. Although the DEGs in neurotrophin-MAPK signaling pathway are all located in autosome, caution should still be taken since only female subjects were involved in the present study, and more experiments are required to confirm it in male patients.

Neurotrophic factors are essential molecules that develop and maintain the nervous system by promoting the growth and survival of neurons. The neurotrophin family of growth factors includes nerve growth factor (NGF), brain-derived neurotrophic factor (BDNF), and neurotrophin- (NT-) 3/4/5. Glial cell-derived neurotrophic factors (GDNF) form a second family and include GDNF, neurturin, artemin, and persephin [35, 36]. Deficiencies in NGF and NT-3 have long been reported in both the tissue and sera of DPN patients. Diabetes also decreases the anterograde and retrograde axonal transport of BDNF, NGF, and NT-3 in peripheral nerves [37–39]. In the current study, the expression levels of NGF, NT-3, and NT-4 remained unchanged. However, the BDNF level decreased significantly. BDNF plays important roles in regulating the survival and growth of neurons and influences synaptic efficiency and plasticity. The human BDNF gene consists of 11 exons, and the majority of the BDNF transcripts are detected not only in the brain but also in blood cells [40]. BDNF mediates neuronal differentiation and survival by binding and activating tropomyosin receptor kinase B (TrkB), an important member of the larger Trk family [41]. In the current study, the *NTRK2* gene, which encodes TrkB in humans, was specifically downregulated in DPN patients but not in DM patients, thus strongly suggesting that downregulation of the BDNF-TrkB signaling pathway is associated with DPN.

The binding of BDNF to TrkB leads to the dimerization and autophosphorylation of tyrosine residues in the intracellular domain of the receptor [42], which in turn leads to phosphorylation of tyrosine residues in the juxtamembrane domain or the C-terminus of the receptor [43]. These tyrosine residues serve as docking sites for multiple adaptor molecules, including Shc adaptor proteins, fibroblast growth factor receptor substrate 2 (FRS2), phospholipase Cγ (PLCγ), SH2B adaptor proteins, ankyrin repeat-rich membrane spanning (ARMS), Csk homology kinase (CHK), insulin receptor substrate 1 (IRS1), and c-ABL1 [43]. Among these adaptor molecules, only the expression level of *SH2B2* (also known as rAPS) decreased in DPN patients, probably due to the downregulation of TrkB. TrkB activates three major intracellular signaling cascades: the mitogen-activated protein kinase (MAPK) pathway, phosphatidylinositol 3-kinase (PI3K)-Akt pathway, and the PLCγ-Ca^{2+} pathway [44]. However, in the current study, only the MAPK pathway was affected in DPN patients. Among the three major MAPK family members, the Erk1/2 and p38 pathways were found to be downregulated in our original microarray study. However, after

TABLE 4: Expression of TLR family genes.

Gene symbol	Log$_2$ (ratio) DM/CN	Log$_2$ (ratio) DPN/CN	Log$_2$ (ratio) DPN/DM	P value DM/CN	P value DPN/CN	P value DPN/DM
TLR1	1.744	2.033	0.289	4.40E−04	5.22E−05	0.516
TLR2	2.175	2.056	−0.119	9.34E−04	1.05E−05	0.818
TLR4	2.861	4.254	1.393	1.73E−05	5.71E−09	1.38E−02
TLR5	2.213	3.682	1.469	6.31E−03	2.55E−11	0.054
TLR6	2.908	2.169	−0.738	4.24E−05	5.15E−06	0.213
TLR7	1.677	3.475	1.799	1.44E−02	2.72E−09	6.67E−03
TLR8	2.041	2.785	0.745	1.31E−04	2.61E−06	0.109
TLR9	1.623	1.135	−0.488	3.37E−04	3.82E−04	0.232

TLR3 and *TLR10* were removed after data normalization because of the low fluorescent intensity of probes.

TABLE 5: The significant KEGG pathways for the DEGs of different groups.

	KEGG pathway	Count	Benjamini q value
DM	hsa04210: apoptosis	32	0.009
	hsa04620: Toll-like receptor signaling pathway	35	0.007
	hsa04144: endocytosis	53	0.014
	hsa04666: Fc gamma R-mediated phagocytosis	32	0.014
	hsa04062: chemokine signaling pathway	53	0.013
	hsa04662: B cell receptor signaling pathway	26	0.024
	hsa04910: insulin signaling pathway	39	0.044
DPN	hsa04662: B cell receptor signaling pathway	39	0.000
	hsa04210: apoptosis	40	0.004
	hsa04621: NOD-like receptor signaling pathway	31	0.004
	hsa04144: endocytosis	69	0.009
	hsa04620: Toll-like receptor signaling pathway	41	0.032
	hsa04142: lysosome	46	0.028
	hsa00280: valine, leucine, and isoleucine degradation	22	0.026
	hsa00520: amino sugar and nucleotide sugar metabolism	22	0.026
DPN versus DM	hsa04010: MAPK signaling pathway	53	0.001
	hsa04621: NOD-like receptor signaling pathway	18	0.016
	hsa04722: neurotrophin signaling pathway	27	0.029

qRT-PCR validation, only the expression level of p38 decreased. This result is actually reasonable, because the direct downstream target of p38, MAPKAPK2, was also downregulated, whereas the downstream targets of Erk1/2, MSK1, and p90RSK were unchanged.

In neuronal development and function, neurotrophins activate the p38 MAPK/MAPKAPK2 pathway through Trk receptor-mediated signaling mechanisms [45]. Subsequently, MAPKAPK2 phosphorylates CREB (cAMP response element binding protein) and other transcription factors [46]. These transcription factors in turn regulate the expression of genes whose products are involved in many aspects of neural development and function, including cell fate decisions, axon growth, dendrite pruning, synaptic function, and plasticity [45]. In the present study, 2898 genes exhibited altered expression in DM patients, whereas this number in DPN patients was 4493. Moreover, in DPN patients, compared with DM patients, the number of downregulated genes increased 7 times, possibly because of decreased CREB expression mediated by the downregulation of the neurotrophin-MAPK signaling pathway.

In addition to the "neurotrophin signaling pathway" and "MAPK signaling pathway," the present study also showed that the "NOD-like receptor signaling pathway" was affected in DPN patients. Nucleotide-binding oligomerization domain containing 2 (NOD2), a member of the NOD-like receptor family, has been found to be one of the critical components of a signal transduction pathway linking renal injury to inflammation and podocyte insulin resistance in diabetic nephropathy [47]. A recent study has also suggested that the formation and activation of the NOD-like receptor protein 1 (NLRP1) inflammasome induces neuroinflammation and neuron injury during hyperglycemia, thus representing a novel mechanism of diabetes-associated neuron injury [48]. Interestingly, our microarray data indicated that the expression of *NOD2* and *NLRP1* remained unchanged in DM patients but increased significantly in DPN patients (3.76-fold for *NOD2* and 2.07-fold for *NLRP1*). Therefore, the NOD-like receptor signaling pathway may be an important mechanism in the pathogenesis of diabetic complications.

It is now widely accepted that increased inflammation is a key etiological factor in the development of many chronic diseases, including diabetes [49]. Similar to Nod-like receptors, Toll-like receptors (TLRs) belong to another major family of pattern recognition receptors, which have been demonstrated to play a critical role in the innate immune system [50]. Among these TLRs, TLR4 plays an important role in many inflammatory disorders, and system inflammation facilitated by TLR4 is involved in the pathophysiological process of diabetes [51]. A recent study has further demonstrated that TLR4 may be a potential diagnostic biomarker for DPN [52]. In the current microarray study, *TLR4* expression increased in both DM and DPN patients, and there was even higher expression in the DPN patients (Table 4), in accordance with the results of the abovementioned study [52]. Moreover, it has been suggested that the inflammatory effects of high glucose may be mediated through the modulation of inflammatory responses resulting from TLR activation in diabetes [53]. The present microarray study showed that the "Toll-like receptor signaling pathway" was significantly enriched, and all TLR family genes were upregulated in both DPN and DM patients (Tables 4 and 5). These results strongly suggest that although some TLR genes, such as *TLR4* and *TLR7*, were expressed at much higher levels in DPN patients, they may not be sensitive biomarkers for DPN, because the TLR signaling pathway is involved in diabetes and multiple diabetic complications.

5. Conclusions

In summary, these findings provide the first demonstration that downregulation of the neurotrophin-MAPK signaling pathway may be the major pathogenesis of DPN. The use of growth factors in treating DPN has been extensively explored [54], and NGF, BDNF, and NT-3 have been assessed in various levels of clinical trials of DPN, with limited success [35]. The current study suggests that pharmacological targeting of both the neurotrophin signaling pathway and the MAPK signaling pathway at multiple levels may provide a potential approach for the treatment of DPN.

Abbreviations

BDNF: Brain-derived neurotrophic factor
CREB: cAMP response element binding protein
DAVID: Database for Annotation, Visualization and Integrated Discovery
DEG: Differentially expressed gene
DM: Diabetes mellitus
DPN: Diabetic peripheral neuropathy
GO: Gene Ontology
KEGG: Kyoto Encyclopedia of Genes and Genomes
NGF: Nerve growth factor
OGTT: Oral glucose tolerance test
qRT-PCR: Quantitative real-time PCR
RIN: RNA integrity number
TLR: Toll-like receptor.

Conflicts of Interest

The authors declare that they have no conflicts of interest.

Acknowledgments

The authors thank all the study participants and the clinical staffs from the affiliated hospitals of Ningbo University for their contribution to this research study. This work was supported by the Applied Research Project on Nonprofit Technology of Zhejiang Province (2015C33309), the National Natural Science Foundation of China (81541039, 81402747), the Natural Science Foundation of Ningbo (2016A610085, 2017A610199), and the K.C. Wong Magna Fund of Ningbo University.

References

[1] World Health Organization, *Global Report on Diabetes*, Geneva, 2016.

[2] R. Singh, L. Kishore, and N. Kaur, "Diabetic peripheral neuropathy: current perspective and future directions," *Pharmacological Research*, vol. 80, pp. 21–35, 2014.

[3] J. M. Forbes and M. E. Cooper, "Mechanisms of diabetic complications," *Physiological Reviews*, vol. 93, no. 1, pp. 137–188, 2013.

[4] J. L. Edwards, A. M. Vincent, H. T. Cheng, and E. L. Feldman, "Diabetic neuropathy: mechanisms to management," *Pharmacology & Therapeutics*, vol. 120, no. 1, pp. 1–34, 2008.

[5] S. Tesfaye and D. Selvarajah, "Advances in the epidemiology, pathogenesis and management of diabetic peripheral neuropathy," *Diabetes/Metabolism Research and Reviews*, vol. 28, Supplement 1, pp. 8–14, 2012.

[6] N. E. Cameron, S. E. Eaton, M. A. Cotter, and S. Tesfaye, "Vascular factors and metabolic interactions in the pathogenesis of diabetic neuropathy," *Diabetologia*, vol. 44, no. 11, pp. 1973–1988, 2001.

[7] DCCT Research Group, "The effect of intensive treatment of diabetes on the development and progression of long-term complications in insulin-dependent diabetes mellitus. The Diabetes Control and Complications Trial Research Group," *The New England Journal of Medicine*, vol. 329, no. 14, pp. 977–986, 1993.

[8] W. Duckworth, C. Abraira, T. Moritz et al., "Glucose control and vascular complications in veterans with type 2 diabetes," *The New England Journal of Medicine*, vol. 360, no. 2, pp. 129–139, 2009.

[9] K. Juster-Switlyk and A. G. Smith, "Updates in diabetic peripheral neuropathy," *F1000Res*, vol. 5, 2016.

[10] P. J. Oates, "Polyol pathway and diabetic peripheral neuropathy," *International Review of Neurobiology*, vol. 50, pp. 325–392, 2002.

[11] S. Y. Goh and M. E. Cooper, "Clinical review: the role of advanced glycation end products in progression and complications of diabetes," *The Journal of Clinical Endocrinology and Metabolism*, vol. 93, no. 4, pp. 1143–1152, 2008.

[12] I. G. Obrosova, "Diabetes and the peripheral nerve," *Biochimica et Biophysica Acta*, vol. 1792, no. 10, pp. 931–940, 2009.

[13] I. Vareniuk, I. A. Pavlov, and I. G. Obrosova, "Inducible nitric oxide synthase gene deficiency counteracts multiple manifestations of peripheral neuropathy in a streptozotocin-induced mouse model of diabetes," *Diabetologia*, vol. 51, no. 11, pp. 2126–2133, 2008.

[14] I. G. Obrosova, W. Xu, V. V. Lyzogubov et al., "PARP inhibition or gene deficiency counteracts intraepidermal nerve fiber loss and neuropathic pain in advanced diabetic neuropathy," *Free Radical Biology & Medicine*, vol. 44, no. 6, pp. 972–981, 2008.

[15] N. E. Cameron and M. A. Cotter, "Pro-inflammatory mechanisms in diabetic neuropathy: focus on the nuclear factor kappa B pathway," *Current Drug Targets*, vol. 9, no. 1, pp. 60–67, 2008.

[16] A. M. Vincent, J. W. Russell, P. Low, and E. L. Feldman, "Oxidative stress in the pathogenesis of diabetic neuropathy," *Endocrine Reviews*, vol. 25, no. 4, pp. 612–628, 2004.

[17] P. J. Dyck and C. Giannini, "Pathologic alterations in the diabetic neuropathies of humans: a review," *Journal of Neuropathology and Experimental Neurology*, vol. 55, no. 12, pp. 1181–1193, 1996.

[18] J. Doupis, T. E. Lyons, S. Wu, C. Gnardellis, T. Dinh, and A. Veves, "Microvascular reactivity and inflammatory cytokines in painful and painless peripheral diabetic neuropathy," *The Journal of Clinical Endocrinology and Metabolism*, vol. 94, no. 6, pp. 2157–2163, 2009.

[19] S. C. Apfel, "Nerve growth factor for the treatment of diabetic neuropathy: what went wrong, what went right, and what does the future hold?," *International Review of Neurobiology*, vol. 50, pp. 393–413, 2002.

[20] J. Hur, P. D. O'Brien, V. Nair et al., "Transcriptional networks of murine diabetic peripheral neuropathy and nephropathy: common and distinct gene expression patterns," *Diabetologia*, vol. 59, no. 6, pp. 1297–1306, 2016.

[21] G. K. Smyth, *Limma: Linear Models for Microarray Data. Bioinformatics and Computational Biology Solutions Using R and Bioconductor*, Springer, 2005.

[22] W. Huang da, B. T. Sherman, and R. A. Lempicki, "Systematic and integrative analysis of large gene lists using DAVID bioinformatics resources," *Nature Protocols*, vol. 4, no. 1, pp. 44–57, 2009.

[23] W. Luo and C. Brouwer, "Pathview: an R/Bioconductor package for pathway-based data integration and visualization," *Bioinformatics*, vol. 29, no. 14, pp. 1830-1831, 2013.

[24] J. Lasheras, M. Vila, M. Zamora et al., "Gene expression profiling in hearts of diabetic mice uncovers a potential role of estrogen-related receptor gamma in diabetic cardiomyopathy," *Molecular and Cellular Endocrinology*, vol. 430, pp. 77–88, 2016.

[25] M. L. Caramori, Y. Kim, A. B. Goldfine et al., "Differential gene expression in diabetic nephropathy in individuals with type 1 diabetes," *The Journal of Clinical Endocrinology and Metabolism*, vol. 100, no. 6, pp. E876–E882, 2015.

[26] A. T. Haug, K. F. Braun, S. Ehnert et al., "Gene expression changes in cancellous bone of type 2 diabetics: a biomolecular basis for diabetic bone disease," *Langenbeck's Archives of Surgery*, vol. 399, no. 5, pp. 639–647, 2014.

[27] O. M. Andriankaja, J. Galicia, G. Dong, W. Xiao, F. Alawi, and D. T. Graves, "Gene expression dynamics during diabetic periodontitis," *Journal of Dental Research*, vol. 91, no. 12, pp. 1160–1165, 2012.

[28] J. Hur, K. A. Sullivan, M. Pande et al., "The identification of gene expression profiles associated with progression of human diabetic neuropathy," *Brain*, vol. 134, Part 11, pp. 3222–3235, 2011.

[29] K. M. Irvine, P. Gallego, X. An et al., "Peripheral blood monocyte gene expression profile clinically stratifies patients with recent-onset type 1 diabetes," *Diabetes*, vol. 61, no. 5, pp. 1281–1290, 2012.

[30] T. Takamura, M. Honda, Y. Sakai et al., "Gene expression profiles in peripheral blood mononuclear cells reflect the pathophysiology of type 2 diabetes," *Biochemical and Biophysical Research Communications*, vol. 361, no. 2, pp. 379–384, 2007.

[31] E. C. Kaizer, C. L. Glaser, D. Chaussabel, J. Banchereau, V. Pascual, and P. C. White, "Gene expression in peripheral blood mononuclear cells from children with diabetes," *The Journal of Clinical Endocrinology and Metabolism*, vol. 92, no. 9, pp. 3705–3711, 2007.

[32] D. K. Moczulski, H. Fojcik, A. Wielgorecki et al., "Expression pattern of genes in peripheral blood mononuclear cells in diabetic nephropathy," *Diabetic Medicine*, vol. 24, no. 3, pp. 266–271, 2007.

[33] J. Wada and H. Makino, "Innate immunity in diabetes and diabetic nephropathy," *Nature Reviews Nephrology*, vol. 12, no. 1, pp. 13–26, 2016.

[34] J. Nilsson, E. Bengtsson, G. N. Fredrikson, and H. Bjorkbacka, "Inflammation and immunity in diabetic vascular complications," *Current Opinion in Lipidology*, vol. 19, no. 5, pp. 519–524, 2008.

[35] K. L. Farmer, C. Li, and R. T. Dobrowsky, "Diabetic peripheral neuropathy: should a chaperone accompany our therapeutic approach?," *Pharmacological Reviews*, vol. 64, no. 4, pp. 880–900, 2012.

[36] T. J. Boucher and S. B. McMahon, "Neurotrophic factors and neuropathic pain," *Current Opinion in Pharmacology*, vol. 1, no. 1, pp. 66–72, 2001.

[37] R. Hellweg and H. D. Hartung, "Endogenous levels of nerve growth factor (NGF) are altered in experimental diabetes mellitus: a possible role for NGF in the pathogenesis of diabetic neuropathy," *Journal of Neuroscience Research*, vol. 26, no. 2, pp. 258–267, 1990.

[38] R. Hellweg, G. Raivich, H. D. Hartung, C. Hock, and G. W. Kreutzberg, "Axonal transport of endogenous nerve growth factor (NGF) and NGF receptor in experimental diabetic neuropathy," *Experimental Neurology*, vol. 130, no. 1, pp. 24–30, 1994.

[39] A. P. Mizisin, N. A. Calcutt, D. R. Tomlinson, A. Gallagher, and P. Fernyhough, "Neurotrophin-3 reverses nerve conduction velocity deficits in streptozotocin-diabetic rats," *Journal of the Peripheral Nervous System*, vol. 4, no. 3-4, pp. 211–221, 1999.

[40] A. Cattaneo, N. Cattane, V. Begni, C. M. Pariante, and M. A. Riva, "The human BDNF gene: peripheral gene expression and protein levels as biomarkers for psychiatric disorders," *Translational Psychiatry*, vol. 6, no. 11, article e958, 2016.

[41] B. Xu, W. Gottschalk, A. Chow et al., "The role of brain-derived neurotrophic factor receptors in the mature hippocampus: modulation of long-term potentiation through a presynaptic mechanism involving TrkB," *The Journal of Neuroscience*, vol. 20, no. 18, pp. 6888–6897, 2000.

[42] M. E. Cunningham and L. A. Greene, "A function-structure model for NGF-activated TRK," *The EMBO Journal*, vol. 17, no. 24, pp. 7282–7293, 1998.

[43] L. Minichiello, "TrkB signalling pathways in LTP and learning," *Nature Reviews Neuroscience*, vol. 10, no. 12, pp. 850–860, 2009.

[44] E. J. Huang and L. F. Reichardt, "Trk receptors: roles in neuronal signal transduction," *Annual Review of Biochemistry*, vol. 72, pp. 609–642, 2003.

[45] E. J. Huang and L. F. Reichardt, "Neurotrophins: roles in neuronal development and function," *Annual Review of Neuroscience*, vol. 24, pp. 677–736, 2001.

[46] B. Mayr and M. Montminy, "Transcriptional regulation by the phosphorylation-dependent factor CREB," *Nature Reviews Molecular Cell Biology*, vol. 2, no. 8, pp. 599–609, 2001.

[47] P. Du, B. Fan, H. Han et al., "NOD2 promotes renal injury by exacerbating inflammation and podocyte insulin resistance in diabetic nephropathy," *Kidney International*, vol. 84, no. 2, pp. 265–276, 2013.

[48] X. F. Meng, X. L. Wang, X. J. Tian et al., "Nod-like receptor protein 1 inflammasome mediates neuron injury under high glucose," *Molecular Neurobiology*, vol. 49, no. 2, pp. 673–684, 2014.

[49] M. Y. Donath, "Multiple benefits of targeting inflammation in the treatment of type 2 diabetes," *Diabetologia*, vol. 59, no. 4, pp. 679–682, 2016.

[50] S. Akira and K. Takeda, "Toll-like receptor signalling," *Nature Reviews Immunology*, vol. 4, no. 7, pp. 499–511, 2004.

[51] M. R. Dasu, S. Devaraj, S. Park, and I. Jialal, "Increased Toll-like receptor (TLR) activation and TLR ligands in recently diagnosed type 2 diabetic subjects," *Diabetes Care*, vol. 33, no. 4, pp. 861–868, 2010.

[52] T. Zhu, Q. Meng, J. Ji, X. Lou, and L. Zhang, "Toll-like receptor 4 and tumor necrosis factor-alpha as diagnostic biomarkers for diabetic peripheral neuropathy," *Neuroscience Letters*, vol. 585, pp. 28–32, 2015.

[53] M. R. Dasu, S. Devaraj, L. Zhao, D. H. Hwang, and I. Jialal, "High glucose induces Toll-like receptor expression in human monocytes: mechanism of activation," *Diabetes*, vol. 57, no. 11, pp. 3090–3098, 2008.

[54] N. A. Calcutt, C. G. Jolivalt, and P. Fernyhough, "Growth factors as therapeutics for diabetic neuropathy," *Current Drug Targets*, vol. 9, no. 1, pp. 47–59, 2008.

20

Enhancing Exercise Responsiveness across Prediabetes Phenotypes by Targeting Insulin Sensitivity with Nutrition

Julian M. Gaitan,[1] Arthur Weltman,[1,2] and Steven K. Malin[1,2,3]

[1]Department of Kinesiology, University of Virginia, Charlottesville, VA, USA
[2]Division of Endocrinology and Metabolism, University of Virginia, Charlottesville, VA, USA
[3]Robert M. Berne Cardiovascular Research Center, University of Virginia, Charlottesville, VA, USA

Correspondence should be addressed to Steven K. Malin; skm6n@virginia.edu

Academic Editor: Maria Pia Francescato

Exercise is a cornerstone therapy for chronic diseases related to multiorgan insulin resistance. However, not all individuals show the anticipated improvement in insulin sensitivity following exercise and these individuals are considered exercise resistant. Caloric restriction is an approach to enhance the effect of exercise on increasing peripheral and hepatic insulin sensitivity, as replenishing expended calories blunts these benefits. Alternatively, restricting carbohydrate intake, independent of energy balance, following exercise provides an additive effect on peripheral insulin sensitivity when compared to refeeding carbohydrate. Although carbohydrate composition modulates insulin sensitivity, few have studied effects of low glycemic index or whole-grain diets following exercise across prediabetes phenotypes on insulin sensitivity. Herein, we propose the novel hypothesis that the combination of individualized nutrition therapy and exercise should be based on the clinical pathology of prediabetes to overcome exercise resistance and improve responsiveness in people at risk for type 2 diabetes and cardiovascular disease.

1. Introduction

Approximately 382 million adults worldwide have type 2 diabetes (T2D), and this figure is projected to rise to 592 million by the year 2035 [1]. Prediabetes is characterized by blood glucose levels above normal but below the diagnostic criteria for T2D [2]. The etiology of prediabetes is primarily skeletal muscle, liver, and/or adipose tissue insulin resistance that, in time, promotes oversecretion of insulin from the β-cell and results in pancreatic exhaustion that leads to severe hyperglycemia [3].

Skeletal muscle insulin resistance is primarily responsible for impaired glucose tolerance (IGT; 2 hr postprandial glucose > 140 mg/dL). In contrast, hepatic insulin resistance manifests mainly as impaired fasting glucose (IFG; fasting plasma glucose > 100 mg/dL) because glucose production is excessive despite normal insulinemia [4]. Individuals with both IFG and IGT (i.e., IFG + IGT) have peripheral and hepatic insulin resistance. Obesity is considered a chief factor promoting this insulin resistance, and many individuals with IFG and/or IGT are advised to lose approximately 5–10% of body weight by consuming a low-fat diet and participating in at least 150 min/week of moderate or 75 min/week of vigorous intensity exercise [5]. However, there is substantial intersubject variability for glycemic control [6, 7], cardiometabolic health [8, 9], and skeletal muscle hypertrophy [10] in response to lifestyle intervention, despite exercise intensity influencing these fitness-related insulin sensitivity adaptations [11]. Those who respond with little improvement, or even with adverse response, are often termed "nonresponders" or "exercise resistant." With regard to prediabetes, individuals with IFG + IGT have attenuated insulin sensitivity responses to high-volume (300 min/wk)/high-intensity (85% HR_{max}) exercise with approximately 7% weight loss treatment as compared to IFG or IGT alone [6, 7]. This phenomenon represents a specific case of intersubject variability in response to a high dose of exercise. Interestingly, ad libitum changes in diet behavior were recently suggested to have tissue-specific effects on insulin sensitivity [12]. As IFG generally develops due to hepatic insulin resistance and IGT emerges from skeletal muscle insulin resistance, we propose the novel hypothesis that applying individualized dietary prescription may enable the insulin-sensitizing effects of exercise in exercise-resistant individuals based on the underlying hyperglycemic phenotype [6, 7, 9].

This review will examine the potential for diet to augment the benefits of exercise on glucose regulation in people with insulin resistance in the liver and skeletal muscle. In particular, attention will focus on the impact of energy balance, carbohydrate balance, and carbohydrate type (i.e., low glycemic index (GI) and whole grain) in conjunction with exercise on multiorgan insulin resistance and glycemic control. Acute exercise interventions consist of 1–10 days to reflect metabolic responsiveness, while chronic (~>8 weeks exposure) exercise studies are used to understand adaptations to the stimuli. These exercise conditions are discussed separately because insulin sensitivity effects may differ based on the length of exposure.

2. Energy Deficit

2.1. Acute Exercise. Energy deficit following acute exercise contributes to increased postexercise insulin sensitivity. In fact, an energy deficit of 6.5 kcal/kg body weight following an acute exercise bout resulted in a 22% lower postprandial insulin incremental area under the curve (AUC) during an oral glucose tolerance test (OGTT) compared with an 11% decrease when expended calories were replenished [13]. This suggests that approximately 50% of the exercise effect on insulin sensitivity is due to the exercise-induced energy deficit. Although use of an OGTT limits the ability to discern whether skeletal muscle or liver is responsible for the improvement, earlier work using clamp or stable isotope approaches confirm that energy deficit is at least partially responsible for increased insulin sensitivity. Assali et al. prescribed hypocaloric diets in two groups of obese individuals by caloric restriction of 33 or 66% of the habitual energy intake [14]. Peripheral insulin sensitivity as measured by the euglycemic clamp increased significantly in the first week of the intervention, before any documented change in weight. In 2 subsequent weeks when subjects were prescribed an isoenergetic diet, the same improvements in insulin sensitivity were lost. Consistent with these observations, Black et al. studied the effects of an energy deficit (500 kcal/day) induced by 6 days of exercise training on isotope-derived insulin sensitivity in overweight and obese adults in comparison to a group who had calories replenished following exercise [15]. After training, the energy deficit intervention increased peripheral glucose disposal and suppressed hepatic glucose production compared to energy repletion. In another acute study, a 10-day energy deficit via either moderate aerobic exercise training or a low-calorie diet (50% of kcal needed to maintain energy balance) in obese, IGT, and T2D subjects significantly increased insulin action as determined by a modified hyperglycemic clamp [16]. Despite similar energy deficits, exercise training had a significantly greater effect on improving insulin action than the low-calorie diet. Together, these studies support that energy deficit is an important mechanism accounting for increased skeletal muscle and hepatic insulin sensitivity, but that exercise training confers additional improvement. Thus, combining exercise with diet-induced energy deficit could be a manner of alleviating exercise resistance in groups such as IFG + IGT, but this remains to be tested.

2.2. Exercise Training. Long-term studies ranging from 6–12 months report that exercise-induced energy deficit is responsible for increasing insulin sensitivity. Weiss et al. demonstrated that energy deficit via caloric restriction or exercise after 12 months improved insulin sensitivity comparably [17]. This is consistent with work by Larson-Meyer et al. showing that when energy deficit was held constant through 25% caloric restriction or 12.5% caloric restriction plus 12.5% energy expenditure from aerobic exercise, there was no difference between groups in skeletal muscle insulin sensitivity improvements [18]. Moreover, in obese, nondiabetic African American women who underwent 14 weeks of high-intensity interval training (HIIT) with a weight-maintenance diet [19], there was no significant increase in insulin sensitivity when calories were refed. Collectively these studies suggest that energy deficit is important for explaining the improved insulin sensitivity seen with chronic exercise training. Indeed, when lean, obese, and T2D men underwent 12 weeks of aerobic exercise training and were refed sufficient calories (55% carbohydrate, 21% fat, and 24% protein) to maintain body weight, no group experienced improvements in peripheral insulin sensitivity as measured by the clamp, despite increased oxidative glucose disposal [20]. Nonetheless, basal hepatic glucose production was reduced in subjects with T2D following exercise plus diet, indicating an independent effect of exercise on liver glucose metabolism in people with T2D. More recent work suggests that an energy deficit of about 700 kcal/day by either restricting caloric intake (diet-induced weight loss) or 60 min/day of moderate intensity aerobic exercise (exercise-induced weight loss) resulted in similar increases in glucose tolerance and nonoxidative glucose disposal [21]. These findings are similar to those of Solomon et al. [22], who compared a eucaloric diet plus exercise (i.e., energy deficit by exercise) or a hypocaloric diet plus exercise (i.e., diet-imposed 500 kcal/day deficit plus exercise-induced energy deficit) in older, obese, sedentary adults. Individuals in the hypocaloric diet group lost approximately 4 kg more weight compared with people in the eucaloric group. Clamp-derived peripheral insulin sensitivity improved similarly in both groups following the 12 weeks of aerobic exercise training regardless of eucaloric or hypocaloric diet, suggesting that above a given threshold of weight loss, there may be no further improvement in insulin sensitivity. However, subsequent work by the same group showed that hepatic insulin sensitivity improved to a greater extent following exercise training with hypocaloric diet than with a eucaloric diet during lipid-infused conditions [23]. This suggests that in addition to exercise, calorie restriction may protect the liver from obesity-driven insulin resistance more so than training alone, despite comparable peripheral insulin sensitivity. These findings may suggest that people with hepatic insulin resistance derive more benefit by focusing on energy deficit than those people with IGT alone [23].

A confounding factor when interpreting the collective findings from the effects of acute and long-term energy deficit on insulin sensitivity is that a carbohydrate deficit is often induced concurrently. This raises the possibility that carbohydrate deficit (e.g., low-glycogen concentrations), and not energy deficit per se, regulates insulin sensitivity postexercise (see Carbohydrate Availability). Further work awaits investigation to elucidate the optimal nutrition program for maximizing improvements in hepatic and/or skeletal muscle insulin resistance during exercise interventions across the prediabetes phenotypes.

3. Carbohydrate Availability

3.1. Acute Exercise. Skeletal muscle glycogen concentration is a driver of insulin-stimulated glucose uptake [24], and exercise and dietary carbohydrate intake both affect muscle glycogen. In healthy young men, exercise-induced glycogen depletion combined with dietary carbohydrate restriction promotes insulin sensitivity [25], but no studies have tested this effect in subjects with hyperglycemia. Nonetheless, Holtz et al. [26] studied overweight, sedentary, normoglycemic adults and found that carbohydrate restriction after moderate exercise increased nonoxidative glucose disposal during glucose infusion to a greater extent than carbohydrate replenishment. This higher degree of carbohydrate restriction was strongly correlated with enhanced insulin action, suggesting that exercise-mediated glycogen depletion modulates the insulin-stimulated effect on skeletal muscle glucose uptake. In addition to the degree of carbohydrate restriction, the timing of nutrient intake may affect peripheral insulin sensitivity. After an exercise session, insulin action improved to the greatest extent when subjects were refed the expended calories and carbohydrate immediately after the exercise bout, as opposed to immediately before or 3 hr after exercise [27]. However, insulin-mediated hepatic glucose production was significantly suppressed with preexercise or 3 hrs delayed feeding compared with immediately postexercise feeding. Although these findings may not generalize to individuals with hyperglycemia, as the subjects tested were fit and of normal weight, the results suggest that the timing of energy and/or carbohydrate intake relative to exercise may alter whether peripheral or hepatic insulin sensitivity are most affected. If true in individuals with prediabetes, this would have implications for augmenting insulin sensitivity using exercise and nutrition prescriptions categorized by prediabetes phenotype.

To gain insight into the importance of carbohydrate restriction on enhancing exercise-induced insulin sensitivity, it is necessary to compare energy deficit and replenishment models that are matched for carbohydrate intake [25, 26, 28]. Studies on dietary energy deficit cannot distinguish whether exercise-induced insulin sensitivity is augmented by global calorie reduction or a specific effect of carbohydrate deficit. Those that compare postexercise dietary energy restriction plus carbohydrate balance, energy restriction plus carbohydrate restriction, and energy restriction plus carbohydrate balance are useful for understanding the importance of carbohydrate. They establish that carbohydrate is a key dietary variable for augmenting insulin sensitivity following exercise [29, 30]. Nevertheless, energy deficit even with carbohydrate replenishment enhances fat oxidation [29, 30], which may be advantageous for improving clamp and OGTT-derived insulin sensitivity during periods of energy deficit [31–33]. Similar to the study of Holtz et al. [26], greater improvement in insulin sensitivity coincided with greater reductions in skeletal muscle glycogen [30]. Given that chronic hyperglycemia attenuates skeletal muscle glycogen utilization during exercise [34–36], this observation of glycogen depletion could be important for individualizing exercise prescription if these results hold true in adults with T2D or IFG + IGT. Furthermore, this may explain to some extent why people with IFG + IGT appear exercise resistant and respond to exercise with smaller rises in insulin sensitivity [37]. Thus, adults with IFG + IGT could benefit from restricted postexercise carbohydrate intake of approximately 3 to 12 hrs [27, 30]. Further work is required to identify specific postexercise carbohydrate manipulations to increase insulin sensitivity among different prediabetes phenotypes.

Since insulin suppresses lipolysis via adipocyte insulin action, diets high in carbohydrate could reduce circulating lipids (barring high dietary fat intake) and diminish lipid-induced impairments on hepatic and/or skeletal muscle insulin sensitivity. This may be important for individuals with IGT, who tend to have more severe adipose insulin resistance than individuals with IFG [38]. Carbohydrate restriction after an exercise bout may enhance adipocyte insulin sensitivity. Harrison et al. [39] reported that circulating triglycerides (TG) were lower and free fatty acids (FFA) were higher during an oral fat tolerance test (OFTT) after an exercise bout and carbohydrate restriction. The effect as absent when carbohydrate was refed to replenish the exercise expenditure, suggesting adipocyte insulin sensitivity, was enhanced by dietary restriction after exercise. While muscle glycogen was substantially reduced by carbohydrate restriction, the study design makes it unclear whether carbohydrate deficit per se or energy deficit was responsible for reducing circulating TG. In either case, other work indicates that energy deficit decreases circulating TG in response to a high-fat meal thereby minimizing deleterious effects of lipids on insulin action [40]. To date, few data exist examining the impact of refeeding with or without carbohydrate on lipid availability as a result of insulin sensitivity. Further work is needed to understand the interaction among exercise, carbohydrate restriction, insulin sensitivity, and lipid availability, particularly in individuals with IGT who have adipose insulin resistance.

A final consideration with regard to restricting carbohydrate intake is that limiting one nutrient could be compensated by increased intake of another, such as fat. High dietary fat intake is thought to decrease insulin-stimulated skeletal muscle glucose uptake because of a rise in circulating lipids [41–44]. However, exercise may offer some protection. Several studies [45, 46] suggest that a 90 min aerobic exercise bout enhances peripheral and hepatic insulin sensitivity regardless of high- or low-fat feeding after the bout. Since skeletal muscle lipid oxidation capacity is correlated with insulin sensitivity in subjects with a high VO_2peak and high IMTG content [47], these subjects' tolerance to high-fat meals may be partly explained by their aerobic fitness (VO_2peak = 55.5 ± 1.6 mL/kg/min) [45] or the high oxidative capacity of females [46]. Further studies are needed to understand effects in clinical populations. Nonetheless, carbohydrate intake and muscle glycogen content were similar across conditions in these studies, thereby reinforcing the hypothesis that carbohydrate, and not fat, is a key dietary variable for enhancing exercise-induced insulin sensitivity in short term.

3.2. Exercise Training. While acute studies suggest that exercise with carbohydrate restriction may be effective for enhancing the insulin-sensitizing effect of exercise at the level of skeletal muscle and the liver, it is currently unknown whether this nutritional strategy is effective in conjunction with chronic exercise training in clinical populations. Subsequently, we can only speculate that since individuals with IFG + IGT tend to have blunted insulin sensitivity and fuel selection exercise responses to training [6, 7], carbohydrate restriction could be a strategy to enhance exercise-related mitochondrial adaptations in this population that relate to insulin sensitivity [48]. The mechanism by which low carbohydrate availability confers metabolic adaptation has been shown to act through targeting glycogen depletion to upregulate mitochondrial oxidative enzymes (e.g., citrate synthase, β-HAD) involved in glucose tolerance and insulin action [49, 50]. Further work is needed to determine whether exercise training with carbohydrate restriction is feasible in individuals across the prediabetes phenotypes.

4. Glycemic Index

4.1. Acute Exercise. The glycemic index (GI) of a food is characterized by the resulting blood glucose excursion with reference to a standardized meal (e.g., white bread or glucose) [51]. On the other hand, the glycemic load (GL) is determined by the GI of the food multiplied by the amount of carbohydrate (i.e., grams) in that serving, also described by the area under the curve of the GI response. It is worth acknowledging, however, that GI and GL are independent of dietary energy, which has been an important topic of this review. Nevertheless, the purpose of a low-GI or low-GL diet is to manage circulating glucose levels (and by association, insulin levels), which in turn, may contribute to healthier body weight, reduced appetite cravings, and improved cardiometabolic health [51, 52]. Although few studies have systematically compared the effect of low versus high GI food following an acute bout of exercise on insulin sensitivity, it should be noted that many of the acute exercise studies examined in this review utilized a high content of simple carbohydrates, which have a high GI index. In one of the few acute studies conducted, Solomon et al. [53] examined older, obese adults after 7 days of moderate intensity aerobic exercise together with a low- or high-GI diet. Exercise combined with low- and high-GI diets enhanced insulin-stimulated glucose disposal and hepatic glucose production (markers of peripheral and hepatic insulin sensitivity). Since these two diets improved insulin sensitivity in both tissues, further work is warranted to determine whether IFG, IGT, and IFG + IGT phenotypes respond differently to each diet. Although the low-GI diet did not improve insulin sensitivity more than high GI following acute exercise, the low-GI group reduced systolic blood pressure to a greater extent. Thus, a low-GI diet with exercise may contribute to short-term cardiovascular benefits, presenting a possible strategy to mitigate cardiovascular disease if exercise is performed regularly. This may be clinically important for the prediabetes phenotypes since individuals with IFG + IGT have higher CVD risk than those with IGT or IFG [54].

4.2. Exercise Training. Exercise training and a eucaloric low-GI diet have been suggested to synergistically enhance glucose regulation in older adults with prediabetes [55]. Despite comparable improvements in peripheral and hepatic insulin sensitivity, exercise training combined with a low-GI diet can preserve β-cell function and reduce insulin secretion demand to a greater extent than a high-GI diet [56]. Preserving β-cell function is relevant to all three prediabetes phenotypes (IFG, IGT, and IFG + IGT), since pancreatic dysfunction is differentially implicated in the progression to T2D [57]. On the other hand, Malin et al. [58] showed that 12 weeks of either a low- or high-GI diet and supervised exercise training was effective in lowering HbA_{1c} and body fat as well as increasing peripheral insulin sensitivity in adults with metabolic syndrome, without change in resting fat oxidation. Consistent with this observation, a low-GI food consumption combined with increased walking in adults with T2D resulted in reductions of HbA_{1c} that were similar to increased walking alone [59]. When drawing on these observations, there does not appear to be clear evidence that a eucaloric low-GI diet confers benefit above that of a high-GI diet when combined with increased physical activity and/or exercise training. Additional research is needed to understand differential responses in each prediabetic phenotype to better understand personalizing diets with exercise on insulin sensitivity and/or secretion.

5. Whole Grains

To date, there are no systematic acute or long-term exercise interventions combined with whole-grain consumption examining effects on insulin sensitivity in hyperglycemic individuals. However, epidemiological data suggest that dietary whole-grain intake (e.g., oats and barely) is associated with a lower incidence of T2D compared with refined-grain intake [60]. Whole-grain consumption (~30–60 g/d) may also reduce the risk of progression from normal glucose tolerance to prediabetes [61]. Indeed, Kirwan et al. [62] recently demonstrated that 8 weeks of whole-grain diet (consisting of mainly wheat and rice) feeding decreased HbA_{1c}, fasting insulinemia, and insulin resistance (HOMA-IR) in overweight/obese subjects. The reason whole-grain intake lowers T2D risk is an area ready for investigation as preliminary work suggests that short-chain fatty acid release in the gut mediates the effect of whole-grain (bran and germ

Table 1: Summary of exercise plus diet effects compared with preintervention.

	Insulin-stimulated muscle glucose uptake	Nonoxidative glucose disposal	Glycogen concentration	Hepatic insulin sensitivity	Fat oxidation
Caloric restriction	↑ [15, 22]	↑ [15]	↔ [30]	↓ [16]	↑ [22, 29, 30]
Caloric replacement	↑ ↔ [15, 20–22, 75]	↓↔ [15, 20]	↔ [30, 39, 46]	↑↔ [15, 20]	↑↔ [13, 19, 30]
CHO restriction	↑↑ [26, 30]	↑↑ [26]	↓ [30, 39]	↔ [26]	↑↔ [30]
CHO Replacement	↔ [30]	↑↔ [26, 27]	↔ [30]	↔ [27]	↑ [27]
Low GI	↑ [56]	↑ [52]	?	↑ [52]	?
High GI	↑ [52]	↑ [52]	?	↑ [52]	?
Whole grain	?	?	?	?	?
Refined grain	?	?	?	?	?

↑ indicates an increase. ↓ indicates a decrease. ↔ indicates no substantial change. ? indicates inconsistent findings or no available data across studies. ↑↑ indicates a substantial change.

with high fiber) intake on clamp-derived insulin sensitivity in overweight adults with or without metabolic syndrome [63]. This suggests that whole-grain intake may improve skeletal muscle glucose uptake or reduce hepatic glucose production regardless of the metabolic derangement. However, whole grains have little effect on rates of meal glucose appearance from the gut in response to a standard OGTT with the dual-tracer technique [64, 65]. A single meal consisting of whole grains (barley-based meals rich in the soluble fiber β-glucan) results in better glycemic control than refined grains due to lower hepatic glucose production [65]. In addition, longitudinal data support that whole-grain consumption (rye bread based) may result in improved β-cell function [66]. It is worth recognizing though that dietary fiber is often associated with whole-grain intake and has shown independent effects on insulin sensitivity [67, 68]. Collectively, these studies support that whole-grain intake can improve peripheral and hepatic insulin sensitivity, along with pancreatic function. The results are thus relevant to IFG, IGT, and IFG + IGT populations, and particular attention should be paid to IFG + IGT since these individuals are most at risk for progression to T2D and may benefit from the combined peripheral and hepatic effects of whole-grain intake. However, whether adding whole grains and/or fiber augments, exercise effects above remain to be seen. This could be of clinical interest since exercise is a significant variable when studying the relationship between fiber intake and insulin resistance [67]. Future research is needed to examine responses in each obese prediabetic phenotype to the interaction between whole grains with acute and long-term exercise on insulin sensitivity for T2D prevention/treatment.

6. Conclusions

Modifying dietary energy and nutrient intake is an appropriate tool to enhance the effectiveness of exercise on insulin sensitivity. Various dietary strategies appear to have independent effects on targeting skeletal muscle versus hepatic insulin sensitivity (Table 1). For instance, inducing an energy deficit improves skeletal muscle and hepatic insulin sensitivity following acute and chronic exercise interventions, which has implications for individuals with IFG, IGT, and IFG + IGT. Carbohydrate restriction is primarily responsible for depleting and maintaining low skeletal muscle glycogen, which enhances peripheral glucose uptake further than energy deficit with carbohydrate balance. Individuals with IGT, and especially IFG + IGT (as this group is more resistant to insulin sensitizing effects of exercise [6, 7]), may benefit from restricting carbohydrate intake following exercise bouts. Increased fasting fat oxidation is also consistently observed after exercise with calorie and/or carbohydrate restriction, suggesting that enhanced mitochondrial reliance on fat may contribute to improved insulin sensitivity. Effects of low- versus high-GI carbohydrates are unclear, but the literature supports that exercise followed by high-GI carbohydrate intake increases pancreatic insulin secretion. The pancreas is thus potentially subjected to additional burden in order to maintain normal glycemia. This is undesirable in IFG, IGT, and IFG + IGT phenotypes as pancreatic β-cell dysfunction contributes in the progression to T2D [69]. Whether whole grains modulate exercise adaption also remains to be seen. This is important as nutritional interventions suggest that adherence to low or high carbohydrate-based diets overtime may be most important for weight loss and glycemic control [70, 71].

A substantial number of the studies on interaction of nutrition and exercise for insulin action have been conducted in nonclinical populations. Clinical trials are needed to determine the efficacy of diet plus exercise for T2D prevention, particularly across the prediabetes phenotypes. Although individuals are often advised to consume nutrients at specific times before and after exercise to stimulate physiological adaptation and maximize athletic performance [72–74], the implication of nutrient composition and timing for individuals with IFG, IGT, and IFG + IGT remains largely unknown. Furthermore, no data exist examining the interaction between exercise intensity and nutrient composition and timing. These are significant knowledge gaps to fill since the pathophysiology of prediabetes differs among the clinical phenotypes. Addressing these questions will eventually allow individualized diet and exercise prescription and inform clinical and public health recommendations for optimizing the prevention and/or delay of T2D onset.

Conflicts of Interest

All authors declare that they have no competing interests.

Authors' Contributions

Julian M. Gaitan and Steven K. Malin shared responsibility for writing the manuscript. Arthur Weltman reviewed and provided edits to the manuscript.

Acknowledgments

The authors thank the members of the Applied Metabolism & Physiology Laboratory for helpful discussion on the manuscript. In particular, the authors thank Dr. Sibylle Kranz, PhD, RDN, for constructive feedback.

References

[1] L. Guariguata, D. R. Whiting, I. Hambleton, J. Beagley, U. Linnenkamp, and J. E. Shaw, "Global estimates of diabetes prevalence for 2013 and projections for 2035," *Diabetes Research and Clinical Practice*, vol. 103, no. 2, pp. 137–149, 2014.

[2] American Diabetes Association, "2. Classification and Diagnosis of Diabetes," *Diabetes Care*, vol. 38, Supplement 1, pp. S8–S16, 2015.

[3] V. A. Fonseca, "Defining and characterizing the progression of type 2 diabetes," *Diabetes Care*, vol. 32, Supplement 2, pp. S151–S156, 2009.

[4] C. Meyer, W. Pimenta, H. J. Woerle et al., "Different mechanisms for impaired fasting glucose and impaired postprandial glucose tolerance in humans," *Diabetes Care*, vol. 29, no. 8, pp. 1909–1914, 2006.

[5] W. C. Knowler, E. Barrett-Connor, S. E. Fowler et al., "Reduction in the incidence of type 2 diabetes with lifestyle intervention or metformin," *The New England Journal of Medicine*, vol. 346, no. 6, pp. 393–403, 2002.

[6] S. K. Malin, J. M. Haus, T. P. J. Solomon, A. Blaszczak, S. R. Kashyap, and J. P. Kirwan, "Insulin sensitivity and metabolic flexibility following exercise training among different obese insulin-resistant phenotypes," *American Journal of Physiology - Endocrinology and Metabolism*, vol. 305, no. 10, pp. E1292–E1298, 2013.

[7] T. P. J. Solomon, S. K. Malin, K. Karstoft, J. M. Haus, and J. P. Kirwan, "The influence of hyperglycemia on the therapeutic effect of exercise on glycemic control in patients with type 2 diabetes mellitus," *JAMA Internal Medicine*, vol. 173, no. 19, pp. 1834–1836, 2013.

[8] C. Bouchard, S. N. Blair, T. S. Church et al., "Adverse metabolic response to regular exercise: is it a rare or common occurrence?," *PLoS One*, vol. 7, no. 5, article e37887, 2012.

[9] D. J. Green, T. Eijsvogels, Y. M. Bouts et al., "Exercise training and artery function in humans: nonresponse and its relationship to cardiovascular risk factors," *Journal of Applied Physiology*, vol. 117, no. 4, pp. 345–352, 2014.

[10] A. Thalacker-Mercer, M. Stec, X. Cui, J. Cross, S. Windham, and M. Bamman, "Cluster analysis reveals differential transcript profiles associated with resistance training-induced human skeletal muscle hypertrophy," *Physiological Genomics*, vol. 45, no. 12, pp. 499–507, 2013.

[11] C. Alvarez, R. Ramirez-Campillo, R. Ramirez-Velez, and M. Izquierdo, "Prevelance of non-responders for glucose control markers after 10 weeks of high intensity interval training in adult women with higher and lower insulin resistance," *Frontiers in Physiology*, vol. 8, p. 479, 2017.

[12] R. Blanco-Rojo, J. F. Alcala-Diaz, S. Wopereis et al., "The insulin resistance phenotype (muscle or liver) interacts with the type of diet to determine changes in disposition index after 2 years of intervention: the CORDIOPREV-DIAB randomised clinical trial," *Diabetologia*, vol. 59, no. 1, pp. 67–76, 2016.

[13] F. L. Burton, D. Malkova, M. J. Caslake, and J. M. R. Gill, "Energy replacement attenuates the effects of prior moderate exercise on postprandial metabolism in overweight/obese men," *International Journal of Obesity*, vol. 32, no. 3, pp. 481–489, 2008.

[14] A. R. Assali, A. Ganor, Y. Beigel, Z. Shafer, T. Hershcovici, and M. Fainaru, "Insulin resistance in obesity: body-weight or energy balance?," *The Journal of Endocrinology*, vol. 171, no. 2, pp. 293–298, 2001.

[15] S. E. Black, E. Mitchell, P. S. Freedson, S. R. Chipkin, and B. Braun, "Improved insulin action following short-term exercise training: role of energy and carbohydrate balance," *Journal of Applied Physiology*, vol. 99, no. 6, pp. 2285–2293, 2005.

[16] P. J. Arciero, M. D. Vukovich, J. O. Holloszy, S. B. Racette, and W. M. Kohrt, "Comparison of short-term diet and exercise on insulin action in individuals with abnormal glucose tolerance," *Journal of Applied Physiology*, vol. 86, no. 6, pp. 1930–1935, 1999.

[17] E. P. Weiss, S. B. Racette, D. T. Villareal et al., "Improvements in glucose tolerance and insulin action induced by increasing energy expenditure or decreasing energy intake: a randomized controlled trial," *The American Journal of Clinical Nutrition*, vol. 84, no. 5, pp. 1033–1042, 2006.

[18] D. E. Larson-Meyer, L. K. Heilbronn, L. M. Redman et al., "Effect of calorie restriction with or without exercise on insulin sensitivity, β-cell function, fat cell size, and ectopic lipid in overweight subjects," *Diabetes Care*, vol. 29, no. 6, pp. 1337–1344, 2006.

[19] A. D. Arad, F. J. DiMenna, N. Thomas et al., "High-intensity interval training without weight loss improves exercise but not basal or insulin-induced metabolism in overweight/obese African American women," *Journal of Applied Physiology*, vol. 119, no. 4, pp. 352–362, 2015.

[20] K. R. Segal, A. Edano, A. Abalos et al., "Effect of exercise training on insulin sensitivity and glucose metabolism in lean, obese, and diabetic men," *Journal of Applied Physiology*, vol. 71, no. 6, pp. 2402–2411, 1991.

[21] R. Ross, D. Dagnone, P. J. Jones et al., "Reduction in obesity and related comorbid conditions after diet-induced weight loss or exercise-induced weight loss in men: a randomized, controlled trial," *Annals of Internal Medicine*, vol. 133, no. 2, pp. 92–103, 2000.

[22] T. P. J. Solomon, S. N. Sistrun, R. K. Krishnan et al., "Exercise and diet enhance fat oxidation and reduce insulin resistance in older obese adults," *Journal of Applied Physiology*, vol. 104, no. 5, pp. 1313–1319, 2008.

[23] J. M. Haus, T. P. Solomon, C. M. Marchetti, J. M. Edmison, F. Gonzalez, and J. P. Kirwan, "Free fatty acid-induced hepatic insulin resistance is attenuated following lifestyle intervention in obese individuals with impaired glucose tolerance," *The Journal of Clinical Endocrinology & Metabolism*, vol. 95, no. 1, pp. 323–327, 2010.

[24] J. F. P. Wojtaszewski, J. N. Nielsen, and E. A. Richter, "Invited review: effect of acute exercise on insulin signaling and action in humans," *Journal of Applied Physiology*, vol. 93, no. 1, pp. 384–392, 2002.

[25] A. Sparti and J. Decombaz, "Effect of diet on glucose tolerance 36 hours after glycogen-depleting exercise," *European Journal of Clinical Nutrition*, vol. 46, no. 6, pp. 377–385, 1992.

[26] K. A. Holtz, B. R. Stephens, C. G. Sharoff, S. R. Chipkin, and B. Braun, "The effect of carbohydrate availability following exercise on whole-body insulin action," *Applied Physiology, Nutrition, and Metabolism*, vol. 33, no. 5, pp. 946–956, 2008.

[27] B. R. Stephens, J. M. Sautter, K. A. Holtz, C. G. Sharoff, S. R. Chipkin, and B. Braun, "Effect of timing of energy and carbohydrate replacement on post-exercise insulin action," *Applied Physiology, Nutrition, and Metabolism*, vol. 32, no. 6, pp. 1139–1147, 2007.

[28] G. D. Cartee, D. A. Young, M. D. Sleeper, J. Zierath, H. Wallberg-Henriksson, and J. O. Holloszy, "Prolonged increase in insulin-stimulated glucose transport in muscle after exercise," *American Journal of Physiology - Endocrinology and Metabolism*, vol. 256, no. 4, pp. E494–E499, 1989.

[29] J. F. Horowitz, A. E. Kaufman, A. K. Fox, and M. P. Harber, "Energy deficit without reducing dietary carbohydrate alters resting carbohydrate oxidation and fatty acid availability," *Journal of Applied Physiology*, vol. 98, no. 5, pp. 1612–1618, 2005.

[30] S. A. Newsom, S. Schenk, K. M. Thomas et al., "Energy deficit after exercise augments lipid mobilization but does not contribute to the exercise-induced increase in insulin sensitivity," *Journal of Applied Physiology*, vol. 108, no. 3, pp. 554–560, 2010.

[31] B. H. Goodpaster, A. Katsariaras, and D. E. Kelley, "Enhanced fat oxidation through physical activity is associated with improvements in insulin sensitivity in obesity," *Diabetes*, vol. 52, no. 9, pp. 2191–2197, 2003.

[32] G. Lattuada, F. Costantino, A. Caumo et al., "Reduced whole-body lipid oxidation is associated with insulin resistance, but not with intramyocellular lipid content in offspring of type 2 diabetic patients," *Diabetologia*, vol. 48, no. 4, pp. 741–747, 2005.

[33] M. C. Venables and A. E. Jeukendrup, "Endurance training and obesity: effect on substrate metabolism and insulin sensitivity," *Medicine and Science in Sports and Exercise*, vol. 40, no. 3, pp. 495–502, 2008.

[34] B. Braun, C. Sharoff, S. R. Chipkin, and F. Beaudoin, "Effects of insulin resistance on substrate utilization during exercise in overweight women," *Journal of Applied Physiology*, vol. 97, no. 3, pp. 991–997, 2004.

[35] J. Kang, D. E. Kelley, R. J. Robertson et al., "Substrate utilization and glucose turnover during exercise of varying intensities in individuals with NIDDM," *Medicine & Science in Sports & Exercise*, vol. 31, no. 1, pp. 82–89, 1999.

[36] S. K. Malin, R. Viskochil, C. Oliver, and B. Braun, "Mild fasting hyperglycemia shifts fuel reliance toward fat during exercise in adults with impaired glucose tolerance," *Journal of Applied Physiology*, vol. 115, no. 1, pp. 78–83, 2013.

[37] S. K. Malin, T. P. J. Solomon, A. Blaszczak, S. Finnegan, J. Filion, and J. P. Kirwan, "Pancreatic β-cell function increases in a linear dose-response manner following exercise training in adults with prediabetes," *American Journal of Physiology - Endocrinology and Metabolism*, vol. 305, no. 10, pp. E1248–E1254, 2013.

[38] M. A. Abdul-Ghani, M. Molina-Carrion, R. Jani, C. Jenkinson, and R. A. DeFronzo, "Adipocytes in subjects with impaired fasting glucose and impaired glucose tolerance are resistant to the anti-lipolytic effect of insulin," *Acta Diabetologica*, vol. 45, no. 3, pp. 147–150, 2008.

[39] M. Harrison, D. J. O'Gorman, N. McCaffrey et al., "Influence of acute exercise with and without carbohydrate replacement on postprandial lipid metabolism," *Journal of Applied Physiology*, vol. 106, no. 3, pp. 943–949, 2009.

[40] E. C. Freese, A. S. Levine, D. P. Chapman, D. B. Hausman, and K. J. Cureton, "Effects of acute sprint interval cycling and energy replacement on postprandial lipemia," *Journal of Applied Physiology*, vol. 111, no. 6, pp. 1584–1589, 2011.

[41] G. Boden, "Role of fatty acids in the pathogenesis of insulin resistance and NIDDM," *Diabetes*, vol. 46, no. 1, pp. 3–10, 1997.

[42] G. Boden and X. Chen, "Effects of fat on glucose uptake and utilization in patients with non-insulin-dependent diabetes," *The Journal of Clinical Investigation*, vol. 96, no. 3, pp. 1261–1268, 1995.

[43] G. Boden, X. Chen, J. Ruiz, J. V. White, and L. Rossetti, "Mechanisms of fatty acid-induced inhibition of glucose uptake," *The Journal of Clinical Investigation*, vol. 93, no. 6, pp. 2438–2446, 1994.

[44] C. Yu, "Mechanism by which fatty acids inhibit insulin activation of insulin receptor substrate-1 (IRS-1)-associated phosphatidylinositol 3-kinase activity in muscle," *The Journal of Biological Chemistry*, vol. 277, no. 52, pp. 50230–50236, 2002.

[45] A. K. Fox, A. E. Kaufman, and J. F. Horowitz, "Adding fat calories to meals after exercise does not alter glucose tolerance," *Journal of Applied Physiology*, vol. 97, no. 1, pp. 11–16, 2004.

[46] S. Schenk, J. N. Cook, A. E. Kaufman, and J. F. Horowitz, "Postexercise insulin sensitivity is not impaired after an overnight lipid infusion," *American Journal of Physiology - Endocrinology and Metabolism*, vol. 288, no. 3, pp. E519–E525, 2004.

[47] B. H. Goodpaster, J. He, S. Watkins, and D. E. Kelley, "Skeletal muscle lipid content and insulin resistance: evidence for a paradox in endurance-trained athletes," *The Journal of Clinical Endocrinology and Metabolism*, vol. 86, no. 12, pp. 5755–5761, 2001.

[48] D. E. Kelley and L. J. Mandarino, "Fuel selection in human skeletal muscle in insulin resistance: a reexamination," *Diabetes*, vol. 49, no. 5, pp. 677–683, 2000.

[49] K. Van Proeyen, K. Szlufcik, H. Nielens et al., "Training in the fasted state improves glucose tolerance during fat-rich diet," *The Journal of Physiology*, vol. 588, no. 21, pp. 4289–4302, 2010.

[50] A. E. Jeukendrup, "Periodized nutrition for athletes," *Sports Medicine*, vol. 47, Supplement 1, pp. 51–63, 2017.

[51] A. B. Evert, J. L. Boucher, M. Cypress et al., "Nutrition therapy recommendations for the management of adults with diabetes," *Diabetes Care*, vol. 37, Supplement 1, pp. S120–S143, 2014.

[52] C. Visuthranukul, P. Sirimongkol, A. Prachansuwan, C. Pruksananonda, and S. Chomtho, "Low-glycemic index diet may improve insulin sensitivity in obese children," *Pediatric Research*, vol. 78, no. 5, pp. 567–573, 2015.

[53] T. P. Solomon, J. M. Haus, K. R. Kelly et al., "Randomized trial on the effects of a 7-d low-glycemic diet and exercise intervention on insulin resistance in older obese humans," *The American Journal of Clinical Nutrition*, vol. 90, no. 5, pp. 1222–1229, 2009.

[54] M. Abdul-Ghani, R. A. DeFronzo, and J. Amin, "Prediabetes and risk of diabetes and associated complications," *Current Opinion in Clinical Nutrition and Metabolic Care*, vol. 19, no. 5, pp. 394–399, 2016.

[55] J. P. Kirwan, H. Barkoukis, L. M. Brooks, C. M. Marchetti, B. P. Stetzer, and F. Gonzalez, "Exercise training and dietary glycemic load may have synergistic effects on insulin resistance in older obese adults," *Annals of Nutrition & Metabolism*, vol. 55, no. 4, pp. 326–333, 2009.

[56] T. P. Solomon, J. M. Haus, K. R. Kelly et al., "A low-glycemic index diet combined with exercise reduces insulin resistance, postprandial hyperinsulinemia, and glucose-dependent insulinotropic polypeptide responses in obese, prediabetic humans," *The American Journal of Clinical Nutrition*, vol. 92, no. 6, pp. 1359–1368, 2010.

[57] K. Færch, K. Borch-Johnsen, J. J. Holst, and A. Vaag, "Pathophysiology and aetiology of impaired fasting glycaemia and impaired glucose tolerance: does it matter for prevention and treatment of type 2 diabetes?," *Diabetologia*, vol. 52, no. 9, pp. 1714–1723, 2009.

[58] S. K. Malin, N. Niemi, T. P. J. Solomon et al., "Exercise training with weight loss and either a high- or low-glycemic index diet reduces metabolic syndrome severity in older adults," *Annals of Nutrition & Metabolism*, vol. 61, no. 2, pp. 135–141, 2012.

[59] S. H. Cheong, L. J. McCargar, B. W. Paty, C. Tudor-Locke, and R. C. Bell, "The first step first bite program: guidance to increase physical activity and daily intake of low-glycemic index foods," *Journal of the American Dietetic Association*, vol. 109, no. 8, pp. 1411–1416, 2009.

[60] E. Q. Ye, S. A. Chacko, E. L. Chou, M. Kugizaki, and S. Liu, "Greater whole-grain intake is associated with lower risk of type 2 diabetes, cardiovascular disease, and weight gain," *The Journal of Nutrition*, vol. 142, no. 7, pp. 1304–1313, 2012.

[61] T. Wirstrom, A. Hilding, G. HF, C.-G. Ostenson, and A. Bjorklund, "Consumption of whole grain reduces risk of deteriorating glucose tolerance, including progression to prediabetes," *The American Journal of Clinical Nutrition*, vol. 97, no. 1, pp. 179–187, 2013.

[62] J. P. Kirwan, S. K. Malin, A. R. Scelsi et al., "A whole-grain diet reduces cardiovascular risk factors in overweight and obese adults: a randomized controlled trial," *The Journal of Nutrition*, vol. 146, no. 11, pp. 2244–2251, 2016.

[63] M. A. Pereira, D. R. Jacobs, J. J. Pins et al., "Effect of whole grains on insulin sensitivity in overweight hyperinsulinemic adults," *The American Journal of Clinical Nutrition*, vol. 75, no. 5, pp. 848–855, 2002.

[64] M. G. Priebe, H. Wang, D. Weening, M. Schepers, T. Preston, and R. J. Vonk, "Factors related to colonic fermentation of nondigestible carbohydrates of a previous evening meal increase tissue glucose uptake and moderate glucose-associated inflammation," *The American Journal of Clinical Nutrition*, vol. 91, no. 1, pp. 90–97, 2010.

[65] A. Thorburn, J. Muir, and J. Proietto, "Carbohydrate fermentation decreases hepatic glucose output in healthy subjects," *Metabolism*, vol. 42, no. 6, pp. 780–785, 1993.

[66] K. S. Juntunen, D. E. Laaksonen, K. S. Poutanen, L. K. Niskanen, and H. M. Mykkänen, "High-fiber rye bread and insulin secretion and sensitivity in healthy postmenopausal women," *The American Journal of Clinical Nutrition*, vol. 77, no. 2, pp. 385–391, 2003.

[67] C. B. Breneman and L. Tucker, "Dietary fibre consumption and insulin resistance – the role of body fat and physical activity," *The British Journal of Nutrition*, vol. 110, no. 02, pp. 375–383, 2013.

[68] H. M. Heikkilä, B. Krachler, R. Rauramaa, and U. S. Schwab, "Diet, insulin secretion and insulin sensitivity – the dose-responses to exercise training (DR's EXTRA) study (ISRCTN45977199)," *The British Journal of Nutrition*, vol. 112, no. 09, pp. 1530–1541, 2014.

[69] M. Kanat, D. Winnier, L. Norton et al., "The relationship between β-cell function and glycated hemoglobin: results from the veterans administration epidemiology study," *Diabetes Care*, vol. 34, no. 4, pp. 1006–1010, 2011.

[70] C. L. Rock, S. W. Flatt, B. Pakiz et al., "Weight loss, glycemic control, and cardiovascular disease risk factors in response to differential diet composition in a weight loss program in type 2 diabetes: a randomized controlled trial," *Diabetes Care*, vol. 37, no. 6, pp. 1573–1580, 2014.

[71] F. M. Sacks, V. J. Carey, C. A. M. Anderson et al., "Effects of high vs low glycemic index of dietary carbohydrate on cardiovascular disease risk factors and insulin sensitivity," *Journal of the American Medical Association*, vol. 312, no. 23, pp. 2531–2541, 2014.

[72] J. L. Ivy, M. C. Lee, J. T. Brozinick, and M. J. Reed, "Muscle glycogen storage after different amounts of carbohydrate ingestion," *Journal of Applied Physiology*, vol. 65, no. 5, pp. 2018–2023, 1988.

[73] R. Jentjens and A. E. Jeukendrup, "Determinants of post-exercise glycogen synthesis during short-term recovery," *Sports Medicine*, vol. 33, no. 2, pp. 117–144, 2003.

[74] J. D. MacDougall, G. R. Ward, and J. R. Sutton, "Muscle glycogen repletion after high-intensity intermittent exercise," *Journal of Applied Physiology*, vol. 42, no. 2, pp. 129–132, 1977.

[75] R. Ross, I. Janssen, J. Dawson et al., "Exercise-induced reduction in obesity and insulin resistance in women: a randomized controlled trial," *Obesity Research*, vol. 12, no. 5, pp. 789–798, 2004.

21

Intravitreal Bevacizumab Injection Attenuates Diabetic Retinopathy in Adult Rats with Experimentally Induced Diabetes in the Early Stage

Jiao Lv,[1] Miao-Miao Chen,[2] Zhi-Hao Mu,[1] Fang Wang,[1] Zhong-Yi Qian,[3] Lei Zhou,[4] Qiu-Ting Guo,[1] Zhi-Min Zhao,[1] Yu-Ping Pan,[1] Xin-Yu Liao,[1] Zhi-Hong Yang,[1] Ning Cai,[2] Shu-De Li,[5] and Ying-Ying Zou[1]

[1]*Department of Pathology and Pathophysiology, Faculty of Basic Medical Sciences, Kunming Medical University, 1168 West Chunrong Road, Kunming 650500, China*
[2]*Department of Ophthalmology, First Affiliated Hospital of Kunming Medical University, 295 Xi Chang Road, Kunming 650032, China*
[3]*Department of Morphological Laboratory, Faculty of Basic Medical Sciences, Kunming Medical University, 1168 West Chunrong Road, Kunming 650500, China*
[4]*The Key Laboratory of Stem Cell and Regenerative Medicine of Yunnan Province, Kunming Medical University, 1168 West Chunrong Road, Kunming 650500, China*
[5]*Department of Biochemistry and Molecular Biology, Faculty of Basic Medical Sciences, Kunming Medical University, 1168 West Chunrong Road, Kunming 650500, China*

Correspondence should be addressed to Shu-De Li; shudeli006@vip.sina.com and Ying-Ying Zou; zouyingyingzyy@126.com

Academic Editor: Patrizio Tatti

Diabetic retinopathy is the leading cause of blindness, yet its treatment is very limited. Anti-VEGF drug has been widely applied in ocular disease, but its effects on diabetic retinopathy and the underlying mechanism have remained to be fully explored. To elucidate the role of anti-VEGF treatment, we sought to determine the effects of bevacizumab on diabetic neurovascular changes extending from the 3rd to 9th week with induced diabetes in adult rats. The retinal neurovascular changes included increased expression of VEGF, nNOS, iNOS, eNOS, and NO in the course of diabetes progression. In diabetic rats given bevacizumab injection, the ganglion cell loss and alterations of retinal thickness were ameliorated. In this connection, the immunofluorescence labeling of the above biomarkers was noticeably decreased. Along with this, Western blotting confirmed that bevacizumab treatment was associated with a decrease of VEGF, Flk-1, and cAMP response element binding and protein kinase C protein expression. The present results suggest that bevacizumab treatment in the early stage of the retinopathy may ameliorate the lesions of retinopathy, in which VEGF/Flk-1 signaling has been shown here to play an important role.

1. Introduction

Diabetic retinopathy (DR) is the commonest complication of diabetes and the leading cause of blindness in developed countries [1–3]. Although laser therapy and vitreoretinal surgery have been widely adopted, their effectiveness is limited and they mainly target at the later stages of the disease [1]. The control of the risk factors for diabetes in the early stage is therefore desirable to find new ways to identify, to prevent, and, hopefully, to eventually cure the diabetic retinopathy [2, 4].

The retina is a highly vascularized neural tissue [4]. Traditional treatments have focused on pathological changes of vasculature and intervention in the later stages. Recent studies have shifted the focus to the role of nonvascular cells, such as neurons, astrocytes, and Müller cells, in the progression of

DR and accompanying molecular changes [5]. Further understanding of the biology of DR, especially the relationship between vascular and neural changes, would contribute to the development of novel treatments [4].

Vascular endothelial growth factor (VEGF) has been reported to play a pivotal role in the development of DR [3, 6, 7]. VEGF levels are increased in animals with experimental diabetes and patients with diabetic retinopathy [3]. Previous studies have reported that inhibition of VEGF with anti-VEGF drugs could reduce retinal permeability and neovascularization [8, 9]. These results have resulted in the development of anti-VEGF strategies such as bevacizumab as potential new therapies [10, 11]. Bevacizumab has been shown to ameliorate rapid regression of retinal neovascularization and improve visual acuity and decrease retinal thickness [3, 12]. There is ample evidence supporting its effect on preventing retinal angiogenesis in DR [13]. Though many clinical studies have confirmed its efficacy [14–16], it remains to be fully explored how bevacizumab might affect both neuronal and vascular changes and contributes to functional improvement. Treating DR using bevacizumab at a late stage while lesion is severe is often unsatisfactory.

cAMP response element binding (CREB), a cellular transcription factor important to angiogenesis, could be activated by VEGF through phosphorylation of VEGF receptor 2 (Flk-1) tyrosine kinase. Protein kinase C (PKC) is an important mediator of CREB phosphorylation [17]. In light of this, we hypothesized that CREB-induced angiogenesis might play an important role in DR.

This study was therefore aimed to ascertain whether bevacizumab may be applied in the early stage to improve its efficacy. Meanwhile, we also aimed to determine on how bevacizumab might influence the neuronal and vascular changes in the early stage of DR. The efficacy of bevacizumab on these changes, including some signaling pathways, is therefore explored.

In consideration of the above, we have carried out this study in two phases. Firstly, the neuronal and vascular changes during the development of diabetes were examined. This was to determine the critical stage for intravitreal bevacizumab injection. Secondly, we sought to determine how bevacizumab treatment might reduce retinal pathological damage in the early stage of diabetes.

2. Material and Methods

2.1. Induction of Diabetes. Animal experiment protocols were performed in accordance with the National Institutes of Health Guide for the Care and Use of Laboratory Animals (NIH publication number 80-23) revised 1996. One hundred and twenty adult male Sprague Dawley rats (Dashuo, Chengdu, China), weighing 300–340 g, were divided into 8 groups according to duration of diabetes mellitus (DM) since its induction, including normal control (NC and NC11w) group ($n = 12$), DM3w, DM6w, DM9w, and DM11w groups ($n = 16$), and different treatments, including diabetes with a single intravitreal injection of sodium lactate Ringer's (DM11w + LR) group ($n = 16$) and diabetes with a single intravitreal injection of bevacizumab (DM11w + B) group ($n = 16$).

Diabetes was induced by a bolus intraperitoneal injection of streptozotocin (STZ, 65 mg/kg in citrate buffer; Sigma, St. Louis, MO, USA), while the normal control group received the same volume of citrate buffer. The body weight was recorded, likewise, for the fasting blood glucose level at 4 days after STZ injection. Diabetes was defined by a fasting blood glucose concentration of over 16.67 mmol/L. In our previous study, we have monitored the blood glucose level and found it maintained at a high level [18].

2.2. Intravitreal Injection. Intravitreal injection was administered at 6 weeks after diabetes induction. Rats were anaesthetized by an intraperitoneal injection of 10% chloral hydrate (0.35 ± 0.05 mL/100 g, Hengtai Chemical Co. Ltd., Jiangsu, China). The pupil was dilated by Tropicamide (Bausch & Lomb Freda Pharmaceutical Co. Ltd., Shandong, China) topically anesthetized by Benoxil (Santen Pharmaceutical Co. Ltd., Osaka, Japan). The injection site was located temporal at 3 o'clock of corneal limbal and 1.0–1.5 mm to the limbus. Firstly, we used a NovoPen (Novo Nordisk Pharmaceutical Co. Ltd., Denmark) to pierce into the vitreous cavity. Next, 3 μL of sodium lactate Ringer's or bevacizumab (25 mg/mL, Roche Pharmaceutical Co. Ltd., Schweiz) was injected into the vitreous body with a microsyringe (YuanQuan Biological Technology Co. Ltd., Shanghai, China). After the needle was withdrawn, pressure was applied at the injection site with a cotton swab, and Chloramphenicol Eye Drop (Medco Huakang Pharmaceutical Co. Ltd., Sichuan, China) was applied for the following three days. Rats with any postoperative complications, for example, cataract, were excluded from the study.

2.3. Paraffin Embedding and Sectioning. For histology and immunohistochemistry and double immunofluorescence labeling, four rats in each group were anesthetized with 10% chloral hydrate (4 mL/kg body weight) and perfused with filtered saline (150 mL and 12 mL/min), followed by 4% paraformaldehyde in phosphate-buffered saline (PBS), pH 7.4 (500 mL and 12 mL/min). The eyeballs were removed, dehydrated, embedded in paraffin, and cut into 4 μm thick sections. The sections were transferred to silane-coated microscope slides and dewaxed.

2.4. H&E Staining. After dewaxing and hydration, the paraffin sections were processed for routine hematoxylin and eosin (H&E) staining.

2.5. Double Immunofluorescence Labeling. Normal control rats, rats of the diabetes groups (DM3, 6, and 9w), and different treatments groups (DM11w + LR and DM11w + B) were used for immunofluorescence studies. Paraffin coronal sections of the eyeball derived from different time points were incubated in primary antibodies including rat-specific vascular endothelial growth factor (VEGF, 1 : 150, Santa Cruz Biotechnology, Dallas, TX), rat-specific Flk-1 (1 : 150, Santa Cruz Biotechnology, Dallas, TX), rabbit-specific cAMP-response

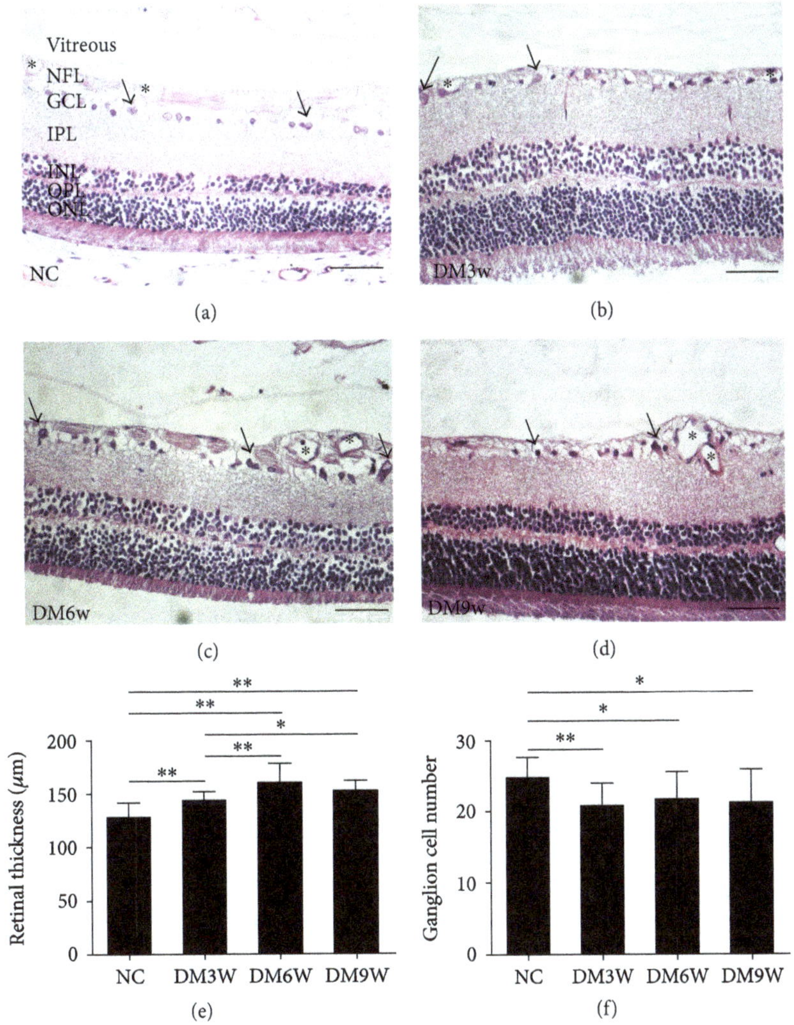

FIGURE 1: Neuronal and vascular changes in the early stage of diabetes. (a–d) H&E staining of the retina in the NC, DM3w, DM6w, and DM9w groups. Black arrow indicates neuronal changes in which the ganglion cells appeared to be enlarged at the DM3w group but were condensed at the DM6w and DM9w groups. Blood vessels were dilated in diabetic retina notably at the DM6w and DM9w groups (asterisk). (e, f) Quantification of retinal thickness and ganglion cell number in the NC, DM3w, DM6w, and DM9w groups. Bar = 50 μm. $^{*}p < 0.05$ and $^{**}p < 0.01$.

element binding protein (CREB, 1 : 150, Millipore, Darmstadt, Germany), and rat-specific PKC (1 : 150, Abcam, Cambridge, UK). NeuN (1 : 250, Abcam/Millipore) was used for neuronal labeling and GFAP (1 : 500, Abcam) for astrocyte labeling. After incubation and washing, FITC-conjugated and Cy3-conjugated secondary antibodies were added. After mounting, images representing at least one eyeball section each from four rats at different time points were captured under a confocal fluorescence microscope (Olympus, Tokyo, Japan). Immunofluorescence labeling for the various antibodies directed against the respective cell types was consistent and reproducible across different rats.

Semiquantification of CREB and Flk-1 by immunofluorescence was conducted with ImageJ (version 1.50i software; ImageJ, National Institutes of Health, Bethesda, MD, USA). Immunofluorescent images were transformed into 16-bit grayscale images. Areas with immunofluorescence expression were selected, and integrated density was measured. The background immunofluorescence intensity was also measured in an area without immunofluorescence. The data of corrected integrated density was gained by subtracting the background intensity from the integrated density.

2.6. Western Blot. Fresh tissue samples were collected from the retina. To analyze the expression levels of respective proteins, equal amounts of total proteins were subjected to 10% (*w*/*v*) SDS-PAGE and transferred onto polyvinylidene fluoride (PVDF) membranes (Millipore, Darmstadt, Germany). Membranes were then blocked with 5% skim milk for 2 hours at room temperature and probed with anti-VEGF (1 : 500; Santa Cruz Biotechnology, Dallas, TX), anti-Flk-1 (1 : 1000; Santa Cruz Biotechnology, Dallas, TX), anti-CREB (1 : 1000; Millipore, Darmstadt, Germany), anti-PKC (1 : 750; Abcam, Cambridge, UK), anti-β actin (1 : 1000; Santa Cruz Biotechnology, Dallas, TX), anti-GAPDH (Abcam, Cambridge, UK), anti-nNOS (1 : 1000, BD Biosciences, USA), anti-iNOS

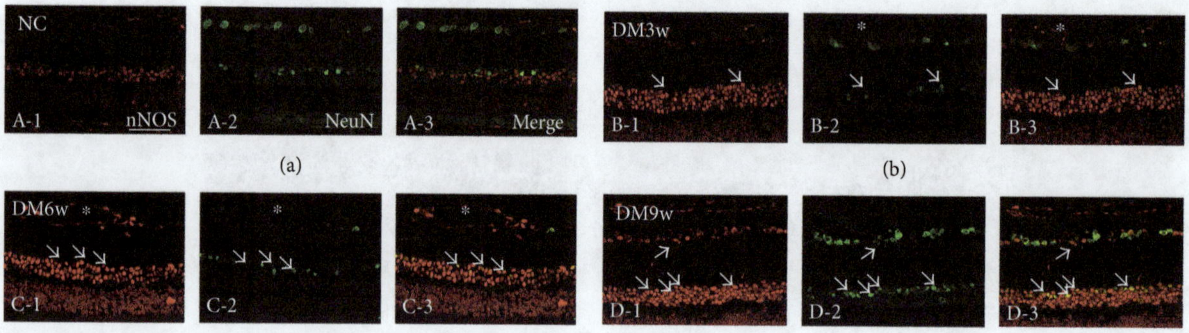

(a) (b) (c) (d)

FIGURE 2: Representative photomicrographs of nNOS (red) and NeuN (green) double staining of the retina in the NC and DM6w groups. nNOS immunoreactivity was localized in NeuN-labeled neurons (single arrow) and blood vessels (asterisk), and it was relatively higher in the DM6w group (B-1) than in the NC group (A-1). Moreover, coexpression of nNOS and NeuN was apparent in the DM6w group (B-3) compared to the NC group (A-3). Blood vessels appeared to be dilated in diabetic retina at the DM6w group (asterisk). Note the enhanced nNOS staining and smaller size of NeuN-positive neurons at the DM6w group compared with the control group. Bar = 50 μm.

(1 : 750, Santa Cruz Biotechnology, Dallas, TX), and anti-eNOS (1 : 750, Santa Cruz Biotechnology, Dallas, TX) antibodies at 4°C overnight. Subsequently, membranes were incubated with horseradish peroxidase- (HRP-) conjugated goat anti-rabbit (Thermo Fisher Scientific, Waltham, MA) or rabbit anti-rat (Thermo Fisher Scientific, Waltham, MA) IgG for 2 hours at room temperature after three times TBST washing and then reacted with a prolight HRP agent (Santa Cruz Biotechnology, Dallas, TX). The result of chemiluminescence was recorded with an imaging system and semi-quantified using the ImageJ software (National Institutes of Health, Bethesda, MD).

2.7. Nitrite Assay. The total amount of NO (mM) in the retina was assessed with a colorimetric assay kit (US Biological, Swampscott, MA) by the Griess reaction, detecting nitrite a stable reaction product of NO and NO^{2-}. Briefly, 85 μL of each sample was added to 5 μL of nitrate reductase followed by 5 μL of enzyme cofactor according to the manufacturer's instructions and incubated for 1 h at room temperature. Five microliters of enhancer was then added and incubated for 10 min. Following this, 50 μL of Griess reagent R1 and R2 was added to the above solution and the color could develop at room temperature for 10 min. The optical density of the samples was measured at 540 nm using the GENios microplate reader (Tecan, Austria GmbH, Salzburg, Austria). Nitrite concentration was determined from a nitrite standard curve.

2.8. Retinal Thickness Assay and Ganglion Cell Counting. The sections for the quantitative measurement of the retinal thickness were from the same eyes used in the H&E staining. Quantification of the retinal thickness was performed in 4 μm thick sagittal sections of the eyeball. Three intact sections were evaluated at 3 sites 52 μm adjacent to the optic nerve head and along the periphery, each separated by a distance of 20 μm. In each selected section under 40x objective, the retinal thickness at three sites per section was measured by ImageJ. The thickness was measured across the different retinal layers including the nerve fiber layer (NFL), ganglion cell layer (GCL), inner plexiform layer (IPL), inner nuclear layer (INL), outer plexiform layer (OPL), and outer nuclear layer (ONL).

The sections for the quantitative counting of the ganglion cells were the same used in retinal thickness assay. Three intact sections were evaluated in each eye, and ganglion cells were counted under 20x objective. The linear length of retina measured was about 600 μm.

2.9. Statistical Analysis. Data were presented as mean ± SD and percentage. Data obtained in diverse groups were assessed with an unpaired Student *t*-test using SPSS 16.0 (SPSS Inc., Armonk, NY). One-way ANOVA was carried out to assess within-group differences of immunofluorescence intensity. A probability value of $p < 0.05$ was considered significant.

3. Results

3.1. Neuronal and Vascular Changes during Diabetes Progression

3.1.1. Animals: Physical and Clinical Observations. The body weight of diabetic rats in the DM3w group was significantly lower than that in the NC group (325 ± 16 versus 294 ± 44; $p < 0.01$). The blood glucose level was maintained at a high level after diabetes induction.

3.1.2. H&E Staining. H&E staining showed that the retina of diabetic rats did not present obvious structural changes at 3w after diabetes induction. Nevertheless, retinal thickness was increased in the DM3w, DM6w, and DM9w groups. When compared with the DM3w group, the retinal thickness was significantly higher in the DM6w and DM9w groups (Figure 1(e)). The results of enumeration of ganglion cells showed that the cell number was decreased in the DM3w, DM6w, and DM9w groups (Figure 1(f)).

Compared with the NC and DM3w groups, the retina in the DM6w group exhibited edema and retinovascular

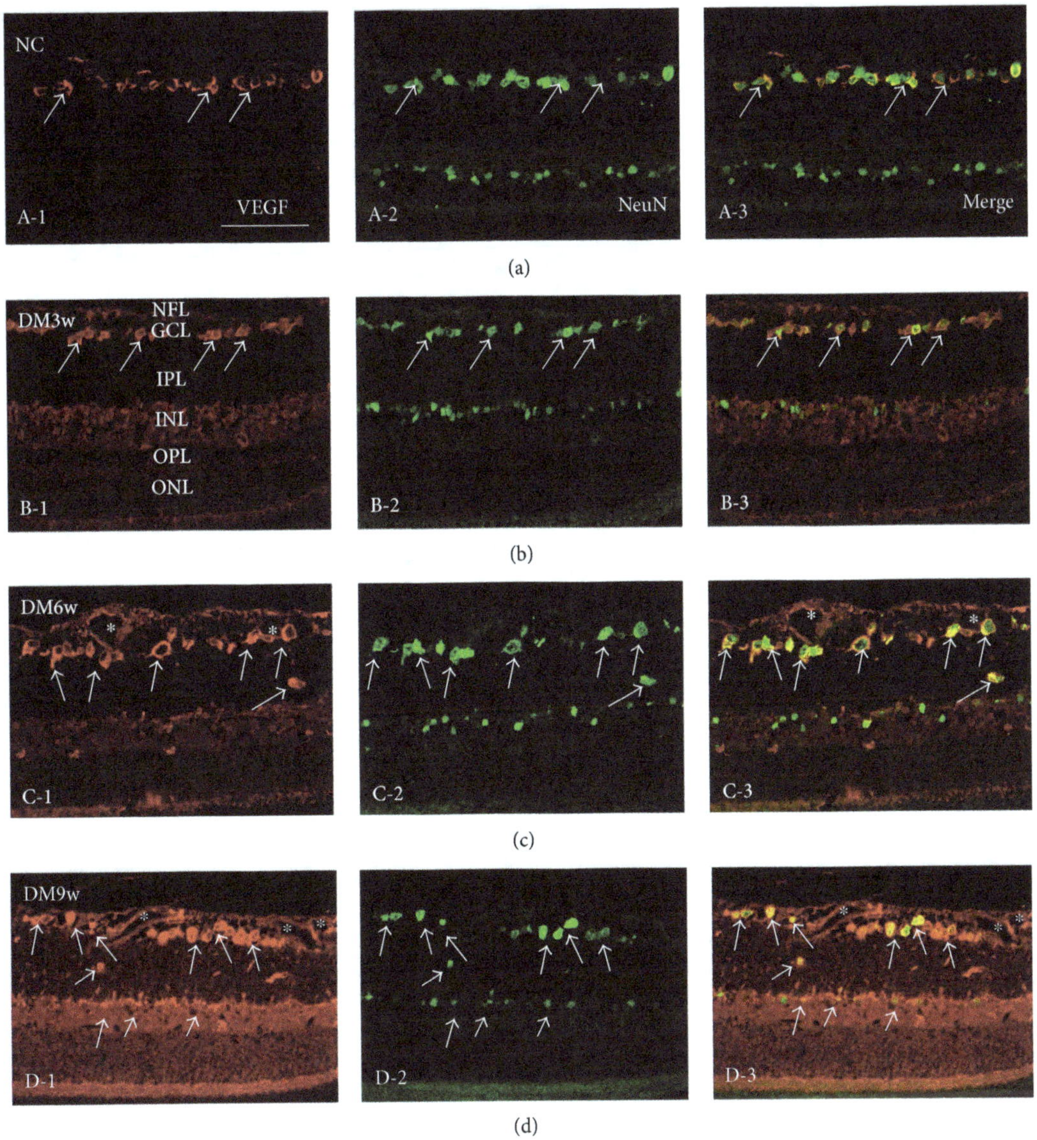

FIGURE 3: Representative photomicrographs of VEGF (red) and NeuN (green) double staining of the retina in the NC, DM3w, DM6w, and DM9w groups. VEGF immunoreactivity was localized in NeuN-labeled neurons (single arrow) and blood vessels (asterisk). VEGF staining appeared to be enhanced with the progress of diabetes (a, b, c, D-1), while the size of NeuN-labeled neurons became smaller (a, b, c, D-2). Bar = 50 μm.

dilation, while neural and endothelial cells remained relatively normal (Figures 1(a)–1(c)). In the DM9w group, the retinal vasculature underwent more pathological changes such as vitreous degeneration, thickening of vascular wall, and luminal stenosis. In addition, the nerve fiber layer (NFL) of the retina became thinner (Figure 1(d)).

3.1.3. Double Immunofluorescence Labeling. In the control rats, a moderate nNOS labeling was detected in different layers of the retina (Figure 2). nNOS expressing cells were identified to be the neurons as they coexpressed NeuN (Figure 2(a), A-1). In the DM3w, DM6w, and DM9w groups, the incidence of nNOS expressing neurons was increased and nNOS immunofluorescence was more intense in comparison with the matching control (Figures 2(a) and 2(b), B-1).

In the control rats, VEGF labeling was detected in the NFL, ganglion cell layer (GCL), and inner plexiform layer (IPL) (Figure 3(a), A-1). In the DM3w, DM6w, and DM9w groups, VEGF expression was conspicuously augmented in various retinal layers. VEGF immunoreactivity was most intense in the ganglion cells, whose identification was confirmed by double labeling with anti-VEGF and anti-NeuN (Figures 3(a)–3(d), D-3). Some neurons in the inner nuclear layer (INL) also exhibited colocalization of VEGF and NeuN at the DM6w and DM9w groups (Figures 3(c) and 3(d), D-3).

In the normal control rats, astrocytes were confined to the NFL and GCL and emitted GFAP immunofluorescence (Figure 4(a), A-2). Colocalization of VEGF labeling with GFAP was evident, but it was only detected in the GCL (Figure 4(a), A-3). In the DM3w, DM6w, and DM9w groups, the incidence of VEGF expressing astrocytes was increased

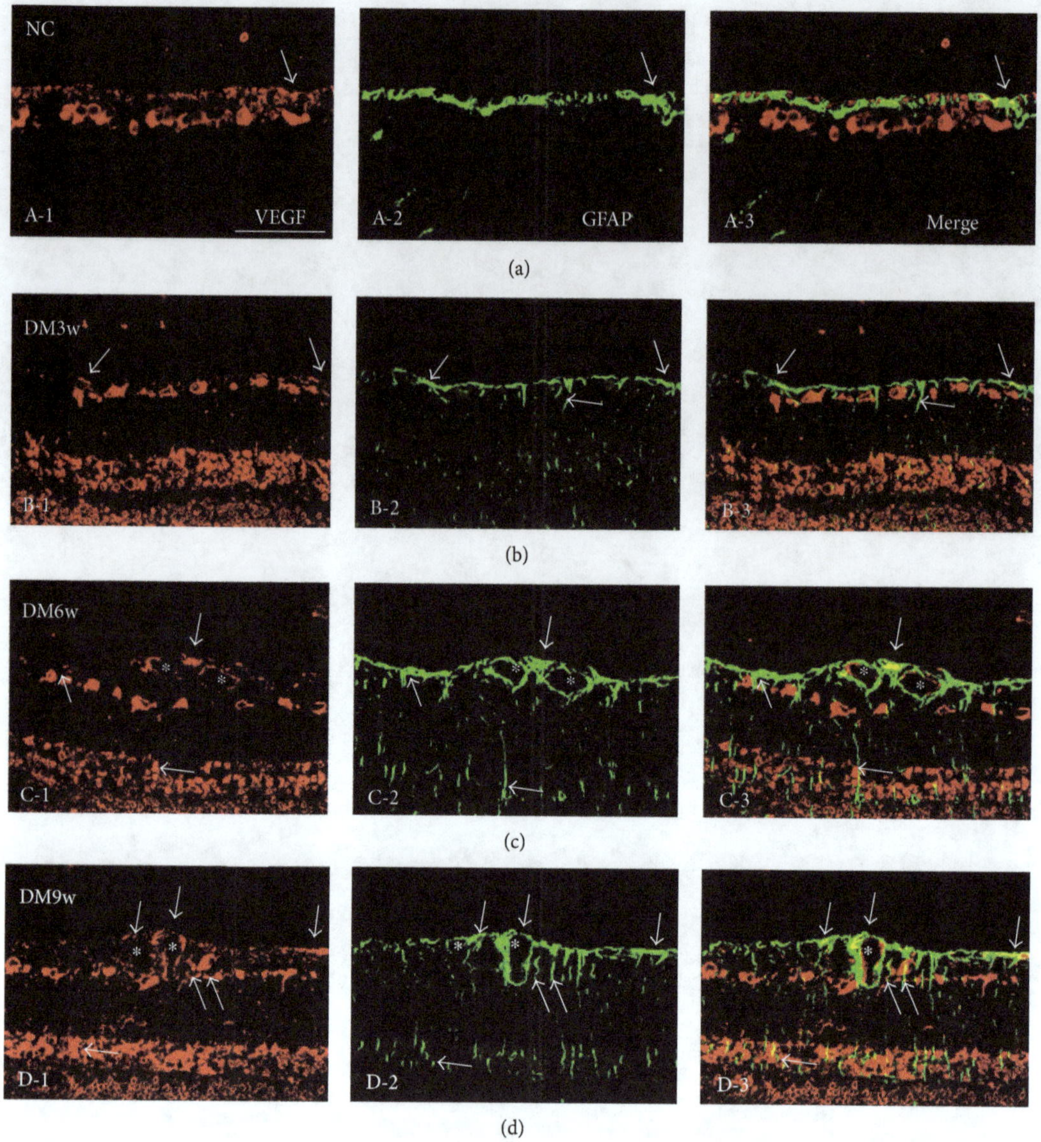

FIGURE 4: Representative photomicrographs of VEGF (red) and GFAP (green) double staining of the retina in the NC, DM3w, DM6w, and DM9w groups. VEGF immunoreactivity was localized in GFAP-labeled astrocytes (single arrow), blood vessels (asterisk), and Müller cells with their processes spanning across different retinal layers (double arrows). Bar = 50 μm.

(Figures 4(b)–4(d), D-3), and their long extending and hypertrophic processes were intensely stained with GFAP (Figures 4(b)–4(d), D-2). Müller cell processes in palisade spanned the different retinal layers (Figures 4(c) and 4(d), D-2); such a configuration was especially pronounced at the DM9w group. Enhanced VEGF expression was most conspicuous at 9w (Figure 4(d), D-1), in comparison with other time points (Figures 4(b) and 4(c), C-1). Except for some vascular profiles, GFAP-positive astrocytes in NFL were colocalized with VEGF immunofluorescence (Figures 4(c) and 4(d), D-3). Both VEGF and GFAP immunoreactivity in astrocytes or associated with the blood vessels were markedly enhanced after disease exposure (Figures 4(c) and 4(d), D-3).

Western blot analysis showed that VEGF and NOS proteins were increased after diabetes induction (Figures 5(a)–5(d)). Compared with the NC group, densitometry of the VEGF immunoreactive band showed a significant increase at the DM3w ($p < 0.01$), DM6w ($p < 0.01$), and DM9w groups ($p < 0.01$). VEGF expression level was significantly higher in the DM6w ($p < 0.01$) and DM 9w ($p < 0.01$) groups than that in the DM3w group. nNOS expression level was also increased at the DM3w ($p < 0.01$), DM6w ($p < 0.01$), and DM9w groups ($p < 0.01$). Among the three groups, protein expression was the highest in the DM9w group than that in the DM3w ($p < 0.01$) group and the DM6w group ($p < 0.05$). The expression level of iNOS was increased in the DM3w ($p < 0.05$), DM6w ($p < 0.01$), and DM9w groups ($p < 0.01$), while the difference between the DM6w and DM9w groups was insignificant. The expression changes in pattern of eNOS followed that of iNOS, except that eNOS expression in the DM9w group was significantly higher than that in the DM3w group ($p < 0.05$).

Measurement of NO production showed that it was increased with the progression of diabetes (Figure 5(e)).

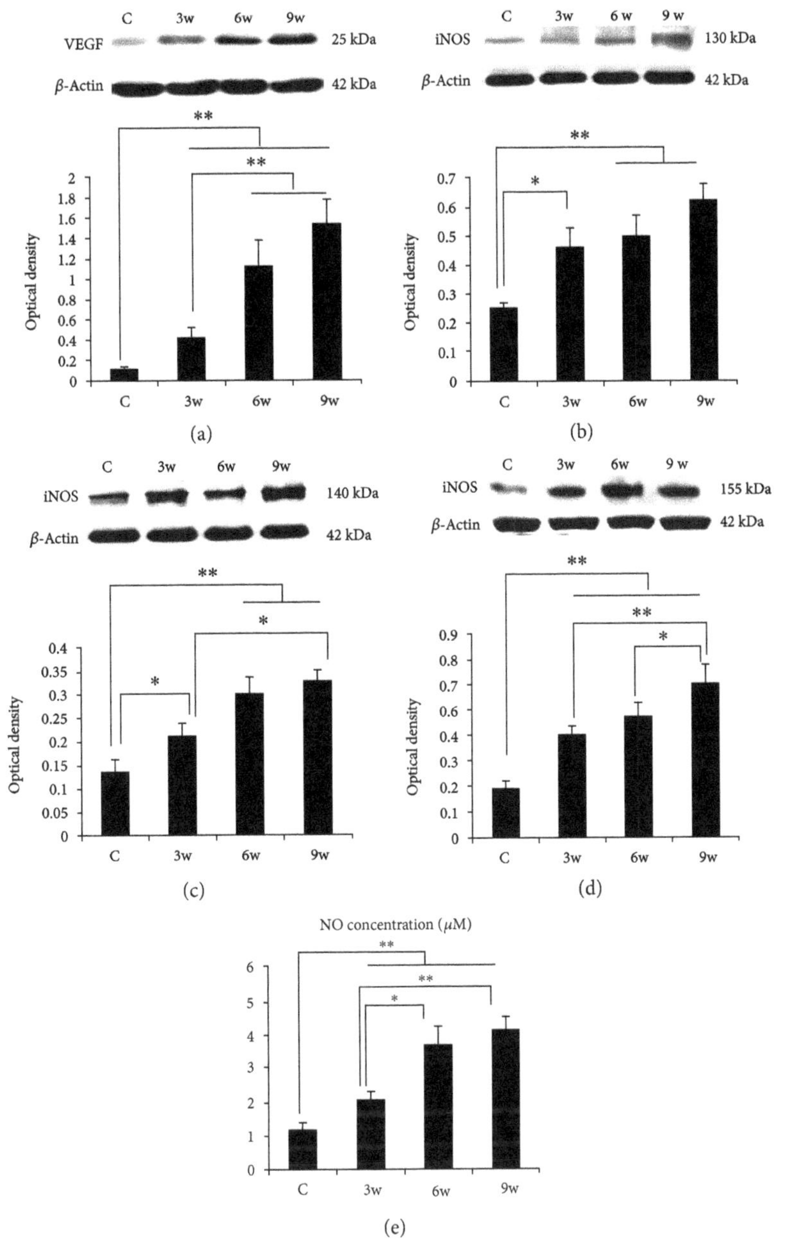

Figure 5: Western blot analysis of VEGF (a), iNOS (b), eNOS (c), and nNOS (d) protein expression levels in the retina in the NC, DM3w, DM6w, and DM9w groups, including the immunoreactive bands of VEGF (21 kDa), iNOS (130 kDa), eNOS (140 kDa), nNOS (155 kDa), and β-actin (42 kDa). Bar graphs representing optical density (mean ± SD). The expression levels were all increased after diabetes induction. (e) NO concentration in the NC, DM3w, DM6w, and DM9w groups. NO concentration was significantly increased in the retina at 3w, 6w, and 9w after diabetes induction when compared with that of control rats. $^{*}p < 0.05$ and $^{**}p < 0.01$.

It was significantly higher in the DM3w ($p < 0.01$), DM6w ($p < 0.01$), and DM9w groups ($p < 0.01$). Compared with the DM3w group, NO level was increased significantly in the DM6w ($p < 0.05$) and DM9w groups ($p < 0.01$).

3.2. Bevacizumab Treatment Ameliorated Retinal Pathological Changes in the Early Stage of Diabetes

3.2.1. H&E Staining. To study the effect and mechanism of anti-VEGF treatment on the early stage of DR, we adopted intravitreous injection of bevacizumab at 6 weeks after diabetes induction and evaluated its effect at 11w after diabetes induction. H&E staining showed that the retina from the DM11w and DM11w + LR groups exhibited structural alterations, such as decrease in ganglion cells, vascular dilation in both the inner limiting membrane (ILM) and NFL, and thickening of inner plexiform layer (Figures 6(a)–6(c)). By contrast, the retina in the diabetic rats from the DM11w + B group did not show significant changes; rather, it appeared to be comparable to the NC11w group (Figure 6(d)). When compared with the NC and DM11w + B groups, the retinal thickness was increased in the DM11w and DM11w + LR groups (Figure 6(e)). Furthermore, quantification of ganglion cells showed that the

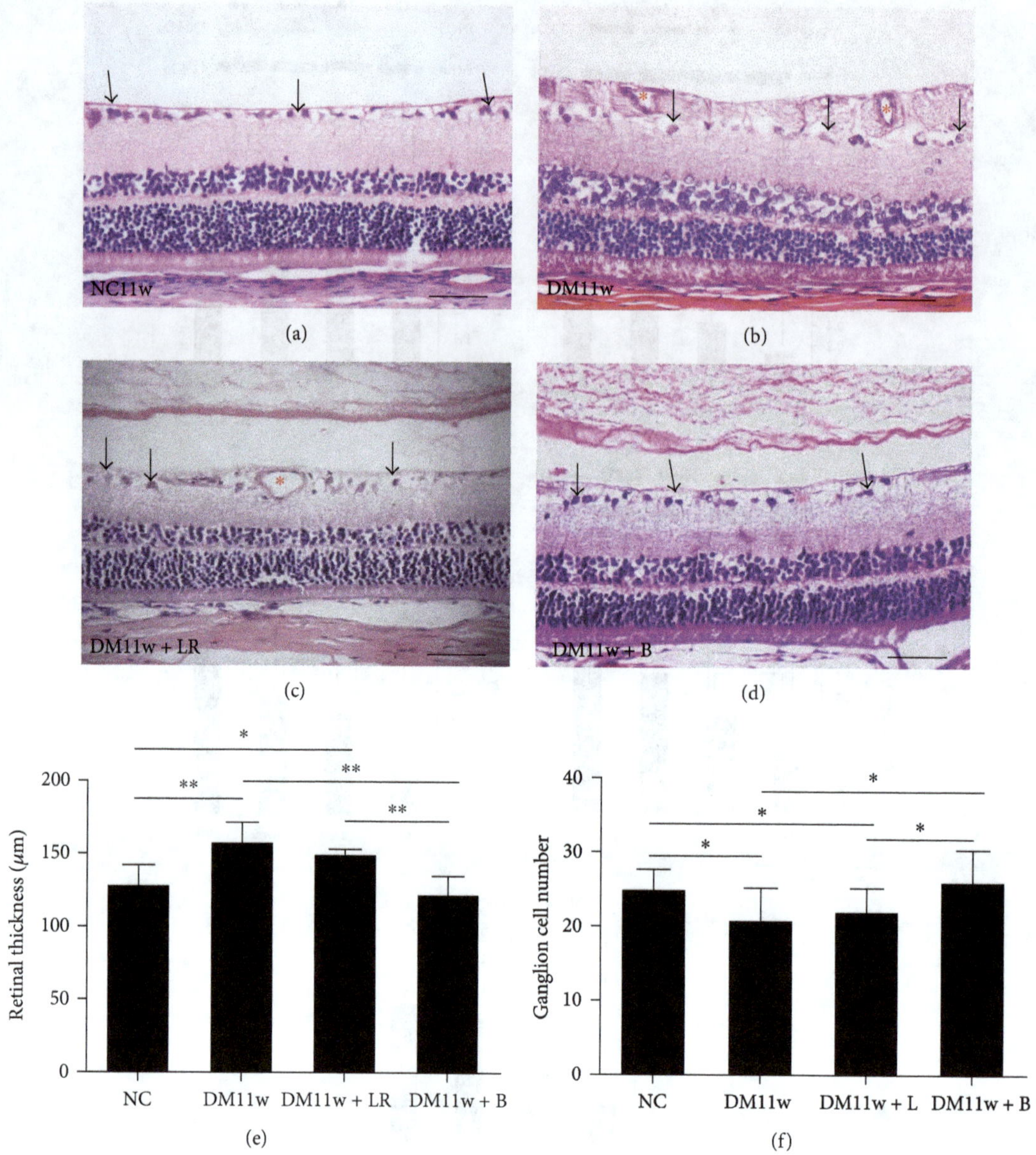

Figure 6: H&E staining of the retina in the NC11w, DM11w, DM11w + LR, and DM11w + B groups. (a–d) Note the cellular morphological changes (single arrow) in the DM11w and DM11w + LR groups compared with the NC11w and DM11w + B groups. Blood vessels were dilated in diabetic retina notably at the DM11w and DM11w + LR (asterisk). (e, f) Quantification of retinal thickness and ganglion cell number each group. Bar = 50 μm. $^{*}p < 0.05$ and $^{**}p < 0.01$.

ganglion cell number was decreased in the DM11w and DM11w + LR groups (Figure 6(f)).

3.2.2. Double Immunofluorescence Labeling. Immunostaining showed that VEGF, Flk-1, CREB, and PKC proteins were mainly expressed in GCL, INL, and outer nuclear layer (ONL). The protein expression of these proteins was higher in the DM11w and DM11w + LR groups than in the NC11w and DM11w + B groups. However, Flk-1 and CREB expression was mainly localized within GCL in the retina of normal rats, while PKC expression was spread into INL. In the DM11w + B group, CREB expression was reduced in GCL, while Flk-1 and PKC expression remained in INL and ONL (Figures 7–11).

Immunostaining results showed that the DM11w and DM11w + LR groups had more VEGF-positive cells than the NC11w group localized mainly in GCL and ONL. Furthermore, in the DM11w + LR group, the blood vessels in the ILM and NFL appeared to be dilated. VEGF expression was localized in the endothelial cells. After treatment with bevacizumab, VEGF expression was evidently decreased. Along with this, the structural integrity of blood vessels was relatively intact in the DM11w + B (Figure 7).

In the control rats, Flk-1 immunofluorescence was evident in NFL and GCL and relatively weak in INL (Figure 8(a)). Cells expressing Flk-1 were colocalized with neurons expressing NeuN (Figures 8(a)–8(d), D-3). Compared with the NC11w group, Flk-1 expression was

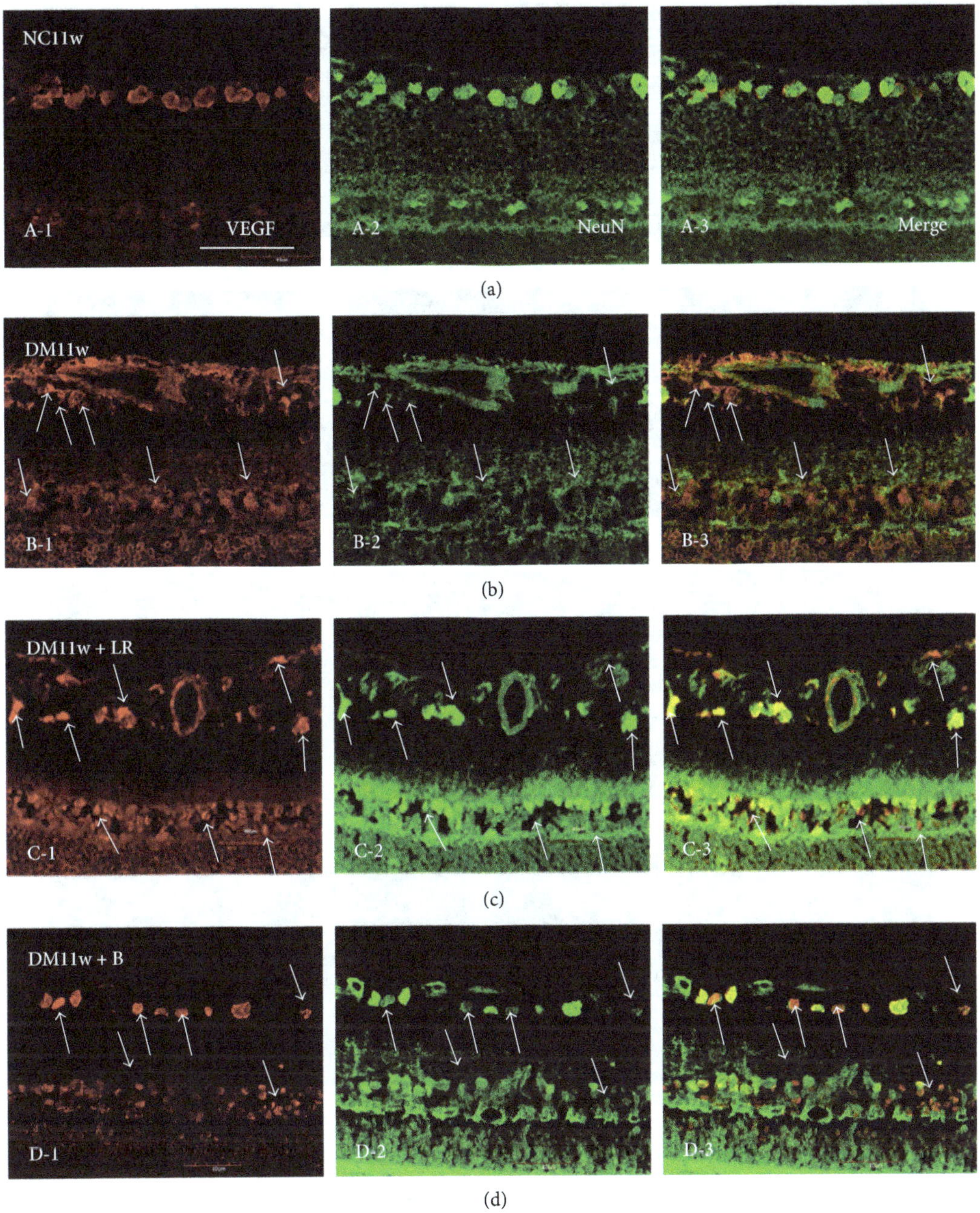

FIGURE 7: Representative photomicrographs of VEGF (red) and NeuN (green) double staining of the retina in the NC11w, DM11w, DM11w + LR, and DM11w + B groups. VEGF immunoreactivity was localized in NeuN-labeled neurons (single arrow) and blood vessels (asterisk). (a, b, c, D-1) The expression of VEGF was notably enhanced in the DM11w and DM11w + LR groups compared with the NC11w and DM11w + B groups. (a, b, c, D-2) Moreover, NeuN-labeled neurons appeared to be condensed and exhibit morphological changes in the DM11w and DM11w + LR groups, in comparison with the NC11w and DM11w + B groups. Bar = 50 μm.

significantly increased in the DM11w group and the DM11w + LR group (Figures 8(b), 8(c), C-1, and 8(e)). In these two groups, Flk-1/NeuN coexpressing cells were distributed in GCL and IPL. And Flk-1 expression was significantly decreased in the DM11w + B group compared with the DM11w group (Figures 8(d), D-3 and 8(e)).

CREB immunofluorescence was evident in NFL, GCL, and ONL in control rats (Figure 9(a), A-1). In diabetes-induced rats, CREB expression was noticeably increased in ONL and coexpressed with neurons expressing NeuN (Figures 9(a)–9(d), D-3). After bevacizumab treatment, CREB immunofluorescence was limited to NFL and GCL (Figure 9(d), D-3). Compared with the control rats, CREB expression in all three diabetes groups overlapped with NeuN expression (Figures 9(b)–9(d), D-3). Semiquantification of its fluorescent intensity showed that CREB expression was significantly increased in the DM11w and DM11w + LR groups (Figure 9(e)).

Moderate PKC immunoreactivity was detected in ONL, GCL, and NFL in control rats (Figure 10(a), A-1). In

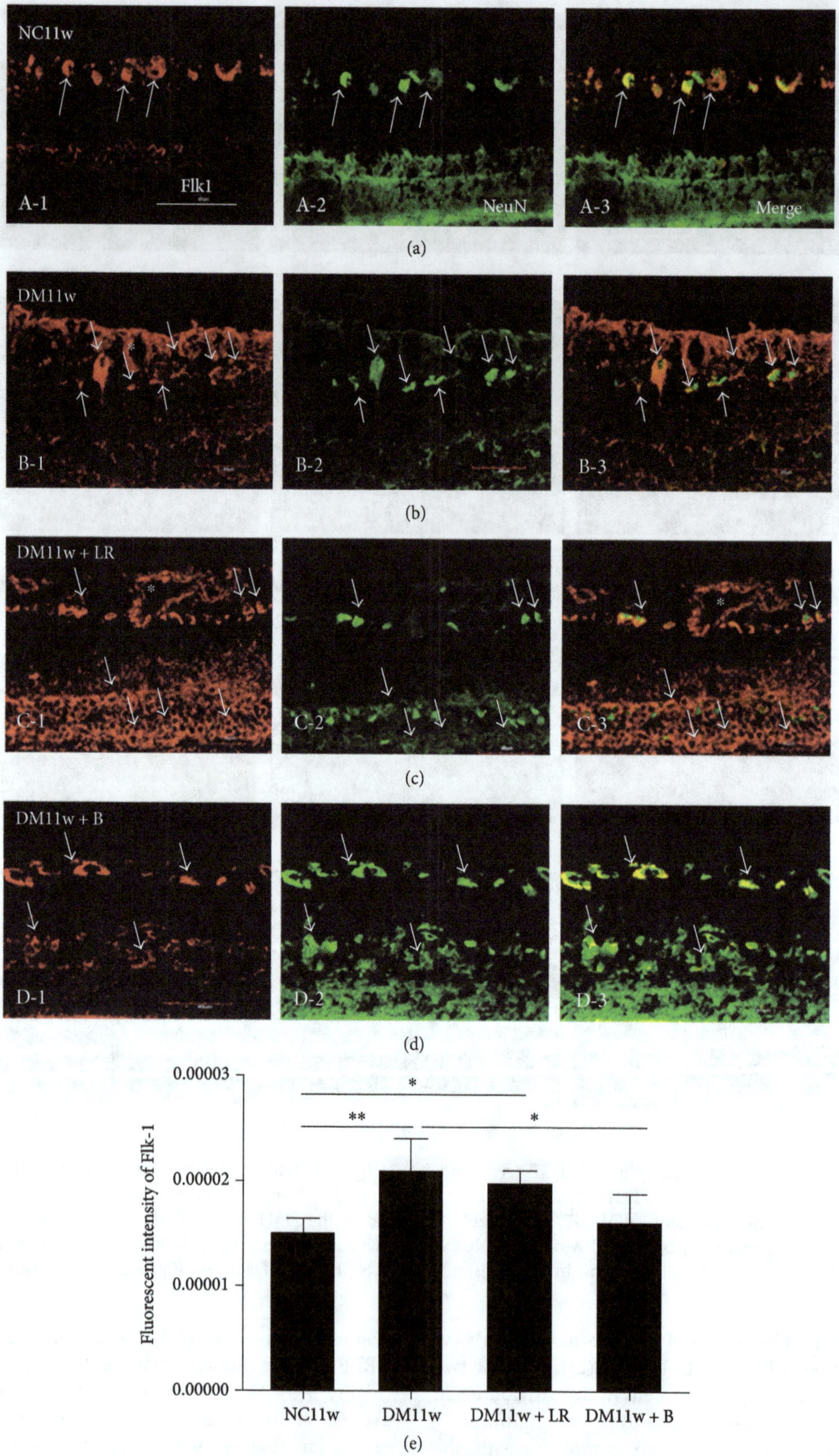

FIGURE 8: Representative photomicrographs of Flk-1 (red) and NeuN (green) double staining of the retina in the NC11w, DM11w, DM11w + LR, and DM11w + B groups. (a, b, c, D-1) Flk-1 immunoreactivity appeared to maintain its structural integrity and to be lower in the NC11w and NC11w + B groups (single arrow). (e) Semiquantification of Flk-1 by immunofluorescence. Note the dilated blood vessels in diabetic retina at the DM11w and DM11w + LR (asterisk). Bar = 50 μm. $^{*}p < 0.05$ and $^{**}p < 0.01$.

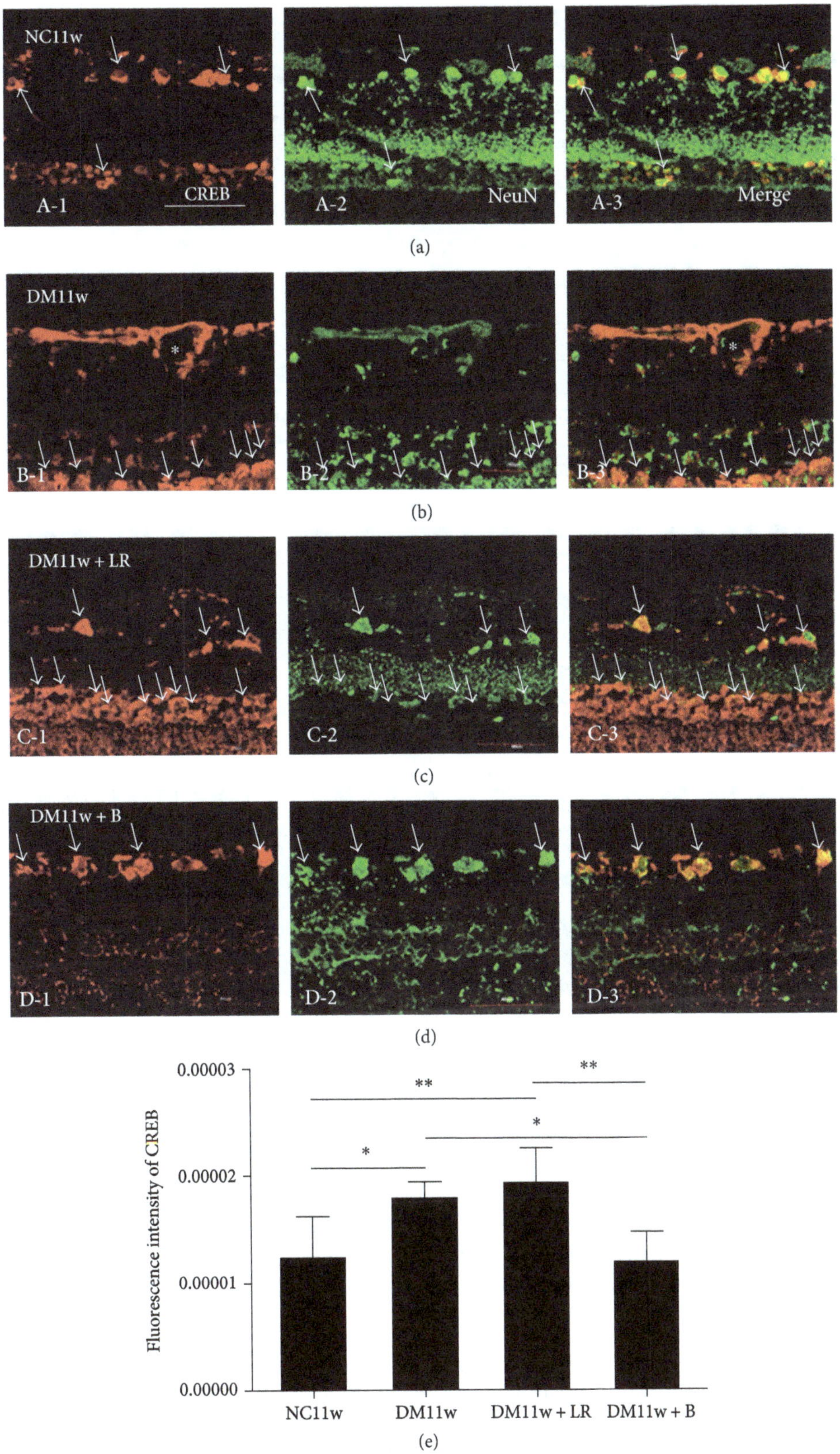

FIGURE 9: Representative photomicrographs of CREB (red) and NeuN (green) double staining of the retina in the NC11w, DM11w, DM11w + LR, and DM11w + B groups. CREB immunoreactivity is localized in NeuN-labeled neurons (single arrow) and blood vessels (asterisk). (b, C-1) In the DM11w and DM11w + LR groups, CREB expression was notably increased and even could be found in IPL. (D-1) However, CREB almost expressed only in GCL in the DM11w + B group. (e) Semiquantification of CREB by immunofluorescence. Bar = 50 μm. $^{*}p < 0.05$ and $^{**}p < 0.01$.

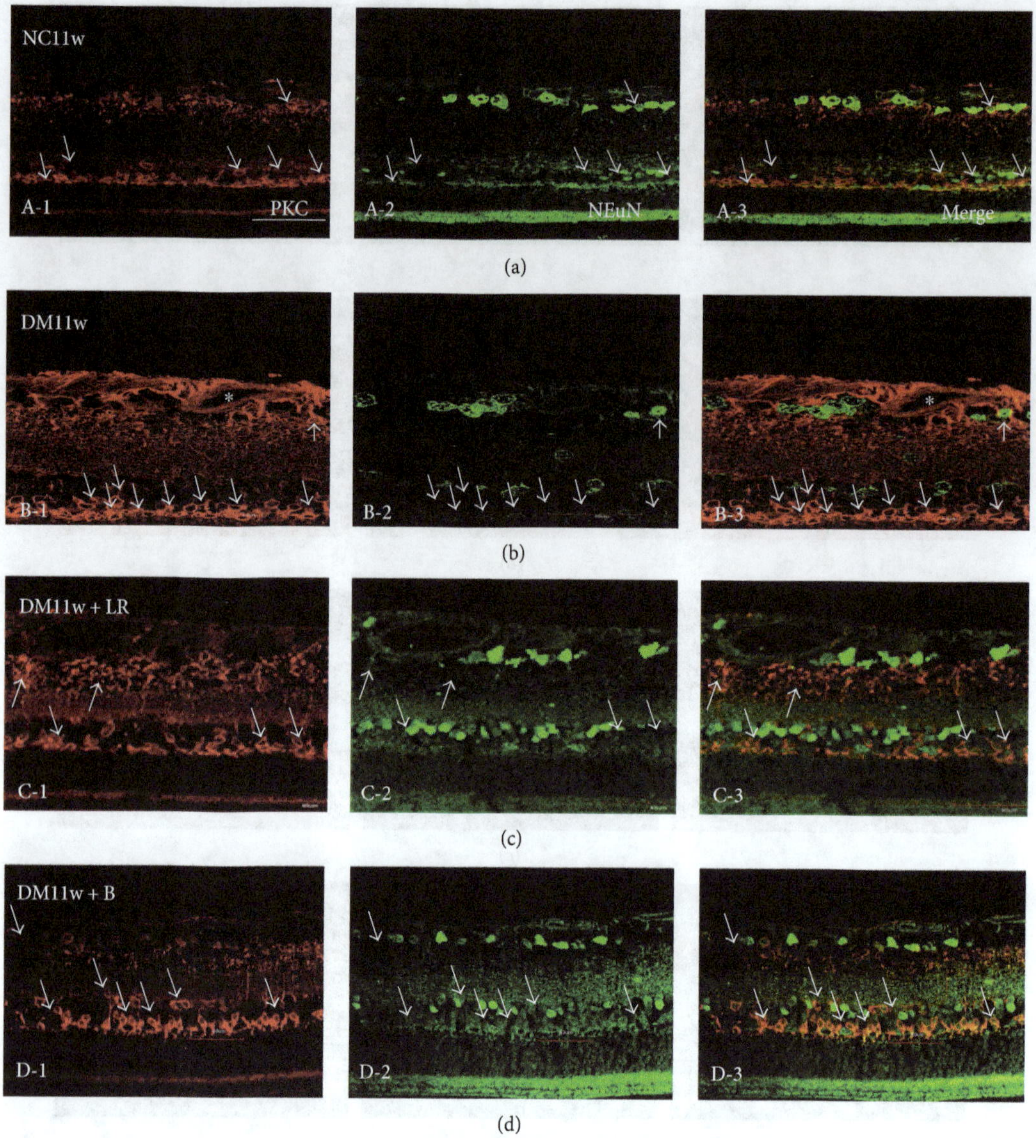

FIGURE 10: Representative photomicrographs of PKC (red) and NeuN (green) double staining of the retina in the NC11w, DM11w, DM11w + LR, and DM11w + B groups. PKC immunoreactivity was localized in NeuN-labeled neurons (single arrow) and blood vessels (asterisk). Bar = 50 μm.

diabetes-induced rats, PKC expression was markedly augmented; moreover, it was also expressed in neurons in INL (Figures 10(b)–10(d), D-3). After bevacizumab treatment, PKC expression was noticeably reduced that was localized mainly in ONL (Figure 10(d), D-3).

In the control rats, astrocytes confined to the NFL and ganglion cell layer (GCL) exhibited GFAP immunofluorescence (Figure 11(a), A-2). A moderate VEGF labeling was detected in the NFL, GCL, INL, and ONL (Figure 11(a), A-1). Colocalization of GFAP and VEGF was very minimal that was detected in the GCL only (Figure 11(a), A-3). In the DM11w and DM11w + LR groups, Müller cells intensely stained for GFAP and whose cell bodies residing in the GCL were hypertrophied (Figures 11(b), B-2 and 11(c), C-2). The cells exhibited long extending processes (Figures 11(b), B-2 and 11(c), C-2), but they appeared attenuated at the DM11w + B group (Figure 11(d), D-2). Double labeling with anti-VEGF and anti-GFAP had revealed that the VEGF-positive cells were astrocytes (Figures 11(b)–11(d), D-3).

Western blot analysis showed that VEGF protein expression in the DM11w ($p < 0.05$) and DM11w + LR groups ($p < 0.01$) was significantly higher than that in the NC11w group. In the DM11w + B group, VEGF protein expression level was higher than that in the NC11w group, but it was lower than that in the DM11w and DM11w + LR groups; however, the difference was not significant (Figure 12(a)).

Flk-1 protein expression of the retina in the DM11w ($p < 0.05$) and DM11w + LR groups ($p < 0.01$) was significantly higher than that in the NC11w group. In the DM11w + B group, Flk-1 protein expression was significantly lower than that in the DM11w + LR group ($p < 0.01$) (Figure 12(b)).

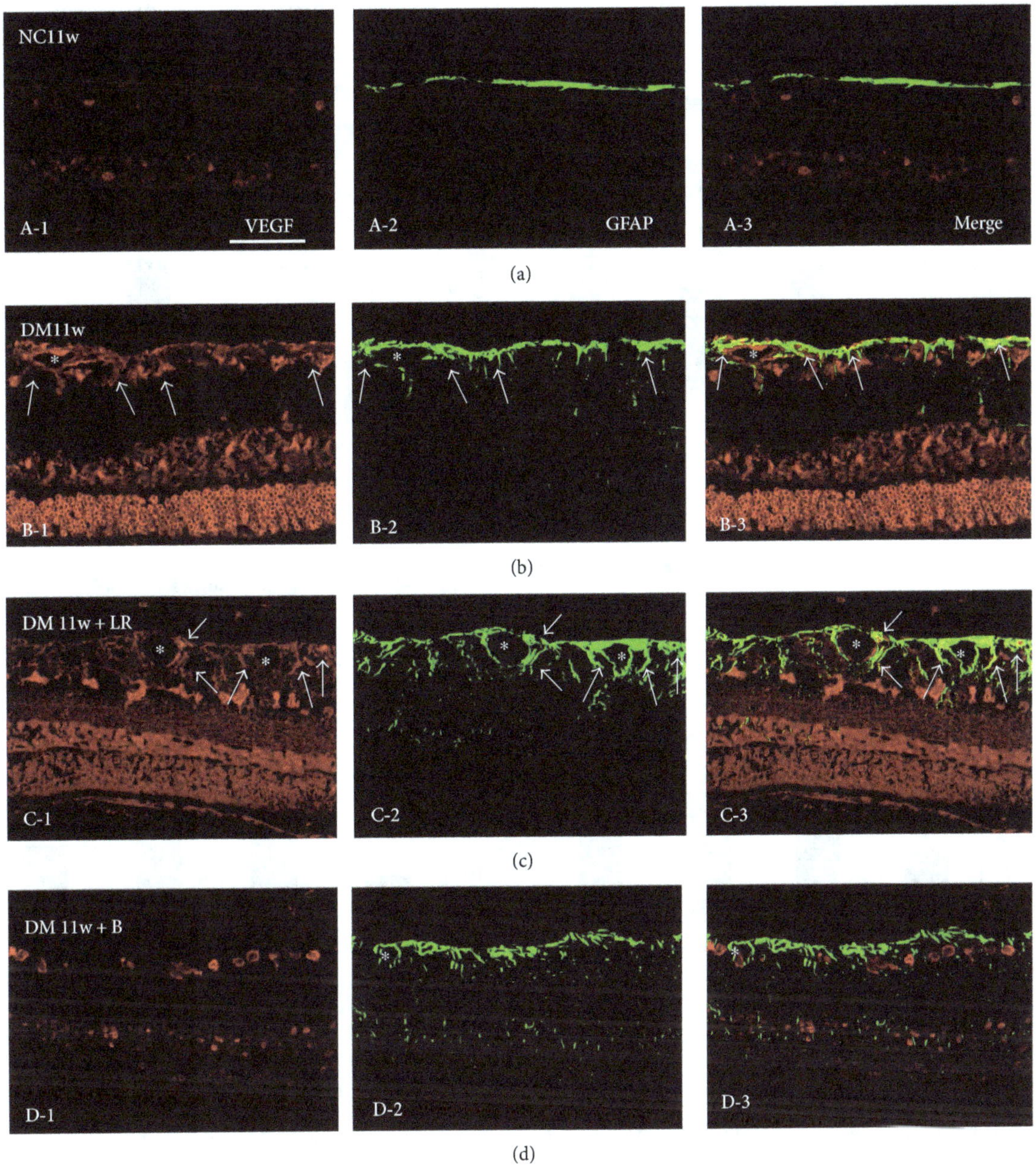

Figure 11: Representative photomicrographs of VEGF (red) and GFAP (green) double staining of the retina in the NC11w, DM11w, DM11w + LR, and DM11w + B groups. VEGF immunoreactivity was localized in GFAP-labeled astrocytes (single arrow) and blood vessels (asterisk). (b, C-2) GFAP expression appeared to be enhanced in the DM11w and DM11w + LR, consistent with the expression of VEGF in these two groups. (A-1, 2, D-1, 2) By contrast, both VEGF and GFAP expressions were relatively lower in the NC11w and DM11w + B groups. Note the dilated blood vessels in diabetic retina at the DM11w + LR group (asterisk). Bar = 50 μm.

CREB protein expression of retina in the DM11w ($p < 0.05$) and DM11w + LR groups ($p < 0.01$) was significantly higher than that in the NC11w group. In the DM11w + B group ($p < 0.01$) and the DM11w group ($p < 0.05$), it was significantly lower than that in the DM11w + LR group (Figure 12(c)).

PKC protein expression of the retina in the DM11w ($p < 0.01$) and DM11w + LR groups ($p < 0.01$) was significantly higher than that in the NC11w group. In the DM11w + B group, it was higher than that in the NC11w ($p < 0.05$) and DM11w + LR groups ($p < 0.01$) (Figure 12(d)).

4. Discussion

The present results have shown that diabetes could result in progressive neuronal and vascular damage in the retina from 3 to 9 weeks after diabetes induction. We have shown that anti-VEGF treatment using bevacizumab could not only prevent retinal pathological changes but also exert beneficial effects on the underlying molecular mechanism, mainly through limiting an undesirable increase in VEGF. In this connection and although other experimental studies have shown the protective effect of anti-VEGF

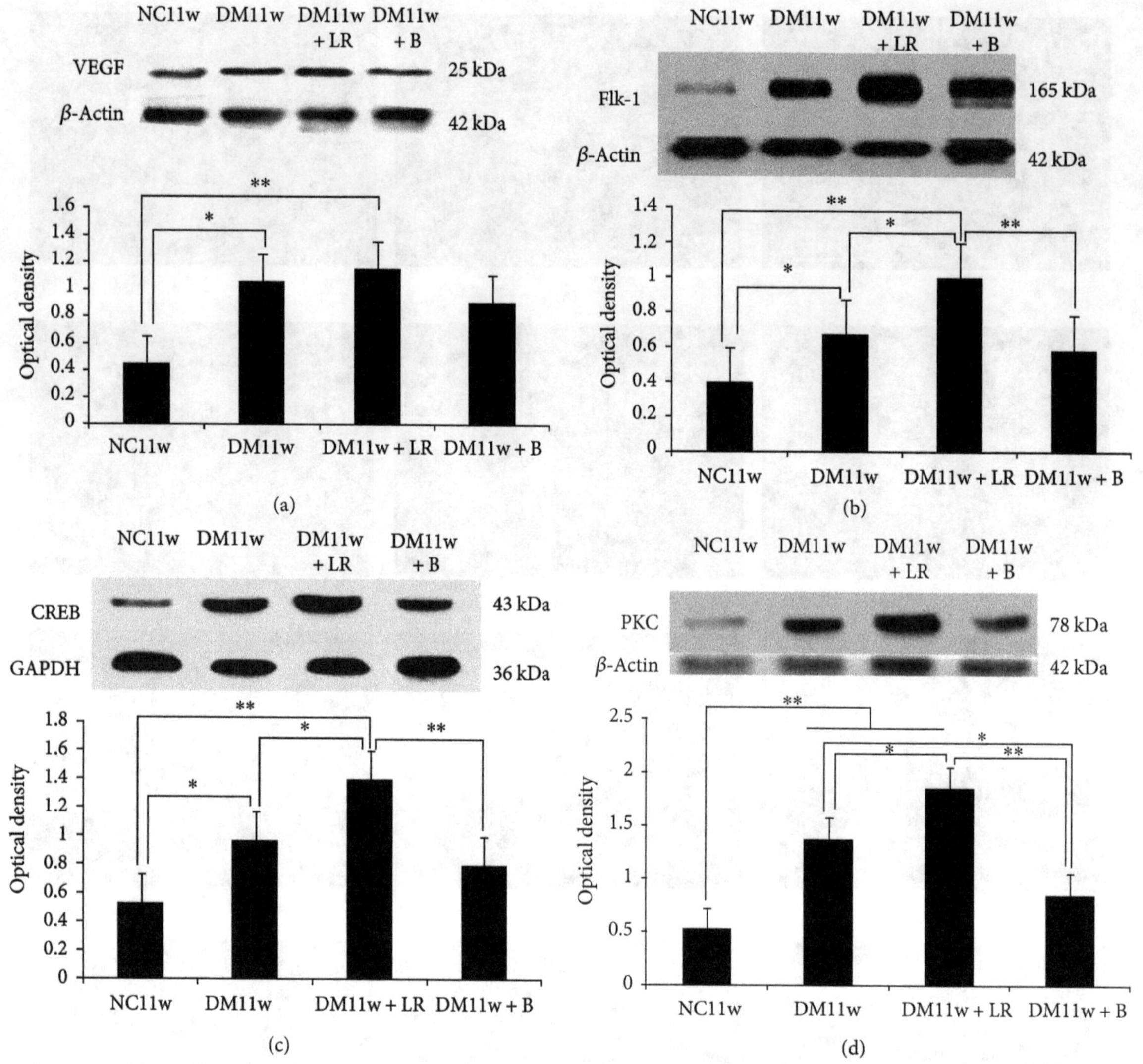

Figure 12: (a) Western blot analysis showed the expression of VEFG, Flk-1, CREB, and PKC in the NC11w, DM11w, DM11w + LR, and DM11w + B groups, including the immunoreactive bands of VEGF (21 kDa), iNOS (130 kDa), eNOS (140 kDa), nNOS (155 kDa), and β-actin (42 kDa). Bar graph showed the semiquantitative data of Western blot analysis of VEGF (a), Flk-1 (b), CREB (c), and PKC (d). (a) VEGF showed an evident increase in the DM11w and DM11w + LR groups compared with the NC11w group. (b–d) Flk-1, CREB, and PKC showed significant increase in the DM11w and DM11w + LR groups compared with the NC11w group, which was attenuated in the DM11w + B group. $^{*}p < 0.05$ and $^{**}p < 0.01$.

treatment [13, 19–22], the changes of neural and vascular elements of retinopathy pathogenesis after VEGF inhibition have remained uncertain. Therefore, clarifying how diabetes might affect the neural retina is crucial to the development of new therapeutic agents. Compared with previous studies, here, we have examined both neuronal and vascular changes in DR. In the latter, and importantly, we showed here that VEGF maybe involved in the neuronal damage through NOS. To ascertain this, we have adopted the application of bevacizumab as a preventive strategy for DR. Thus, in this study, we have closely monitored the diabetes-induced pathological changes and intervened at the early phase of diabetes with bevacizumab. Additionally, we measured the VEGF and NOS protein expression before and after bevacizumab treatment and explored their mutual role in anti-VEGF treatment. Finally, we tested changes of some relevant factors and their possible involvement in DR.

4.1. VEGF, NOS, and Inflammation. VEGF has long been regarded as an important factor of DR [23], and its relationship with nitric oxide has been extensively investigated. VEGF could activate eNOS in vascular endothelial cells, which could then change the vascular permeability and stimulate angiogenesis [24]. Flk-1, which is a vascular endothelial growth factor receptor 2 (VEGFR2), plays a key role in these processes, activating eNOS with its autophosphorylation [25], and topical application of a novel VEGFR2/Src kinase inhibitor could suppress retinal vascular permeability in mice and rabbits [19]. In turn, NO could induce VEGF synthesis [26]. Previous study found that VEGF and eNOS were increased in the retina of diabetic rats and VEGF inhibitor could potently suppress the increase of eNOS and thus reduce retinal inflammation [27]. In addition to eNOS, iNOS was critical in the early pathogenesis of vascular lesions of DR. Using iNOS-deficient mice, it was reported that mice lacking iNOS were protected from the diabetes-induced degeneration of retinal capillaries [28]. Moreover, the upregulation of iNOS, not eNOS and nNOS, accounts for the compromised retinal function in DR through increasing NO levels [5]. Therefore, iNOS has been identified as one of the most important culprits in vascular changes associated with the early stages of DR [29]. Our previous studies have found that VEGF and NOS protein expression was increased under hypoxia condition both in the brain [30] and the retina [31] and NOS inhibitors effectively reduced the vascular leakage.

VEGF is reported to be chemotactic for monocytes *in vitro* [32] and to significantly enhance recruitment of monocytes *in vivo* [33]. Furthermore, VEGF is a potent enhancer of vascular permeability [34], and thus resulting in increased leukocyte recruitment [35]. The effect of VEGF on inflammation is thought to be important for angiogenesis [36, 37].

In this study, we found that VEGF protein expression was elevated with the progression of diabetes from 3 to 9 weeks. VEGF protein was mainly expressed in the blood vessels and cells in the ganglion cell layer and ONL. Meanwhile, the protein level of iNOS, eNOS, and nNOS and production of NO was increased. Remarkably, in DR rats given treatment with bevacizumab, the preservation and integrity of cellular and vascular structure appeared to correlate with decrease in VEGF and NOS protein expression. It stands to the reason therefore that NOS proteins are important factors regulated by VEGF which can cause neuronal damage in the retina of diabetic rats.

4.2. Bevacizumab Treatment. Many studies supported that the inhibition of VEGF bioactivity could be an effective treatment for the early diabetic retinopathy [27, 38]. Bevacizumab has been approved for the treatment of metastatic colorectal cancer [39] and become a current off-label treatment by ophthalmologists for neovascular age-related macular disease [3]. Several clinical trials have confirmed the effect of bevacizumab on ocular disease, especially on proliferative diabetic retinopathy [10, 15, 16].

Here, we present evidence supporting that bevacizumab can maintain the structural integrity in the diabetic retina. It has been reported that widened retinal venular caliber is independently associated with prevalence and progression of diabetic retinopathy and predicts risk of proliferative retinopathy [40]; we postulate that bevacizumab treatment as shown in this study has a preventive effect on DR.

4.3. The Underlying Mechanism of Anti-VEGF Therapy. To gain a better understanding of the underlying molecular mechanism that may be involved in bevacizumab treatment, we have explored for some crucial factors. To this end, the expression levels of PKC, VEGF, Flk-1, and CREB proteins were significantly increased in the diabetic rats; more strikingly, the expression was suppressed after anti-VEGF treatment. Concurrent to this, the neuronal and vascular changes in DR were restored showing histological features that were comparable to those of the control rats.

We next evaluated the protein expression of PKC because diacylglycerol- (DAG-) protein kinase (PK) C pathway is a very important pathway in cellular signaling induced by diabetes [41, 42]. During the pathogenesis of DR, PKC, activated by DAG, causes retinal vascular dysfunction by changing NO and VEGF enzyme activities in both endothelial cells and pericytes [43]. Moreover, it has been documented that inhibition of PKC could protect ECs from the damage of high glucose [29]. In the present study, we found that PKC protein expression was increased in diabetic rats and was significantly higher than that in normal rats. As a corollary, we hypothesized that bevacizumab treatment may exert its effects through DAG-PKC pathway.

Flk-1 (VEGFR2) is a decisive factor in the induction of angiogenesis and PKC activation [44]. Previous study has found that VEGF/Flk-1 signaling could phosphorylate CREB and exert protective effect on neurons and endothelial cells. We also found that anti-VEGF treatment decreased the expression of CREB [45]. Though CREB may be beneficial for hypoxic damage, it may contribute to the pathogenesis of diabetic retinopathy. Previous study has found that blocking CREB will affect the high glucose-induced VEGF expression, thus preventing activation of retinal Müller cells and enhanced angiogenesis [46]. In view of the above, it is suggested that anti-VEGF therapy may attenuate diabetic retinopathy through inhibiting NO production as well as affecting PKC and CREB expression.

4.4. Some Considerations about Anti-VEGF Therapy. Despite all these existing positive results, it needs to be cautioned that there remain some issues concerning the use of anti-VEGF therapy [44]. For example, the half-life of bevacizumab is short. To elicit and retain the required therapeutic response, repeated maintenance doses are required. In our study, we also found that intravitreal injection of sodium lactate Ringer's led to more severe retinovascular changes and higher expression of Flk-1, CREB, and PKC compared with the DM11w group. It is also noteworthy that the cognitive function of diabetic rats was not aggravated by an intravitreal injection of bevacizumab (data not shown). Although there are reports of the adverse effects following anti-VEGF therapy, such as tractional retinal detachment, macular hole formation, and foveal avascular zone enlargement [38], these have not been noted in our DR model; moreover, clinical trials on the use of intravitreal anti-VEGF therapy for treatment of diabetic retinopathy generally show low rates of side-effects [14, 16, 47].

All in all, our study still has some limitations. Firstly, for clinical relevance, we should have considered applying glycemic control to diabetic rats. However, our study focused mainly on the early pathogenesis of the diabetic retinopathy and studied its progression without interference. In addition, we found that retinal thickening and RGC loss occurred much earlier than in other studies [48]. We attribute the difference to the factor of insulin therapy. We postulated that diabetic pathological changes progressed rapidly without insulin intervention. Our previous study has supported this postulation, finding that diabetes caused arteries narrowing in the circle of Willis under synchrotron radiation angiography as early as 2 weeks [18].

Conflicts of Interest

The authors declare no competing financial interest.

Authors' Contributions

Ying-Ying Zou is the corresponding author and Shu-De Li is the co-corresponding author of this article. Jiao Lv and Miao-Miao Chen contributed equally to this work. Ying-Ying Zou and Shu-De Li designed the project and contributed to the analysis of data and the finalization of the manuscript. Jiao Lv and Miao-Miao Chen conducted most of the experiments and participated in the discussion and analysis of data. Zhi-Hao Mu prepared the first draft of the manuscript and analysis of data as well as conducted part of the experiments. Fang Wang conducted part of the experiments and participated in the discussion and analysis of data. Zhong-Yi Qian carried out the paraffin embedding, sectioning, and H&E staining. Lei Zhou guided the molecular biology experiment and the analysis of data. Qiu-Ting Guo and Zhi-Min Zhao carried out part of the immunofluorescence double staining. Yu-Ping Pan, Xin-Yu Liao, and Zhi-Hong Yang carried out the part of taking tissue samples and taking care of the rats. Ning Cai guided the intravitreal injections of bevacizumab. All authors have read and approved the final version of the manuscript.

Acknowledgments

This study was supported in part by grants (81760149, 81360176, 81200840, 81260361, and 81360128) from the National Natural Sciences Foundation of China, the grant (2013HB078) from the Yunnan Provincial Science and Technology Department, the grants (2017FE468 (-171) and 2014FZ007) from the Joint Special Funds for Yunnan Provincial Science and Technology Department-Kunming Medical University, and the grants (2018JS156, 2013Z105, and 2014C037Y) from the Project of Yunnan Provincial Education Commission.

References

[1] R. Simo and C. Hernandez, "Novel approaches for treating diabetic retinopathy based on recent pathogenic evidence," *Progress in Retinal and Eye Research*, vol. 48, pp. 160–180, 2015.

[2] O. Simo-Servat, R. Simo, and C. Hernandez, "Circulating biomarkers of diabetic retinopathy: an overview based on physiopathology," *Journal of Diabetes Research*, vol. 2016, Article ID 5263798, 13 pages, 2016.

[3] R. Simo and C. Hernandez, "Advances in the medical treatment of diabetic retinopathy," *Diabetes Care*, vol. 32, no. 8, pp. 1556–1562, 2009.

[4] D. A. Antonetti, A. J. Barber, S. K. Bronson et al., "Diabetic retinopathy: seeing beyond glucose-induced microvascular disease," *Diabetes*, vol. 55, no. 9, pp. 2401–2411, 2006.

[5] A. Mishra and E. A. Newman, "Inhibition of inducible nitric oxide synthase reverses the loss of functional hyperemia in diabetic retinopathy," *Glia*, vol. 58, no. 16, pp. 1996–2004, 2010.

[6] R. B. Caldwell, M. Bartoli, M. A. Behzadian et al., "Vascular endothelial growth factor and diabetic retinopathy: pathophysiological mechanisms and treatment perspectives," *Diabetes/Metabolism Research and Reviews*, vol. 19, no. 6, pp. 442–455, 2003.

[7] D. N. Sang and P. A. D'Amore, "Is blockade of vascular endothelial growth factor beneficial for all types of diabetic retinopathy?," *Diabetologia*, vol. 51, no. 9, pp. 1570–1573, 2008.

[8] B. Wirostko, T. Wong, and R. Simo, "Vascular endothelial growth factor and diabetic complications," *Progress in Retinal and Eye Research*, vol. 27, no. 6, pp. 608–621, 2008.

[9] L. P. Aiello, R. L. Avery, P. G. Arrigg et al., "Vascular endothelial growth factor in ocular fluid of patients with diabetic retinopathy and other retinal disorders," *The New England Journal of Medicine*, vol. 331, no. 22, pp. 1480–1487, 1994.

[10] R. F. Spaide and Y. L. Fisher, "Intravitreal bevacizumab (Avastin) treatment of proliferative diabetic retinopathy complicated by vitreous hemorrhage," *Retina*, vol. 26, no. 3, pp. 275–278, 2006.

[11] R. L. Avery, J. Pearlman, D. J. Pieramici et al., "Intravitreal bevacizumab (Avastin) in the treatment of proliferative diabetic retinopathy," *Ophthalmology*, vol. 113, no. 10, pp. 1695–1705.e6, 2006.

[12] R. L. Avery, "Regression of retinal and iris neovascularization after intravitreal bevacizumab (Avastin) treatment," *Retina*, vol. 26, no. 3, pp. 352–354, 2006.

[13] J. Ma, T. Zhu, X. Tang, P. Ye, and Z. Zhang, "Effect of an intravitreal injection of bevacizumab on the expression of VEGF and CD34 in the retina of diabetic rats," *Clinical & Experimental Ophthalmology*, vol. 38, no. 9, pp. 875–884, 2010.

[14] J. F. Arevalo, J. G. Sanchez, A. F. Lasave et al., "Intravitreal bevacizumab (Avastin®) for diabetic retinopathy at 24-months: The 2008 Juan Verdaguer-Planas Lecture," *Current Diabetes Reviews*, vol. 6, no. 5, pp. 313–322, 2010.

[15] J. F. Arevalo, L. Wu, J. G. Sanchez et al., "Intravitreal bevacizumab (Avastin) for proliferative diabetic retinopathy: 6-months follow-up," *Eye*, vol. 23, no. 1, pp. 117–123, 2009.

[16] L. P. Cintra, R. A. Costa, J. A. S. Ribeiro et al., "Intravitreal bevacizumab (Avastin) for persistent new vessels in diabetic retinopathy (IBEPE study): 1-year results," *Retina*, vol. 33, no. 6, pp. 1109–1116, 2013.

[17] L. D. Mayo, K. M. Kessler, R. Pincheira, R. S. Warren, and D. B. Donner, "Vascular endothelial cell growth factor activates CRE-binding protein by signaling through the KDR receptor tyrosine kinase," *Journal of Biological Chemistry*, vol. 276, no. 27, pp. 25184–25189, 2001.

[18] Z. H. Mu, Z. Jiang, X. J. Lin et al., "Vessel dilation attenuates endothelial dysfunction following middle cerebral artery

occlusion in hyperglycemic rats," *CNS Neuroscience & Therapeutics*, vol. 22, no. 4, pp. 316–324, 2016.

[19] L. Scheppke, E. Aguilar, R. F. Gariano et al., "Retinal vascular permeability suppression by topical application of a novel VEGFR2/Src kinase inhibitor in mice and rabbits," *The Journal of Clinical Investigation*, vol. 118, no. 6, pp. 2337–2346, 2008.

[20] P. Zhang and Z. Zhou, "Combination of bevacizumab and NGF reduces the risk of diabetic retinopathy," *Cell Biochemistry and Biophysics*, vol. 73, no. 1, pp. 79–85, 2015.

[21] Y. Lu, N. Zhou, X. Huang et al., "Effect of intravitreal injection of bevacizumab-chitosan nanoparticles on retina of diabetic rats," *International Journal of Ophthalmology*, vol. 7, no. 1, pp. 1–7, 2014.

[22] F. Celik, F. Ulas, Z. G. Ozunal, T. Firat, S. Celebi, and U. Dogan, "Comparison of the effect of intravitreal bevacizumab and intravitreal fasudil on retinal VEGF, TNFα, and caspase 3 levels in an experimental diabetes model," *International Journal of Ophthalmology*, vol. 7, no. 1, pp. 57–61, 2014.

[23] E. Duh and L. P. Aiello, "Vascular endothelial growth factor and diabetes: the agonist versus antagonist paradox," *Diabetes*, vol. 48, no. 10, pp. 1899–1906, 1999.

[24] M. Ziche, L. Morbidelli, R. Choudhuri et al., "Nitric oxide synthase lies downstream from vascular endothelial growth factor-induced but not basic fibroblast growth factor-induced angiogenesis," *The Journal of Clinical Investigation*, vol. 99, no. 11, pp. 2625–2634, 1997.

[25] D. Thuringer, L. Maulon, and C. Frelin, "Rapid transactivation of the vascular endothelial growth factor receptor KDR/Flk-1 by the bradykinin B2 receptor contributes to endothelial nitric-oxide synthase activation in cardiac capillary endothelial cells," *Journal of Biological Chemistry*, vol. 277, no. 3, pp. 2028–2032, 2002.

[26] H. Kimura and H. Esumi, "Reciprocal regulation between nitric oxide and vascular endothelial growth factor in angiogenesis," *Acta Biochimica Polonica*, vol. 50, no. 1, pp. 49–59, 2003.

[27] A. M. Joussen, V. Poulaki, W. Qin et al., "Retinal vascular endothelial growth factor induces intercellular adhesion molecule-1 and endothelial nitric oxide synthase expression and initiates early diabetic retinal leukocyte adhesion *in vivo*," *The American Journal of Pathology*, vol. 160, no. 2, pp. 501–509, 2002.

[28] L. Zheng, Y. Du, C. Miller et al., "Critical role of inducible nitric oxide synthase in degeneration of retinal capillaries in mice with streptozotocin-induced diabetes," *Diabetologia*, vol. 50, no. 9, pp. 1987–1996, 2007.

[29] E. C. Leal, A. Manivannan, K.-I. Hosoya et al., "Inducible nitric oxide synthase isoform is a key mediator of leukostasis and blood-retinal barrier breakdown in diabetic retinopathy," *Investigative Ophthalmology & Visual Science*, vol. 48, no. 11, pp. 5257–5265, 2007.

[30] Y. Y. Zou, E. M. Kan, Q. Cao, J. Lu, and E. A. Ling, "Combustion smoke-induced inflammation in the cerebellum and hippocampus of adult rats," *Neuropathology and Applied Neurobiology*, vol. 39, no. 5, pp. 531–552, 2013.

[31] Y. Y. Zou, J. Lu, D. J. F. Poon et al., "Combustion smoke exposure induces up-regulated expression of vascular endothelial growth factor, aquaporin 4, nitric oxide synthases and vascular permeability in the retina of adult rats," *Neuroscience*, vol. 160, no. 3, pp. 698–709, 2009.

[32] B. Barleon, S. Sozzani, D. Zhou, H. A. Weich, A. Mantovani, and D. Marme, "Migration of human monocytes in response to vascular endothelial growth factor (VEGF) is mediated via the VEGF receptor flt-1," *Blood*, vol. 87, no. 8, pp. 3336–3343, 1996.

[33] S. I. Zittermann and A. C. Issekutz, "Endothelial growth factors VEGF and bFGF differentially enhance monocyte and neutrophil recruitment to inflammation," *Journal of Leukocyte Biology*, vol. 80, no. 2, pp. 247–257, 2006.

[34] S. M. Weis and D. A. Cheresh, "Pathophysiological consequences of VEGF-induced vascular permeability," *Nature*, vol. 437, no. 7058, pp. 497–504, 2005.

[35] A. C. Issekutz, "Effect of vasoactive agents on polymorphonuclear leukocyte emigration in vivo," *Laboratory Investigation*, vol. 45, no. 3, pp. 234–240, 1981.

[36] S. D. Croll, R. M. Ransohoff, N. Cai et al., "VEGF-mediated inflammation precedes angiogenesis in adult brain," *Experimental Neurology*, vol. 187, no. 2, pp. 388–402, 2004.

[37] C. G. Lee, H. Link, P. Baluk et al., "Vascular endothelial growth factor (VEGF) induces remodeling and enhances T_H2-mediated sensitization and inflammation in the lung," *Nature Medicine*, vol. 10, no. 10, pp. 1095–1103, 2004.

[38] R. Simo and C. Hernandez, "Intravitreous anti-VEGF for diabetic retinopathy: hopes and fears for a new therapeutic strategy," *Diabetologia*, vol. 51, no. 9, pp. 1574–1580, 2008.

[39] J. C. Yang, L. Haworth, R. M. Sherry et al., "A randomized trial of bevacizumab, an anti–vascular endothelial growth factor antibody, for metastatic renal cancer," *The New England Journal of Medicine*, vol. 349, no. 5, pp. 427–434, 2003.

[40] R. Klein, B. E. Klein, S. E. Moss et al., "The relation of retinal vessel caliber to the incidence and progression of diabetic retinopathy: XIX: the Wisconsin epidemiologic study of diabetic retinopathy," *Archives of Ophthalmology*, vol. 122, no. 1, pp. 76–83, 2004.

[41] D. Koya and G. L. King, "Protein kinase C activation and the development of diabetic complications," *Diabetes*, vol. 47, no. 6, pp. 859–866, 1998.

[42] P. Geraldes and G. L. King, "Activation of protein kinase C isoforms and its impact on diabetic complications," *Circulation Research*, vol. 106, no. 8, pp. 1319–1331, 2010.

[43] K. J. Way, N. Katai, and G. L. King, "Protein kinase C and the development of diabetic vascular complications," *Diabetic Medicine*, vol. 18, no. 12, pp. 945–959, 2001.

[44] T. Behl and A. Kotwani, "Exploring the various aspects of the pathological role of vascular endothelial growth factor (VEGF) in diabetic retinopathy," *Pharmacological Research*, vol. 99, pp. 137–148, 2015.

[45] H. T. Lee, Y. C. Chang, Y. F. Tu, and C. C. Huang, "VEGF-A/VEGFR-2 signaling leading to cAMP response element-binding protein phosphorylation is a shared pathway underlying the protective effect of preconditioning on neurons and endothelial cells," *Journal of Neuroscience*, vol. 29, no. 14, pp. 4356–4368, 2009.

[46] J. Li, S. Z. Zhao, P. P. Wang, S. P. Yu, Z. Zheng, and X. Xu, "Calcium mediates high glucose-induced HIF-1α and VEGF expression in cultured rat retinal Müller cells through CaMKII-CREB pathway," *Acta Pharmacologica Sinica*, vol. 33, no. 8, pp. 1030–1036, 2012.

Frequency and Predictors of Self-Reported Hypoglycemia in Insulin-Treated Diabetes

Samir Malkani[1] and Anupam Kotwal[2]

[1]Division of Diabetes, Department of Medicine, University of Massachusetts Medical School, Worcester, MA 01655, USA
[2]Division of Endocrinology, Diabetes, Metabolism, and Nutrition, Mayo Clinic, 200 First Street SW, Mayo 18, Rochester, MN 55905, USA

Correspondence should be addressed to Anupam Kotwal; Kotwal.Anupam@mayo.edu

Academic Editor: Konstantinos Papatheodorou

Aims. Hypoglycemia is a limiting factor for achieving stringent glycemic control in diabetes. This study analyzes the frequency and predictors of hypoglycemia in insulin-treated diabetes in an ambulatory setting. *Methods.* A retrospective chart review was performed to study self-monitored blood glucose (SMBG) data for 3 months prior to a patient's HbA1c test. *Results.* Hypoglycemia occurred more frequently in type 1 than in type 2 diabetes; however, 19% of type 2 diabetes patients did experience at least one episode of severe hypoglycemia. For type 1 diabetes, hypoglycemia had a positive association with glycemic variability and duration of diabetes and a negative association with HbA1c and lowest blood glucose (BG). For type 2 diabetes, a positive association was noted with glycemic variability and a negative association with age and lowest BG. *Conclusions.* Delineating factors predisposing to hypoglycemia in type 2 diabetes is difficult. Lower HbA1c is a potential predictor of hypoglycemia in type 1 but not in type 2 diabetes. Longer duration of diabetes for type 1 and younger age for type 2 are associated with more hypoglycemia. Glycemic variability portends increased risk for hypoglycemia and should be a focus of further research.

1. Introduction

Hypoglycemia is a major limiting factor for achieving stringent glycemic control in diabetes. It influences self-management of diabetes with some patients accepting suboptimal glycemic control to reduce the risk of hypoglycemia [1]. Moreover, hypoglycemia is associated with significant morbidity. Severe hypoglycemia can cause seizures and arrhythmias. It is associated with dementia [2], and it has been linked with poor cardiovascular outcomes [3] and death [4]. Hypoglycemia has also been shown to trigger adrenergic discharge and the expression of proinflammatory cytokines [5].

Hypoglycemia is common in type 1 diabetes, and its occurrence increases with insulin use in type 2 diabetes [6–10]. It is a common and potentially dangerous side effect of insulin therapy; however, its occurrence is not easy to predict. The majority of our knowledge about severe hypoglycemia comes from type 1 diabetes. Data on rates and potential risk factors for severe hypoglycemia in insulin-treated type 2 diabetes are relatively scarce and conflicting. Clinical trials have reported low rates of severe hypoglycemia in type 2 diabetes [11, 12], and population-based studies have reported highly variable rates [13, 14]. The reported frequency of severe hypoglycemia in clinical trials may represent only the "tip of the iceberg" in terms of all episodes. In the case of severe hypoglycemia, most studies have used its clinical definition that was first described by the Diabetes Control and Complications Trial (DCCT), as any hypoglycemia that requires external assistance [15]. However, reporting of such episodes by patients, especially those with hypoglycemia unawareness, can be unreliable. Data derived from the frequency of treated episodes of severe hypoglycemia by emergency services are similarly inadequate to quantify the overall incidence, as only 10% of severe episodes are treated in the hospital. Data from continuous glucose monitoring (CGM) studies reveal that even asymptomatic hypoglycemia is associated with the risk of cardiac arrhythmias [16].

In patients on insulin therapy, inadequate caloric intake, exercise, renal insufficiency, and alcohol ingestion can precipitate hypoglycemia. In many episodes of hypoglycemia, a precipitating factor cannot be identified. Although some phenotypic markers are known to predispose patients to hypoglycemia, its predictors in insulin-treated diabetes have not been well studied, especially when these patients are followed on an ambulatory basis and have not been actively enrolled in a study. Hypoglycemia unawareness is common in longstanding diabetes and can lead to serious consequences in spite of lack of symptoms, and blood glucose testing or CGM can identify such episodes more reliably. To try and fill the gaps in knowledge, we conducted this study to analyze the frequency and potential predictors of self-monitored hypoglycemia in type 1 and insulin-treated type 2 diabetes in an ambulatory setting.

2. Material and Methods

2.1. Subjects with Diabetes Mellitus. We performed a cross-sectional chart review study utilizing the electronic database of the University of Massachusetts Medical School Diabetes Clinic. The clinic, which serves residents of central Massachusetts, uses an electronic diabetes management system, My Care Team™ (MCT) that captures all the patients' self-monitored blood glucose (SMBG) data. The system is able to upload readings from most commercial blood glucose monitors; data from blood glucose meters is uploaded at each clinic visit. Diabetic adults who were seen at the clinic between October 1, 2012, and September 30, 2013, were eligible if they were on insulin treatment, and their meter download on MCT showed a SMBG testing frequency of 3 times or more daily. Pregnant women were excluded. The UMass IRB approved the study proposal. Of the total sample of 3000 patients, 298 were included in the study based on the eligibility criteria. Each patient had a hemoglobin A1c (HbA1c) tested at the visit, and the SMBG data for a 3-month period prior to the clinic visit was collected. For patients who had more than one clinic visit during the study period, the most recent one was used for the purpose of data collection. Categorical variables assessed were gender, race, and presence or absence of depression, coronary artery disease (CAD), hypertension (HTN), nephropathy, and retinopathy. Nephropathy was defined as albuminuria (spot urine albumin : creatinine ratio > 300 mcg/mg) or progressive chronic kidney disease, and presence of retinopathy included all classes of detectable retinopathy. Continuous variables assessed were age, body mass index (BMI), duration of diabetes, HbA1c, daily insulin dose, number of daily injections, and SMBG data including minimum SMBG value and standard deviation (SD) around mean SMBG.

2.2. Identification of Hypoglycemic Episodes. Hypoglycemia was defined as a SMBG reading $\leq$ 70 mg/dL [17], and severe hypoglycemia as a SMBG reading $\leq$ 45 mg/dL. All commercial SMBG monitors provide glucose readings such that the reported result most closely matches that of a laboratory method measuring serum or plasma glucose [18]. No distinction was made between asymptomatic and symptomatic hypoglycemic episodes. We calculated the number hypoglycemic episodes for each patient from their home glucose meter upload for a 3-month period prior to their clinic visit. Sequential SMBG readings meeting hypoglycemia criteria recorded within a 2-hour period were considered as a single episode.

2.3. Statistical Analysis. A database was created with data for all the variables, and statistical analysis was performed using the software SPSS. As the independent variables were not distributed normally, nonparametric tests of significance were utilized. Mann–Whitney *U* test was used to assess the association of categorical independent variables with dependent variables (frequency of hypoglycemia and severe hypoglycemia). For continuous variables, Spearman's correlation and Wilcoxon signed-rank test were used for univariate analysis. p value ≤ 0.05 was considered significant. All probabilities were two tailed. Multivariate linear regression (as dependent variables were continuous) was then used for all the associations that were significant on univariate analysis to remove the effect of confounders. Two separate models were created using the frequencies of all hypoglycemic episodes and severe hypoglycemic episodes as dependent variables.

3. Results

3.1. Study Sample. A total of 298 patients with diabetes on insulin were included for analysis. This included 133 patients with type 1 and 165 patients with type 2 diabetes. Of the 133 subjects with type 1 diabetes, 47 (35.3%) were using an insulin pump and the rest were on multiple daily injections (MDI). The characteristics of the subjects including mean age, gender distribution, and diabetes duration are shown in Table 1. The group with type 1 diabetes had a significantly lower age, BMI, and duration of diabetes as well as a significantly lower percentage of individuals suffering from hypertension, CAD, and nephropathy as compared to the group with type 2 diabetes. This group had a significantly higher mean HbA1c, number of daily insulin injections, daily insulin dose, and SD around mean SMBG (indicator of glycemic variability) as compared to the group with type 2 diabetes. There was no statistically significant difference in regard to gender, daily insulin dose adjusted for BMI, and the percentage of individuals with depression or retinopathy between the two groups. The characteristics of the individuals with insulin-treated diabetes that were excluded from the study were similar to those that were included.

3.2. Frequency of Hypoglycemia. All patients with type 1 diabetes and 82% of patients with type 2 diabetes experienced at least one episode of hypoglycemia. The corresponding numbers for severe hypoglycemia were 68% for type 1 and 19% for type 2 diabetes. 88% of those with type 1 experienced more than 10 hypoglycemic episodes compared to 30% with type 2 diabetes. Those with type 1 diabetes recorded a total of 4583 hypoglycemic episodes that corresponds to a rate of 137.8 (95% CI 135.9 and 139.8) episodes per person per year.

TABLE 1: Characteristics of patients with insulin-treated diabetes participating in the study.

Patient characteristics	All patients Mean ± SD, range or n (%) patients	Type 1 diabetes Mean ± SD, range or n (%) patients	Type 2 diabetes Mean ± SD, range or n (%) patients	p value
Number of patients (%)	298 (100)	133 (44.6)	165 (55.4)	—
Age (years)	60.54 ± 16.64	52.11 ± 17.19	67.33 ± 12.63	0.001
Males	153/145	62 (46.6)	83 (50)	0.606
BMI (kg/m^2) [mean ± SD]	30.38 ± 7.45	26.38 ± 4.66	33.58 ± 7.73	0.001
Known duration of diabetes (years) [mean ± SD]	21.43 ± 14.62	25.26 ± 16.75	18.11 ± 11.58	0.001
Daily insulin dose (units/day) [mean ± SD]	66.48 ± 56.05	49.04 ± 26.91	74.59 ± 63.80	0.001
Daily insulin dose/BMI (units/kg/m^2/day) [mean ± SD]	2.06 ± 1.35 (n = 210)	1.84 ± 0.91 (n = 66)	2.16 ± 1.52 (n = 144)	0.307
HbA1c (%) [mean ± SD]	7.77 ± 1.25	7.94 ± 1.94	7.64 ± 1.27	
<7		31 (23.3)	48 (28.9)	
7-8		36 (27.1)	59 (35.5)	0.032
>8		66 (49.6)	58 (34.9)	
SD around mean SMBG	68.71 ± 17.04	78.93 ± 2.04	60.47 ± 1.69	0.001
Lowest SMBG reading [mean ± SD]	49.69 ± 15.78	40.98 ± 9.54	56.71 ± 16.33	0.001
Number of daily insulin injections [mean ± SD]	3.87 ± 0.93 (median 4, range 1–6)	4.12 ± 0.48 (median 4, range 2–6)	3.73 ± 1.08 (median 4, range 1–5)	0.001
MDI		86 (64.7)	165 (100)	—
Insulin pump		47 (35.3)	None	
HTN	170 (57.0)	47 (35.3)	123 (74.5)	0.001
CAD	74 (24.8)	19 (14.3)	55 (33.3)	0.001
Nephropathy	102 (34.2)	27 (20.3)	75 (45.2)	0.001
Retinopathy (n, %)	63 (21.1)	32 (24.1)	31 (18.8)	0.334
Depression (n, %)	49 (16.4)	16 (12.0)	33 (20.0)	0.091
Caucasians (n, %)	265 (88.9)	128 (96.2)	137 (83.1)	0.001
All hypoglycemic episodes	6100 events	4583 events in 133 (100%) patients	1517 events in 136 (82%) patients	0.000
All hypoglycemic episodes per person per year [OR (95% CI)]	81.9 (80.0 to 82.9)	137.8 (135.9 to 139.8)	36.8 (35.9 to 37.7)	0.000
No hypoglycemic episodes	29 (9.7%)	0 (0%)	29 (17.6%)	—
1–10 hypoglycemic episodes in 3 months	269 (90.3%)	16 (12%)	86 (52.1%)	—
>10 hypoglycemic episodes in 3 months	167 (56.0%)	117 (88%)	50 (30.3%)	—
Severe hypoglycemic episodes	762	643 events in 91 (68%) patients	119 events in 32 (19%) patients	0.000
Severe hypoglycemic episodes per person per year [OR (95% CI)]	10.2 (9.9 to 10.6)	19.3 (18.6 to 20.1)	2.9 (2.6 to 3.2)	0.000
No severe hypoglycemic episodes	175 (58.7%)	42 (31.6%)	133 (80.6%)	—
1–10 severe hypoglycemic episodes in 3 months	123 (41.3%)	73 (54.9%)	31 (18.8%)	—
>10 severe hypoglycemic episodes in 3 months	19 (6.4%)	18 (13.5%)	1 (0.6%)	—

643 (14%) of these were severe, corresponding to 19.3 (95% CI 18.6 and 20.1) severe episodes per person per year. In those with type 2 diabetes, a total of 1517 hypoglycemic episodes were recorded; of which, 119 (8%) were severe. This corresponds to an event rate per person per year for hypoglycemia and severe hypoglycemia of 36.8 (95% CI 35.9, 37.7) and 2.9 (95% CI 2.6, 3.2), respectively. Less than 1% of individuals with type 2 diabetes reported greater than 10 severe

TABLE 2: Results of nonparametric test (Mann–Whitney U test) for association of categorical independent variables with frequencies of hypoglycemia and severe hypoglycemia.

Categorical variables	Type 1 diabetes				Type 2 diabetes			
Mann–Whitney U test	Hypoglycemia [mean ± SD]	p value	Severe hypoglycemia [mean ± SD]	p value	Hypoglycemia [mean ± SD]	p value	Severe hypoglycemia [mean ± SD]	p value
Females	37.96 ± 26.40	0.188	5.69 ± 7.99	0.523	8.16 ± 9.96	0.617	0.88 ± 2.66	0.412
Males	30.45 ± 19.31		3.85 ± 5.22		10.22 ± 11.91		0.57 ± 1.72	
Nephropathy absent	36.45 ± 24.62	0.089	5.10 ± 7.08	0.162	9.57 ± 11.84	0.581	0.91 ± 2.69	0.487
Nephropathy present	26.63 ± 17.16		3.78 ± 6.02		8.75 ± 9.95		0.49 ± 1.50	
Retinopathy absent	35.85 ± 24.14	0.258	4.94 ± 7.03	0.524	9.22 ± 11.68	0.109	0.81 ± 2.43	0.551
Retinopathy present	30.06 ± 21.49		4.50 ± 6.46		9.06 ± 7.53		0.35 ± 1.02	
On MDI	32.92 ± 23.43	0.224	4.85 ± 7.24	0.543	9.30 ± 11.02	0.085	0.73 ± 2.25	—
On insulin pump	37.28 ± 23.84		4.81 ± 6.23		0.50 ± 0.71		0.00	
HTN absent	35.23 ± 24.09	0.648	5.08 ± 6.94	0.377	10.48 ± 11.60	0.324	0.74 ± 1.81	0.647
HTN present	33.04 ± 22.79		4.38 ± 6.80		8.76 ± 10.80		0.71 ± 2.37	
CAD absent	35.69 ± 23.23	0.063	5.12 ± 7.09	0.132	9.50 ± 11.08	0.367	0.76 ± 2.42	0.783
CAD present	27.05 ± 24.92		3.10 ± 5.22		8.58 ± 10.91		0.64 ± 1.83	
Other race	24.60 ± 11.33	0.435	1.40 ± 1.34	0.284	10.11 ± 12.25	0.913	1.28 ± 2.92	0.326
Caucasians	34.84 ± 23.87		4.97 ± 6.97		9.01 ± 10.76		0.60 ± 2.06	
Depression absent	34.63 ± 24.07	0.912	4.69 ± 6.86	0.484	8.56 ± 10.72	0.047	0.67 ± 2.29	0.366
Depression present	33.19 ± 20.21		5.87 ± 7.13		11.73 ± 11.89		0.94 ± 2.03	
Different categories of A1c (<7, 7-8, >8)		0.001		0.052		0.507		0.363

TABLE 3: Results of nonparametric tests Spearman's correlation (to calculate correlation coefficient) and Wilcoxon signed-rank test (to assess significance with p value) for association of continuous independent variables with frequencies of hypoglycemia and severe hypoglycemia.

Continuous variables	Type 1 diabetes: Hypoglycemia		Type 1 diabetes: Severe hypoglycemia		Type 2 diabetes: Hypoglycemia		Type 2 diabetes: Severe hypoglycemia	
	Correlation coefficient ρ	p value	Correlation coefficient ρ	p value	Correlation coefficient ρ	p value	Correlation coefficient ρ	p value
Age (years)	−0.2	0.000	−0.2	0.000	−0.03	0.000	−0.01	0.000
BMI	−0.1	0.005	−0.1	0.000	−0.1	0.000	−0.2	0.000
Duration of diabetes	+0.2	0.000	+0.2	0.000	+0.2	0.000	+0.2	0.000
Daily insulin dose	0.1 ($n = 66$)	0.003	0.1 ($n = 46$)	0.000	0.1 ($n = 119$)	0.000	0.01 ($n = 29$)	0.000
Daily insulin injections	+0.2	0.000	+0.2	0.14	+0.04	0.000	+0.1	0.000
Lowest BG reading	−0.7	0.006	−0.9	0.000	−0.8	0.000	−0.7	0.000
SD around mean BG	+0.1	0.000	+0.2	0.000	+0.2	0.000	+0.2	0.000
HbA1c	−0.4	0.000	−0.2	0.000	−0.1	0.456	−0.04	0.000

hypoglycemic episodes compared to almost 14% with type 1 diabetes. The frequencies of both all and severe hypoglycemic episodes were significantly higher for type 1 as compared to type 2 diabetes ($p = 0.000$ for both).

3.3. Predictors of Hypoglycemia in Type 1 Diabetes. On univariate analysis initially by correlation (for continuous variables) and then tests of significance (Tables 2 and 3), the frequencies of all and severe hypoglycemia had a significant negative association with the mean HbA1c ($p = 0.000$ for both), the lowest BG reading recorded ($p = 0.000$ for both), BMI ($p = 0.000$ for both), and age ($p = 0.000$ for both). The frequencies of all and severe hypoglycemia demonstrated a significant positive association with the duration of diabetes ($p = 0.000$ for both), daily insulin dose ($p = 0.003$ and 0.000, resp.), and glycemic variability ($p = 0.000$ for both). There was a positive association with the number of daily insulin injections that was statistically significant only for all hypoglycemia ($p = 0.000$).

Multivariate linear regression analysis (Table 4) which adjusted for independently associated variables revealed a significant positive association of the frequencies of all and severe hypoglycemia with glycemic variability and duration of diabetes and a significant negative association with HbA1c. When the lowest BG reading was included in this analysis, it continued to be significantly negatively associated

TABLE 4: Multivariate regression analysis using hypoglycemic episodes and severe hypoglycemic episodes as dependent variables and variables that achieved significance on univariate analysis as independent variables.

Variables significant on univariate analysis	Type 1 diabetes Hypoglycemia (beta; p value)	Type 1 diabetes Severe hypoglycemia (beta; p value)	Type 2 diabetes Hypoglycemia (beta; p value)	Type 2 diabetes Severe hypoglycemia (beta; p value)
Age	−0.25; 0.28	−0.09; 0.23	−0.26; 0.032	−0.01; 0.84
BMI	1.27; 0.14	0.11; 0.71	−0.27; 0.10	−0.03; 0.41
Duration of diabetes	0.46; 0.042	0.16; 0.037	0.18; 0.11	−0.01; 0.65
Total insulin dose	0.24; 0.11	0.02; 0.72	0.01; 0.74	0.002; 0.79
Number of daily injections	1.95; 0.76	—	−0.89; 0.44	0.05; 0.84
SD around mean BG	0.43; 0.022	0.15; 0.023	0.07; 0.22	0.01; 0.50
HbA1c	−9.69; 0.010	−3.19; 0.015	—	−0.09; 0.71
Depression	—	—	−1.63; 0.61	—

with both all and severe hypoglycemia. The association with other variables like age, BMI, number of daily insulin injections, and daily insulin dose did not achieve significance in the regression analysis.

3.4. Predictors of Hypoglycemia in Insulin-Treated Type 2 Diabetes. On univariate analysis, the frequencies of all and severe hypoglycemia had a significant negative association with the lowest BG reading recorded ($p = 0.000$ for both), BMI ($p = 0.000$ for both), and age ($p = 0.000$ for both). There was a negative association with HbA1c that was statistically significant only for severe hypoglycemia ($p = 0.000$). The frequencies of all and severe hypoglycemia had a significant positive association with the duration of diabetes ($p = 0.000$ for both), daily insulin dose ($p = 0.000$ for both), number of daily insulin injections ($p = 0.000$ for both), and glycemic variability ($p = 0.000$ for both). The frequency of all hypoglycemia had a significant positive association with the presence of depression ($p = 0.047$).

Multivariate linear regression analysis (Table 4), which adjusted for independently associated variables, revealed a significant negative association of the frequency of all hypoglycemia with age. The association with other variables seen on univariate analysis did not achieve significance during regression analysis. However, when the lowest BG reading was included in this analysis, it continued to be significantly negatively associated with both all and severe hypoglycemia, and the positive association of all hypoglycemia with glycemic variability achieved statistical significance.

When comparing individuals with type 1 diabetes using an insulin pump versus those on MDI, there was no statistically significant difference between the frequencies of all or severe hypoglycemia and mean HbA1C value. In regard to different therapeutic regimens, there was no statistically significant difference in hypoglycemia frequency when comparing different MDI regimens for either type 1 or type 2 diabetes.

4. Discussion

Although hypoglycemia is a common complication of insulin treatment in diabetes, very few studies have evaluated the frequency and predictors of self-reported hypoglycemia on an ambulatory basis, especially in insulin-treated type 2 diabetes. The present study examined self-reported hypoglycemia in a sample of patients with insulin-treated diabetes who were being managed at a university hospital diabetes clinic and accurately represented the population base. Our results are based on hypoglycemia recorded by the subject whether or not they experienced symptoms. SMBG frequency of at least 3 times a day reduced the likelihood of missing any episodes of hypoglycemia. The over recording of hypoglycemia in the initial data was corrected by counting SMBG readings ≤ 70 mg/dL recorded within a 2-hour period as one hypoglycemic episode unless there was a reading > 70 mg/dL in between them. It is not surprising that our patients with type 1 diabetes reported more hypoglycemic episodes as compared to those with type 2 diabetes. However, compared with previous studies of both type 1 [19, 20] and type 2 diabetes [11, 14, 21], the event rates and the proportion of subjects experiencing hypoglycemic events in our study were higher, especially in type 2 diabetes with 19% experiencing an episode of severe hypoglycemia. The possible reasons for this could be the longer duration of diabetes in our patients, being followed on an ambulatory basis as compared to being enrolled in a clinical trial, and the fact that many other studies have defined severe hypoglycemia on symptoms and not BG values. The rates of severe hypoglycemia in insulin-treated type 2 diabetes are reported to be low [11, 14, 21], but these have been recorded in the context of clinical trials and often in people with a short duration of insulin therapy.

Insulin use has been linked to higher likelihood of experiencing hypoglycemia; however, within the group of insulin-treated diabetes, the predictors of hypoglycemia remain unclear. In type 1 diabetes, a negative association of hypoglycemia with HbA1c has been reported by several studies [15, 22, 23]. In type 2 diabetes, either no association or a positive association of hypoglycemia with HbA1c has been reported [8, 20, 24] except in the PREDICTIVE trial which demonstrated a negative association between the two in both type 1 and type 2 diabetes [23]. Within the intensive treatment arm of the ACCORD trial for type 2 diabetes, a higher HbA1c and lower change in HbA1c from baseline were associated with a higher rate of occurrence of hypoglycemia [25]. In our study, after adjusting for independent variables, lower HbA1c was a potential predictor of hypoglycemia in type 1 but not in type 2 diabetes. Glycemic variability has been assessed by studies using different parameters, SD around mean BG being the best demonstrated for SMBG data. In our study, this was a significant predictor for hypoglycemia. A history of previous severe hypoglycemia has been reported to be a risk factor for severe hypoglycemia [15, 26]. Similarly, our study found a significant association between experiencing a low PG reading and increased frequency of all and severe hypoglycemic episodes in both type 1 and type 2 diabetes. Also, the distribution of hypoglycemia in our study was highly skewed with a small proportion of patients accounting for the majority of episodes.

In the UKPDS trial, hypoglycemia was more frequent in younger patients, females, non-obese patients and those with positive islet cell antibodies [11]. Our study also showed a higher frequency of hypoglycemia in younger type 2 diabetes patients, but there was no significant association with gender or BMI in regression analysis. However these two studies are not exactly comparable as we studied only insulin-treated diabetics with longer diabetes duration. Other studies have reported hypoglycemia in type 2 diabetes to be linked to longer duration of diabetes [7, 20] which we found on univariate but not multivariate analysis. The increased occurrence of hypoglycemia in patients with longer duration of diabetes could be related to the accompanying hypoglycemia-associated autonomic failure (HAAF). Depression has been associated with severe hypoglycemia in type 2 diabetes [27]; in our study, this association was observed on univariate analysis but did not hold up in multivariate regression analysis. In type 2 diabetes, a lower BMI is associated with hypoglycemia in some studies [23], and in our cohort, this relationship was observed only in univariate, but not in multivariate analysis. Our observation of higher rates of hypoglycemia in younger type 2 diabetes patients can be explained by the higher insulin sensitivity in this group. There was no significant difference in the frequency of hypoglycemia or mean HbA1c between those with type 1 diabetes that were on an insulin pump versus those on MDI; however the study was not powered to assess this. Similar findings have been reported by a recent meta-analysis [28].

5. Conclusions

Insulin treatment of diabetes increases the likelihood of experiencing hypoglycemia. We studied a cohort of patients with relatively well-controlled diabetes in terms of their HbA1c values, who had diabetes for a long duration thus increasing their risk of HAAF. Even though hypoglycemia is more common in type 1 diabetes, it continues to remain an important complication of insulin treatment in type 2 diabetes. In type 1 diabetes, striving for a lower HbA1c increases the risk of hypoglycemia. In addition, increased glycemic variability and longer duration of diabetes are significant potential predictors of hypoglycemia. In type 2 diabetes, factors predisposing to hypoglycemia are interdependent and we found it difficult to delineate them separately. However, we did find higher glycemic variability to be associated with a higher frequency of hypoglycemic episodes in this group. There seems to be a positive association of hypoglycemia with depression in type 2 diabetes, which needs to be further explored. In our study, younger insulin-treated type 2 diabetics experienced more hypoglycemic episodes, which is contrary to some other studies. Experiencing a hypoglycemic episode increases the risk of more hypoglycemia in both type 1 and type 2 diabetes. Very frequent hypoglycemia occurs in a small proportion of patients, and these are the ones that require the greatest attention to avoid hypoglycemia. Glycemic variability, which is an indicator of poor glycemic control rather than tight glycemic control, portends increased risk for hypoglycemia. Studies that focus on glycemic variability and interventions to prevent hypoglycemia in high-risk patients are needed.

Disclosure

The initial abstract for this study was published as part of ADA 75th scientific sessions [29].

Conflicts of Interest

The authors have no conflicts of interest to disclose.

Authors' Contributions

Anupam Kotwal researched the data, performed data analysis, and prepared the manuscript. Samir Malkani supervised the project and reviewed and edited the manuscript.

Acknowledgments

The authors thank Louise Maranda for her help with data analysis.

References

[1] C. J. Thompson, J. F. Cummings, J. Chalmers, C. Gould, and R. W. Newton, "How have patients reacted to the implications of the DCCT?," *Diabetes Care*, vol. 19, pp. 876–879, 1996.

[2] R. A. Whitmer, A. J. Karter, K. Yaffe, C. P. Quesenberry Jr., and J. V. Selby, "Hypoglycemic episodes and risk of dementia in older patients with type 2 diabetes mellitus," *JAMA*, vol. 301, pp. 1565–1572, 2009.

[3] A. Goto, O. A. Arah, M. Goto, Y. Terauchi, and M. Noda, "Severe hypoglycaemia and cardiovascular disease: systematic review and meta-analysis with bias analysis," *BMJ (Clinical Research Edition)*, vol. 347, article f4533, 2013.

[4] P. E. Cryer, "Severe hypoglycemia predicts mortality in diabetes," *Diabetes Care*, vol. 35, pp. 1814–1816, 2012.

[5] L. Razavi Nematollahi, A. E. Kitabchi, F. B. Stentz et al., "Proinflammatory cytokines in response to insulin-induced hypoglycemic stress in healthy subjects," *Metabolism*, vol. 58, pp. 443–448, 2009.

[6] W. Duckworth, C. Abraira, T. Moritz et al., "Glucose control and vascular complications in veterans with type 2 diabetes," *The New England Journal of Medicine*, vol. 360, pp. 129–139, 2009.

[7] L. Monnier, A. Wojtusciszyn, C. Colette, and D. Owens, "The contribution of glucose variability to asymptomatic hypoglycemia in persons with type 2 diabetes," *Diabetes Technology & Therapeutics*, vol. 13, pp. 813–818, 2011.

[8] T. M. Davis, S. G. Brown, I. G. Jacobs, M. Bulsara, D. G. Bruce, and W. A. Davis, "Determinants of severe hypoglycemia complicating type 2 diabetes: the Fremantle diabetes study," *The Journal of Clinical Endocrinology and Metabolism*, vol. 95, pp. 2240–2247, 2010.

[9] D. Tschope, P. Bramlage, C. Binz, M. Krekler, E. Deeg, and A. K. Gitt, "Incidence and predictors of hypoglycaemia in type 2 diabetes - an analysis of the prospective DiaRegis registry," *BMC Endocrine Disorders*, vol. 12, pp. 1472–6823, 2012.

[10] ORIGIN Trial Investigators, "Predictors of nonsevere and severe hypoglycemia during glucose-lowering treatment with insulin glargine or standard drugs in the ORIGIN trial," *Diabetes Care*, vol. 38, pp. 22–28, 2015.

[11] A. D. Wright, C. A. Cull, K. M. Macleod, and R. R. Holman, "Hypoglycemia in type 2 diabetic patients randomized to and maintained on monotherapy with diet, sulfonylurea, metformin, or insulin for 6 years from diagnosis: UKPDS73," *Journal of Diabetes and Its Complications*, vol. 20, pp. 395–401, 2006.

[12] K. Akram, U. Pedersen-Bjergaard, K. Borch-Johnsen, and B. Thorsteinsson, "Frequency and risk factors of severe hypoglycemia in insulin-treated type 2 diabetes: a literature survey," *Journal of Diabetes and Its Complications*, vol. 20, pp. 402–408, 2006.

[13] C. D. Miller, L. S. Phillips, D. C. Ziemer, D. L. Gallina, C. B. Cook, and I. M. El-Kebbi, "Hypoglycemia in patients with type 2 diabetes mellitus," *Archives of Internal Medicine*, vol. 161, pp. 1653–1659, 2001.

[14] C. Abraira, J. A. Colwell, F. Q. Nuttall et al., "Veterans affairs cooperative study on glycemic control and complications in type II diabetes (VA CSDM). Results of the feasibility trial. Veterans affairs cooperative study in type II diabetes," *Diabetes Care*, vol. 18, pp. 1113–1123, 1995.

[15] "The effect of intensive treatment of diabetes on the development and progression of long-term complications in insulin-dependent diabetes mellitus. The Diabetes Control and Complications Trial Research Group," *The New England Journal of Medicine*, vol. 329, pp. 977–986, 1993.

[16] E. Chow, A. Bernjak, S. Williams et al., "Risk of cardiac arrhythmias during hypoglycemia in patients with type 2 diabetes and cardiovascular risk," *Diabetes*, vol. 63, pp. 1738–1747, 2014.

[17] E. R. Seaquist, J. Anderson, B. Childs et al., "Hypoglycemia and diabetes: a report of a workgroup of the American Diabetes Association and the Endocrine Society," *Diabetes Care*, vol. 36, pp. 1384–1395, 2013.

[18] K. Tonyushkina and J. H. Nichols, "Glucose meters: a review of technical challenges to obtaining accurate results," *Journal of Diabetes Science and Technology*, vol. 3, pp. 971–980, 2009.

[19] U. Pedersen-Bjergaard, S. Pramming, S. R. Heller et al., "Severe hypoglycaemia in 1076 adult patients with type 1 diabetes: influence of risk markers and selection," *Diabetes/Metabolism Research and Reviews*, vol. 20, pp. 479–486, 2004.

[20] L. A. Donnelly, A. D. Morris, B. M. Frier et al., "Frequency and predictors of hypoglycaemia in type 1 and insulin-treated type 2 diabetes: a population-based study," *Diabetic Medicine*, vol. 22, pp. 749–755, 2005.

[21] UK Hypoglycaemia Study Group, "Risk of hypoglycaemia in types 1 and 2 diabetes: effects of treatment modalities and their duration," *Diabetologia*, vol. 50, pp. 1140–1147, 2007.

[22] E. S. Kilpatrick, A. S. Rigby, K. Goode, and S. L. Atkin, "Relating mean blood glucose and glucose variability to the risk of multiple episodes of hypoglycaemia in type 1 diabetes," *Diabetologia*, vol. 50, pp. 2553–2561, 2007.

[23] H. J. Luddeke, S. Sreenan, S. Aczel et al., "PREDICTIVE - a global, prospective observational study to evaluate insulin detemir treatment in types 1 and 2 diabetes: baseline characteristics and predictors of hypoglycaemia from the European cohort," *Diabetes, Obesity & Metabolism*, vol. 9, pp. 428–434, 2007.

[24] M. E. Miller, D. E. Bonds, H. C. Gerstein et al., "The effects of baseline characteristics, glycaemia treatment approach, and glycated haemoglobin concentration on the risk of severe hypoglycaemia: post hoc epidemiological analysis of the ACCORD study," *BMJ*, vol. 8, 2010.

[25] M. E. Miller, D. E. Bonds, H. C. Gerstein et al., "The effects of baseline characteristics, glycaemia treatment approach, and glycated haemoglobin concentration on the risk of severe hypoglycaemia: post hoc epidemiological analysis of the ACCORD study," *BMJ*, vol. 340, article b5444, 2010.

[26] S. Bott, U. Bott, M. Berger, and I. Muhlhauser, "Intensified insulin therapy and the risk of severe hypoglycaemia," *Diabetologia*, vol. 40, pp. 926–932, 1997.

[27] Y. Kikuchi, M. Iwase, H. Fujii et al., "Association of severe hypoglycemia with depressive symptoms in patients with type 2 diabetes: the Fukuoka Diabetes Registry," *BMJ Open Diabetes Research & Care*, vol. 3, article e000063, 2015.

[28] M. M. Fatourechi, Y. C. Kudva, M. H. Murad, M. B. Elamin, C. C. Tabini, and V. M. Montori, "Clinical review: hypoglycemia with intensive insulin therapy: a systematic review and meta-analyses of randomized trials of continuous subcutaneous insulin infusion versus multiple daily injections," *The Journal of Clinical Endocrinology and Metabolism*, vol. 94, pp. 729–740, 2009.

[29] A. Kotwal, T. English, and S. Malkani, "Potential predictors of hypoglycemia in type 1 and type 2 diabetes," *Diabetes*, vol. 64, Supplement 1, article A102, 2015.

23

Levels of Urinary Trypsin Inhibitor and Structure of its Chondroitin Sulphate Moiety in Type 1 and Type 2 Diabetes

Antonio Junior Lepedda,[1] Gabriele Nieddu,[1] Silvia Rocchiccioli,[2] Nadia Ucciferri,[2] Michela Idini,[1] Pierina De Muro,[1] and Marilena Formato[1]

[1]*Dipartimento di Scienze Biomediche, University of Sassari, Sassari, Italy*
[2]*Istituto di Fisiologia Clinica, National Research Council, Pisa, Italy*

Correspondence should be addressed to Antonio Junior Lepedda; ajlepedda@uniss.it and Marilena Formato; formato@uniss.it

Academic Editor: Tuomas O. Kilpeläinen

Background. Diabetes mellitus is a global health problem representing the fifth leading cause of mortality and a major risk factor for cardiovascular diseases. In the last years, we reported an association among urinary trypsin inhibitor (UTI), a small proteoglycan that plays pleiotropic roles in many inflammatory processes, and both type 1 and 2 diabetes and developed a method for its direct quantitation and structural characterization. *Methods.* Urine from 39 patients affected by type 1 diabetes, 32 patients with type 2 diabetes, and 52 controls were analysed. UTI was separated from the main glycosaminoglycans physiologically present in urine by anion exchange chromatography, treated for chondroitin sulphate (CS) chain complete depolymerisation, and analysed for both UTI content and CS structure. UTI identification was performed by nano-LC-MS/MS analysis. *Results.* We evidenced increased UTI levels, as well as reduced sulphation of its CS moiety in association with diabetes, regardless of both age and medium-term glycaemic control. Furthermore, no association between UTI and albumin excretion rate was found. *Conclusions.* Evidences suggest that UTI levels are not directly correlated with renal function or, otherwise, that they may increase before the onset of renal impairment in diabetes, representing a potential marker for the underlying inflammatory condition.

1. Introduction

Urinary trypsin inhibitor (UTI) is a small proteoglycan (PG), with inhibitory activity against serine proteases, resulting from excretion of plasma bikunin into urine [1]. Despite that UTI was purified in 1955 for the first time [2] and several studies on its structure and levels have been performed since the 1950s, its biological function has not been fully understood yet [3]. It is composed of a protein moiety, a low-sulphated chondroitin sulphate (CS) chain, O-linked to the serine 10, as well as an oligosaccharide, N-linked to the asparagine 45 of the protein moiety (Figure 1). The polypeptide portion consists of 147 amino acid residues folded in two Kunitz-type domains (7 kDa each) containing three disulphide bonds, a connecting peptide as well as N- and C-terminal moieties of 10–25 amino acid residues each [4]. The molecular mass of the whole proteoglycan is about 25-26 kDa, being the protein core, the CS moiety, and the oligosaccharide chains 16 kDa, 7 kDa, and 2 kDa, respectively, as reported by various studies and confirmed by ultracentrifugation methods [1, 3–5]. However, because of CS chain extended conformation, bikunin behaves like a globular protein of about 67 kDa by gel filtration and has an apparent molecular mass of 35–45 kDa by SDS-PAGE [6]. CS chain is composed of 12–18 disaccharide repeating units, consisting of glucuronic acid and N-acetyl galactosamine (GalNAc), which may be sulphated either in position C4 or in C6 [7, 8]. Four monosaccharides (Xyl-Gal-Gal-GlcA) connect this glycosaminoglycan (GAG) to bikunin [8].

About 90–98% of bikunin occurs in plasma as a subunit of interalpha inhibitor family molecules, linked via an ester bond between C6 of a nonsulphated GalNAc residue of the

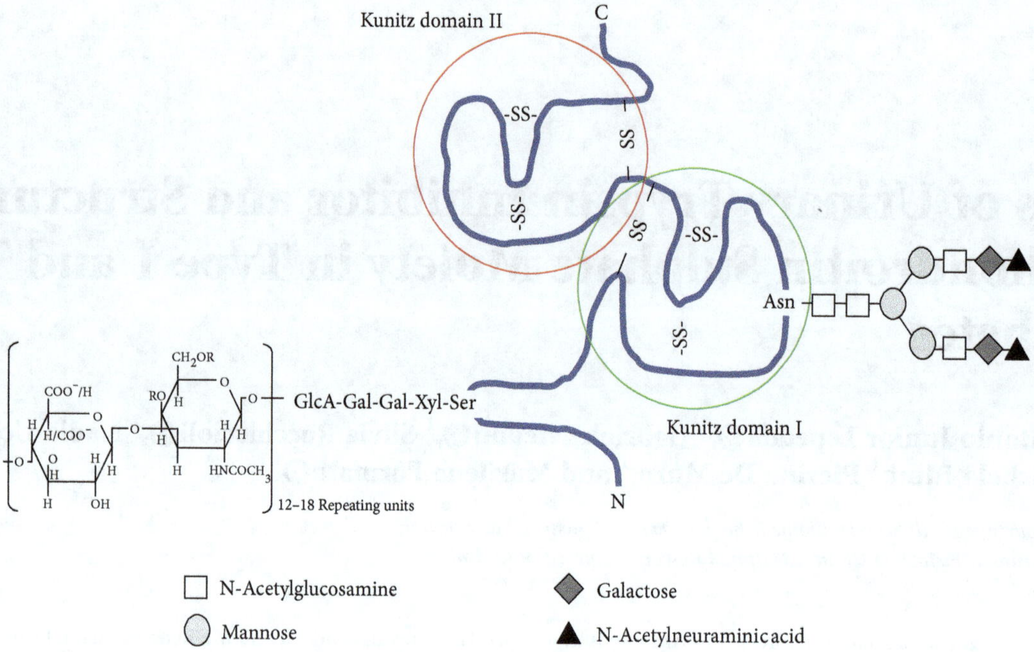

FIGURE 1: Schematic drawing of urinary trypsin inhibitor structure. R=H/SO_3^-.

CS chain and the α-carbon of the C-terminal amino acid residue of one or two polypeptides [9], called the heavy chains, to form interalpha inhibitor and prealpha inhibitor, respectively [1].

Although its main activity is the inhibition of various serine proteases such as trypsin, chymotrypsin, elastase, granzyme K, cathepsin G, acrosin, and plasmin [3, 4, 10], many studies provided evidences also on its role in many regulatory mechanisms, such as inhibition of IL-8 gene expression induced by lipopolysaccharide [10], neutrophil release of elastase [11], mast cell release of histamine [12], urolithiasis [13], stabilization of the lysosomal membrane [14], stimulation of fibroblast growth [15], and regulation of smooth muscle contraction by modulating calcium intracellular levels [16], as well as in supporting the formation of the hyaluronan-containing extracellular matrix [17] and in inhibiting the formation of kidney stone [18].

Furthermore, bikunin was proven to have a protective role in several inflammatory processes, by preventing protease-activated receptor activation on cell surfaces [19], by inhibiting blood coagulation through its action on plasmin and blood coagulation factors [20], and by protecting acinar and endocrine pancreatic cells from self-digestion [21], thus providing protection against pathologies such as diabetes, kidney diseases, cancer, bacterial and viral infections, and vascular diseases [21].

Several studies reported that UTI/bikunin levels can increase up to 10-fold following both acute and chronic inflammatory diseases [22], bladder carcinoma [23], brain contusion [24], disseminated cancers [25], acute hepatitis [26], Fabry's disease [27], Crohn's disease, arthritis, pericarditis, deep vein thrombosis, fibromyalgia, asthmatiform bronchitis [28, neoplasia, and kidney diseases [4]. Besides, we reported variations of UTI/GAGs levels in pathological conditions such as chronic glomerulonephritis [29, 30], type 1 and 2 diabetes [31–35], systemic lupus erythematosus [36] and following kidney transplantation [37]. In human plasma, the concentration of bikunin is 4–7 μM, of which only 2–10% is in free form, while in urine UTI levels are about 0.03–0.05 μM [4].

To date, UTI quantitation in urine is performed mainly by means of enzyme inhibition assays or immunological detection [38]. Both approaches may be affected by low specificity and/or sensibility. Recently, we developed a method for a direct quantitation and structural characterization of UTI protein moiety, starting from very low quantities of specimen. To achieve this goal, we merged classical chromatographic methods, applied for GAG/PG purification [27, 30, 31, 33, 34, 36], with image analysis of SDS-PAGE profiles, which had been proven useful in quantifying protein microquantities from different sources [39]. Furthermore, nano-LC-MS/MS analysis on tryptic-digested UTI bands was performed for protein identification and characterization.

The aim of the present study was to characterize the CS moiety of UTI in diabetic patients by fluorophore-assisted carbohydrate electrophoresis (FACE) analysis, applying a preanalytical step for UTI purification. Furthermore, the obtained results allowed us to validate previous preliminary data on both type 1 and 2 diabetes mellitus (T1DM and T2DM) suggesting UTI as a potential useful marker of these two chronic inflammatory conditions [32].

2. Methods

2.1. Sample Collection. Twenty-four-hour urine samples were collected from 39 patients affected by type 1 diabetes (age 31.79 ± 10.90), 32 patients with type 2 diabetes (age

64.50 ± 7.50), and 52 controls (age 36.25 ± 19.34) and immediately centrifuged at 5000 ×g for 15 minutes before storing at −20°C until analysis. Each sample was assessed for both urinary creatinine, carried out by the Jaffè method (Sentinel Diagnostics, Italy), and twenty-four-hour albumin excretion rate (AER), assessed by an immunoturbidimetric method (Roche Diagnostics, Germany). All diabetic patients were normoalbuminuric with an AER lower than 30 mg/24 hours except for three microalbuminuric patients. Fasting glycaemia was outside the target range (70–130 mg/dL) being 163.44 ± 29.99 mg/dL and 145.10 ± 22.78 mg/dL for T1DM and T2DM, respectively, whereas glycated haemoglobin (HbA1c%) was 7.51 ± 0.95 and 6.70 ± 0.86, indicating a poor long-term control of blood glucose in both groups.

Informed consent was obtained before enrolment. Institutional Review Board approval was obtained. The study was conducted in accordance with the ethical principles of the current Declaration of Helsinki.

2.2. UTI Purification and Analysis. UTI was purified according to a method recently developed by our research group [32] with slight modifications (Figure 2). Briefly, two elution fractions were obtained by anion exchange chromatography; the first one contained UTI and UTI derivatives, while the latter contained free highly charged GAGs, that is, HS and CS, as assessed by electrophoresis on cellulose acetate plates. Following chondroitin ABC lyase (Chase-ABC) depolymerisation of CS moiety, UTI fraction was analysed for both UTI content, by SDS-PAGE, and CS detailed structure, by FACE. UTI band obtained by SDS-PAGE was identified by MS analysis.

2.3. Anion Exchange Chromatography. A volume of urine corresponding to 5 mg of creatinine (usually ranging from 2 to 8 mL) was loaded into a chromatography column (Econo-Column Chromatography Columns, 0.5 × 20 cm, Bio-Rad Laboratories, California, USA) packed with DEAE-Sephacel anion exchange resin (GE Healthcare Life Sciences, United Kingdom) and equilibrated with 0.02 M Tris buffer, pH 8.6, containing 0.15 M NaCl, which was also used to wash away from the column all the by-products and impurities contained in urine samples until absorbance at 280 nm was lower than 0.05. Two consecutive gravity feed elution steps were performed using 0.02 M Tris buffer, pH 8.6, containing 0.45 M LiCl, and 0.02 M Tris buffer, pH 8.6, containing 2 M LiCl, to elute separately UTI-containing fraction (first elution) from highly charged urinary GAGs (second elution). Both fractions were immediately concentrated and dialysed by means of Amicon Ultra-0.5 Centrifugal Filter Units (Millipore, MA, USA), according to the manufacturer's instructions, for further analyses.

2.4. Cellulose Acetate Electrophoresis Analysis. To evaluate GAG composition, aliquots of both eluted fractions were resolved by discontinuous electrophoresis on Titan III-H cellulose acetate plates (6.0 × 7.5 cm, Helena BioSciences, United Kingdom), according to Cappelletti et al. [40]. This technique, combined with the differential susceptibility of GAGs to precipitation by organic solvents, allows for optimal and rapid separation of intact GAGs with high resolution and sensitivity (10 ng detection limit). GAG separation was carried out in 0.25 M barium acetate buffer, pH 5.0, by three electrophoretic steps as previously described [27]. Electrophoretic profiles were detected following 0.1% (*w*/*v*) alcian blue staining. Images were acquired by means of a GS-800 calibrated densitometer (Bio-Rad Laboratories, California, USA) and analysed by using Quantity One v4.6.3 software (Bio-Rad Laboratories, California, USA).

2.5. Chondroitin Sulphate Depolymerisation. Following concentration and dialysis, UTI fraction was diluted with 0.5 M ammonium acetate 5X buffer, pH 8.0, and incubated overnight at 37°C with 0.025 U of Chase-ABC (Sigma-Aldrich, MO, USA), allowing for chondroitin sulphate complete depolymerisation into constituent disaccharide units with an unsaturation between C4 and C5 of hexuronic acid (Δ-disaccharides). Subsequently, samples were split in two aliquots and analysed for both UTI content, by SDS-PAGE, and CS detailed structure, by FACE.

2.6. SDS-PAGE Analysis. Samples were diluted with 4X Laemmli buffer, consisting of 250 mM Tris, pH 6.8, 8% SDS (*w*/*v*), 8% dithiothreitol (DTT) (*w*/*v*), 40% glycerol (*v*/*v*), and 0.0008% bromophenol blue (*w*/*v*), boiled for 5 minutes, and resolved by Tris-glycine SDS-PAGE, through 1 mm thick 15% T and 3% C running gel. Electrophoresis was carried out at 50 V for 15 minutes and then at 150 V, until the bromophenol dye front reached the lower limit of the gel, in a Mini-Protean II cell vertical slab gel electrophoresis apparatus (Bio-Rad Laboratories, California, USA). Following Coomassie brilliant blue G-250 staining, gels were acquired at 63 μm resolution using a GS-800 calibrated densitometer (Bio-Rad Laboratories, California, USA) and analysed by means of Quantity One software, v 4.6.3 (Bio-Rad Laboratories, California, USA) [39]. For UTI quantitation, a calibration curve was set ($y = 1.337x - 0.1868$, $R^2 = 0.9943$) by loading known quantities of highly purified CS-free UTI, ranging from 0.25 to 4 μg. The linear response between band intensity, expressed as optical density, and UTI levels allowed for accurate quantitation in the considered range. UTI concentration in each sample was normalized for creatinine content.

2.7. UTI Identification by Nano-LC-MS/MS Analysis. Nano-LC-MS/MS analysis on tryptic-digested UTI bands was performed for protein identification and characterization as previously described [31, 32]. Briefly, spots were excised, destained, and dehydrated. Rehydrated spots were in gel reduced, alkylated, and trypsin digested. Recovered peptides were purified through a C18 column, and 2 μL was injected into a nano-HPLC system (Eksigent, ABSciex, USA). Peptides were separated through a C18 PepMap-100 column (3 μm, 75 μm × 250 mm, Thermo Scientific, USA) in a 70-minute linear gradient from 5% of 0.1% formic acid to 40% of acetonitrile/0.1% formic acid. HPLC was directly coupled to a TripleTOF™ 5600 mass spectrometer (ABSciex, USA), and MS/MS data were processed with ProteinPilot™ Software (ABSciex, USA).

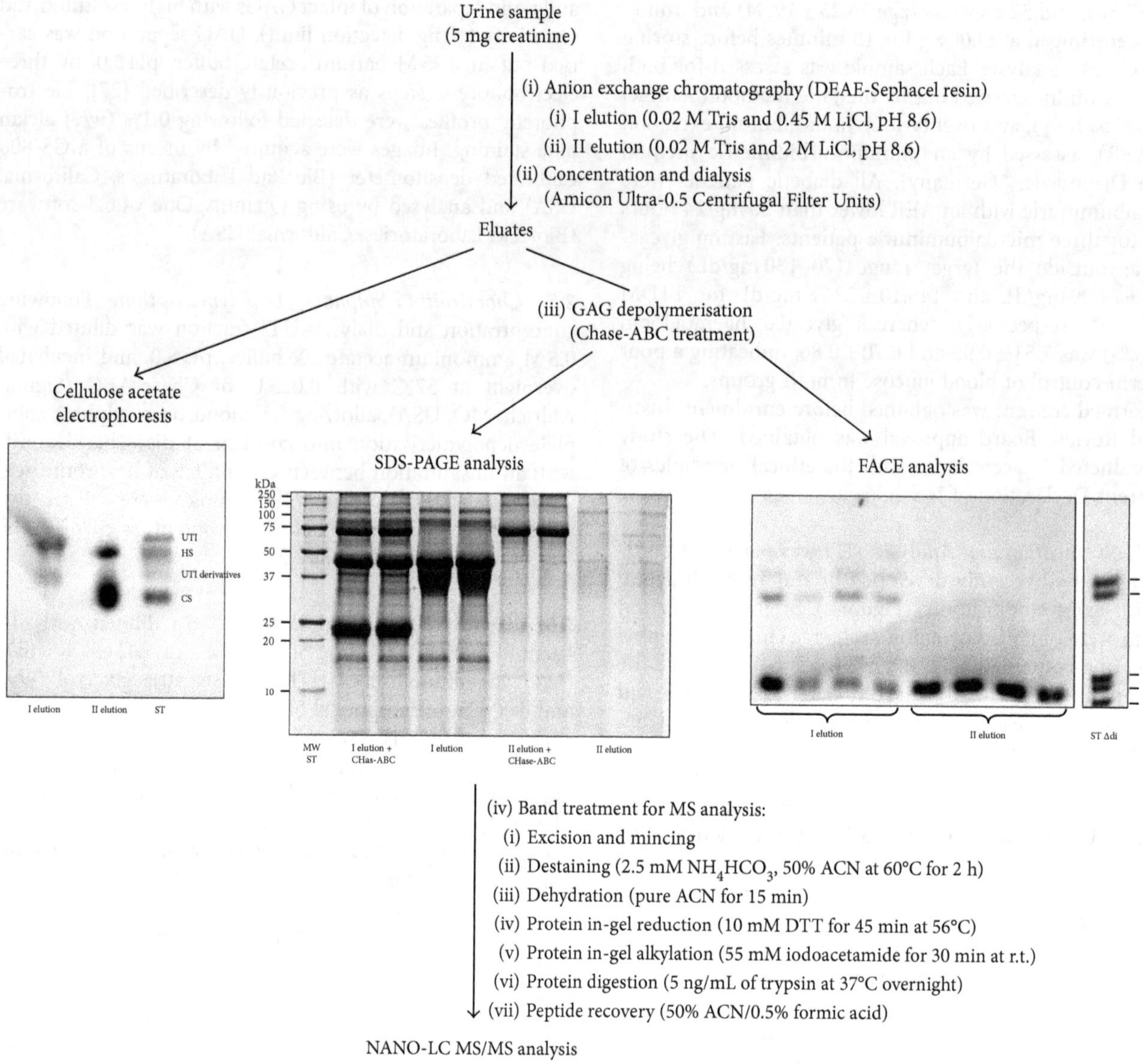

FIGURE 2: Flow chart showing the adopted methods for UTI purification (anion exchange chromatography) and analysis of both protein core (SDS-PAGE followed by MS analysis) and chondroitin sulphate moiety (fluorophore-assisted carbohydrate electrophoresis analysis). Cellulose acetate electrophoresis was performed to assess effectiveness of UTI purification. I elution: UTI and UTI derivatives; II elution: heparan sulphate (HS) and free highly charged chondroitin sulphate (CS).

2.8. FACE Analysis. Structural analysis on CS moiety was performed on samples from 10 T1DM and 10 T2DM patients and 10 healthy controls, as previously described [41]. Δ-Disaccharide units obtained by depolymerisation of CS chain from UTI fraction were fluorotagged by reductive amination with 2-aminoacridone (AMAC), in the presence of sodium cyanoborohydride ($NaBH_3CN$), as previously described by Calabro et al. [42]. Briefly, 40 μL of 12.5 mM AMAC solution in glacial acetic acid/DMSO (3 : 17 *v*/*v*) was added to Chase-ABC-treated lyophilized sample and incubated for 15 minutes, at room temperature, followed by 40 μL of 1.25 M $NaBH_3CN$ and overnight incubation at 37°C. After derivatization, 20 μL of glycerol was added to each sample prior to electrophoresis, which was performed in a MiniProtean II cell vertical slab gel electrophoresis apparatus (Bio-Rad Laboratories, California, USA) as previously described by Karousou et al. [43]. 5 μL of each sample was resolved through 25% T and 7.5% C polyacrylamide running gels prepared in 187.5 mM Tris-borate and 187.5 mM Tris-HCl buffer, pH 8.8. 5% T and 15% C stacking gels were prepared in 0.36 M Tris-HCl buffer, pH 8.8. 5 μL of bromophenol blue dye was run in the first lane to monitor the electrophoresis front. The run was carried out in 0.15 M Tris-borate buffer, pH 8.8, at 400 V and 4°C until the dye reached the bottom of the gel. Gels were then acquired by UV transillumination using the Gel Doc XR System (Bio-Rad) and analysed with Quantity One 4.6.3 (Bio-Rad Laboratories, California, USA). Band identification was achieved by comparing their electrophoretic mobility with standard Δ-disaccharides, run in the same gel. A

Table 1: UTI identification by nano-LC-MS/MS analysis in the 3 groups analysed.

	Paragon score	% Cov (95)	Accession number	Entry name	Protein name	Species	Peptides (95%)
Controls	110.11	38.64	P02760	AMBP_HUMAN	Protein AMBP	HUMAN	149
T1DM	167.84	57.1	P02760	AMBP_HUMAN	Protein AMBP	HUMAN	337
T2DM	123.92	41.76	P02760	AMBP_HUMAN	Protein AMBP	HUMAN	218

Each spot was analysed separately and MS/MS data from the same group were treated as replicates for database analysis. % Cov = coverage percentage with at least 95% confidence. Peptides = identified peptides with at least 95% confidence. AMBP = alpha-1-microglobulin/bikunin precursor.

calibration curve was set up ($y = 909.14x - 9891.9$, $R^2 = 0.9996$), allowing for accurate Δ-disaccharide quantitation in each sample, by loading known quantities (from 25 to 800 ng) of AMAC-derivatized Δ-disaccharides obtained by depolymerisation of a highly purified UTI sample assayed for uronic acid (UA) content, according to the carbazole method by Bitter and Muir [44]. CS concentration in each sample was normalized for creatinine content.

2.9. Statistical Analysis. Statistical analyses were performed using Sigma Stat 3 software package (Systat Software). UTI concentration values were reported as median and interquartile range, as normality test failed. Mann–Whitney rank sum test was performed to evaluate differences among the three groups, while correlations between UTI levels and age, UTI levels and glycated haemoglobin, and UTI levels and microalbuminuria were assessed by Spearman's correlation. Significance was set at $p < 0.05$.

3. Results

Both purification and quantitation of UTI were performed according to a method recently published [31, 32], with some modifications (Figure 2). In particular, as the purpose of this work was to analyse at a structural level UTI-CS moiety, we performed two elution steps that allowed the separation of UTI fraction (first elution) from the highly charged GAG fraction (second elution), containing HS and a normo-sulphated CS with different origin from UTI-CS. Then, both fractions were concentrated, dialysed, and treated with Chase-ABC for CS complete depolymerisation into Δ-disaccharide units.

A half of each sample was subjected to SDS-PAGE analysis for UTI quantitation and identification by nano-LC-MS/MS analysis (Table 1, see Supplementary Material 1 for complete MS information), while the other one, following AMAC derivatization, was analysed by means of FACE for CS content and structure. Since all data were normalized for creatinine content, the method was effective in analysing also randomly collected urine samples in a wide range of concentrations. Furthermore, an estimation of UTI-CS chain length was performed as the ratio between the moles of disaccharides and the moles of UTI, considering 15.974 kDa as UTI molecular weight calculated through ExPASy Compute pI/Mw tool (http://www.expasy.org), according to the sequence reported by Xu et al. [45].

Data obtained from patients affected by both type 1 and type 2 diabetes were compared with those from a healthy control group (Table 2). We evidenced higher levels of UTI, expressed as μg protein/mg creatinine, in both T1DM and T2DM patients with respect to controls ($p = 0.001$ and $p = 0.006$, resp.), whereas no differences were found between the two groups of patients ($p = 0.160$) (Figure 3). With regard to the glycosaminoglycan moiety of UTI, CS levels, expressed as μg UA/mg creatinine, were found significantly higher in both T1DM and T2DM patients with respect to controls ($p = 0.005$ and $p = 0.041$, resp.). Besides, a lower sulphation degree of CS chains, expressed as ratio between Δdi-mono 4S and total disaccharides (Δdi-mono 4S + Δdi-non S), was observed in both classes of patients compared to controls ($p = 0.046$ and $p = 0.021$ for T1DM and T2DM, resp.), while no differences were found between T1DM and T2DM patients ($p = 0.873$). Finally, no differences in CS chain length were evidenced between both classes of patients and controls ($p = 0.967$, $p = 0.096$, and $p = 0.473$, for T1DM versus controls, T2DM versus controls, and T1DM versus T2DM, resp.) as further corroborated by the strict positive correlation between levels of UTI protein core and CS reported for T1DM ($p < 0.001$), T2DM ($p < 0.001$), and the totality of samples (including controls) (Table 3).

To evaluate any possible association among UTI and medium-term glycaemic control or renal function, we performed Spearman's correlation tests evidencing no correlation neither with glycated haemoglobin nor with albumin excretion rate (Table 4). Finally, no correlation was evidenced between UTI levels and age in controls, T1DM, and T2DM and in the totality of samples (Table 5).

4. Discussion

Diabetes mellitus is a huge global health problem representing the fifth leading cause of mortality and a major risk factor for cardiovascular diseases, such as coronary artery disease, stroke, and peripheral vascular disease [46]. T1DM results from the autoimmune destruction of the insulin-producing β cells of Langerhans islets; it is usually diagnosed in children and young adults and represents less than 10% of all cases of diabetes. T2DM, or adult-onset diabetes, represents over 90% of cases of diabetes mellitus and is characterized by hyperglycaemia caused by insulin resistance. A major issue of T2DM is that its diagnosis is frequently made years after disease onset, when vascular complications are already present in most patients [47]. Since patients with diabetes are at increased risk of microvascular and macrovascular complications [47], identification of early diagnostic markers to be

TABLE 2: UTI levels and CS moiety structure in T1DM, T2DM, and healthy controls.

	Controls	T1DM	T2DM	T1DM versus controls	T2DM versus controls	T1DM versus T2DM
UTI protein core levels (μg prot./mg creatinine)[a]	4.093[d] (2.326–9.920)	9.612[d] (5.532–22.738)	7.792[d] (4.304–16.181)	**0.001**[b]	**0.006**[b]	0.160[b]
CS levels (μg UA/mg creatinine)[a]	1.251[e] (1.041–1.413)	1.940[e] (1.459–5.949)	1.514[e] (1.315–2.286)	**0.005**[b]	**0.041**[b]	0.162[b]
Sulphation degree (Δdi-mono 4S/Δdi-mono 4S + Δdi-non S)[a]	53.113%[e] (47.360–55.338)	42.612%[e] (35.734–49.263)	44.712%[e] (36.633–50.073)	**0.046**[c]	**0.021**[c]	0.873[c]
Chain length (moles of Δdi/moles of UTI)[a]	10.951[e] (9.010–12.780)	8.967[e] (8.498–23.598)	12.764[e] (12.212–15.502)	0.967[b]	0.096[b]	0.473[b]

[a]Median and interquartile ranges (in parenthesis) are reported. [b]p values, obtained by the Mann–Whitney Rank Sum tests, are reported. [c]p values, obtained by t-tests, are reported. [d]Data obtained from 52 controls, 39 type 1 diabetics, and 32 type 2 diabetics. [e]Data obtained from 10 controls, 10 type 1 diabetics, and 10 type 2 diabetics. Significant differences are reported in bold ($p < 0.05$).

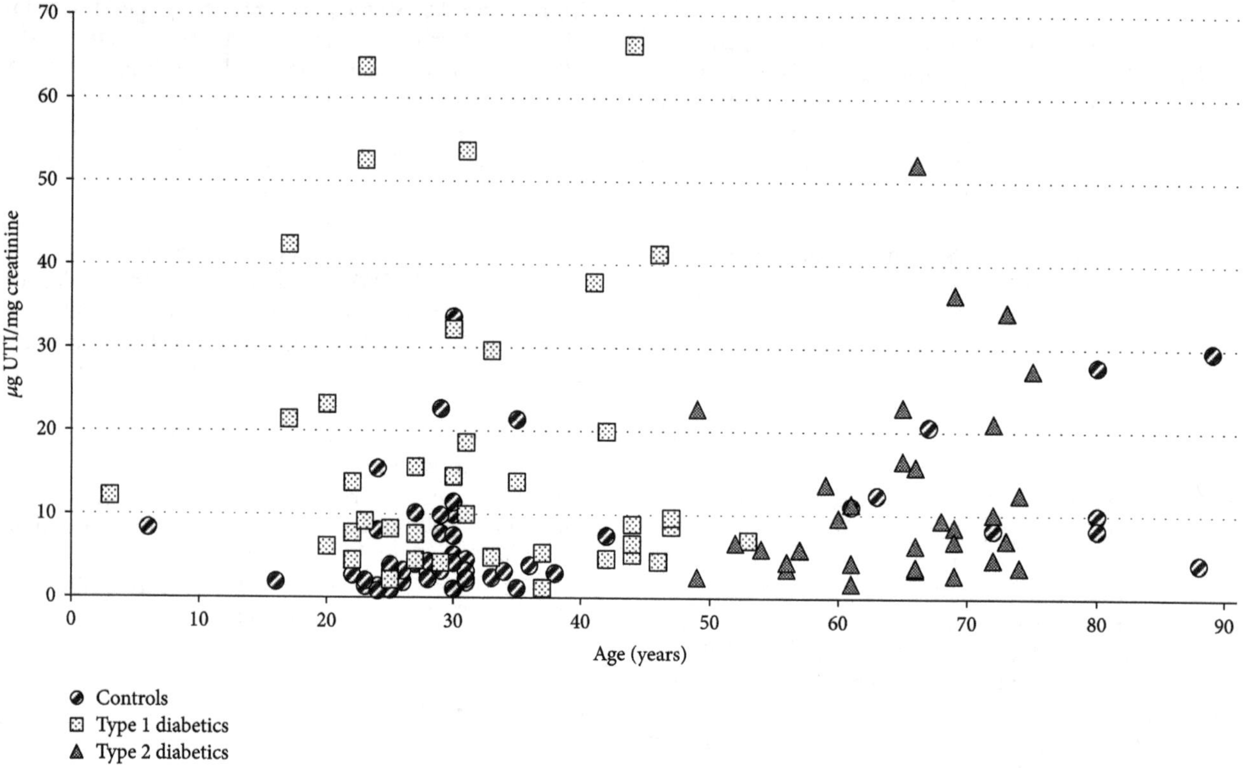

FIGURE 3: Scatter plot showing UTI levels in patients with type 1 diabetes (⊠) and type 2 diabetes (▲) and healthy controls (●) in relation to age.

TABLE 3: Spearman's correlation tests between levels of UTI protein core and CS moiety.

UTI protein core versus CS	Corr. coefficient	p value
Controls	0.376	0.284
Type 1 diabetics	**0.897**	<0.001
Type 2 diabetics	**0.911**	<0.001
All (including controls)	**0.763**	<0.001

Positive correlation between values that tend to increase together is indicated in bold.

TABLE 4: Spearman's correlation tests between UTI protein core levels and glycated haemoglobin and between UTI protein core levels and AER.

UTI versus HbA1c%	Corr. coefficient	p value
T1DM	0.318	0.087
T2DM	−0.152	0.500
UTI versus AER		
T1DM	−0.156	0.457
T2DM	−0.004	0.986

TABLE 5: Spearman's correlation tests between UTI protein core levels and age.

UTI versus age	Corr. coefficient	p value
Controls (under 50 years old)	0.103	0.510
Controls (over 50 years old)	0.178	0.646
Type 1 diabetics	−0.070	0.673
Type 2 diabetics	0.243	0.181
All (including controls)	0.088	0.330

associated with the current standard tests is mandatory to slow disease progression and reduce adverse outcomes.

The association between diabetes and GAG/PG excretion in urine has been extensively studied [48]. Except for a few studies that report no change or even a reduced excretion of GAGs/PGs, a plethora of papers evidence an increased excretion as a whole (in most of them only a quantitative analysis was performed) and in particular of HS in both type 1 and 2 diabetes, often in association with diabetic nephropathy [48]. In the last years, we reported an association among UTI and both type 1 and 2 diabetes [31–35] suggesting UTI as a promising marker for the chronic inflammation resulting from diabetic condition [31, 32]. Despite the numerous studies on both UTI structure and function, several aspects related to its structural modifications following inflammation and their relevance for a biological and diagnostic point of view remain to be elucidated. In this respect, Mizon et al. demonstrated that the CS chain of bikunin increases in size in inflammatory diseases [49]. Furthermore, Capon et al. evidenced that, in acute inflammation, the CS chain is both longer and undersulphated [50].

The aims of this study were both to characterize at a structural level the CS moiety of UTI, which has not been analysed so far in relation to diabetic condition, and to strengthen our previous preliminary results on both T1DM and T2DM, suggesting UTI as a potential useful marker of these two chronic inflammatory conditions.

Hence, we evidenced that diabetes may result in UTI levels increase, as well as in changes in CS chain sulphation degree. In this respect, we did not evidence any correlation among UTI levels, age and glycated haemoglobin ruling out these parameters from the potential confounders. Furthermore, no association between UTI and albumin excretion rate was found, suggesting that UTI levels are not directly correlated with renal function or, otherwise, that they may increase before the onset of renal impairment.

With regard to CS chain sulphation degree, UTI was undersulphated in both T1DM and T2DM patients. The sulphation balance and pattern of CS on specific carbon residues are tightly regulated during development, injury, and disease, with the temporal and spatial expression of different chondroitin sulfotransferase isoforms [51].

Glycosaminoglycan/proteoglycan biosynthesis and turnover require many enzymatic activities and are finely regulated by molecules such as hormones, cytokines, and growth factors [52, 53]. In particular, it is known that in diabetic patients, there is an increased renal production of TGF-β that is a potent modulator of extracellular matrix (ECM) proteoglycan synthesis and represents a potential link between hyperglycaemia and the accelerated development of atherosclerosis in diabetes [54].

Improving diagnosis and follow-up of both T1DM and T2DM is mandatory, as they may result in microvascular and macrovascular complications, as well as in a significant increase in cardiovascular risk [47]. In this study, both levels and structure of UTI have been found associated with T1DM and T2DM and may represent potential markers for the underlying inflammatory condition. As far as we know, the relationship between UTI-CS structure and diabetes has not been investigated yet. Therefore, we can only speculate that similar pathways involved in ECM proteoglycan remodelling could affect UTI biosynthesis in the liver. The applied method was proven valuable in both UTI purification from free highly charged CS and quantitative/structural analyses, also starting from small sample volumes or randomly collected samples. Therefore, it may represent a promising tool in monitoring the onset and the progression of type 1 and type 2 diabetes. The mechanisms underlying UTI modifications in diabetes as well as their pathophysiological role are not yet known and surely deserve further studies.

Conflicts of Interest

The authors declare that they have no conflicts of interest.

Authors' Contributions

Antonio Junior Lepedda and Gabriele Nieddu contributed equally to this work.

Acknowledgments

The authors wish to thank Dr. Pietro Fresu (Unità Operativa di Diabetologia e Malattie del Ricambio, AOU-Sassari, Sassari, Italy) who provided clinical support. This study was funded by Fondazione di Sardegna, Sassari, Italy (Grant no. 2014.0220).

References

[1] M. J. Pugia and J. A. Lott, "Pathophysiology and diagnostic value of urinary trypsin inhibitors," *Clinical Chemistry and Laboratory Medicine (CCLM)*, vol. 43, no. 1, pp. 1–16, 2005.

[2] N. R. Shulman, "A proteolytic inhibitor with anticoagulant activity separated from human urine and plasma," *The Journal of Biological Chemistry*, vol. 213, no. 2, pp. 655–671, 1955.

[3] A. Kaczmarczyk, A. M. Blom, J. Alston-Smith, M. Sjöquist, and E. Fries, "Plasma bikunin: half-life and tissue uptake," *Molecular and Cellular Biochemistry*, vol. 271, no. 1-2, pp. 61–67, 2005.

[4] E. Fries and A. M. Blom, "Bikunin–not just a plasma proteinase inhibitor," *The International Journal of Biochemistry & Cell Biology*, vol. 32, no. 2, pp. 125–137, 2000.

[5] K. E. Lindström, A. Blom, E. Johnsson, B. Haraldsson, and E. Fries, "High glomerular permeability of bikunin despite similarity in charge and hydrodynamic size to serum albumin," *Kidney International*, vol. 51, no. 4, pp. 1053–1058, 1997.

[6] A. Slota, M. Sjöquist, M. Wolgast, J. Alston-Smith, and E. Fries, "Bikunin in rat plasma, lymph and bile," *Biological Chemistry Hoppe-Seyler*, vol. 375, no. 2, pp. 127–134, 1994.

[7] J. E. Silbert and G. Sugumaran, "Biosynthesis of chondroitin/dermatan sulfate," *IUBMB Life (International Union of Biochemistry and Molecular Biology: Life)*, vol. 54, no. 4, pp. 177–186, 2002.

[8] H. Toyoda, T. Ikei, Y. Demachi, T. Toida, and T. Imanari, "Structural analysis of the N-linked oligosaccharides from human urinary trypsin inhibitor," *Chemical & Pharmaceutical Bulletin*, vol. 40, no. 10, pp. 2882–2884, 1992.

[9] W. Morelle, C. Capon, M. Balduyck et al., "Chondroitin sulphate covalently cross-links the three polypeptide chains of inter-α-trypsin inhibitor," *European Journal of Biochemistry*, vol. 221, no. 2, pp. 881–888, 1994.

[10] K. Maehara, N. Kanayama, A. Halim et al., "Down-regulation of interleukin-8 gene expression in HL60 cell line by human Kunitz-type trypsin inhibitor," *Biochemical and Biophysical Research Communications*, vol. 206, no. 3, pp. 927–934, 1995.

[11] A. Hiyama, J. Takeda, Y. Kotake, H. Morisaki, and K. Fukushima, "A human urinary protease inhibitor (ulinastatin) inhibits neutrophil extracellular release of elastase during cardiopulmonary bypass," *Journal of Cardiothoracic and Vascular Anesthesia*, vol. 11, no. 5, pp. 580–584, 1997.

[12] H. Kobayashi, K. Shibata, M. Fujie, and T. Terao, "Urinary trypsin inhibitor reduces the release of histamine from rat peritoneal mast cells," *Journal of Laboratory and Clinical Medicine*, vol. 131, no. 4, pp. 375–385, 1998.

[13] F. Atmani, P. A. Glenton, and S. R. Khan, "Role of inter-α-inhibitor and its related proteins in experimentally induced calcium oxalate urolithiasis. Localization of proteins and expression of bikunin gene in the rat kidney," *Urological Research*, vol. 27, no. 1, pp. 63–67, 1999.

[14] Y. Kato, M. Kudo, T. Shinkawa et al., "Role ofO-linked carbohydrate of human urinary trypsin inhibitor on its lysosomal membrane-stabilizing property," *Biochemical and Biophysical Research Communications*, vol. 243, no. 2, pp. 377–383, 1998.

[15] J. K. Perry, G. K. Scott, and C. A. Tse, "Modulation of proliferation of cultured human cells by urinary trypsin inhibitor," *Biochimica et Biophysica Acta (BBA) - Molecular Cell Research*, vol. 1221, no. 2, pp. 145–152, 1994.

[16] N. Kanayama, K. Maehara, L. She et al., "Urinary trypsin inhibitor suppresses vascular smooth muscle contraction by inhibition of Ca^{2+} influx," *Biochimica et Biophysica Acta (BBA) - General Subjects*, vol. 1381, no. 2, pp. 139–146, 1998.

[17] A. Blom, H. Pertoft, and E. Fries, "Inter-α-inhibitor is required for the formation of the hyaluronan-containing coat on fibroblasts and mesothelial cells," *Journal of Biological Chemistry*, vol. 270, no. 17, pp. 9698–9701, 1995.

[18] J. Médétognon-Benissan, S. Tardivel, C. Hennequin, M. Daudon, T. Drüeke, and B. Lacour, "Inhibitory effect of bikunin on calcium oxalate crystallization in vitro and urinary bikunin decrease in renal stone formers," *Urological Research*, vol. 27, no. 1, pp. 69–75, 1999.

[19] G. S. Cottrell, A. M. Coelho, and N. W. Bunnett, "Protease-activated receptors: the role of cell-surface proteolysis in signalling," *Essays in Biochemistry*, vol. 38, pp. 169–183, 2002.

[20] A. Nii, H. Morishita, T. Yamakawa et al., "Design of variants of the second domain of urinary trypsin inhibitor (R-020) with increased factor Xa inhibitory activity," *The Journal of Biochemistry*, vol. 115, no. 6, pp. 1107–1112, 1994.

[21] M. J. Pugia, R. Valdes, and S. A. Jortani, "Bikunin (urinary trypsin inhibitor): structure, biological relevance, and measurement," *Advances in Clinical Chemistry*, vol. 44, pp. 223–245, 2007.

[22] S. A. Jortani, M. J. Pugia, R. J. Elin et al., "Sensitive noninvasive marker for the diagnosis of probable bacterial or viral infection," *Journal of Clinical Laboratory Analysis*, vol. 18, no. 6, pp. 289–295, 2004.

[23] K. H. Tsui, P. Tang, C. Y. Lin, P. L. Chang, C. H. Chang, and B. Y. M. Yung, "Bikunin loss in urine as useful marker for bladder carcinoma," *The Journal of Urology*, vol. 183, no. 1, pp. 339–344, 2010.

[24] K. Sakai, H. Okudera, and K. Hongo, "Significant elevation of urinary trypsin inhibitor in patients with brain contusion - a preliminary report," *Journal of Clinical Neuroscience*, vol. 10, no. 6, pp. 677–679, 2003.

[25] S. D. Lin, R. Endo, H. Kuroda et al., "Plasma and urine levels of urinary trypsin inhibitor in patients with chronic liver diseases and hepatocellular carcinoma," *Journal of Gastroenterology and Hepatology*, vol. 19, no. 3, pp. 327–332, 2004.

[26] S. D. Lin, R. Endo, A. Sato, Y. Takikawa, K. Shirakawa, and K. Suzuki, "Plasma and urine levels of urinary trypsin inhibitor in patients with acute and fulminant hepatitis," *Journal of Gastroenterology and Hepatology*, vol. 17, no. 2, pp. 140–147, 2002.

[27] A. J. Lepedda, L. Fancellu, E. Zinellu et al., "Urine bikunin as a marker of renal impairment in Fabry's disease," *BioMed Research International*, vol. 2013, Article ID 205948, 9 pages, 2013.

[28] C. Mizon, F. Piva, V. Queyrel, M. Balduyck, E. Hachulla, and J. Mizon, "Urinary bikunin determination provides insight into proteinase/proteinase inhibitor imbalance in patients with inflammatory diseases," *Clinical Chemistry and Laboratory Medicine*, vol. 40, no. 6, pp. 579–586, 2002.

[29] P. De Muro, R. Faedda, A. Satta et al., "Urinary glycosaminoglycan composition in chronic glomerulonephritis," *Journal of Nephrology*, vol. 18, no. 2, pp. 154–160, 2005.

[30] P. De Muro, R. Faedda, A. E. Satta et al., "Quali-quantitative analysis of urinary glycosaminoglycans for monitoring glomerular inflammatory activity," *Scandinavian Journal of Urology and Nephrology*, vol. 41, no. 3, pp. 230–236, 2007.

[31] G. Nieddu, *Identification and characterization of biomarkers in atherosclerosis and diabetes, International PhD School in Biomolecular and Biotechnological Sciences, [Ph.D. thesis]*, University of Sassari, 2015.

[32] A. J. Lepedda, G. Nieddu, S. Rocchiccioli, P. Fresu, P. de Muro, and M. Formato, "Development of a method for urine bikunin/urinary trypsin inhibitor (UTI) quantitation and structural characterization: application to type 1 and type 2 diabetes," *Electrophoresis*, vol. 34, no. 22-23, pp. 3227–3233, 2013.

[33] P. De Muro, P. Fresu, M. Formato et al., "Urinary glycosaminoglycan and proteoglycan excretion in normoalbuminuric patients with type 1 diabetes mellitus," *Journal of Nephrology*, vol. 15, no. 3, pp. 290–296, 2002.

[34] P. De Muro, P. Fresu, G. Tonolo et al., "A longitudinal evaluation of urinary glycosaminoglycan excretion in normoalbuminuric type 1 diabetic patients," *Clinical Chemistry and Laboratory Medicine*, vol. 44, no. 5, pp. 561–567, 2006.

[35] P. De Muro, A. J. Lepedda, G. Nieddu et al., "Evaluation of early markers of nephropathy in patients with type 2 diabetes mellitus," *Biochemistry Research International*, vol. 2016, Article ID 7497614, 6 pages, 2016.

[36] P. De Muro, R. Faedda, M. Formato et al., "Urinary glycosaminoglycans in patients with systemic lupus erythematosus," *Clinical and Experimental Rheumatology*, vol. 19, no. 2, pp. 125–130, 2001.

[37] P. De Muro, R. Faedda, A. Masala et al., "Kidney post-transplant monitoring of urinary glycosaminoglycans/proteoglycans and monokine induced by IFN-γ (MIG)," *Clinical and Experimental Medicine*, vol. 13, no. 1, pp. 59–65, 2013.

[38] M. J. Pugia, S. A. Jortani, M. Basu et al., "Immunological evaluation of urinary trypsin inhibitors in blood and urine: role of N- & O-linked glycoproteins," *Glycoconjugate Journal*, vol. 24, no. 1, pp. 5–15, 2007.

[39] A. Zinellu, A. Lepedda, S. Sotgia et al., "Albumin-bound low molecular weight thiols analysis in plasma and carotid plaques by CE," *Journal of Separation Science*, vol. 33, no. 1, pp. 126–131, 2010.

[40] R. Cappelletti, M. Del Rosso, and V. P. Chiarugi, "A new electrophoretic method for the complete separation of all known animal glycosaminoglycans in a monodimensional run," *Analytical Biochemistry*, vol. 99, no. 2, pp. 311–315, 1979.

[41] A. Zinellu, S. Pisanu, E. Zinellu et al., "A novel LIF-CE method for the separation of hyaluronan- and chondroitin sulfate-derived disaccharides: application to structural and quantitative analyses of human plasma low- and high-charged chondroitin sulfate isomers," *Electrophoresis*, vol. 28, no. 14, pp. 2439–2447, 2007.

[42] A. Calabro, M. Benavides, M. Tammi, V. C. Hascall, and R. J. Midura, "Microanalysis of enzyme digests of hyaluronan and chondroitin/dermatan sulfate by fluorophore-assisted carbohydrate electrophoresis (FACE)," *Glycobiology*, vol. 10, no. 3, pp. 273–281, 2000.

[43] E. G. Karousou, M. Militsopoulou, G. Porta, G. de Luca, V. C. Hascall, and A. Passi, "Polyacrylamide gel electrophoresis of fluorophore-labeled hyaluronan and chondroitin sulfate disaccharides: application to the analysis in cells and tissues," *Electrophoresis*, vol. 25, no. 17, pp. 2919–2925, 2004.

[44] T. Bitter and H. M. Muir, "A modified uronic acid carbazole reaction," *Analytical Biochemistry*, vol. 4, no. 4, pp. 330–334, 1962.

[45] Y. Xu, P. D. Carr, J. M. Guss, and D. L. Ollis, "The crystal structure of bikunin from the inter-α-inhibitor complex: a serine protease inhibitor with two Kunitz domains," *Journal of Molecular Biology*, vol. 276, no. 5, pp. 955–966, 1998.

[46] O. H. Franco, E. W. Steyerberg, F. B. Hu, J. Mackenbach, and W. Nusselder, "Associations of diabetes mellitus with total life expectancy and life expectancy with and without cardiovascular disease," *Archives of Internal Medicine*, vol. 167, no. 11, pp. 1145–1151, 2007.

[47] F. Paneni, J. A. Beckman, M. A. Creager, and F. Cosentino, "Diabetes and vascular disease: pathophysiology, clinical consequences, and medical therapy: part I," *European Heart Journal*, vol. 34, no. 31, pp. 2436–2443, 2013.

[48] A. J. Lepedda, P. De Muro, G. Capobianco, and M. Formato, "Significance of urinary glycosaminoglycans/proteoglycans in the evaluation of type 1 and type 2 diabetes complications," *Journal of Diabetes and its Complications*, vol. 31, no. 1, pp. 149–155, 2017.

[49] C. Mizon, C. Mairie, M. Balduyck, E. Hachulla, and J. Mizon, "The chondroitin sulfate chain of bikunin-containing proteins in the inter-α-inhibitor family increases in size in inflammatory diseases," *European Journal of Biochemistry*, vol. 268, no. 9, pp. 2717–2724, 2001.

[50] C. Capon, C. Mizon, J. Lemoine, P. Rodié-Talbère, and J. Mizon, "In acute inflammation, the chondroitin-4 sulphate carried by bikunin is not only longer; it is also undersulphated," *Biochimie*, vol. 85, no. 1-2, pp. 101–107, 2003.

[51] M. Klüppel, "The roles of chondroitin-4-sulfotransferase-1 in development and disease," *Progress in Molecular Biology and Translational Science*, vol. 93, pp. 113–132, 2010.

[52] E. Schönherr, H. T. Järveläinen, L. J. Sandell, and T. N. Wight, "Effects of platelet-derived growth factor and transforming growth factor-beta 1 on the synthesis of a large versican-like chondroitin sulfate proteoglycan by arterial smooth muscle cells," *The Journal of Biological Chemistry*, vol. 266, no. 26, pp. 17640–17647, 1991.

[53] E. Tufvesson and G. Westergren-Thorsson, "Alteration of proteoglycan synthesis in human lung fibroblasts induced by interleukin-1β and tumor necrosis factor-α," *Journal of Cellular Biochemistry*, vol. 77, no. 2, pp. 298–309, 2000.

[54] S. N. Yang, M. L. Burch, L. R. Tannock, S. Evanko, N. Osman, and P. J. Little, "Transforming growth factor-β regulation of proteoglycan synthesis in vascular smooth muscle: contribution to lipid binding and accelerated atherosclerosis in diabetes," *Journal of Diabetes*, vol. 2, no. 4, pp. 233–242, 2010.

24

Classification and Differential Diagnosis of Diabetic Nephropathy

Chenyang Qi,[1] Xing Mao,[1] Zhigang Zhang,[1,2] and Huijuan Wu[1,2]

[1]Department of Pathology, Shanghai Medical College, Fudan University, Shanghai, China
[2]Shanghai Institute for Kidneys and Dialysis, Shanghai, China

Correspondence should be addressed to Huijuan Wu; hjwu@shmu.edu.cn

Academic Editor: Carlos Martinez Salgado

Diabetic nephropathy (DN) is a major cause of end-stage renal disease throughout the world in both developed and developing countries. This review briefly introduces the characteristic pathological changes of DN and Tervaert pathological classification, which divides DN into four classifications according to glomerular lesions, along with a separate scoring system for tubular, interstitial, and vascular lesions. Given the heterogeneity of the renal lesions and the complex mechanism underlying diabetic nephropathy, Tervaert classification has both significance and controversies in the guidance of diagnosis and prognosis. Applications and evaluations using Tervaert classification and indications for renal biopsy are summarized in this review according to recent studies. Meanwhile, differential diagnosis with another nodular glomerulopathy and the situation that a typical DN superimposed with a nondiabetic renal disease (NDRD) are discussed and concluded in this review.

1. Introduction

Diabetic nephropathy (DN) caused by diabetes mellitus is one of the major causes of end-stage renal failure worldwide [1]. Clinically, microalbuminuria is an important index to assess the progression of DN [2]. However, it is not accurate to evaluate the severity or prognosis simply based on the degree of proteinuria. It is now well recognized that not all diabetic patients who develop renal function failure have massive albuminuria [3]. Therefore, nephrologists and endocrinologists should be aware of the significance of pathological changes of DN in their clinical practice. Specifically, nondiabetic renal disease (NDRD), which might commonly be superimposed with diabetic renal lesions in some patients with type 2 diabetes, could only be confirmed and excluded by biopsy [4].

2. Pathological Changes of DN

The most significant and consistent pathological changes identified in renal biopsies of clinical DN patients are the glomerular lesions [5] which are, especially, diffuse and nodular mesangial expansion and Glomerular Basement Membrane (GBM) thickening [6]. Diffuse mesangial expansion, which develops at as early as 5th year since the onset of diabetes, is the earliest observable change by light microscopy [7]. The mesangial fractional volume [Vv(Mes/glom)] is correlated with albumin excretion rate (AER) and Glomerular Filtration Rate (GFR) in both type 1 [8] and type 2 diabetes [9]. As the disease advances, diffuse mesangial expansion progressively develops into nodular accumulations of mesangial matrix in the late stage of the DN. These nodular lesions, also known as Kimmelstiel-Wilson nodules, can be observed in about 25% of patients with advanced DN [10]. Nodular lesions and diffuse lesions are two stages of DN. Compared to the patients with diffuse mesangial expansion, those patients with nodular diabetic glomerulosclerosis present more severe renal damage, longer diabetic durations, and poorer renal prognosis [11].

GBM thickening can be observed within 2–8 years after the onset of diabetes. It is an early lesion which could be detected and measured by electron microscopy (EM) [12]. GBM width tends to increase linearly according to diabetes

TABLE 1: Diabetic nephropathy is divided into four hierarchical glomerular lesions.

Class	Description and criteria
I	Mild or nonspecific changes on light microscopy and conformed GBM thickening proven by electron microscopy: GBM > 395 nm (female), GBM > 430 nm (male).
IIa	Mild mesangial expansion in >25% of the observed mesangium; area of mesangial proliferation < area of capillary cavity.
IIb	Severe mesangial expansion in >25% of the observed mesangium. Area of mesangial proliferation < area of capillary cavity.
III	At least one convincing nodular sclerosis (Kimmelstiel-Wilson lesion).
IV	Advanced diabetic glomerulosclerosis in >50% of glomeruli.

TABLE 2: Separate scoring system of interstitial and vascular lesions of DN.

Lesion	Criteria	Score
Tubulointerstitial lesions	No IFTA	0
	IFTA < 25%	1
	25% < IFTA < 50%	2
	IFTA > 50%	3
Interstitial inflammation	Absent	0
	Relate to IFTA	1
	In areas without IFTA	2
Arteriolar hyalinosis	Absent	0
	One hyaline arteriole	1
	More than one hyaline arteriole	2
Arteriosclerosis (most severely affected artery)	No intimal thickening is observed	0
	Intimal thickening is less than the thickness of the media	1
	Intimal thickening is more than the thickness of the media	2

Note. IFTA: tubulointerstitial fibrosis and tubular atrophy.

duration in type 1 diabetes [13]. Vv(Mes/glom) and GBM width together explain 59% of the AER variability in a group of 125 patients of type 1 diabetes [8].

Although diabetic glomerular lesions have been the focus of the investigation on DN, the extraglomerular lesions are also involved in the progression of the disease. Tubulointerstitial lesions, including tubular atrophy, interstitial inflammation, and tubulointerstitial fibrosis, are closely related to renal function loss in the progression towards ESRD in patients with preexisting renal insufficiency [14]. Since DN is a kind of diabetic microangiopathy, hyalinosis occurs in both afferent and efferent arterioles. The hyalinosis of the efferent arteriole is a typical lesion by which diabetic nephropathy could be differentiated from hypertensive nephropathy [15].

There is increasing recognition of lesions like glomerular endothelial injury [5], podocyte impairment [16], and glomerulotubular junctions abnormalities in DN [17]. Given that the detection methods of these lesions are difficult to generalize in clinical practice, for now their value in diagnosis and classification is not as important as glomerular, tubulointerstitial, and vascular lesions.

3. Tervaert Classification of Diabetic Nephropathy

Journal of the American Society of Nephrology published pathological classification of DN by Tervaert et al. in 2010 (Tables 1 and 2) [10].

4. The Application and Evaluation of Tervaert Classification of DN

4.1. Contribution to the Early Diagnosis of Diabetic Nephropathy and Guiding Significance for Renal Prognosis in Patients with Diabetes. The classification outlined in Tervaert et al. is based on glomerular lesions, which best reflect the course of progressive DN. This is an important first step to set up an evaluable scheme of clinical value. Patients with typical DN show a longer impairment duration, worse metabolic control, and higher prevalence of diabetic retinopathy [18]. Diabetic patients with microalbuminuria without glomerulopathy are more likely to either regress to normoalbuminuria or remain with microalbuminuria with a slower rate of decline in renal function [19].

Using Tervaert pathological classification, Zhu et al. rediagnosed 37 cases of renal biopsies obtained from patients with type 2 diabetes manifesting microalbuminuria or clinical albuminuria and found that 6 out of 11 patients who were previously diagnosed with nondiabetic nephropathy actually belonged to class I~class II DN [20]. To explore the significance of this classification on prognosis, one group analyzed the relationship between structural changes and clinical features in 50 patients with type 2 diabetic and found that, as the glomerular lesions advanced from classes I to IV, the average GFR and 5-year renal survival decreased (100% of renal survived in classes I and IIa patients and 75% and 66.7% in classes IIb and III patients, respectively, whereas only 38.1% in class IV patients) [21]. Furthermore, another large-scale follow-up study of 396 patients with type 2 diabetes also revealed that the severity of glomerular and interstitial lesions had a significant impact on renal prognosis and could be used as an independent risk factor for renal outcomes [22]. Studies mentioned above all employed Tervaert pathological classification of DN, which suggested that this method can help to increase the accuracy of diagnosis, the possibility of an early diagnosis, and treatment of DN, as well as the prediction of renal prognosis.

As interstitial lesions also contribute to the impairment in renal function and may be an independent factor involved in the progression of DN, the classification scheme has put the extraglomerular lesions into consideration and introduces a separate scoring system for interstitial and vascular lesions.

4.2. Requirements to Involve Tubular, Interstitial, and Vascular Lesions into the Classification. Although the severity of tubular, interstitial, and vascular lesions has been taken into consideration by Tervaert classification, it is still not enough to meet practical requirements. Before Tervaert classification, Fioretto classification has been used for a long time, which included tubular, interstitial, and vascular lesions and divided DN into 3 categories according to the pathological changes under light microscope: C1, normal/near normal; C2, typical diabetic nephropathy with predominantly glomerular changes; and C3, atypical patterns of injury, associated with disproportionately damage including tubulointerstitial or arteriolar hyalinosis and with absent or only mild diabetic glomerular changes [23]. By using Fioretto classification, 31 patients with type 2 diabetes accompanied with normo-, micro-, or macroalbuminuria were investigated, and GFR lower than 60 mL/min/1.73 m^2 was considered as the decline of renal function [24]. Majority of patients (22 of 23) with micro- or macroalbuminuria were diagnosed as typical glomerular changes (C2) of Fioretto classification, and only one patient was diagnosed as atypical pattern of renal damage (C3). Notably, among patients with normoalbuminuria, 3 of 8 were diagnosed as C3 according to the tubular, interstitial, and vascular lesions [24]. When compared to Fioretto classification, Tervaert classification was only based on glomerular lesions, which is not sufficient for clinical application, which failed to classify tubular, interstitial, and vascular lesions belonging to Fioretto C3, due to the heterogeneity of the renal lesions and the complicated mechanism underlying diabetic nephropathy.

4.3. The Complexity and Heterogeneity of Type 2 Diabetes Should be Involved in Classification. Renal lesions in type 2 diabetes are much more complex than those in type 1 diabetes. There are more challenges to reach a correlation or predictive accuracy in renal function with glomerular structural variables in type 2 diabetes than in type 1 diabetes [19]. Tervaert et al. suggested that their classification can be used for both type 1 and type 2 diabetic patients, because of the substantial overlaps between these two types in histologic changes and clinical complications [10]. However, failure to distinguish the patients with type 1 diabetes or with type 2 diabetes in Tervaert classification might limit its significance on clinical practice [25]. There are two points worth taking into account for type 2 diabetes.

The first point is the high prevalence of nondiabetic superimposed renal lesions in type 2 diabetes. In many clinical cases, renal biopsies are usually performed in patients with an atypical manifestation of DN. There is no wonder that nondiabetic renal lesions in proteinuric type 2 diabetic patients have a prevalence as high as approximately 30% [18].

The second point is the heterogeneity in renal structure and pathogenesis of type 2 diabetes. Due to the heterogeneity of type 2 diabetes, a minority of type 2 diabetic patients have typical histopathological patterns resembling those present in type 1 diabetes, due to the heterogeneity of type 2 diabetes. Only 30% of type 2 diabetic patients with microalbuminuria and 50% of patients with proteinuria demonstrate typical diabetic glomerulopathy [23]. Atypical patterns of renal injury account for 35% of those with microalbuminuria and proteinuria. These patients exhibiting mild or atypical diabetic glomerular lesions usually present severe tubulointerstitial lesions which include tubular atrophy, TBM thickening and reduplication, advanced glomerular arteriolar hyalinosis associated with atherosclerosis of large vessels, interstitial fibrosis, and global glomerular sclerosis. These tubulointerstitial lesions not only are related to hyperglycemia, but also reflect the contributions from various causes predated type 2 diabetes, such as ageing, atherosclerosis, and systemic hypertension [23].

5. Differential Diagnosis of DN with another Nodular Glomerulopathy

Nodular diabetic glomerulosclerosis has a variety of pathological features but still should be differentiated from another mesangial nodular sclerosing glomerulopathy, which usually has similar light microscopic manifestations. It is necessary and essential to include manifestations, immunofluorescence staining (IF), and EM into the distinction of lesions caused by immune complex or monoclonal protein [26].

Nodular lesions could be observed in various renal primary and secondary diseases, such as membranoproliferative glomerulonephritis, renal amyloidosis, type III collagen glomerulopathy, monoclonal immunoglobulin or light chain deposition disease, fibronectin nephropathy, and cryoglobulinemia glomerulosclerosis [6, 27–29]. Table 3 shows the

TABLE 3: Differential diagnosis of DN with another nodular glomerulopathy.

Disease	Clinical manifestations	Light microscopy	Immunofluorescence microscopy	Electron microscopy
Diabetic nephropathy	Long duration of diabetes	Mesangial nodular sclerosis; PAS (+); silver (+)	Linear deposition of immunoglobulin (Ig) G, with or without IgM and C3 in sclerotic nodules	Mesangial expansion; diffuse GBM thickening; nonspecific fibrillar deposition
Membranoproliferative glomerulonephritis	Chronic nephritis, nephrotic syndrome, hypertension, hypocomplementemia	Mesangial nodular sclerosis; mesangial insertion; double contouring; PAS (+); silver (+)	Granular deposition of multiple immunoglobulin deposition and complement components	Subendothelial (type I), intramembranous, often ribbon-like or nodular (type II), subepithelial (type III) electron-dense deposits
Renal amyloidosis	Chronic infection, systemic amyloidosis, lymphoproliferative disease, long-term dialysis, family inheritance	Mesangial nodular sclerosis; Congo red (+)	Light chain λ (+) in the mesangium, GBM, tubulointerstitium, and blood vessel wall	Amyloid fibrils (randomly oriented, nonbranching, 9–11 nm in diameter)
Monoclonal immunoglobulin/light chain deposition disease	Ageing, plasma cell dyscrasia, idiopathic	Mesangial nodular sclerosis; PAS (+); silver (−)	Monoclonal light chain κ (+) in the GBM, TBM, and vascular wall basement membranes	Granular, powdery deposits
Type III collagen glomerulopathy	Persistent proteinuria, nephrotic syndrome	Mesangial nodular sclerosis; PAS (weak +)	Collagen III (+)	Parallel collagen fibers (100 nm in diameter)
Fibronectin nephropathy	A rare autosomal dominant disease, nephrotic syndrome	Mesangial nodular sclerosis; PAS (+); Congo red (−)	Fibronectin (+)	Granular deposits with short fibers (10–14 nm in diameter)
Cryoglobulinemia glomerulosclerosis	Proteinuria, nephrotic syndrome, high serum cryoglobulins, lymphoproliferative disorders	Intracapillary proliferation and inflammatory cell infiltrates, intracapillary thrombi, nodular glomerulosclerosis; double contouring; PAS (+)	Monoclonal or polyclonal immunoglobulin (IgM, IgG and C3), rheumatoid factor	Organized electron-dense deposits (microtubular, 30 nm in diameter)
Idiopathic nodular glomerulosclerosis	Smoking, long-standing hypertension; normal glucose metabolism	Similar to those of nodular diabetic glomerulosclerosis,	IgG and albumin	No electron-dense or fibrillar deposits

differential diagnosis of several mesangial nodular sclerosing glomerulopathy based on clinical manifestations, periodic acid Schiff (PAS) stain, methenamine silver stain, IF, and EM.

6. DM Accompanied with Nondiabetic Renal Disease (NDRD)

DM patients generally do not receive renal biopsy, unless there is a need to make an exclusive or differential diagnosis due to the complicated clinical situation. Because most of the DM patients undergoing renal biopsy show compound clinical manifestations, it is easy for pathologists to find superimposed lesions in renal biopsy in addition to pure pathological changes of DN.

Normally, no immune complexes and obvious complements could be detected by IF and EM in patients with DN. If there is a variety of typical deposition in the glomeruli, such as granular/chunky patterns of immunoglobulin by IF or electron dense deposits by EM, it usually indicates a superimposed nondiabetic renal disease [6].

In China, IgA nephropathy was the most frequently biopsy finding seen in all NDRD patients, followed by membranous nephropathy, mesangial proliferative glomerulonephritis, hypertensive nephrosclerosis, renal damage, minimal-change disease, focal segmental glomerulosclerosis, and crescentic glomerulonephritis [30]. However, the disease spectrum of NDRD varies in different populations. For example, in the United States, unlike in China which has a high prevalence of IgA nephropathy, two large-scale retrospective studies found that focal segmental glomerulosclerosis, acute tubular necrosis, and IgA nephropathy were the most common lesions found in patients with NDRD. Hypertensive nephrosclerosis, minimal-change disease, and membranous nephropathies were also common NDRDs of diabetic patients in the United States [31, 32]. In this review, we focus on the prevalence of NDRD in China. Table 4

TABLE 4: Literature review of NDRD in China.

Author	Year of publication	References	Number of patients	Pathological diagnosis			Statistical analysis of NDRD (alone and coexistent with DN)
				DN	NDRD	DN plus NDRD	
Mak et al.	1997	[35]	51	67	16	17	IgAN (59%), HTN (24%)
Wong et al.	2002	[36]	68	35	46	19	IgAN (29.5%), HTN (20.4%), MN (18.2%), MCD (9%)
Cao et al.	2007	[37]	120	85.8	—	14.2	IgAN (41.2%), MN (17.6%), HTN (11.7%), TIN (11.7%), RA (5.9%), FSGS (5.9%), micropolyarteritis (5.9%)
Zhou et al.	2008	[38]	110	54.5	—	45.5	IgAN (34%), MN (22%), MPGN (14%), HBV-associated GN (8%), MCD (4%), HTN (4%), MPGN (4%), CrGN (2%)
Lin et al.	2009	[39]	50	48	22	30	MN (19.23%), IgAN (11.54%), MCD (3.85%), HTN (3.85%), ATN (3.85%), CIN (7.69%)
Mou et al.	2010	[40]	69	47.8	52.2	—	FSGS (37.7%), IgAN (15.9%), MCD (15.9%), MN (8.7%)
Bi et al.	2011	[41]	220	54.5	—	45.5	IgAN (34%), MN (22%), MPGN (14%), HBV-associated GN (8%), MCD (4%), HTN (4%), MPGN (4%), CrGN (2%)
Zhang et al.	2011	[42]	130	73.9	26.1	—	IgAN (16.9%), MN (6.15%)
Zhuo et al.	2013	[43]	216	6.5	82.9	10.7	17–35 years (group I): IgAN (29%), MN (11.8%), FSGS (8.8%), MPGN (8.8%), APGN (5.9%), CrGN (5.9%); 36–59 years (group II): IgAN (34.7%), MN (15%), FSGS (1.4%), MPGN (6.1%), APGN (0.7%), CrGN (1.4%); 60 years (group III): IgAN (2.9%), FSGS (2.9%), MN (25.7%), CrGN (8.6%), MPGN (11.4%), RA (5.7%)
Peng and Wang	2013	[44]	61	52.5	—	47.5	IgAN (31%), MN (17.2%), MPGN (13.8%), HTN (13.8%), FSGS (10.3%), MCD (6.9%), APGN (3.5%)
Wang	2015	[45]	56	57.1		42.9	IgAN (33.3%), MN (25.0%), MPGN (20.8%), HTN (8.3%), FSGS (4.2%), MCD (4.2%)

Note. IgAN, primary IgA nephropathy; HTN, hypertensive nephrosclerosis; MN, membranous nephropathy; MCD, minimal change disease; TIN, tubulointerstitial nephritis; RA, renal amyloidosis; MPGN, mesangial proliferative glomerulonephritis; CrGN, crescentic glomerulonephritis; ATN, acute tubular necrosis; CIN, chronic interstitial nephritis; FSGS, focal segmental glomerular sclerosis.

summarizes recent studies on NDRD which include both NDRD alone and alongside concomitant DN in China.

As the DN and NDRD have different causes, their relationship, synergistic or independent, remains to be further studied. Given the fact that there is a wide clinical variation of DN patients combined with NDRD, the renal biopsy is an important method to improve the detection rate of NDRD. A clear diagnosis of the renal disease and proactive treatment meanwhile can stabilize or even reverse the renal function and improve the long-term prognosis of patients.

7. The Indications for Renal Biopsy

Although renal biopsy is the gold standard of DN diagnosis, the majority of diabetic patients with renal involvement are not biopsied. Some scholars believe that most diabetic glomerular changes are nonspecific in the early stage of diabetes, so there is no need to expand the indications of renal biopsy blindly. The bleeding risk of renal biopsy should be carefully considered in patients who have been suffering from hypertension, renal dysfunction, or anemia [33].

Moreover, microalbuminuria is clinically considered as a major index to judge the progression of DN. However, it is not as accurate as expected. For example, type 1 diabetes usually develops into DN within 10 to 15 years after diagnosis, while microalbuminuria may occur as early as 2 to 5 years after diagnosis. Some patients with type 2 diabetes may already have microalbuminuria at the time of diagnosis, but without DN. Thus, renal biopsy and morphological changes may offer important insights into the understanding of the complex course of diabetes and help to classify, diagnose, prognose, and manage the disease. Indications for renal biopsy in DN are as follows [30, 34]:

(1) Proteinuria of nephrotic range with diabetes less than 5 years or normal kidney functions

(2) An unexplained microscopic hematuria (especially acanthocytosis and cellular cast)

(3) An unexplained rapidly worsening renal function in patients with a previously stable renal function

(4) Application of angiotensin converting enzyme inhibitor (ACEI)/angiotensin receptor antagonist (ARB) for 2~3 months, while GFR decreased by more than 30%

(5) Failure to exclude renal diseases in the absence of diabetic retinopathy, with or without systemic diseases

8. Conclusion

DN has a pathological diversity and affects all structural components of the kidney. Recognition of these lesions and their morphological characteristics in renal biopsy may aid in preventing, slowing down, or even reversing the processes of diabetic nephropathy. Tervaert classification of DN has a positive meaning in developing novel strategies for an early diagnosis and treatment of DN. However, the complexity and heterogeneity of type 2 diabetes, different from type 1 diabetes, along with tubular, interstitial, and vascular lesions should be taken into consideration in new classification methods in the future. Regardless of its limitations, the Tervaert classification represents a very meaningful step towards the establishment of a DN classification scheme with clinical utility. When the pathologist observes the pathological changes of DN, they still need to make a differential diagnosis with another nodular glomerulopathy and clarify whether it is a typical DN complicated with NDRD or not. Furthermore, the indications and risks of renal biopsy should be prudently taken into consideration.

Competing Interests

The authors declare that there is no conflict of interests regarding the publication of this paper.

Acknowledgments

This work was supported by a grant from the Science and Technology Commission of Shanghai Municipality (no. 15140902900).

References

[1] W. Zou and H. Wang, *Pathology of Renal Biopsy*, Peking University Medical Press, 2nd edition, 2009.

[2] KDOQI, "KDOQI clinical practice guidelines and clinical practice recommendations for diabetes and chronic kidney disease," *American Journal of Kidney Diseases*, vol. 49, no. 2, supplement 2, pp. S12–S154, 2007.

[3] N. J. Radcliffe, J.-M. Seah, M. Clarke, R. J. Macisaac, G. Jerums, and E. I. Ekinci, "Clinical predictive factors in diabetic kidney disease progression," *Journal of Diabetes Investigation*, 2016.

[4] Y. An and Z. Liu, "Relationship between pathological changes and prognosis in diabetic nephropathy," *Chinese Journal of Nephrology, Dialysis & Transplantation*, vol. 22, no. 4, pp. 368–372, 2013.

[5] Y. Maezawa, M. Takemoto, and K. Yokote, "Cell biology of diabetic nephropathy: roles of endothelial cells, tubulointerstitial cells and podocytes," *Journal of Diabetes Investigation*, vol. 6, no. 1, pp. 3–15, 2015.

[6] B. Najafian, C. E. Alpers, and A. B. Fogo, "Pathology of human diabetic nephropathy," *Diabetes and the Kidney*, vol. 170, pp. 36–47, 2011.

[7] M. Pourghasem, H. Shafi, and Z. Babazadeh, "Histological changes of kidney in diabetic nephropathy," *Caspian Journal of Internal Medicine*, vol. 6, no. 3, pp. 120–127, 2015.

[8] M. L. Caramori, Y. Kim, C. Huang et al., "Cellular basis of diabetic nephropathy: 1. Study design and renal structural-functional relationships in patients with long-standing type 1 diabetes," *Diabetes*, vol. 51, pp. 506–513, 2002.

[9] R. Nosadini, M. Velussi, E. Brocco et al., "Course of renal function in type 2 diabetic patients with abnormalities of albumin excretion rate," *Diabetes*, vol. 49, no. 3, pp. 476–484, 2000.

[10] T. W. C. Tervaert, A. L. Mooyaart, K. Amann et al., "Pathologic classification of diabetic nephropathy," *Journal of the American Society of Nephrology*, vol. 21, no. 4, pp. 556–563, 2010.

[11] D. Hong, T. Zheng, S. Jia-qing, W. Jian, L. Zhi-hong, and L. Lei-shi, "Nodular glomerular lesion: a later stage of diabetic nephropathy?" *Diabetes Research and Clinical Practice*, vol. 78, no. 2, pp. 189–195, 2007.

[12] P. Fioretto and M. Mauer, "Histopathology of diabetic nephropathy," *Seminars in Nephrology*, vol. 27, no. 2, pp. 195–207, 2007.

[13] K. N. Drummond, M. S. Kramer, S. Suissa et al., "Effects of duration and age at onset of type 1 diabetes on preclinical manifestations of nephropathy," *Diabetes*, vol. 52, no. 7, pp. 1818–1824, 2003.

[14] R. E. Gilbert and M. E. Cooper, "The tubulointerstitium in progressive diabetic kidney disease: more than an aftermath of glomerular injury?" *Kidney International*, vol. 56, no. 5, pp. 1627–1637, 1999.

[15] W. Min and N. Yamanaka, "Three-dimensional analysis of increased vasculature around the glomerular vascular pole in diabetic nephropathy," *Virchows Archiv A Pathological Anatomy and Histopathology*, vol. 423, no. 3, pp. 201–207, 1993.

[16] K. E. White and R. W. Bilous, "Structural alterations to the podocyte are related to proteinuria in type 2 diabetic patients," *Nephrology Dialysis Transplantation*, vol. 19, no. 6, pp. 1437–1440, 2004.

[17] B. Najafian, J. T. Crosson, Y. Kim, and M. Mauer, "Glomerulotubular junction abnormalities are associated with proteinuria

in type 1 diabetes," *Journal of the American Society of Nephrology*, vol. 17, no. 2, pp. S53–S60, 2006.

[18] H.-H. Parving, M.-A. Gall, P. Skøtt et al., "Prevalence and causes of albuminuria in non-insulin-dependent diabetic patients," *Kidney International*, vol. 41, no. 4, pp. 758–762, 1992.

[19] P. Fioretto, M. L. Caramori, and M. Mauer, "The kidney in diabetes: dynamic pathways of injury and repair. The Camillo Golgi Lecture 2007," *Diabetologia*, vol. 51, no. 8, pp. 1347–1355, 2008.

[20] X. Zhu, F. Liu, Y. Peng et al., "New pathologic classification of diabetic nephropathy (retrospective study of 37 cases)," *Journal of Central South University (Medical Sciences)*, vol. 37, no. 2, pp. 185–189, 2012.

[21] S. W. Oh, S. Kim, K. Y. Na et al., "Clinical implications of pathologic diagnosis and classification for diabetic nephropathy," *Diabetes Research and Clinical Practice*, vol. 97, no. 3, pp. 418–424, 2012.

[22] Y. An, F. Xu, W. Le et al., "Renal histologic changes and the outcome in patients with diabetic nephropathy," *Nephrology Dialysis Transplantation*, vol. 30, no. 2, pp. 257–266, 2015.

[23] P. Fioretto, M. Mauer, E. Brocco et al., "Patterns of renal injury in NIDDM patients with microalbuminuria," *Diabetologia*, vol. 39, no. 12, pp. 1569–1576, 1996.

[24] E. I. Ekinci, G. Jerums, A. Skene et al., "Renal structure in normoalbuminuric and albuminuric patients with type 2 diabetes and impaired renal function," *Diabetes Care*, vol. 36, no. 11, pp. 3620–3626, 2013.

[25] P. Fioretto and M. Mauer, "Diabetic nephropathy: diabetic nephropathy-challenges in pathologic classification," *Nature Reviews Nephrology*, vol. 6, no. 9, pp. 508–510, 2010.

[26] G. S. Markowitz, J. Lin, A. M. Valeri, C. Avila, S. H. Nasr, and V. D. D'Agati, "Idiopathic nodular glomerulosclerosis is a distinct clinicopathologic entity linked to hypertension and smoking," *Human Pathology*, vol. 33, no. 8, pp. 826–835, 2002.

[27] M. Guo, *Pathology of Renal Biopsy*, Fudan University Press, 2007.

[28] V. Kumar, A. K. Abbas, and J. C. Aster, *Robbins Basic Pathology*, W.B. Saunders, 9th edition, 2012.

[29] K. O. Alsaad and A. M. Herzenberg, "Distinguishing diabetic nephropathy from other causes of glomerulosclerosis: an update," *Journal of Clinical Pathology*, vol. 60, no. 1, pp. 18–26, 2007.

[30] M. Fiorentino, D. Bolignano, V. Tesar et al., "Renal biopsy in 2015—from epidemiology to evidence-based indications," *American Journal of Nephrology*, vol. 43, no. 1, pp. 1–19, 2016.

[31] S. G. Sharma, A. S. Bomback, J. Radhakrishnan et al., "The modern spectrum of renal biopsy findings in patients with diabetes," *Clinical Journal of the American Society of Nephrology*, vol. 8, no. 10, pp. 1718–1724, 2013.

[32] T. T. Pham, J. J. Sim, D. A. Kujubu, I.-L. A. Liu, and V. A. Kumar, "Prevalence of nondiabetic renal disease in diabetic patients," *American Journal of Nephrology*, vol. 27, no. 3, pp. 322–328, 2007.

[33] E. Espinel, I. Agraz, M. Ibernon, N. Ramos, J. Fort, and D. Serón, "Renal biopsy in type 2 diabetic patients," *Journal of Clinical Medicine*, vol. 4, no. 5, pp. 998–1009, 2015.

[34] J. Chen, "Early diagnosis of diabetic nephropathy and indications of renal biopsy," *Nephrology Dialysis Transplantation*, pp. 349–351, 2011 (Chinese).

[35] S. K. Mak, E. Gwi, K. W. Chan et al., "Clinical predictors of non-diabetic renal disease in patients with non-insulin dependent diabetes mellitus," *Nephrology Dialysis Transplantation*, vol. 12, no. 12, pp. 2588–2591, 1997.

[36] T. Y. H. Wong, P. C. L. Choi, C. S. Chun et al., "Renal outcome in type 2 diabetic patients with or without coexisting nondiabetic nephropathies," *Diabetes Care*, vol. 25, no. 5, pp. 900–905, 2002.

[37] S. Cao, M. Fang, Y. Sun, Y. Fang, and Z. Liu, "Clinical and pathological analysis of diabetic nephropathy combined with non-diabetic nephropathy," *Clinical Focus*, vol. 22, pp. 1580–1582, 2007 (Chinese).

[38] J. Zhou, X. Chen, Y. Xie, J. Li, N. Yamanaka, and X. Tong, "A differential diagnostic model of diabetic nephropathy and non-diabetic renal diseases," *Nephrology Dialysis Transplantation*, vol. 23, no. 6, pp. 1940–1945, 2008.

[39] Y.-L. Lin, S.-J. Peng, S.-H. Ferng, C.-Y. Tzen, and C.-S. Yang, "Clinical indicators which necessitate renal biopsy in type 2 diabetes mellitus patients with renal disease," *International Journal of Clinical Practice*, vol. 63, no. 8, pp. 1167–1176, 2009.

[40] S. Mou, Q. Wang, J. Liu et al., "Prevalence of non-diabetic renal disease in patients with type 2 diabetes," *Diabetes Research and Clinical Practice*, vol. 87, no. 3, pp. 354–359, 2010.

[41] H. Bi, N. Chen, G. Ling, S. Yuan, G. Huang, and R. Liu, "Nondiabetic renal disease in type 2 diabetic patients: a review of our experience in 220 cases," *Renal Failure*, vol. 33, no. 1, pp. 26–30, 2011.

[42] P.-P. Zhang, Y.-C. Ge, S.-J. Li, H.-L. Xie, L.-S. Li, and Z.-H. Liu, "Renal biopsy in type 2 diabetes: timing of complications and evaluating of safety in Chinese patients," *Nephrology*, vol. 16, no. 1, pp. 100–105, 2011.

[43] L. Zhuo, W. Ren, W. Li, G. Zou, and J. Lu, "Evaluation of renal biopsies in type 2 diabetic patients with kidney disease: a clinicopathological study of 216 cases," *International Urology and Nephrology*, vol. 45, no. 1, pp. 173–179, 2013.

[44] L. Peng and Y. Wang, "Pathological analysis of diabetic nephropathy and non-diabetic renal disease in patients with type 2 diabetes mellitus," *Chinese and Foreign Medical Research*, vol. 11, no. 35, pp. 7–9, 2013 (Chinese).

[45] X. Wang, "Pathological and clinical characteristics of diabetic nephropathy and diabetic nephropathy combined with non-diabetic nephropathy," *Journal of Clinical Research*, pp. 151–152, 2015 (Chinese).

Permissions

All chapters in this book were first published in JDR, by Hindawi Publishing Corporation; hereby published with permission under the Creative Commons Attribution License or equivalent. Every chapter published in this book has been scrutinized by our experts. Their significance has been extensively debated. The topics covered herein carry significant findings which will fuel the growth of the discipline. They may even be implemented as practical applications or may be referred to as a beginning point for another development.

The contributors of this book come from diverse backgrounds, making this book a truly international effort. This book will bring forth new frontiers with its revolutionizing research information and detailed analysis of the nascent developments around the world.

We would like to thank all the contributing authors for lending their expertise to make the book truly unique. They have played a crucial role in the development of this book. Without their invaluable contributions this book wouldn't have been possible. They have made vital efforts to compile up to date information on the varied aspects of this subject to make this book a valuable addition to the collection of many professionals and students.

This book was conceptualized with the vision of imparting up-to-date information and advanced data in this field. To ensure the same, a matchless editorial board was set up. Every individual on the board went through rigorous rounds of assessment to prove their worth. After which they invested a large part of their time researching and compiling the most relevant data for our readers.

The editorial board has been involved in producing this book since its inception. They have spent rigorous hours researching and exploring the diverse topics which have resulted in the successful publishing of this book. They have passed on their knowledge of decades through this book. To expedite this challenging task, the publisher supported the team at every step. A small team of assistant editors was also appointed to further simplify the editing procedure and attain best results for the readers.

Apart from the editorial board, the designing team has also invested a significant amount of their time in understanding the subject and creating the most relevant covers. They scrutinized every image to scout for the most suitable representation of the subject and create an appropriate cover for the book.

The publishing team has been an ardent support to the editorial, designing and production team. Their endless efforts to recruit the best for this project, has resulted in the accomplishment of this book. They are a veteran in the field of academics and their pool of knowledge is as vast as their experience in printing. Their expertise and guidance has proved useful at every step. Their uncompromising quality standards have made this book an exceptional effort. Their encouragement from time to time has been an inspiration for everyone.

The publisher and the editorial board hope that this book will prove to be a valuable piece of knowledge for researchers, students, practitioners and scholars across the globe.

List of Contributors

Bogdan Mircea Mihai, Elena-Daniela Grigorescu and Cristina Mihaela Lăcătuşu
"Grigore T. Popa" University of Medicine and Pharmacy, Clinical Centre of Diabetes, Nutrition and Metabolic Diseases, "Sf. Spiridon" Clinical Hospital, Iaşi, Romania

Cătălina Mihai, Cristina Cijevschi-Prelipcean, Mihaela Dranga and Vasile Drug
"Grigore T. Popa" University of Medicine and Pharmacy, Institute of Gastroenterology and Hepatology, "Sf. Spiridon" Clinical Hospital, Iaşi, Romania

Ioan Sporea
Gastroenterology, "Victor Babes" University of Medicine and Pharmacy Timişoara, Romania

Rasmus Bo Jansen and Ole Lander Svendsen
Copenhagen Diabetes Foot Center (CODIF), Bispebjerg Hospital, University of Copenhagen, 2400 Copenhagen NV, Denmark
Department of Endocrinology, Bispebjerg Hospital, University of Copenhagen, 2400 Copenhagen NV, Denmark

Tomas Møller Christensen
Department of Endocrinology, Bispebjerg Hospital, University of Copenhagen, 2400 Copenhagen NV, Denmark

Jens Bülow and Lene Rørdam
Department of Clinical Physiology and Nuclear Medicine, Bispebjerg Hospital, University of Copenhagen, 2400 Copenhagen NV, Denmark

Niklas Rye Jørgensen
Department of Clinical Biochemistry, Rigshospitalet, University of Copenhagen, 2600 Glostrup, Denmark
Odense Patient data Explorative Network (OPEN), Odense University Hospital/Institute of Clinical Research, University of Southern Denmark, Odense, Denmark

Alberto López-Delis
Medical Biophysics Center, University of Oriente, Santiago de Cuba, Cuba
Biomedical Engineering Program, University of Brasilia, Brasilia, DF, Brazil

Suélia de S. Rodrigues Fleury Rosa, Yasmin Carneiro Lobo Macedo and Adson Ferreira da Rocha
Biomedical Engineering Program, University of Brasilia, Brasilia, DF, Brazil

Paulo Eduardo Narcizo de Souza
Laboratory of Electron Paramagnetic Resonance, Institute of Physics, University of Brasilia, Brasilia, DF, Brazil

Marcella Lemos Brettas Carneiro
Faculty of Planaltina, University of Brasilia, Planaltina, GO, Brazil

Mário Fabrício Fleury Rosa
Biomedical Engineering Program, University of Brasilia, Brasilia, DF, Brazil
Policy-Making in Collective Health, Faculty of Ceilândia, University of Brasilia, Ceilândia, DF, Brazil

Fabiane Hiratsuka Veiga-Souza
Laboratory of Biochemistry and Protein Chemistry, Institute of Biological Sciences, University of Brasilia, Brasilia, DF, Brazil
Faculty of Ceilândia, University of Brasilia, Ceilândia, DF, Brazil

Michał Bulc, Katarzyna Palus and Jarosław Całka
Department of Clinical Physiology Faculty of Veterinary Medicine, University of Warmia and Mazury in Olsztyn, Oczapowskiego Str. 13, 10-719 Olsztyn, Poland

Łukasz Zielonka
Department of Veterinary Prevention and Feed Hygiene, Faculty of Veterinary Medicine, University of Warmia and Mazury in Olsztyn, 10-718 Olsztyn, Poland

Daisuke Aono, Mitsuhiro Kometani, Yoshimichi Takeda, Shigehiro Karashima, Yoshiyu Takeda and Takashi Yoneda
Department of Cardiovascular and Internal Medicine, Kanazawa University Graduate School of Medicine, Kanazawa, Japan

Rie Oka
Department of Cardiovascular and Internal Medicine, Kanazawa University Graduate School of Medicine, Kanazawa, Japan
Department of Internal Medicine, Hokuriku Central Hospital, Oyabe, Japan

Kenichi Yoshimura
Department of Biostatistics, Innovative Clinical Research Center (iCREK), Kanazawa University Hospital, Kanazawa, Japan

Janneth Bermeo-Cabrera and Josefa Riofrios-Palacios
Departamento de Endocrinología y Metabolismo, Instituto Nacional de Ciencias Médicas y Nutrición Salvador Zubirán, Mexico City, Mexico

Paloma Almeda-Valdes, Carlos A. Aguilar-Salinas and Roopa Mehta
Departamento de Endocrinología y Metabolismo, Instituto Nacional de Ciencias Médicas y Nutrición Salvador Zubirán, Mexico City, Mexico
Unidad de Investigación de Enfermedades Metabólicas, Instituto Nacional de Ciencias Médicas y Nutrición Salvador Zubirán, Mexico City, Mexico

Romina Bertinat and Francisco Nualart
Centro de Microscopía Avanzada (CMA BIO-BIO), Universidad de Concepción, Concepción, Chile

Francisco Westermeier
Institute of Biomedical Science, FH Joanneum Gesellschaft mbH University of Applied Sciences, Eggenberger Allee 13, 8020 Graz, Austria
Facultad de Ciencia, Universidad San Sebastián, Santiago, Chile

Pamela Silva
Facultad de Salud, Universidad Santo Tomás, Osorno, Chile

Rodrigo Gatica
Escuela de Veterinaria, Facultad de Ciencias, Universidad Mayor, Santiago, Chile

Joana Moitinho Oliveira
CIBER de Diabetes y Enfermedades Metabólicas Asociadas (CIBERDEM), Barcelona, Spain
Diabetes and Obesity Research Laboratory, IDIBAPS, Barcelona, Spain

Ramón Gomis
CIBER de Diabetes y Enfermedades Metabólicas Asociadas (CIBERDEM), Barcelona, Spain
Diabetes and Obesity Research Laboratory, IDIBAPS, Barcelona, Spain
Department of Endocrinology and Nutrition, Hospital Clinic, Barcelona, Spain
Faculty of Medicine, University of Barcelona, Barcelona, Spain

Alejandro J. Yáñez
Facultad de Ciencias, Universidad Austral de Chile, Valdivia, Chile

Kimberly Wallace
School of Nursing, West Virginia University, Morgantown 26506, USA

Xiaohui Zhao and Usha Sambamoorthi
School of Pharmacy, West Virginia University, Morgantown, 26506 WV, USA

Ranjita Misra
School of Public Health, West Virginia University, Morgantown, 26506 WV, USA

Rebecca Paprott, Christa Scheidt-Nave and Christin Heidemann
Department of Epidemiology and Health Monitoring, Robert Koch Institute, 12101 Berlin, Germany

Khadijah Saeed Balamash, Elham Hamed Al Gahdali and Sawsan Omer Khoja
Department of Biochemistry, Faculty of Science, King Abdulaziz University, Jeddah, Saudi Arabia

Huda Mohammed Alkreathy
Department of Pharmacology, Faculty of Medicine, King Abdulaziz University, Jeddah, Saudi Arabia

Aftab Ahmad
Health Information Technology Department, Jeddah Community College, King Abdulaziz University, Jeddah 21589, Saudi Arabia

Theresa Leyco and Chin Meng Khoo
Department of Medicine, National University Hospital, Singapore

Davin Ryanputra and Ray Peh
Yong Loo Lin School of Medicine, National University of Singapore, Singapore

Alexphil Ponce
Higher Education Department, Centre for International Education, Cebu, Philippines

Pınar Korkmaz and Duru Mıstanoğlu Özatağ
Department of Clinical Microbiology and Infectious Diseases, Dumlupınar University Faculty of Medicine, 43020 Kutahya, Turkey

Havva Koçak
Department of Biochemistry, Dumlupınar University Faculty of Medicine, Kutahya, Turkey

Kevser Onbaşı
Department of Endocrinology and Metabolism, Dumlupınar University Faculty of Medicine, Kutahya, Turkey

Polat Biçici
Department of Plastic Surgery, Kütahya Dumlupınar Training and Research Hospital, Kutahya, Turkey

Ahmet Özmen and Cemile Uyar
Department of Clinical Microbiology and Infectious Diseases, Kütahya Dumlupınar Training and Research Hospital, Kutahya, Turkey

Qiaoyun Gong, Jia'nan Xie, Yang Liu, Ying Li and Guanfang Su
Eye Center, The Second Hospital of Jilin University, No. 218 Ziqiang Street, Changchun, Jilin 130021, China

Shivangini Singh, Sahana Devadasa Acharya, Ashwin Kamath and Sheetal D. Ullal
Department of Pharmacology, Kasturba Medical College, Mangalore, Manipal Academy of Higher Education, Karnataka 575001, India

Rathnakar P. Urval
Department of Pharmacology, Kanachur Institute of Medical Sciences, Mangalore, Karnataka, India

John Winkler and Sanjoy Ghosh
Department of Biology, IKBSAS, University of British Columbia-Okanagan, Canada

Benjamin T. Maatman, Glen Schmeisser and Rolf P. Kreutz
Krannert Institute of Cardiology, Indiana University School of Medicine, Indianapolis, IN, USA

Anelisiwe Siboto, Ntethelelo Sibiya, Andile Khathi and Phikelelani Ngubane
School of Laboratory Medicine and Medical Sciences, University of KwaZulu-Natal, Durban, South Africa

Bernardo Nuche-Berenguer
National Institute of Diabetes and Digestive and Kidney Diseases, National Institutes of Health, Bethesda, MD 20892-1804, USA

Linda E. Kupfer
Fogarty International Center, National Institutes of Health, Bethesda, MD 20814, USA

Lin Luo and Jiang-Jia Cai
Zhejiang Key Laboratory of Pathophysiology, Medical School of Ningbo University, Ningbo 315211, China

Jin Xu
Zhejiang Key Laboratory of Pathophysiology, Medical School of Ningbo University, Ningbo 315211, China
Department of Preventive Medicine, Medical School of Ningbo University, Ningbo 315211, China

Wen-Hua Zhou
Laboratory of Behavioral Neuroscience, Ningbo Addiction Research and Treatment Center, Medical School of Ningbo University, Ningbo 315211, China

Mei Feng and Mi Zhou,
Department of Preventive Medicine, Medical School of Ningbo University, Ningbo 315211, China

Su-Pei Hu
Department of Research and Teaching, Ningbo No. 2 Hospital, Ningbo 315010, China

Lin-Dan Ji
Zhejiang Key Laboratory of Pathophysiology, Medical School of Ningbo University, Ningbo 315211, China
Department of Biochemistry, Medical School of Ningbo University, Ningbo 315211, China

Julian M. Gaitan
Department of Kinesiology, University of Virginia, Charlottesville, VA, USA

Arthur Weltman
Department of Kinesiology, University of Virginia, Charlottesville, VA, USA
Division of Endocrinology and Metabolism, University of Virginia, Charlottesville, VA, USA

Steven K. Malin
Department of Kinesiology, University of Virginia, Charlottesville, VA, USA
Division of Endocrinology and Metabolism, University of Virginia, Charlottesville, VA, USA
Robert M. Berne Cardiovascular Research Center, University of Virginia, Charlottesville, VA, USA

Jiao Lv, Zhi-Hao Mu, Fang Wang, Qiu-Ting Guo, Zhi-Min Zhao, Yu-Ping Pan, Xin-Yu Liao, Zhi-Hong Yang and Ying-Ying Zou
Department of Pathology and Pathophysiology, Faculty of Basic Medical Sciences, Kunming Medical University, 1168 West Chunrong Road, Kunming 650500, China

Miao-Miao Chen and Ning Cai
Department of Ophthalmology, First Affiliated Hospital of Kunming Medical University, 295 Xi Chang Road, Kunming 650032, China

Zhong-Yi Qian,
Department of Morphological Laboratory, Faculty of Basic Medical Sciences, Kunming Medical University, 1168 West Chunrong Road, Kunming 650500, China

Lei Zhou
The Key Laboratory of Stem Cell and Regenerative Medicine of Yunnan Province, Kunming Medical University, 1168 West Chunrong Road, Kunming 650500, China

Shu-De Li
Department of Biochemistry and Molecular Biology, Faculty of Basic Medical Sciences, Kunming Medical University, 1168 West Chunrong Road, Kunming 650500, China

Samir Malkani
Division of Diabetes, Department of Medicine, University of Massachusetts Medical School, Worcester, MA 01655, USA

Anupam Kotwal
Division of Endocrinology, Diabetes, Metabolism and Nutrition, Mayo Clinic, 200 First Street SW, Mayo 18, Rochester, MN 55905, USA

Antonio Junior Lepedda, Gabriele Nieddu, Michela Idini, Pierina De Muro and Marilena Formato
Dipartimento di Scienze Biomediche, University of Sassari, Sassari, Italy

Silvia Rocchiccioli and Nadia Ucciferri
Istituto di Fisiologia Clinica, National Research Council, Pisa, Italy

Chenyang Qi and Xing Mao
Department of Pathology, Shanghai Medical College, Fudan University, Shanghai, China

Zhigang Zhang and Huijuan Wu
Department of Pathology, Shanghai Medical College, Fudan University, Shanghai, China
Shanghai Institute for Kidneys and Dialysis, Shanghai, China

Index

www.ingramcontent.com/pod-product-compliance
Lightning Source LLC
LaVergne TN
LVHW060547210926
848485LV00005B/1275